Sociology in medicine

Sociology in medicine

Third edition

Mervyn Susser, William Watson,
Kim Hopper

New York   Oxford
Oxford University Press
1985

Oxford University Press

Oxford   London   New York   Toronto
Delhi   Bombay   Calcutta   Madras   Karachi
Kuala   Lumpur   Singapore   Hong Kong   Tokyo
Nairobi   Dar es Salaam   Cape Town
Melbourne   Auckland

and associated companies in
Beirut   Berlin   Ibadan   Mexico City   Nicosia

Library of Congress Cataloging in Publication Data

Susser, Mervyn W.
Sociology in medicine.

Includes bibliographical references and index.
1. Social medicine. I. Watson, William,
1917 Jan. 5–   . II. Hopper, Kim. III. Title.
[DNLM: 1. Social medicine. 2. Sociology. 3. Family. W 322 S964s]
RA418.S88   1984   306'.46   83-23649
ISBN 0-19-503444-9

Printing (last digit):   9 8 7 6 5 4 3 2 1

Printed in the United States of America

A new edition for a new generation:

Jude, Leah, Philip, and Zoë

New discoveries of the Earth discover new diseases: for besides the common swarm, there are endemial and local infirmities proper unto certain Regions, which in the whole Earth make no small number; and if Asia, Africa and America should bring in their list, Pandora's Box would swell, and there must be a strange Pathology.

Sir Thomas Browne
(1605–1682)

Preface

In this third edition, the character and the structure of this book in essence remain unchanged. Although the book has continued in use for more than 20 years in only two editions, and we claim this as a virtue, in fact new content and ideas pervade the persisting core. A rapidly growing subject matter, and the rapidly changing world that lies at the heart of that subject matter, could not otherwise be accommodated.

In the second edition of 1971 much was added, part was revised, and a little was subtracted. Aside from rewriting throughout, the third edition has undergone additions and revisions at least as great, with somewhat more subtraction. The more notable additions include an introductory chapter that frames the contribution of the book in terms of human ecology, and an expansion and pulling together of scattered notes on problems of methods in the description of health in populations in a separate chapter (Chapter 2). Substantial pieces have been added on the modern world economic system (Chapter 3); on theories of social class (Chapter 5); on psychosocial stress and disease (Chapter 8); and on the problems of separating heredity and environment in the study of disease (Chapter 9).

The most notable subtraction is the omission of the chapter on "Medicine and Bureaucracy," which had as its centerpiece a Weberian analysis of the British National Health Service. This subtraction allows us to evade the extensive subject of the organization of medical care, as well as to avoid unwelcome expansion. Many pages would be required to keep the evolving forms of health organization in their sociological and anthropological contexts. Moreover, the deletion of the chapter does not result in a loss that cannot be redeemed, as once it might have done. Readers can find other excellent and more systematic sources that cover the relevant topics. Thus comprehensiveness and omniscience are not what we seek. Indeed, an advantage in coherence and focus follows from the deletion of the chapter.

What we believe remains unique to the book stands out more clearly, namely the demonstration of the uses of social science in interpreting the manifestations of health and disease. The way we approach this demonstration has not changed and, as before, the book falls naturally into two parts. The first part (eight chapters) takes as its theme several aspects of society—economy, culture, social class, and social mobility—and relates them to the health of populations. The second part (four chapters) has as its theme the family life cycle and individual development, beginning with the family as an institution, and going on to family formation and the successive stages of life.

In general, we have tried first to explicate the concept under examination and, second, to outline its uses in the health field. Our aim has always been to exemplify by specific, concrete instances and, where the available data would serve, to use only well-founded material. We have not hesitated to draw on our own personal experience. Our approach is on the one side to provide a text that addresses basic issues of social science and, on the other side, to do the same for epidemiology, health, and disease. The fusion of the two fields becomes, we dare to believe, more than the sum of the parts.

From the first we made a strenuous effort to compile a wide-ranging bibliography from many disparate sources. One object was to counter in advance the charges of windiness so often levelled at the social sciences, regardless of quality. We wanted to show that the field could be grounded in sound scientific work. We still find that rationale attractive; we make no defense for our scientific rationalism, although we may open ourselves to charges of positivism and the like from the opposite direction. The bibliographic effort has continued into the third edition; the book has accumulated close to 3000 references.

We should perhaps explain our mode of citing references. To avoid a degree of clutter that many readers might find unbearable, we chose not to back up every point made with specific documentation. Instead, we often provide a sheaf of references from which a coherent idea has been synthesized, or from which an array of data has been compiled. To assist readers in tracing a given author, a separate author index lists the page numbers on which the author's name is cited, and the reference numbers on those pages direct the search to those sections of the bibliography which cite the particular author.

Although we cannot guarantee the quality of every work cited—indeed in many early instances rigorous work was simply not available—we have tried to be selective. Still, we have kept many references from previous editions. As a result, the bibliography in some degree documents the historical unfolding of the field of interest over the past three decades. The textual exposition also, having evolved through the same period, provides a view of the historical unfolding of the issues and concerns of the social sciences related to medicine. Not infrequently, formulations and concepts that in the first or second editions could be supported only by assertion have since been given attention in reports in the literature. Such references supercede the earlier editions of the book in our current citations.

The result of our work is precisely defined by the choice of preposition in our title. We have written a sociology *in* medicine, and not a sociology *of* medicine.° That is, we use social science to inform our understanding of problems of health and disease

---

° R. Strauss (1957) The nature and status of medical sociology, *Amer. Sociol. Rev.*, 22, 200–204.

and the ways of society in coping with them, as opposed to using social science to try and describe health and health care as dimensions of the society. In its earliest manifestations, social science in the health field was an instrument of the health professions, that is, it was social science *in* health. It could not become a fully developed instrument, however, until it also covered the sociology of health organizations and of the health professions, the social relations of the exchanges and transactions around health, and the health system in social context. This is the social science *of* health. Thus there is blurring at the edges between the two areas. The crucial distinction is less in the context or in the problems addressed, and more in the reference group of the users of social science. Where the reference group is within the health field, the task is approached as a health problem, and the solutions sought aim ultimately to improve states of health. Where the reference group is in the social science field, the problems are those of the social science discipline, and the solutions sought aim to advance social science theory.

Social analysis of the place of health in society was under way by the seventeenth century, with the precursor of the analysis of the sociodemographic distribution of mortality in the work of John Graunt (*Natural and Political Observations Mentioned in a Following Index Made Upon the Bills of Mortality*, 1662), and the precursor of cost-benefit analysis in the work of Graunt's friend William Petty (*Political Arithmetick*, 1617). The theme was developed in the eighteenth century by Peter Johann Franck (*System of a Complete Medical Police*, 1st volume° 1779) and much expanded during the nineteenth century by, among others, Pierre-Louis René Villermé, ("Memoire sur la mortalité en France, dans la classe aisee et dans la classe indigente," 1828), Edwin Chadwick (*Report on Sanitary Conditions of the Labouring Population of Great Britain*, 1842), Florence Nightingale (see her *Observations on the British Army in India*, 1863), and John Simon (*English Sanitary Institutions*, 1890). In mid-nineteenth century Germany, Rudolph Virchow roundly declared that medicine was a social science. This nineteenth-century trend expressed itself essentially in terms of social medicine (see Alfred Grotjahn's *Soziale Pathologie* of 1911, and many writers since).

Although Petty and Chadwick addressed economics, and Franck political organization, sociological rather than social analysis began to appear in medicine only in the 1920s, for instance, in the papers of Henry Sigerist (see his 1929 essay on "The Special Position of the Sick"). By the 1930s, explicitly sociological analysis had begun to be made, notably by Bernhard J. Stern (*Social Factors and Medical Progress*, 1927), and L. J. Henderson (see his essay "Doctor and Patient as a Social System," *New England Journal of Medicine*, 1935). Shortly thereafter, Robert Faris and Warren Dunham reported their work on the social situation of patients hospitalized for schizophrenia (*Mental Disorders in Urban Areas*, 1939), and H. Rowland described social relations on the schizophrenic wards of a mental hospital (*Psychiatry*, 1938, 1939).

Following an interim for World War II, there has been what we guess to be an exponential increase in the field of medical sociology. However, by the late 1950s there was as yet no thoroughgoing and effective single attempt to interpret health and

---

° 8 more were to follow; 3 of them appeared posthumously.

health care within a social science framework. Interesting works on the interaction of the agents of disease with society had appeared, such as René Dubos's *Mirage of Health*, (1959); Talcott Parsons had further refined Sigerist's analysis of the "sick role" in *The Social System*, (1951); N. G. Hawkins had made a premature effort—one that would be premature even today—to provide a comprehensive theory of disease in society in *Medical Sociology* (1958). In *Social Science in Medicine* (1954) by Leo W. Simmons and Harold G. Wolff, an anthropologist and an internist placed their parallel interpretations of health and society in counterpoint. In *Health, Culture and Community*, (1955), Benjamin Paul had collected a fascinating set of anthropological studies illuminated by his own insightful commentary; and in *The Student Physician* (1957), R. K. Merton and his colleagues left the lasting imprint on social theory of their studies of the socialization of medical students to the medical profession. There were others and, of course, many individual papers had appeared in medical and social science journals. By the mid 1950s in the United States, more than two hundred members belonged to the medical sociology section of the American Sociological Association (although in Britain, hardly more than five or six social scientists would accept the qualifier "medical"). But in 1959 when the writing of this book began, there was as yet no attempt to synthesize within a single text the material from the fields of social science and medicine.

In 1958 at Manchester University, Zena Stein observed that what were then innovations in teaching by the two future authors of this book were running on convergent lines. One of us (William Watson, lecturer in the Department of Social Anthropology having recently returned from some years of field work in Zambia—then Northern Rhodesia) had been asked by the late Professor Max Gluckman to take responsibiliy for teaching a course in anthropology to physicians in the postgraduate public health program. The other (myself, a displaced South African newly appointed lecurer in the Department of Social and Preventive Medicine, and a person with whom Zena Stein was intimately acquainted in several capacities) in 1957 had been given responsibility by Professor C. Fraser Brockington for teaching the major course in social and preventive medicine to medical students in their penultimate year. Following my own bent and understanding, I had given the course a predominantly sociological and anthropological cast. While I was able to place disease and medical care in their social context, my explication of social science concepts necessarily bore the amateurish mark of the autodidact. We stumbled in the new-ploughed field. But Zena Stein saw that the strengths and deficiencies of the two lecturers complemented each other. Together they should be capable, she concluded, of more fully realizing a new synthesis of social science with medicine and public health. Recklessly (I have always thought, not measuring the possible costs to her own family), she persuaded the two lecturers to undertake the writing of a book. In due course, it was published as the first edition of *Sociology in Medicine* in 1962.

A great part of the book was written jointly. Over a period of three years we sequestered ourselves for weeks on end, threshed issues one after another, and pushed on together page by page, and sometimes line by line. When it came to a second edition, although in the medieval way of modern academics both authors had moved from Manchester, we found ourselves at least on the same continent. In the late 1970s, the time came to consider a third edition, this remained true but the undertaking was more difficult. A stage had been reached at which a number of texts on social science in the health field existed and, besides, we both had numerous other interests that engaged us. Our publishers were kind enough to suggest that the book, having helped to shape the scope and nature of the subject, had an established place that they would like to see maintained. Zena Stein again entered the lists, to argue that the book remained unique, and deserved a longer life, and that to revise it was the responsible thing to do.

It was with trepidation—Sisyphus in mind—that we essayed the task of revision. The difficulties were overcome by the recruitment after several attempts of a third author (Kim Hopper), by the dogged assistance of Robert P. Montera in all aspects (in addition to his contribution to the chapter "Health and Disease in the World Economy"), and by the contributions of Carole Vance, and of Maureen Durkin-Longley in particular, to the chapter entitled "Infant to Adult." It goes without saying that without the contributions of Leslie Dwelle, Barbara Godlesky, Ruth Reich, and Barbara Wright to the typescript, the work would never have been completed.

To our regret, William Watson found himself unable to participate fully in this revision. He therefore properly expressed his reluctance to continue as co-author. Against his judgment, I persuaded him to allow his name to stand on the grounds that his original mark on this book cannot be leached away.

M.S.

New York
April 1985

Preface to the second edition

The need for a second edition of this book stems from a wider and clearer recognition of the place of social science in medicine and public health than existed when the book was first published. The first edition has been read in Europe and Latin America as well as in the English-speaking world. In the United States, social science finds a place in the curricula of many medical schools and of all the schools of public health. In Britain, the Royal Commission on Medical Education, 1965–68, gave official sanction to the inclusion of social science in basic medical education.

Two major influences contribute to the new content of the second edition. First, both authors have added some years of personal experience of the United States to the storehouse of African and British experience on which we drew for the first edition. In this new edition, first-hand knowledge of the American social system and its health patterns has exemplified many concepts, and adumbrated or tempered others. We hope that the book will thereby acquire greater universality and validity.

Secondly, in the years since the first edition appeared, the literature of the field that the book synthesized and demarcated has enormously expanded. This expanded bibliography has brought refinement of concepts, testing of hypotheses, verification of predictions, and sophistication of methods. We have tried to take account of these advances, and to include what seemed most valuable and relevant.

We have not found it necesary to alter the plan, nor the selected field of interest, of the book. The basic concepts and hypotheses of the first edition, and its factual foundation, have proved sufficiently durable to require only elaboration and additions. Nonetheless, in order to incorporate the new material from different sources of experience and scholarship, the entire book has been rewritten. A new feature is the addition of diagrams and tables taken from many sources. These aim to illuminate the written page, and to convey graphically and simply some complex relationships.

New York   M.W.S.
June 1970   W.W.

Preface to the first edition

During the last three centuries, medicine has come to recognize that many diseases
are not natural calamities that strike in a haphazard way, but are injuries inflicted on
people by the nature of their daily occupations and their customary modes of life.
That some diseases are associated with specific occupations, as silicosis is with mining,
is now well established, and as a result many such disorders have been brought under
medical and legal control, and some, like "phossy-jaw," entirely abolished. Other diseases are associated with particular social environments; gastroenteritis of infants in
the past was related to poor housing and inadequate diet, while today poliomyelitis
most affects those who live under hygienic conditions. In many disorders, the occupation and social circumstances of the victim are important in the onset and diagnosis
of the disease as well as in determining the chances of successful treatment.

In other words, man's economic and social environment is part of his natural environment and helps to determine the incidence and prognosis of disease. Hence we
observe distinctive patterns of health in societies with disparate economies and modes
of life. In our own industrial society the conquest of disease has gone hand in hand
with changes in the economic and social environment, as shown, for instance, in the
fall in death rates in Great Britain during the nineteenth century. Disorders which
formerly were mortal or incapacitating are today amenable to treatment; many diabetics, for example, can live busy and useful lives with routine treatment and a mod-
icum of care. The expectation of life has increased, and life itself is easier and more
comfortable for the mass of people than at any time in the past. At the same time,
however, these advances in themselves have produced a population with a high proportion of old and ageing people who have specific medical and social probelms. In
addition, the elaborate division of labour, and the multifarious economic and social
activities of immense urban populations with their resulting social stresses and strains
has accompanied the subsidence of the old "social" and infectious diseases. This has

brought about a new interest in nervous and social disorders, which absorb more and more medical care and attention.

On the other hand, in underdeveloped countries such as Africa, medicine is confronted with quite different problems. There medicine is concerned with the health of peoples who are emerging from tribal societies in which the whole population, with the exception of a few chiefs and specialists, worked at the same tasks, and shared similar housing, diet, and exposure to disease and danger: a common low standard of living. Such tribal societies, where both mortality rates and birth rates are high, have populations in which the young preponderate. All of them are caught up in the immense and rapid transformation of their economic and social environment brought about by industrial enterprise and political development. Not least among these changes is the "population explosion" already triggered off by medical intervention. As a result, these populations are beginning to experience conditions of health and disease similar to those extant in Great Britain at the time of our own industrial revolution, but which we have now surmounted. Indeed, modern medical textbooks are often unsuitable for doctors intending to practise medicine in underdeveloped countries, in that these books reflect the probelms of health and disease current in industrial societies, and deal superficially, if at all, with the major medical problems experienced by transitional societies.

Thus scientific and technical advances, although they provide medicine with weapons with which to attack existing patterns of health and disease, in themselves help to bring about new social conditions and disorders, and in turn these challenge medical science to provide new solutions.

These are some of the problems of social medicine, which concerns itself particularly with the study of the social context of disease and health, that is, with the influence of social and cultural phenomena on sickness and on the effectiveness of medical care and organization. Social medicine is therefore a complex and difficult branch of medical science in that it attempts to grapple both with the nature of social processes and with their complicated relation to health and disease. In consequence, social medicine, if it is to be effective, must draw on the concepts and methods of disciplines other than biology and the natural sciences, on epidemiolqgy, demography, sociology, social anthropology, and social psychology. Epidemiology and demography are both firmly based on the population and vital statisics that have been available in Great Britain and other industrial countries ever since the census was introduced, and since such pioneers as Snow and Farr demonstrated their value, the medical profession has come to recognize their importance. The medical significance of sociological studies has not been so universally accepted, and at present such studies tend to be neglected in the training of doctors. Yet the insights provided by the social sciences into the nature of social processes, and into the structure of society and the relationships between individuals, are a necessary foundation to the effective practice of medicine, whether curative or preventive. The concepts of the social sciences enable us to analyse social relationships in the practice of medicine, and to trace in the patient those social experiences which most affect his behaviour, symptoms, and perception of illness and the form of the illness itself. Moreover, sociological insight assists the clinician to discern those social influences which affect his own behaviour, his interpretation of illness, and his care of patients.

Although the systematic study of medical sociology is new and relatively unorganized, it has already produced an extensive and growing literature, so that distinctive fields of study have been marked out, with specialists, both in medicine and in sociology, devoted to each. Some of these specialists are concerned with epidemiology, with the configuration of disease by social categories; others with the way in which the social environment affects the process of restoring patients to their normal social functions. Other scholars have studied the institutions of medical care, the organization of the medical profession itself, and the systems of medical education. We have not undertaken to give a comprehensive account of all this material, although we have referred to it in many places in the text. Our method has been to begin with sociological concepts and to illustrate these from field studies and documented cases in both medicine and sociology. As each of us has worked in Africa and in Britain, one in epidemiology and clinical practice, the other in sociology and social anthropology, we have drawn our material from these two areas, and attempted to illuminate our general approach to the subject by contrasting them.

We have divided our material into two main parts. In the first part, Chapters 1 to 5, we discuss the significance of demographic studies, the effects on individuals and groups of various social and cultural environments, the importance of epidemiological studies, and the significance for medicine of the division of industrial society into social classes, with the associated problem of social mobility. We attempt here to analyse population trends and their mortality and sickness, as well as social institutions and relationships.

In the second part, Chapters 6 to 9, we concentrate on the contemporary family in Great Britain, particularly as it concerns doctors and others, who, in treating and caring for individual patients, cannot ignore their family backgrounds and personal and social environment. Here we discuss social roles and the special position of the sick, social relationships and the support they give to patients, occupations, and marriage and the founding of a family. We also discuss the growth and development of children, their socialization, behaviour, and various disorders. The perspective here is of clinical and personal medicine, in the light of available field studies in sociology and social anthropology.

The choice of this material is open to criticism, but this seemed to us the most economic use of our resources and the most rewarding way to introduce an extensive subject. We have found this approach useful in our own teaching at Manchester University, one as a physician teaching social medicine to medical students, the other as a sociologist teaching medical postgraduates for the Diploma of Public Health.

This book is intended only as an introduction to the subject, and we have not ventured to prescribe therapeutic action, which would have taken us beyond our aim. As it is, the effort to compress our material within reasonable bounds prevented us from exploring some hypotheses to the extent that they deserve, and if we appear to have dealt arbitrarily with the work of others, we can but plead the necessity of simplified exposition in an endeavour to present a comprehensive account. We have paid particular attention to indicating our sources, although we have not hesitated to reinterpret material in terms of our own hypotheses. The bibliography is therefore extensive, and is intended to provide a guide to the literature and a source for further reading and exploration of the subject.

University of Manchester   M.W.S.
January 1962   W.W.

Contents

Sociology in medicine

1

Economy, ecology, and disease

What most physicians have taken as given about disease, social science makes problematic. For the physician the goal of practice is to cure or care for the individual afflictions caused by disease. The mechanisms and the course of these disruptions of normal bodily functioning are described in standard medical texts, and their treatment requires the sort of attention only a trained specialist can offer.

Social science goes beyond the individual human body and the individual psyche. It inquires into the social dimensions of affliction in two senses: how disease originates, and how it makes its appearance in a society at a given time (1). In the first line of inquiry, the social genesis and mediation of disease are at issue. The form, distribution, and severity of disease are seen as products of the social circumstances under which people live and work. In the second line of inquiry, what is at issue is society's response to disease. Social scientists examine the processes by which disease becomes a social event: the set of symbols by which disease is recognized and made intelligible, the societal agencies and institutions to which the care of disease is tendered, and the techniques and rituals deployed in treating it.

The study of health and its disorders, then, includes but is not limited to fine-grained descriptions of the immediate precursors of the disease and the mechanisms by which they are translated into infirmity and disability. It entails as well analysis of the larger determinants of these precursors, analysis that encompasses the fundamental structures and activities of social life. Societies vary markedly in their supply of food, provision of shelter, organization of work, habits of leisure, assortment of kin ties, networks of communal support, and hierarchies of power—as well as in the range of environmental hazards and constraints they are subject to. So, accordingly, do their respective patterns and burdens and disease (2).

Such an approach broadens the scope of epidemiological inquiry. Conventional analyses of the distribution and determinants of disease often restrict themselves to an examination of the interrelationships within the classic triad: agent, host, and

3

immediate environment. Even after Robert Koch isolated the tubercle bacillus in 1882, some epidemiologists of his day recognized that the microorganism was not the sole and sufficient cause of tuberculosis. To be sure, during the half century of the bacteriological revolution, many behaved as though diseases could be attributed to microbiological agents alone. A few insisted otherwise. For them environmental factors—dirt, deprivation, and dilapidated housing—had to be considered as essential "social allies" of the bacilli, working to ensure their appearance and propagation.

While the broader view represented a decided advance in causal thinking, it fell short of a truly social approach. Missing from most analyses, as well as from present-day investigations in the same tradition, is sustained attention to large-scale social forces. These create the contexts within which the encounters between pathogenic agent and victim take place. Tuberculosis was only one instance of the renewed tide of disease that arose in urban England in the first half of the nineteenth century. The rates of smallpox, typhus, typhoid fever, diphtheria, and scarlet fever all increased; two cholera epidemics had swept through the warrens of the Great Towns, a third was on its way. It is instructive to consider this resurgence, following the lead of a number of contemporary commentators, as a by-product of the rise of industrial capitalism and the reordering of the circumstances of everyday life that ensued. Industrial capitalism gave rise to novel physical arrangements for work and dwelling (the factory, the company town), created new patterns of economic exploitation (mass displacements from land, urban migration in unprecedented numbers, wage-labor), and fueled its own forms of class conflict (Luddism, Chartism, trade unionism, the strike). Hazardous and fatiguing work, damp, cold, and stifling living quarters, cheap gin and adulterated foods, demoralization—the legacy of disease bequeathed by early capitalism stems from such an environment (3).

What is true for the understanding of disease in the nineteenth century will serve as a general principle. In human communities throughout history, the forces mediating the impact of disease have been preeminently social in nature. This recognition is a relatively recent one for Western civilization and has its roots in the Enlightenment.

Historical precursors

When in *The Social Contract* Rousseau wrote that the emergence of civil society transforms natural man "from a stupid ignorant animal into an intelligent being and a Man," he set down in embryonic form a point of departure for modern social science: the recognition of the deep and pervasive influence of culture on individuals in society. The things of culture were things of its own making. At the time, it was an astonishing claim. Not the terms of a divine mandate, not the preordained scheme of a distant providence, but the everyday social round itself was responsible for the collective fate of the members of society. It was there that human nature (and much of nonhuman nature) was shaped. Participation in the human community, Rousseau argued, was at once a socializing and an individualizing experience. In this way human beings were rendered responsible to and dependent upon one another, yet at the same time they were enabled to become uniquely particular. Through the agency of culture, that is, the ranks of *Homo sapiens* were disciplined into the persons of human societies. They become truly human only when their achievements and travails take on an unmistakable social stamp.

In the century following Rousseau, the measure of cultural influence was extended. Not only were the carriers of culture subject to its shaping but so were the seemingly removed and independent conditions under which social life was carried on. The impress of culture, it had long been recognized, could be traced through the design of social settings, the tools and language of social activity and discourse, and the daily habits of men and women as they chatted, worked, prepared food, raised their children, cared for their sick, and worshipped their gods. Long recognized too, as Rousseau reminded us, was the ultimate sway of "invincible nature" over the multiplicities of social forms: only those which "as a result of careful adaptation" observed the inbuilt limits of soil, water, climate, and native food supply could hope for a secure, durable existence. Human industry (in the sense of resourcefulness and activity) might improve upon the store of game and forage, might even persuade nature to yield riches hidden from earlier forms of industry, as the developments of animal husbandry, agriculture, and metallurgy had shown, but nature was still the ultimate arbiter (4).

Developments in the late eighteenth and early nineteenth centuries altered perceptions of the sway of nature. The momentous dislocations—social, economic, and ecologic—of the industrial revolution forced a rethinking of the whole notion of "natural bounds" and of the degree to which "outside" features of the natural environment could be mediated and transformed by the social structures they supported. Among the first subjects to be studied in this way was human disease, one of the most potent of such external forces.

By the middle of the nineteenth century, a new term, "social medicine," had come into use in France. It was meant to designate the coordinated study of the relation of social life and institutions to patterns of health and disease, and the provision of appropriate measures (medical and otherwise) to deal with the problems such study would reveal. The study and practices to which the term referred had had their precursors: William Petty's analysis of the economic costs of disease; John Graunt's studies of the distribution of mortality in London; Johann Peter Frank's efforts to ensure state responsibility for public health under a system of "medical police" in late-eighteenth-century Germany; the far-sighted if only partially implemented social assistance programs proposed by the Convention in postrevolutionary France; the early surveys in Italy, England, France, and Germany of the health of industrial workers and the appalling living and working conditions these surveys had uncovered; and the preliminary investigations of "medical topography" in Europe and the United States, exploring the relationship of physical geography and natural history to endemic and epidemic diseases (5).

The upheavals of the revolutionary period of 1848 created circumstances conducive to rethinking the terms of the social contract. The remedial actions demanded by the French revolutionaries of 1848 were predicated upon new notions of society's proper concern for the health, well-being, and care of the people. Political and economic factors in determining a group's health chances were underlined in studies by

Villermé of textile workers in France, by Virchow of the Silesian typhus epidemic in Germany, and by a small corps of reformist physicians studying the conditions of Manchester's mills. In a statement whose full implications are only today becoming apparent, Rudolf Virchow proclaimed unambiguously: "Medicine is a social science, and politics nothing but medicine on a grand scale" (6).

Eventually, not only collective forces but individual acts would come under the gaze of social analysts. Concentration on the individual morality of social actions would give way to a different orientation, one which insisted that individual actions had to be read within the context of social conditions and were subject to social limits and pressures. Durkheim's landmark study, *Suicide* (1897), in which he interpreted this most private of acts as a "social fact" contingent upon the degree of integration and cohesiveness that exists in a community, charted a course for much subsequent investigation. Observations could be made, data from statistical surveys culled, comparative analyses constructed, and conclusions drawn about the nature of society and its workings. A way of seeing was being invented.

Social science has grown since then, and can count a half dozen contemporary disciplines in its lineage. The generic term remains useful, however, if only to call attention to the wide angle of vision it requires. To demonstrate its analytic power for an understanding of health and disease, we turn first to an examination of society's mode of securing and distributing essential goods and services.

Economy

The manner in which people produce, exchange, and consume goods and the kinds of goods they use set limits to the nature and scope of their social relations. People who live by hunting and gathering tend to have simple forms of social organization; people in industrialized settings tend to have large-scale, settled societies with dense populations and more complex forms of social organization. But though the level of technological development and the endowment of natural resources may limit the range of possible forms of social organization, they do not rigidly determine which one will actually exist. Technology affects social structure, but social structure molds the shape and uses of technology. Highly industrialized societies, to take an obvious example, may be organized along capitalistic or socialistic lines, and so may gear production either to private gain in the market place or to the collective needs of society in the mass. Not only what is produced and by what means, but how it is produced, by what groups, organized in what fashion, coordinated by what integrative principles and to what end: all are crucial questions when examining the organization of production and exchange in a given society (7).

For the Greeks, the work "economy" referred to those activities devoted to household management. Economics had to do with a certain kind of right conduct embedded in the social texture of everyday life. The study of economics, as seen in the works of Aristotle, was considered part of ethics or politics. Following the publication of William Petty's *A Treatise on Taxes and Contributions* in 1662, the concept of economy was gradually transformed into "political economy." The object of study was now seen as a field of social activity with distinctive institutions and laws of its own, and economics could claim an independence that threatened to bring it into conflict with received tradition. Precisely what kind of autonomy economic forces can claim is a major subject of investigation in the historical and comparative study of social institutions.

In its contemporary generic sense, "economy" refers to the process of provisioning a society with the goods and services it requires. Economic activity is thus defined substantively at the level of the collectivity, as something social groups do: the disposing of material resources (including time) needed to realize certain socially prescribed ends. Needs other than survival are always at stake, and their nature and ranking may be a complex function of privilege, custom, and compromise. The operations and ends of the economy are thoroughly enmeshed with the beliefs, practices, and institutions of social life as a whole.

In nonmarket economies (now largely of historical note) the social character of economic activity is readily apparent. On this point the anthropological record is especially revealing. In precapitalist economies the obligations of kinship, requirements of ritual, prerogatives of political power, and dictates of etiquette all command performances or control transactions which are manifestly economic in their effects. While economic activity constitutes the enabling armature of all social activity, it draws its meaning and purpose from the noneconomic provinces of social life. These two spheres animate and reinforce each other. From a social science standpoint, therefore, the word "economy" does more than delimit the social activity of generating the material provisions of a society. It also denotes an "internal" dimension of many social practices whose primary meaning or function may be quite removed from the immediate satisfaction of needs. Anthropologists, concerned with preserving in their accounts the dense and complex layers of ordinary social transactions, consider such practices to have an economic aspect to them.

For any given society, a characteristic way of provisioning itself may be described. This *mode of production* will have a dominant institution for production—the household in a tribal economy, the manor in feudalism, and the corporation in modern capitalism. Each of these employs an appropriate technology and division of labor in the service of a particular economic objective. In practice, a system of production will entail specific forms of property and typical mechanisms of coordination between producing units.

For analytic purposes, these elements can be grouped into two categories: the *forces of production*—those tools and instruments, procedures, kinds of labor, bodies of knowledge and skill, which cultures have devised to ensure their material means of existence; and the *social relations of production*—those arrangements between individuals and social groups that grow out of and make possible the operation of productive techniques. The abstract character of this distinction must be stressed, for in practice there is intimate linkage between tools and social relations. Any productive process, whether agricultural or industrial, is simultaneously a plying of technique and an instance of interpersonal or intergroup cooperation or coercion. The exchange of ceremonial shell ornaments between Trobriand and Dobu islanders, which ostensibly is nothing but ritual, renews ties of reciprocity between these neighboring peoples and provides the occasion for trading crucial necessities as well. When subsistence farmers lose their land or are rendered destitute, they are transformed into wage-laborers on plantation or in the factory, and traditional ways succumb to new ways more suited to the demands of new economic relations. Women provide unremunerated domestic labor where patriarchy rules the hearth. Production is thus as much a social as a technical accomplishment; modes of production are also modes of domination and control.

Systems of production are themselves products of historical development. Thus they are hostage to, even as they strain against, the strictures of politics and the state, social convention, and the resistance of excluded or oppressed groups. There was no economic reason in the 1830s, for example, to restrict the workday to 12 hours; that limit was forced upon textile factory owners as a result of working-class agitation. Tensions and instabilities are thus an inherent feature of any socioeconomic formation. Far from being aberrant or alien, they are indispensable sources of further development and social change (8).

Classically, the domain of economic activity has been divided into four sectors, each with its defining structures. Material provisioning is foremost a problem of *production*—the process by which social groups appropriate and transform natural resources, including labor power, into social goods and services. In order to realize the use-value of the goods so produced—that is, to turn them into objects that satisfy needs—several other operations are necessary. The rules of *distribution* determine the ways in which individuals participate in the productive process, share in its yield, and govern the disposition of the "surplus." Mechanisms of *exchange* enlarge and diversify the supply of goods locally available and enable groups and individuals to convert their share of production into objects tailored to specific wants. *Utilization* either puts the object into immediate use (consumption) or converts it to capital to ensure the continuation of the productive cycle.

As societies become increasingly complex their productive systems do likewise. Within modern economies, ancillary as well as outmoded sectors of economic activity may be found alongside the more advanced sectors. Underground or marginal "economies" may flourish in miniature among socially disenfranchised groups. Poverty-stricken tenants in single-room-occupancy hotels in New York City, for example, have devised their own small-scale versions of a redistributive economy (where communal resources are pooled and then reapportioned), mimicking those of certain primitive communities and operating, in effect, like extended families (on grounds of mutual need rather than kinship). Obviously such anomalous forms are dependent for their existence upon the support, however minimal, of the larger economy (9).

A number of questions, addressed to the four economic domains outlined above, may prove useful for a depiction of the dominant mode of production in any society and the ways in which the economy articulates with other fields of social activity. What techniques and units of production are employed and how effective are they? What are the rules that govern the control and use of the means of production and of their yield? What are the terms and circumstances under which goods are exchanged? What are the corresponding units and types of consumption? And finally, what are the inner connections among these activities and how are they, in turn, related to other activities of social life?

If anthropological research has confirmed the decisive importance of economics in shaping social life in general, it has also shown that such a relationship is neither mechanical nor neat. The substitution of steel axes for stone ones in a New Guinea highland community sharply reduced the amount of time men spent in subsistence activities (though it had little impact on women's work time), increased the power and prestige of already established "big-men," and drew the society into a monetary economy. Yet in the short run, the lineaments of the traditional society were preserved intact (10).

Where economic development clashes with traditional patterns of provisioning, however, it can have momentous effects on the social order. In southern India the establishment of a new irrigation system in a small village led to a reallocation of village resources, redistribution of wealth, and redefinition of the range and relations of economic activity. These changes, in turn, forced accommodations in politics, ritual practice, family structure, and cultural values. Similarly, the introduction of snowmobiles among the reindeer-herding people of Lapland completely altered the technical requirements and the skills needed for productive work. It created a new class of dependent, economically disabled families and intensified a socioeconomic differentiation that had before been little apparent. The society as a whole was made dependent upon outside sources of fuel and cash (11).

When economic exigency requires it, even the strictest conventions may bend, adapt, or disappear. In modern Madras, industrialists recast traditional Hindu ritual obligations to square them with workaday realities. For instance, the traditional pollution taboos and fears of defilement that segregated the higher from the lower castes were dispensed with in the spaces of the factories; rituals were devised to "neutralize" the pollution in order to allow the various castes to work together. Among Mesoamerican Indian communities, the civil-religious ceremonies and ethnic identities originally forged in the context of conquest have both proved adaptive to the changing needs of successive productive systems even up to modern times. Whether Indian labor was employed as subsistence farmer, migrant wage-laborer, or petty shopkeeper, native communities modified their traditional institutions to enable them to take advantage of whatever meager economic opportunities came their way (12).

Appreciation of the structures and functions of economies as social institutions aids appreciation of their relevance to matters of health. Certain connections are readily apparent: precarious productive systems place their populations in constant danger of malnutrition or famine; new trade routes may open a society to unfamiliar and potentially lethal diseases as well as to novel commodities; advanced production techniques may yield toxic by-products. But the true weight of the economy in the distribution of health and disease can only be assessed by examining two cardinal dimensions of social life: the way work is organized and the way social groups are stratified.

Social stratification is largely a function of the relationship of groups to the process of production and distribution. A class is identified by the degree of control exerted over the means and issue of production. For an individual, belonging to a group is an index of social standing and opportunities. Social inequality, as Rousseau recognized, is a social invention. Its epidemiological relevance has long been appreciated: class differences in the distribution and severity of disease are among the oldest and most enduring findings of "political arithmetick"—William Petty's title for his treatise on the economic costs of mortality. Plague was a persisting fact of feudal life, but its flail fell unevenly. Boccacio's *Decameron* and other plague chronicles tell of the wholesale flight out of infected regions by the rich as well as mass destitution and death in the ranks of the poor who remained behind. At the same time, medieval Italian cities created the forerunners of the modern institutions of public health, with methods of inspection and surveillance, warning systems, and quarantine. In London, Bills of Mortality were instituted to provide weekly counts of fatality that would forewarn of the plague, and in the seventeenth century, John Graunt used these to invent epidemiological analysis of vital statistics. In the late eighteenth century, Johann Peter Frank noted that "every social group has its own type of health and disease determined by the mode of living," and christened poverty "the mother of disease." Since then the attendants of poverty—poor hygiene and housing; lack of food, clothing, and fuel; and "vicious" habits—have figured largely in any analysis of the social origins of disease (13). In our own time the association between health disorders and lower-class status has been amply documented; it will be more fully explored in Chapter 6.

The organization of work in a society is a signal feature of the mode of production. The labor process embodies the technical aspects of production (the use of tools, deployment of time, and arrangement of tasks) and is an index of the development of the productive forces. It also embodies the division of labor and patterns of management and control, and thus invariably reflects the social relations of production at large. The relevance of both these dimensions to health has long been recognized (14). In the sixteenth century physicians remarked upon the special dangers of mining and the peculiar ailments that afflicted miners. In Florence in 1700 Ramazzini, in *De morbis artificum diatribe*, examined the health consequences of 41 different trades. Since then, occupations have multiplied and the literature on occupational disease has burgeoned. In addition to the physical demands and imminent dangers of occupation, the life habits and attitudes that grow out of a particular style of work have been the subjects of speculation. As early as 1837 Dr. Benjamin M'Cready warned that Americans were fast becoming "an anxious, careworn people," owing to their incessant "striving after wealth or endeavoring to keep up its appearance." More recent studies in the United States have shown that persons who are driven, competitive, time conscious, and easily provoked are at higher risk for coronary heart disease. Epidemiologically, the impact of work is manifold, and will be further examined in Chapter 6.

Ecology

In the West, at least since the writing of Genesis, reflections on the relations of human society to the natural world have been ruled by two attitudes. The first is the insistence upon the distinctiveness of the human species, upon its special place in the order of creation. To the claim of separateness is added the claim of dominion: not only is "man" distinct from nature, "he" is lord over it. Confronted with a natural order that is taken to be anarchic and cruel, Western thinkers have viewed the human task as one of conquest and mastery over nature. The history of civilization, accordingly, is seen as the story of the gradual freeing of society from the yoke of nature and the subsequent harnessing of nature in the service of "man." Adam and Eve in Eden are succeeded, in the favored parable of the classical economists, by Robinson Crusoe. Abandoned to his own ingenuity and will to survive, Crusoe is entitled to a living only if he can wrest it from the elements. Exploitation of an island has replaced steward-ship of a garden (15).

Ecology, the study of the interplay between all living populations and their environments, is a corrective to the human imperialist view of nature. In the ecological perspective, culture and nature are not antagonists external and alien to one another, but joint participants in the evolution of "living systems." Since the term "ecology" was first introduced by Haeckel in 1868, the concern of ecologists has been with the order of the natural world, its organization and regulation, its interdependence and balance. Deprived by Darwin of the theological device of the "great design" to explain such an order, early ecologists constructed new interpretive schemes. They adopted Darwin's notion of the "web of life" and, tacitly at least, Adam Smith's idea of the "invisible hand of the market." Early Western texts abound with references to the "economy" of nature—"ecology" itself comes from the Greek *oikos*, "household." Another theme of ecology, which in time would prove dominant, was the ancient one of Plato's "dialectic," the sense of "things-in-their-connectedness" (16).

Ecology has expanded beyond its original domains of botany and zoology. As the bounds of the inquiry grew, investigative methods multiplied. Modern ecology is at once a biological, behavioral, and social science: biological because its terms and mea-sures derive from the study of plant and animal populations as trophic units (food and energy converters), and because the numbers and health of these populations are important indices of "success"; behavioral because it is concerned with the regularities of action of diverse groups of organisms; and social not only because human popula-tions are included, but also because within many animal populations relationships are sufficiently complex, organized, and differentiated to warrant the use of the term. Ecology is a communications science as well. Not only matter and energy but infor-mation flows through these integrated complexes of living and nonliving things. Con-stitutive units must be able to make accurate responses to each other's changing con-dition so that appropriate exchanges take place at the proper times (17).

An *ecosystem* is the integrated whole made up by the articulations of animate and inanimate things in a specified region. Within this larger whole, smaller complexes of life-supporting exchanges can be discerned; the set of activities performed by the organism which exploits a given location is called its *niche*. Functionally, any ecosys-tem is the corporate product of a number of linked subsystems, each of which attends to the particular problems of growth and survival of a population of organisms. The modes of subsistence of human cultures comprise one class of such subsystems. Human bodies, in turn, may provide food for another population of organisms, or may serve as a crucial reservoir in its reproductive cycle. The same life form, that is, may be either "organism" or "environment" depending upon the point of view from which its particular life-support system is described.

A key postulate of ecological theory states that living systems tend to be *self-reg-*

ulating. That is, a disturbance in any one part of the system is met by corrective adjustments whose net effect is to restore the original state of the system. In response to enduring changes in the environment, moreover, living systems may modify their organization, structure, and functioning. Where this does not happen, catastrophic changes may be set in motion, and an entirely new system may eventually emerge. Viable habitats may be eliminated and with them their resident populations. New habitats allow for new exploitative modes.

The potential for catastrophic change points up a crucial feature of ecological subsystems: their relative autonomy. There is no guarantee that the short-term interests of subsystems are compatible with the long-term survival of the ecosystem as a whole. This is especially true of human cultures. From an ecological point of view, the distinctive feature of human populations is their power by purpose and will to change the limits and tolerances of a given environment, or to create new environments altogether. The distant consequences of the succession of events which such modifications set in train are seldom apparent. Even where "early warning" signs are detected (as has happened, for example, with the effects of industrial pollutants), the inertia of social orders can block preventive or corrective action. The imperatives of cultural and productive systems may override ecological considerations.

Adaptation is the process of accommodation that takes place between an organism and its environment. Two uses of the term should be distinguished. In evolutionary biology it refers to the goodness of fit between an organism's capacity for survival and the environment in which it is embedded. Biological adaptation is inferred from reproductive success. A given trait is adaptive if it ensures that the surviving offspring of its carriers will outnumber those of competitors in the same habitat. All three components of the Darwinian conception of evolutionary process—the generation of variant forms, environmental pressures that selectively favor some variants over others, and mechanisms for the transmission of the favored variations—are, in principle at least, well understood for biological species.° The matter is far less clear in the case of cultural evolution. There is no such simple measure of the relative viability of particular cultural forms as number of surviving progeny. The cultural mechanisms of innovation and the selection and propagation of traits have been no more than crudely delineated.

Still, the notion of adaptation may serve heuristic purposes in the analysis of cultures. Three features are generally imputed to a population that is said to be well

---

°Darwinian theory is not immune to scientific criticism. Philosophers have charged that the notion of survival of the fittest is merely a tautology: the survivors are those who survive. Others have argued that evolutionary theory presents no testable hypotheses—it is a collection of "just so" stories, *post hoc* reconstructions to fit whatever has in fact occurred. Challenges have come also from within the ranks of evolutionary scientists. Contested questions include the assumption that evolution is a gradual process, proceeding in a step-by-step fashion; the assumption that the current utility of a trait points to selective pressures that operated to bring it into existence; and the assumption that the locus of selection is the individual organism exclusively. Alternative postulates have been proposed that amend, rather than dispose of, the central mechanism of natural selection. In particular, the theory of *punctuated equilibrium* proposes that evolution is better envisioned as a series of radical changes—periods of branching speciation and the exploitation of new survival possibilities—that are relatively compressed in geological time (18).

adapted to its surrounds: that in comparison with earlier or alternative modes of live-lihood, a population is better able to withstand or cope with the stresses of a given environment; that it is better equipped to exploit the life-supporting potential of a given habitat; and that its subsistence activities do not threaten immediate degrada-tion of the environment. The Darwinian index, which is the ability to weather the exigencies of a given setting and to reproduce successfully, may prove useful as a lower limit on successful cultural adaptation. Demographic success, however, may stand in the way of the attainment of a desired quality of life.

Adaptation at the level of the individual, as compared with the population level, is both clearer and more relevant to the study of health and disease. In the strict sense, it refers to those changes in the genetic script which are passed on through successive generations because they confer some selective advantage upon their carriers. But adaptation occurs at other levels as well. Actions, habits, and social routines that enable one to deal with specific environmental hazards may be considered adaptive. So may those increases in red cell production, blood oxygenation, and lung capacity that occur in response to high altitude, or the temporary state of physiological arousal that prepares a threatened animal for fight or flight. In its more encompassing mean-ing, then, adaptation may refer to changes that occur at any of several levels (genetic, physiological, behavioral), which may be reversible or not, and which must be eval-uated with reference to the specific set of problems that are to be solved (19).

The stipulation of the special problems to be solved allows for the possibility that once-effective adaptations—for instance, patterns of autonomic arousal—may become obsolete and even disabling when the original set of circumstances has changed. This situation gives rise to a paradox. The more specialized an organism is to the requirements of a specific habitat, that is, the more closely adapted to it, the less likely it is to be able to survive significant changes in that habitat. Short-run suc-cess may incur long-term disaster. Since fluctuation and change are enduring features of environment, a selective premium is placed on life-forms that retain a plasticity of response. *Adaptability* emerges as a higher-order goal of the evolutionary process (20).

In this view evolution has the character of an "existential game," the aim of which is simply to keep playing. To the degree that survival *tout court* is put forth as the criterion of successful play, this position runs the risk of collapsing into simple tau-tology: anything that exists is adaptive. But all modes of problem-solving are not equally desirable. For instance, in the face of powerful pressures to assimilate, some ethnic minorities by dint of organized resistance have managed to retain their cultural identities. Others have been "acculturated" by dominant groups. An analysis that accords equal value to each is short on discriminant power (21).

Culture includes all learned patterns of behavior such as language, attitudes, and skills, as well as the value systems and ethical judgments that underlie them and the particular material items that people use. Culture, in short, describes an entire way of life. But cultures exist in time, and adaptation refers to a process by which history is transmuted into "second nature." This recognition is behind the great changes in the anthropological assessment of the relation between culture and environment that occurred in the last century. Views on the role of environmental factors have oscillated between two extremes: the one saw environment as an outside limit on what was possible; the other saw it as the crucial, determining factor in what was culturally the case. A more cogent view takes environment as a set both of limits and of pressures which interact with cultural formations. Particular cultural formations may show striking parallels—for example, the resemblances of old Swiss village life to contemporary Nepalese villages, in housing styles, farming and herding techniques, practices of community cooperation, and patterns of land ownership—but they are neither invariant nor inevitable solutions to the environmental problems encountered (22).

Severe environmental pressures, however, may impose strict ecological constraints (23). In the unforgiving habitat of the northern Kalahari desert into which they were driven by colonists, !Kung Bushmen manage to live decently, expending a minimum of energy and using only crude tools. Their successful adaptation depends upon a social ethic of food sharing. A "generalized reciprocity" sees to it that the caloric needs of all members of the band are met, imposes stiff proscriptions against hoarding, and prevents social differences in wealth from developing. When this form of primitive communism breaks down, as it does occasionally, the large territory gives the groups that split off room enough to set up on their own.

In a similar fashion, the Plains tribes of North America adapted their social organization to the migratory and breeding habits of the bison. Authority, the size of social units, and the strength of kin ties varied seasonally with the needs of the hunt. During much of the year, the scattered herds were most effectively pursued by small, loosely knit bands of hunters. In the late summer and early fall, however, bison congregated to breed. Local bands, taking advantage of the transient density of buffalo, then gathered in large encampments; tribal ties were briefly rekindled and hunting became a communal affair. Temporary leaders were designated to quell interband disputes and to supervise the kill.

Much hinges on the strength and constancy of the ecological pressures. The nomadism of Bedouin tribes of northern Arabia is best viewed as an adaptation to the uncertain grazing conditions of desert life. Where pasturage is not scarce, larger units, more extended kinship networks, and more complex social systems may be found. Social forces in turn may mute and even annul environmental hazards; they may also exacerbate them and push a society past a critical threshold into calamity. Disaster in human communities is commonly the dual function of some environmental extremity and a vulnerable social system. The Irish potato famine of the 1840s provides a tragic example.

This disaster owed as much to colonialism as it did to the blight of five successive harvests. Irish agricultural workers and farmers had long been exploited by a system of peonage under the British. Colonial law required equal partition of a farmer's land amongst his heirs. The resulting subdivision of land increased the rent intake of absentee British landlords while diminishing the size of a legally defined working farm. At the same time, it encouraged early marriage by heirs, each of whom was ensured a stake in the family holdings. The impoverishment consequent on subdivision and decreased crop yields and farm size reduced Irish peasants to the status of tenant farmers and crowded them onto ever smaller and poorer plots of land. That the population of Ireland could double in the eighteenth century, in the face of this growing immiseration, was owed in good part to a single imported American crop—the potato. By virtue of its hardiness and nutritional value, the potato had replaced all previous foods cultivated on any scale. Any blight threatened this precarious single-crop system; repeated blight was catastrophic.

Famine was followed closely by disease: typhus, dysentery, and cholera were epidemic, scurvy and other forms of malnutrition widespread. Relief measures were stalled initially; news of the famine was dismissed in England as "the invention of agitators." When eventually enacted, relief measures only compounded the catastrophe. Relief was guided by a blend of the doctrines of Malthus and free enterprise. In the theory of Malthus, misery was to be suffered as a necessary check on population; in the theory of laissez-faire, dependency on relief sapped industry and was to be avoided by all means.

In the first year of the famine Indian corn, unknown as a food in Ireland, was introduced. No provision was made for distributing it, however. The architects of this scheme put their trust in the free play of a market for food which—like the food itself—had ceased to exist. With need at its peak, the English treasury official in charge of relief warned that "dependence on charity is not to be made an agreeable mode of life." Relief was made contingent on work; to enact the plan, workhouses had first to be emptied of their usual residents (the aged and infirm, widows, orphans, and children), who had no place to go.

Between 1846 and 1851, more than two million of Ireland's population of eight million was lost. Approximately one million people emigrated, while another one and a half million died of starvation or of diseases related to famine. Family structure, inheritance patterns, and landlord-peasant relations were irrevocably changed (24).

As this example also suggests, competing logics (or even ethics) of production can be distinguished. In the contemporary world, one crucial distinction is that between productive systems that are ruled chiefly by local exigency and those that are ruled by global market forces. This difference is well illustrated by the contrast between valuations of the native societies and resources of frontier regions given by ecological and by traditional economic perspectives. (25). In these regions, geographically isolated at the edge of what is considered civilization, the ecologists' ideal of a self-regulating ecosystem comes closest to being realized. Remoteness has allowed adaptive processes to evolve undisturbed by outside forces. In the absence of conquest, isolation meant also that cultural integrity could be preserved. In studying tribal communities located in such areas, investigators have been impressed with their careful husbanding of natural resources, their tailoring of the size and mobility of settlements to the shifting state of surrounds, and their flexible response to the vagaries of weather, crop yield, or game distribution.

To expanding mercantilist or industrialist economies, however, frontiers meant vast areas of untapped "natural" resources: abundant cheap labor, seemingly limitless opportunities for cultivation and grazing, for huge mineral, oil, and gas resources. The effects of economic exploitation of such regions are often similar, even when the regions themselves differ markedly. The "economic miracle" of a "developing" country has often been the ethnographic devastation of its indigenous populations. Today, in the Amazon basin and in the Arctic—as in southern Africa, the Americas, and the

Antipodes in earlier centuries—foreign investment ventures have invariably spread disease and debility among native peoples, destroyed their cultures, and sometimes annihilated whole populations. Survivors are brought under external political control, and forced onto "reservations" or drawn into the money economy at the fringes of the dominant culture.

Epidemiology and disease

Since the triad of agent, host, and environment comprises its traditional core, *epidemiology* can be described as that aspect of human ecology that relates to states of health and disease. Epidemiology ("epi" upon, "demos" the people) is the science concerned with the health of populations or communities. The compass of this science is to describe states of health and their variation, to discover the determinants of the variations observed, and to use what is discovered to devise and test ways of preventing and controlling ill health. In the literature, the earliest recognition of the role of the environment can be found in the Hippocratic writings, in the treatise *Airs, Waters and Places*. Here one finds everything from physique and fecundity to sexual practice and warlike temperament ascribed to the influence of the purity of water and violence of seasonal change. Since that time, *personae medicae* of all persuasions—court physician and itinerant healer, philosophe and empirick, chronicler of epidemics and tender of "fluxes, agues, botches and boils," modern scientist and traditional herbalist—have found it necessary to pay heed to environmental influences, however much they may have disagreed as to their consequences (26).

The preceding discussion brings us to the question skirted at the beginning of this chapter: What kind of thing, or fact, is disease? The medical model of the past century viewed disease as an independent, natural entity, a thing unto itself, residing in human bodies. The recognition of the role of social factors and of medical practice itself in constructing concepts and shaping perceptions of disease imposes a broader view of its nature. The definitions of physical disorders, no less than of psychiatric disorders, are influenced by social values sometimes quite removed from the clinical situation (1).

The components of a definition of health will be considered here in the dimension of *depth;* Chapter 4 will consider them in the dimension of *breadth*. By the dimension of depth is meant those components at successive and increasingly complex levels of organization. Each of these levels can be conceived as a subsystem, one encompassing the other. In this way, states of health can be defined at an organic, a functional, and a social level. Discrimination among states of health is aided too by a terminology that distinguishes between conditions that are unstable and in process, whether temporary or progressive, and those that are established, stable, and persistent.

For conditions in process, at the organic level, *disease* is best reserved as a term that describes physiological disorder confined to the individual organism. *Illness* describes a subjective state, a psychological awareness of dysfunction also confined to the individual. *Sickness* describes a state of social dysfunction, a social role assumed by the individual that is defined by the expectations of society and that thereby extends beyond the individual to affect relations with others. For conditions that are

stable and persisting, impairment, disability, and handicap are analogous terms.°
Impairment refers to a persisting physical or psychological defect in the individual
which stems from molecular, cellular, physiological, or structural disorder. *Disability*
refers to persisting physical or psychological dysfunction, also confined to the individual, which stems from the limitations imposed by the impairment and by the individual's psychological reaction to it. *Handicap,* like sickness, refers to persisting social
dysfunction, a social role assumed by the impaired or disabled individual that is
defined by the expectations of society. Handicap stems, not from the individual, but
from the manner and degree in which social expectations alter the performance of
social roles by impaired or disabled persons. Neither the terms that describe disorders
in process, nor those that describe persisting conditions, are synonyms for each other.
That is, they do not necessarily have a one-to-one relationship with each other. A
person may have an organic disorder without feeling ill or being disabled; the sense
of being ill entails neither organic disorder nor the automatic assumption of a social
role appropriate to sickness and the seeking or receiving of care; and a person who
malingers can perform the sick role without being either ill or impaired.

Societies in part create the disease they experience and, futher, they materially
shape the ways in which diseases are to be experienced. Cross-cultural studies of disease consistently show that the varieties of human affliction owe as much to the inven-
tiveness of culture as they do to the vagaries of nature. If disease is seen in its full
dimensions as a phenomenon besetting persons in communities, its status as a culturally constituted reality becomes apparent.

Values and social structure account for much of the lack of correspondence that
exists between the three levels: organic, subjective, and social. Millions of Africans
and Asians suffer from the organic diseases of malaria or severe malnutrition without
assuming the sick-role. Likewise, many working-class Englishmen suffer from bronchitis, and many Puerto Ricans in New York suffer from bilharzia, and have not
assumed the sick-role. Conversely, persons may be assigned the role of sickness or
handicap who have no illness or disability and no organic disease or impairment.
Institutions for mental sickness and mental deficiency provide perhaps the most notorious examples. Two decades ago, about 10 per cent of a sample of inmates of mental
deficiency hospitals in England had IQs above a defined functional threshold of mental subnormality. Many were without organic impairment as well. Moreover, persons
may feel ill, and subcultures may sanction them as such, without showing any organic
disease. Hispanic-Americans may suffer from "soul-loss" produced by fright, called
susto, which disturbs the sufferers' sleep and leaves them listless, disinterested in personal appearance, without appetite, and depressed in waking hours. The syndrome
eludes Western diagnostic categories. Disparities such as these among the three depth
dimensions of disease make cross-cultural epidemiological investigations difficult.

Even within a given society, comparative and historical studies of disease are made
problematic by a number of considerations (27). Changes in medical ideology—in

---

° This terminology, introduced in the previous edition of this text, has since been adopted for the International Classification of Impairments, Disabilities and Handicaps of the World Health Organization.

the conceptual foundations and language of clinical description—may make certain diagnoses unintelligible without a thoroughgoing study of the period. Variations in disease nomenclature may multiply instances of the same disease—modern American historians are confronted by no fewer than seventeen different fever types in the medical annals, all of which we now know denote malaria. Developments in medical diagnostic technology can conjure symptomless "diseases" that previously had escaped clinical detection. Thus, between 15 and 30 million Americans, depending on the diagnostic criterion used, can now be tagged as having mild hypertension that is amenable to treatment. A similar situation holds true for the raised blood sugar of asymptomatic diabetes, or for the cellular dysplasia of the neck of the uterus that may presage cervical cancer. Changes in codification practices may make statistical hash out of data on time-trends. For example, suicide rates in the late nineteenth and early twentieth centuries in a number of European countries leapt 10 to 50 per cent after each major reform in data-collection techniques. And finally, errors in codification pose unknown dangers to miners of official records. A 1966 review of the evidence for deaths attributed to cardiovascular disorders in the United States found that only 12 per cent of them were well established, 41 per cent were reasonable judgments, and fully 20 per cent were unwarranted. These and many other pitfalls make clinical and epidemiological history at times a risky enterprise (28).

From an ecological perspective, evolutionary processes may produce remarkable changes in host-parasite relationships. Selective pressures winnow out the more virulent parasitic types, which lose their purchase by destroying their hosts. They also favor resistant host types who can survive the ordeal of infection. When natural selection operates in both these directions, successive generations of host and parasite will be increasingly well adapted to one another. Myxomatosis in Australia is a well-documented instance of such a process (29). In 1950, the myxomatosis virus was introduced to the continent as a means of controlling the rapidly multiplying wild rabbit population, also introduced from abroad in the previous century. The lethality of the virus and its specificity to rabbits made it seem an ideal rodent control measure. At the outset, 99 per cent of the infections proved fatal. Within three years, though, case fatality rates had fallen to 90 per cent, and mean survival time (between infection and death) had nearly doubled. Viral strains removed from the field were found to be much less virulent than the original strains and survived much longer in the wild. For the virus, clearly, the attenuation of virulence was adaptive. At the same time, though at a slower rate, rabbit resistance was changing. A virus lethal in 90 per cent of infections is a stringent selective sieve. The two processes together altered the balance between mortality and survival. Over a period of seven years (roughly 11 rabbit generations), in areas where rabbits had been exposed to five successive epidemics of myxomatosis, mortality rates fell among the infected from 90 to 25 per cent. The immunity such survivors exhibited was not acquired but innate and inheritable. The case nicely illustrates the simultaneous development of adaptations in both host and agent: the attenuation of a virus whose virulence was too high for its own optimal survival; and the selection of a genetically resistant animal population.

Rapid accommodation between animal host and infectious agent has been recorded in human populations as well. Instances of forced adaptation abound in the history of conquest. The estimated 10 per cent of the Central American Indian population who survived the epidemic onslaught of the Spanish in the sixteenth and seventeenth centuries were surely of a stock more resistant to the European disease pool than their ancestors had been. Similarly, chronic phthisis (pulmonary tuberculosis) appears to be the result of accommodations between host and pathogen worked out over the course of hundreds of years or longer. Its disastrous impact on "virgin soil" populations may be only the first step in the process of accommodation (30).

It is possible also that distinct clinical entities may evolve out of common pathogenic stock, depending upon the circumstances under which the pathogen manifests itself. Just such a development had been hypothesized for the changing patterns of infections by the spirochete *Treponema pallidum*. Four clinical syndromes are manifestations of the treponeme: venereal syphilis, nonvenereal endemic syphilis, yaws, and pinta. The evolutionary thesis is that the clinical gradient among these spirochete infections was established as a consequence of the changing social settings of early human society. Originating in Paleolithic times as an endemic skin infection in tropical regions (as are yaws or pinta in our times), this treponeme accompanied migrating hunter-gatherers northward into drier and colder climes. Under these new conditions, the spirochete retreated to those parts of the body that retained heat and moisture (mouth, axillae, and crotch), where it took the form of a common childhood disease, transmitted by contact in early years. With the development of village life, the place of endemic syphilis was secured. Later, when urban civilizations arose, a minimum of sanitary measures was obligatory if such civilizations were to survive. The hygienic barriers thus erected broke the chain of childhood infection and syphilis took on its familiar, sporadic venereal form (though, worldwide, endemic syphilis is still the most common strain of infection). Nor has the process been run to completion. Changes in the clinical manifestations of syphilis have been observed since the introduction of penicillin; eruptive and ulcerative lesions of the skin and mucous membranes are much less common now and the disease in general is milder.

Since the treponeme in all four syndromes shares a common antigenic structure and cannot be distinguished microscopically, cross-immunization occurs. Survivors of childhood yaws or endemic syphilis are immune to the venereal form. One inadvertent result of the mass campaign against yaws undertaken in 1957 in New Guinea by the World Health Organization was to render an entire population susceptible to syphilitic infection. A new highway was opened shortly thereafter, prostitution flourished along truck routes, and an epidemic of venereal syphilis broke out (31).

Examples such as these call attention to the role of both natural endowment and social environment in shaping the disease experience of human communities. Many infectious diseases in which the organism is dependent on the human host—for instance, smallpox, measles, and poliomyelitis—cannot take hold in human populations until the density of population ensures a frequency of contact that sustains the transmission of the microorganism from person to person. The process of human civilization, from this angle, may be charted as a series of disease transitions (32). The ecological complexity of the tropical African niche occupied by early hominids is presumed to be a critical factor in the development of the relatively robust human form. A wide range of parasitic types and intermediate hosts closely hemmed in the

range of human habitation and exerted pressure for the evolution of resistant phe-
notypes. Migration and the development of skills and tools—symbolic as well as material—made "man the hunter" into a shaper of environments as well. Once crops and
animals had been domesticated, nomadism was no longer obligatory and larger settlements became possible. Disease liability changed accordingly.

For one thing, the colder climates meant a reduction in the variety of parasites.
But settlement brought with it an assortment of hazards of its own making: increased
contact with human feces, greater mobility of certain parasites with more widely
distributed water supplies, intimate association with animals and, where irrigation
was practiced, a transplantation of the parasitic ecology of the tropics. The disease
burden thus incurred was not so great, however, as to curtail population growth. On
the contrary, human communities increased in size and density to a point where viral
and bacterial infections could be sustained without the agency of intermediate, nonhuman hosts. For endemic measles, for example, this population threshold appears to
be in the neighborhood of one million: frequent enough person-to-person encounters
allow the chain of infection to persist indefinitely.

Once a pathogenic microorganism became established in a human community, a
typical pattern of host-parasite relations seems to have ensued (33). Recurrent disease
invasions over time bolstered host resistance and tempered parasite virulence to a
point where the disease was no longer normally lethal. In this way, devastating infections were transformed into familiar childhood afflictions (measles, mumps, whooping
cough, chicken pox). Infected early in life, most children in developed countries will
survive the initial bout with typical symptoms or, for some conditions, with no clinically diagnosable illness at all. Each infectious episode (whether accompanied by illness or not) stimulates immune responses that confer life-long protection against subsequent infection. Many such infections—for example, mumps, chicken pox, and
poliomyelitis—seem to be more dangerous or consequential if they are first met later
in life.

In these ways, disease is domesticated, brought into the human fold, and made a
part of the developmental history of its members. From an economic standpoint, disease represents a cost to society as a whole with loss of productive services and outlay
of technical and professional resources, a benefit to those persons and industries that
treat sickness (the healing professions, hospitals, drug companies), and a liability to
those whose livelihood depends on their work. In societies oriented toward private or
centralized accumulation of capital, health itself is defined functionally as the capacity to work. As illustrated by the great hookworm campaign in the American South
initiated early in this century by the Rockefeller Foundation, philanthropic endeavors
in health may be undertaken to increase the productivity of laborers. As the value of
labor increases as a result of ever more technically specialized skills required in production so, one expects, will the value of human capital (34).

Nature, culture, and human adaptation

Natural environments influence the form of disease in two ways. Environment sets
limiting conditions: for example, trypanosomal infections, which produce sleeping
sickness in Africa and Chagas disease in South America, are not sustained in arctic

environments. Environment is always in some sense a factor in disease. But no less than the genetic make-up of a population every environment has its history, in which social factors may figure highly.

The evolution of the sickle-cell trait in African populations illustrates the historical interplay of environment and genes (35). The presence of this gene can be recognized by the sickle shape of red blood cells, observed under a microscope, when they are deprived of oxygen. Genetically, carriers of the trait are heterozygous for the sickle-cell gene and usually no other blood abnormalities ensue. The homozygous offspring of two heterozygous carriers of the gene, on the other hand, are subject to a severe form of anemia and generally die at an early age. Despite this constant loss of the gene among homozygous individuals, frequencies of 20–40 per cent are regularly recorded among various African people. For the lost genes to have been continually replenished by random mutations would have required an exceedingly high mutation rate. In the late 1940s British researchers working in malarial regions in Africa noted that individuals with sickle-cell trait seemed to be unusually resistant to malarial infections. This resistance suggested that the gene is maintained because it confers a selective advantage on heterozygous carriers of the trait.

By the mid-1950s, several lines of evidence (experimental as well as epidemiological) could be marshaled in support of this hypothesis. Fewer parasites of malignant tertian malaria were found in children heterozygous for the sickle cell trait than in those without the trait, as though carriers were resistant to infection. Proportionately more heterozygous individuals were found in adult age-groups than in children young enough not to have suffered losses either from sickle cell anemia or from malaria, as though carriers had greater power of survival. Most striking was that in every instance studied, a significant difference in malaria mortality rates between sicklers and non-sicklers was observed. Recent laboratory experiments have uncovered a plausible physiological mechanism thought to be the basis for the enhanced resistance of sicklers to the malaria parasite (36).

The selective advantage conferred by the heterozygous carriers of the trait appears to be twofold: on the one hand, it protects the heterozygous carriers against disabling and recurrent infection; on the other, it interrupts the process of parasite multiplication, reducing both the numbers stricken and the numbers of intermediate hosts (mosquitoes) they infect. Risk of infection among even nonresistant people is thereby reduced and the whole population benefits. The sickle-cell gene is thus the prime example of balanced polymorphism. That is, more than one form of a gene occurs at a particular locus, and the "deviant" form maintained by the selective advantage conferred on heterozygotes balances the disadvantage conferred on homozygotes.

Archeological evidence suggests that the areas of sub-Saharan Africa that are hyperendemic for malaria became so some 2000 years ago, when large tracts of tropical rain forest were claimed for agriculture. Newly introduced slash-and-burn cultivation enabled communities to plant root and tree crops which greatly increased their food production and population. At the same time, slash-and-burn cultivation destroyed forest cover, leaving behind standing pools of water directly exposed to sunlight. These were the preferred breeding sites of *Anopheles gambiae*, the mosquito that became the major vector of malaria.

The new productive techniques thus established three new ecological niches. The

larger and surer yield of crops as well as the more demanding husbandry they
required encouraged larger and denser human settlements; favorable breeding conditions increased the numbers of mosquitoes; more people and more mosquitoes
meant that malaria parasitism would thrive since a virtually inexhaustible supply of
new hosts was available. Two countervailing developments were thus set up. As population growth intensified demand for food, death and debility from malaria depleted
the human resources needed to produce it. More labor was needed as less of it was
available. Under such conditions the sickle-cell mutation proved adaptive: it provided
a biological protection against a problem that itself arose from the environmental
modifications inadvertently caused by a productive advance. The gene assisted a new
mode of production to establish itself by removing an environmental limit on the
human population.

References

1. **Dubos, R.** (1959). *The Mirage of Health*, New York.
   Lewis, A. (1963). Health as a social concept, *Brit. J. Sociol.*, 4, 109–124.
   Englehardt, H. T., and **Spicker, S. F.**, eds. (1975). *Evaluation and Explanation in the Biomedical Sciences*, Dordrecht, Holland.
   Engel, G. (1977). The need for a new medical model: A challenge for biomedicine, *Science*, 196, 129–136.
   Eisenberg, L., and **Kleinman, A.**, eds. (1981). *The Relevance of Social Science for Medicine*, Dordrecht, Holland.
2. **Turner, V.** (1964). A Ndembu doctor in practice, in *Magic, Faith and Healing*, ed. Kiev, A., New York, pp. 230–263.
   Dubos, R. (1965). *Man Adapting*, New Haven.
   Fabrega, H. (1976). *Disease and Social Behavior*, Cambridge, Mass.
   Landy, D., ed. (1977). *Culture, Illness, and Healing*, New York.
   Good, B. (1977). The heart of what's the matter: The semantics of illness in Iran, *Culture, Medicine and Psychiatry*, 1, 25–58.
   Kleinman, A., **Eisenberg, L.**, and **Good, B.** (1978). Culture, illness and care, *Annals of Internal Medicine*, 88, 251–258.
   Foster, G. M., and **Anderson, B. G.** (1978). *Medical Anthropology*, New York.
3. **Galdston, I.** (1940). Humanism and public health, *Bull. History of Medicine*, 8, 1032–1039.
   Briggs, A. (1961). Cholera and society in the nineteenth century, *Past and Present, 19*, 76–96.
   Flinn, M. W. (1965). Introduction, in Chadwick, E., *Report on the Sanitary Condition of the Labouring Population of Great Britain* (1842), Edinburgh.
   Stedman Jones, G. (1971). *Outcast London*, London.
   Rosen, G. (1973). Disease, debility and death, in *The Victorian City: Images and Realities*, ed. Dyos, H. J., and Wolf, M., London, vol. 2, pp. 625–667.
   Rosen, G. (1975). *Preventive Medicine in the United States 1900–1975*, New York.
4. **Cassirer, E.** (1954). *The Question of Jean-Jacques Rousseau*, Bloomington, Ind.
   Rousseau, J. J. (1967; first pub. 1755, 1762) *The Social Contract and Discourse on the Origin of Inequality*, trans. Tozer, H. J., New York.
   Colletti, L. (1974). Rousseau as critic of civil society, in his *From Rousseau to Lenin*, New York.

5. **Sigerist, H. E.**, ed. (1956). *Landmarks in the History of Hygiene*, New York.
   Foucault, M. (1973). *The Birth of the Clinic*, New York.
   Frank, J. P. (1976; first pub. 1779). *A System of Medical Police*, trans. Lesky, E., Baltimore.
   Rosen, G. (1979). The evolution of social medicine, in *Handbook of Medical Sociology*, ed. Freeman, H. E., Levine, S., and Reeder, L. G., Englewood Cliffs, N.J.
6. **Rosen, G.** (1941). Disease and social criticism, *Bull. History of Medicine, 10*, 5–15.
   Rosen, G. (1947). What is social medicine? A genetic analysis of the concept, *Bull. History of Medicine, 21*, 674–733.
   Ackerknecht, E. H. (1953). *Rudolf Virchow: Doctor, Statesman, Anthropologist*, Madison, Wis.
   Brockington, C. F. (1961). The history of public health, in *The Theory and Practice of Public Health*, ed. Hobson, W., New York.
   Freyman, J. G. (1975). Medicine's great schism: Prevention vs. care: An historical interpretation, *Medical Care, 13*, 525–536.
   Faris, J. C. (1975). Social evolution, population, and production, in *Population, Ecology and Social Organization*, ed. Polgar, S., The Hague.
   Gorz, A., ed. (1976). *The Division of Labor*, Atlantic Highlands, N.J.
   Seddon, D., ed. (1978). *Relations of Production*, Totowa, N.J.
7. *This discussion of the basic elements of economy is taken from*:
   Polanyi, K. (1944). *The Great Transformation*, Boston.
   Weber, M. (1949). *Methodology of the Social Sciences*, Glencoe, Ill.
   Sahlins, M. (1965). On the sociology of primitive exchange, in *The Relevance of Models for Social Anthropology*, ed. Banton, M., London, pp. 137–227.
   Frankenberg, R. (1967). Economic anthropology: One anthropologist's view, in *Themes in Economic Anthropology*, ed. Firth, R., London, pp. 47–80.
   Sahlins, M. (1969). Economic anthropology and anthropological economics, *Social Science Information, 8*, 13–33.
   Dalton, G. (1969). Theoretical issues in economic anthropology, *Current Anthropology, 10*, 63–80.
   Godelier, M. (1972). *Rationality and Irrationality in Economics*, London.
   Kula, W. (1976). *An Economic Theory of the Feudal System: Towards a Model of the Polish Economy, 1500–1800*, New York.
   Clammer, J., ed., (1978). *The New Economic Anthropology*, New York.
8. **Marx, K.** (1977; orig. publ. 1864) Chapter 10: The working day, in *Capital*, vol. I, trans. Fowkes, B., New York.
   Uberoi, J. S. (1962). *Politics of the Kula Ring*, Manchester.
   Sahlins, M. (1972). *Stone Age Economics*, Chicago.
   Cook, S. (1973). Economic anthropology: Problems in theory, methods and analysis, in *Handbook of Cultural and Social Anthropology*, ed. Honigman, J. J., Chicago, pp. 795–860.
   Godelier, M. (1977). *Perspectives in Marxist Anthropology*, London.
9. **Shapiro, J. H.** (1971). *Communities of the Alone*, New York.
   Lombardi, J. R., and **Stack, C. B.** (1976). Economically cooperating units in an urban black community, in *Anthropology and the Public Interest*, ed. Sanjay, P. R., New York, pp. 205–217.
   Susser, I. (1982). *Norman Street: Poverty and Politics in an Urban Neighborhood*, New York.
10. **Salisbury, R. F.** (1962). *From Stone to Steel*, Melbourne.

11. **Epstein, T. S.** (1962). *Economic Development and Social Change in South India,* Manchester.
Pelto, P. J. (1973). *The Snowmobile Revolution: Technology and Social Change in the Arctic,* Menlo Park, Calif.
12. **Smith, W. R.** (1977). *The Fiesta System and Economic Change,* New York.
Singer, M. (1980). *When a Great Tradition Modernizes,* Chicago.
13. **Frank, J. P.** (1941). The people's misery—mother of disease, *Bull. History of Medicine, 9,* trans., Singer, H., 81–100.
Ziegler, P. (1969). *The Black Death,* New York.
Braudel, F. (1973). *Capitalism and Material Life, 1400-1800,* trans. Kochan, M., New York.
Cipolla, C. M. (1973). *Cristofano and the Plague,* London.
Drietzel, H. P., ed. (1973). *The Social Organization of Health,* New York.
Stark, E. (1977). The epidemic as a social event, *Int. J. Hlth. Serv. 7,* 681–705.
14. **M'Cready, B. W.** (1837). On the influences of trades, professions and occupations in the United States, on the production of disease, *Trans. Med. Soc. State of N.Y., 3,* 91-150.
Sigerist, H. E. (1943). *Civilization and Disease,* Chicago.
Dembroski, T. M., Weiss, S. W., Shields, J. L., Haynes, S. G., and **Feinleib, M.,** eds. (1978). *Coronary-Prone Behavior,* New York.
Hunter, D. (1978). *The Diseases of Occupations,* 6th ed., Boston.
15. **Glacken, C. J.** (1967). *Traces on the Rhodian Shore: Nature and Culture in Western Thought from Ancient Times to the End of the Eighteenth Century,* Berkeley.
White, L. (1968). *Machina Ex Deo: Essays in the Dynamism of Western Culture,* Cambridge, Mass.
Leiss, W. (1974). *The Domination of Nature,* Boston.
16. **Bates, M.** (1961). *Man in Nature.* Englewood Cliffs, N.J.
Hawley, A. H. (1968). Ecology: Human ecology, in *International Encyclopedia of Social Sciences,* ed. Sills, D. L., New York, vol. 4, pp. 328–336.
Anderson, J. M. (1973). Ecological anthropology and anthropological ecology, in *Handbook of Cultural and Social Anthropology,* ed. Honigman, J. J., Chicago, pp. 179–239.
Colinvaux, P. A. (1973). *Introduction to Ecology,* New York.
17. **Rappaport, R. A.** (1971). Nature, culture and ecological anthropology, in *Man, Culture, and Society,* ed. Shapiro, H. L., New York, pp. 237–267.
Odum H. T. (1971). *Environment, Power and Society,* New York.
Bateson, G. (1972). *Steps Toward an Ecology of Mind,* New York.
Bennett, J. W. (1976). *The Ecological Transition,* Elsmford, N.Y.
18. **Kimura, M.** (1960). Optimum mutation rate and the degree of dominance as determined by the principle of minimum of genetic load, *J. Genet., 57,* 21–34.
Brues, A. M. (1969). Genetic load and its varieties. *Science, 164,* 1130–1136.
Gould, S. J., and **Lewontin, R. C.** (1979). The spandrels of San Marco and the Panglossian paradigm: A critique of the adaptationist programme, *Proc. R. Soc. Lond.,* B, *205,* 581–598.
Gould, S. J. (1982). Darwinism and the expansion of evolutionary theory, *Science, 216,* 380–387.
Darlington, P. J. (1983). Evolution: Questions for the modern theory, *Proc. Natl. Acad. Sci. U.S.A., 80,* 1960–1963.
19. **Campbell, D. T.** (1965). Variation and selective retention in sociocultural evolution in *Social Change in Developing Areas: A Re-interpretation of Evolutionary Theory,* ed.

Barringer, H. R., Blanksten, G. I., and Mach, R. W., Cambridge, Mass., pp. 19–48.

Boyden, S. V., ed. (1970). *The Impact of Civilization on the Biology of Man*, Toronto.

Alland, A. (1975). Adaptation, *Annual Review of Anthropology*, 4, 59–73.

Little, M. A., and Morren, G. E. B. (1976). *Ecology, Energetics and Human Variability*, Dubuque, Iowa.

Bodmer, W. F., and Cavalli-Sforza, L. L. (1976). *Genetics, Evolution and Man*, San Francisco.

Durham, W. H. (1976). The adaptive significance of cultural behavior, *Human Ecology*, 4, 89–121.

Hardesty, D. L. (1977). *Ecological Anthropology*, New York.

20. Bateson, G. (1963). The role of somatic change in evolution, *Evolution*, 17, 529–539.

Slobodkin, L. (1964). The strategy of evolution, *American Scientist*, 52, 342–357.

Levins, R. (1968). *Evolution in Changing Environments*, Princeton, N.J.

Slobodkin, L. (1968). Toward a predictive theory of evolution, in *Population Biology and Evolution*, ed. Lewontin, R. C., Syracuse, pp. 187–205.

Holling, C. S. (1973). Resilience and stability of ecological systems, *Annual Review of Ecology and Systematics*, 4, 1–23.

Stini, W. A. (1975). *Ecology and Human Adaptation*, Dubuque, Iowa.

21. Diener, P. (1974). Ecology or evolution? The Hutterite case, *American Ethnologist*, 1, 601–618.

Vayda, A., and McCay, B. (1975). New directions in ecology and ecological anthropology, *Annual Review of Anthropology*, 4, 293–306.

Vayda, A. P., and McCay, B. (1977). Problems in the identification of environmental problems, in *Subsistence and Survival: Rural Ecology in the Pacific*, ed. Bayliss-Smith, T. P., and Feachem, G. A., London.

22. Rhoades, R. E., and Thompson, S. I. (1975). Adaptive strategies in alpine environments: Beyond ecological particularism, *American Ethnologist*, 2, 535–551.

Sahlins, M. (1977). *Culture and Practical Reason*, Chicago.

23. Oliver, S. C. (1962). Ecology and cultural continuity as contributing factors in the social organizations of the Plains Indians, *University of California Publications in American Archeology and Ethnology*, 48.

Sweet L. (1965). Camel raiding of Northern Arabian Bedouin: A mechanism of ecological adaptation, *American Anthropologist*, 67, 1132–1150.

Lee, R. B. (1969). !Kung Bushman subsistence: An input-output analysis, in *Environment and Cultural Behavior*, ed. Vayda, A., Garden City, N.Y., pp. 47–49.

24. Woodham-Smith, C. (1962). *The Great Hunger: Ireland 1845-1849*, New York.

Brody, H. (1973). *Inishkillane*, London.

Marcus, S. (1976). Hunger and ideology, in *Representations*, ed. Marcus, S., New York, pp. 3–16.

O'Keefe, P., Westgate, K., and Wisner, B. (1976). Taking the naturalness out of natural disasters, *Nature*, 260, 556–567.

25. *The examples in this section are culled from:*

Janzen, D. H. (1973). Tropical agro-ecosystems, *Science*, 182, 1212–1219.

Gross, D. R. (1975). Protein capture and cultural development in the Amazon Basin, *American Anthropologist*, 77, 526–549.

Davis, S. H. (1977). *Victims of the Miracle*, Cambridge.

Brody, H. (1978). Ecology, politics and change: The case of the Eskimo, *Development and Change*, 9, 21–40.

Margulies, M. (1977) Historical perspectives on frontier agriculture as an adaptive strategy, *American Ethnologist*, *4*, 42–64.

26. Hippocrates. (1881 ed.). *Airs, Waters, and Places*, trans. Adams, D., London.

King, L. S. (1963). *The Growth of Medical Thought*, Chicago.

Susser, M. (1973). *Causal Thinking in the Health Sciences: Concepts and Strategies in Epidemiology*, New York.

Temkin, O. (1973). Health and disease, in *Dictionary of the History of Ideas*, ed. Wiener, P. P., New York, vol. 2, pp. 395–407.

27. Veith, I. (1965). *Hysteria: The History of a Disease*, Chicago.

Foucault, M. (1967). *Madness and Civilization*, New York.

King, L. S. (1971). *The Medical World of the Eighteenth Century*, Huntington, N.Y.

Susser, M. (1974). Ethical components in the definition of health, *Int. J. Hlth. Serv.*, *4*, 539–48.

Figlio, K. (1978). Chlorosis and chronic disease in nineteenth century Britain: The social constitution of somatic illness in a capitalist society, *Social History*, *3*, 167–197.

Reiser, S. J. (1978). *Medicine and the Reign of Technology*, New York.

Ehrenreich, B., and English, D. (1979). *For Her Own Good: 150 Years of Experts' Advice to Women*, New York.

28. Douglas, J. (1967). *The Social Meanings of Suicide*, Princeton, N.J.

Moriyama, I. M., Dawber, T. R., Kannel, W. B. (1966). Evaluation of diagnostic information supporting medical certification of deaths from cardiovascular disease, *Nat. Cancer Institute Monograph*, *19*, 405–419

Clark, E., ed. (1971). *Modern Methods in the History of Medicine*, Atlantic Highlands, N.J.

Richmond, P. A. (1976). Glossary of historical fever terminology, in *Theory and Practice in American Medicine*, ed. Brieger, G. H., New York.

29. Fenner, F. and Ratcliffe, F. N. (1965). *Myxomatosis*, Cambridge.

Cockburn, T. A., ed. (1967). *Infectious Diseases: Their Evolution and Eradication*, Springfield, Ill.

30. Allen, F. J. (1932). Observations on tuberculo-cutaneous reactions and tuberculosis, *Tubercle*, *13*, 241.

Ferguson, R. G. (1934). Tuberculosis among the Indians of the Great Canadian Plains, *Transactions of the 14th Annual Conference of the National Association for the Prevention of Tuberculosis*.

Dobyns, H. F. (1966). Estimating aboriginal American population, *Current Anthropology*, *7*, 395–416

31. Hudson, E. H. (1965). Treponematosis and man's social evolution, *American Anthropologist*, *67*, 885–901.

Willcox, R. R. (1974). Changing patterns of treponemal disease, *Brit. J. Venereal Disease*, *50*, 169–178.

Wood, C. S. (1978). Syphilis in anthropological perspective, *Social Science and Medicine*, *12*, 147–55.

Hart, G. (1982). Syphilis control in populations previously exposed to yaws, *Int. J. Epidem.*, *11*, 181–187.

32. Polgar, S. (1964). Evolution and the ills of mankind, in Tax, S., ed. *Horizons of Anthropology*, Chicago.

Lasker, G. W. (1969). Human biological adaptability, *Science*, *168*, 1480–1486.

Fenner, F. (1970). The effects of changing social organization on the infectious diseases of man, in *The Impact of Civilization on the Biology of Man,* ed. Boyden, S. V., Toronto.

Neel, J. V. (1970). Lessons from a primitive people, *Science, 170,* 815–822.

Cockburn, T. A. (1971). Infectious diseases in ancient populations, *Current Anthropology, 12,* 45–72.

Brothwell, D. (1971). Disease, micro-evolution and earlier populations: An important bridge between medical history and human biology, in *Modern Methods in the History of Medicine,* ed. Clark, E., Atlantic Highlands, N.J.

Underwood, J. H. (1975). *Biocultural Interactions and Human Variation,* Dubuque, Iowa.

Armelagus, G. T. (1976). Man's changing environment, in *Infectious Diseases: Their Evolution and Eradication,* ed. Cockburn, T. A., Springfield, Ill.

McNeil, W. (1976). *Plagues and Peoples,* New York.

33. **Burnet, M.,** and **White, D. O.** (1972). *Natural History of Infectious Diseases,* 4th ed., Cambridge.

34. **Schatzkin, A.** (1978). Health and labor power: A theoretical investigation, *Int. J. Hlth. Serv. 8,* 213–234.

Tullos, A. (1978). The great hookworm crusade, *Southern Exposure, 6,* 40–49.

Brown, R. (1979). *Rockefeller Medicine Men: Medicine and Capitalism in America,* Berkeley.

Becker, G. S. (1980). *Human Capital,* Chicago.

35. **Beet, E. A.** (1948). The genetics of the sickle-cell trait in a Bantu tribe, *Annals of Eugenics, 14,* 279–284.

Allison, A. C. (1954). Protection afforded by sickle-cell trait against subtertian malarial infection, *Brit. Med. J., 1,* 290–294.

Livingstone, F. B. (1958). Anthropological implications of sickle cell gene distribution in West Africa, *American Anthropologist, 60,* 533–562.

Wiesenfeld, S. L. (1967). Sickle-cell trait in human biological and cultural evolution, *Science, 157,* 1134–1140.

Livingstone, F. B. (1971). Malaria and human polymorphisms, *Annual Review of Genetics, 5,* 33–64.

Livingstone, F. B. (1976). Hemoglobin history in West Africa, *Human Biology, 48,* 487–500.

36. **Luzzatto, L., Nwachuku-Jarrett, E. S.,** and **Reddy, S.** (1970). Increased sickling of parasitised erythrocytes as mechanism of resistance against malaria in the sickle-cell trait, *Lancet, i,* 319–322.

2

The description of states of health in populations: some notes on measures, concepts, and analysis

In the social and population sciences, problems of measurement are notorious. Although many of these problems are shared with all sciences, the difficulty of resolving them is greater in the social sciences because of the scale, the multiplicity, and the complexity as well as the nature of the phenomena to be measured. What is to be measured often lacks concrete physical embodiment. The social sciences must stand on the vital comparisons between the attributes of populations, social groups, and whole societies at different times and places.

It is not our intention here to give a disquisition on the problems of method in social science and epidemiology. Numerous texts are available that treat the relevant subjects at length. Rather, this chapter offers a few guiding ideas on the special problems encountered in measuring and analyzing states of health in populations, problems that recur throughout the material to be discussed.

The attributes and relationships to be measured seldom have determining physical dimensions. For instance, the intelligence quotient is a mental construct, founded on the capacity to perform an array of intellectual tests within the norms established for a given age. A diagnosis of disease is no less a mental construct: diagnosis is founded on the concurrence of a set of symptoms and physical signs and physiological states, a pattern that is inferred to follow from specific antecedent events and that portends a course and a range of outcomes of varying particularity. Likewise, the description of attitudes, beliefs, and behavior each presents its own similar if singular difficulties.

The specification of group membership can be equally abstract: social groups—whether they are social classes, ethnic groups, or "races," occupations, churches, or corporations—do not have physical bounds that contain their members, unless they are the closed systems of such "total institutions" as prisons, warships, or longstay mental hospitals. The membership of an individual in social groups is more or less partial and divided among many other memberships of similar and different groups, and more or less temporary and limited by social mobility among groups. Groups themselves change in character over time and place, and thus seldom conform to a standard that can be generalized across time and place.

The constructs that describe the attributes of individuals and societies, it will be evident, must be reduced in scope and limited by definition if they are to prove measurable. To deploy any such construct in the form of a measure, the salient features of the construct must be identified in a way that has common currency or that can gain the common consent of social scientists. A workable measure will necessarily rest on an *index* of some kind that stands for the construct. The index may depend on one item or on many items in combination. Items may be based on presumed or predetermined knowledge of their significance; or they may be combined to form a statistically derived scale of correlated items to indicate, for example, attitudes, or beliefs, or levels of physical function, or the experience of stressful events.

With a health disorder, any measurable point in its course can be used as an index. The index can be the reports of subjective *symptoms*, some of which would go unmarked unless elicited by interviewers' questions put to persons who feel *ill* but who have not elected to enter medical care; it can be complaints made by those who have declared themselves *sick* and elected to enter care. It can be clinical *disease* discovered by medical examinations or screening tests, either among those who have become patients or in communities at large; it can be those diseases severe enough to lead to hospital admission; it can be one of several consequences of disease, whether impaired physical or psychic function, or disability in social and work performance. Finally, it can be those conditions that apparently cause death, or simply death itself. Some indices are observations, not of disease in its active course, but of stable *impairments* that are the long-term issue of maldevelopment, injury, or disease; others are the functional *disabilities* that attend such impairments, or the social *handicaps* that may characterize the social positions of putatively impaired or functionally disabled persons. (See Chapter 1 for definitions of several of these terms.)

All these constructs are elaborations and specifications of the overarching construct of a state of health. Each construct can be measured by one or several indices, and each index yields complementary but different information. The limits of analysis based on any one index, as in the following pages, must be borne in mind. The essence of a useful index is that it does indeed measure what it purports to measure—that is, it is valid—and that it will reproduce the same result on repetition—that is, it is reliable. Multiple indices may do a better job of producing a valid and reliable measure than does any single index.

The idea of validity is a complex one. *Construct validity* is what the investigator states that the index is measuring, for instance, with a sphygmomanometer reading used to measure a persisting hemodynamic condition described as "blood pressure," or with intelligence tests used to measure "intelligence," or with occupation used to measure social class. *Consensual validity* describes the degree of consensus among experts about such construct validity; the construct is valid because an array of experts agree that the index describes the entity under investigation. *Criterion validity* describes the degree to which such an index is associated with some other index or measure that is taken to be more valid. Class consciousness, if judged more valid as an index of social position than an investigator's ranking of occupations, can thus be used as a criterion for the validity of the occupational ranking. On the other hand, it can also be used to measure predictive validity. *Predictive validity* describes the degree to which a criterion (the "more valid" measure) is associated with an outcome variable. Thus in the class consciousness study cited, occupation could be considered as a criterion that "predicted" attitudes and values. The potential for circularity is evident where the validity of the criterion itself derives from the validity of a construct.

Reliability refers to the degree to which the results obtained by a measurement procedure can be replicated. Unreliability arises from divergences between observers and instruments of measurement. Reliability can be classed in two types and quantified according to whether it relates to "error" between observers or error between instruments. *Intraobserver reliability* is measured by the correspondence between the observations of a single observer at different times; and *interobserver reliability* by the correspondence between the observations of different observers at the same or different times. These are termed "alpha reliabilities." The reliability of instruments and procedures is measured by the correspondence between different procedures and measuring instruments used to acquire the same data. These are termed "beta reliabilities."

Measures of frequency in populations

In the study of the health states of populations, certain measures are basic. Descriptions of health conditions are most usually stated in terms of incidence and prevalence. First we consider incidence.

Incidence describes the frequency with which events occur in a population: an incidence rate describes the frequency with which those events occur over a defined period of time. With health disorders, which may be chronic and longlasting, or episodic and recurrent, as well as acute and once and for all, incidence rates generally refer to the frequency of newly arising disease.

Recurrent *spells* present special problems. Spells of the same disease recurring in the same person may be fresh episodes altogether, as when the many "common cold" or "flu" viruses repeatedly attack an individual. Such spells, on the other hand, may be the recurrent episodes of a chronic disorder, say rheumatoid arthritis or peptic ulcer. Since spells of either kind can recur in the same person, a count of spells may be far from reflecting the count of *persons* affected. Rates for different populations will not be comparable if these distinctions are not made.

The search for those causes of ill health residing in the environment is best pursued by studies of incidence. Incidence relates disorders to circumstances at the time of onset and can obviate some of the crucial uncertainties about the time sequence of events inherent in such observational research. However, most incidence rates must use data gathered in or by health service agencies. The rates based on health services are likely to be unrepresentative of the population as a whole unless the rates reflect serious disease in modern urban societies, or mortality rates of fatal diseases, or total populations under constant surveillance by health services—as in the military and in newborn nurseries in the contemporary United States—or unless they are derived indirectly from repeated prevalence studies. The necessary use of service data sources makes incidence a measure of demand on services rather than a faithful measure of health disorders. A full estimate of health in a community must go beyond the demand for care and seek out the true incidence of disorder, hidden as well as overt.

For uniformly severe or fatal conditions, particularly those where the interval between onset and death is short, the incidence of hospital admission and death can provide useful criteria of need. These rates can be representative of the total population in countries with adequate coverage by health services and universal registration of deaths. Yet even in these circumstances deaths may escape notice, or if noted, may not be accurately certified and tabulated. In places like New York City or London, coronary heart disease is a major cause of death. About half such deaths are sudden and occur outside hospitals, inaccessible to precise diagnosis except at autopsy. Everywhere many old people, whatever the cause, die quietly at home. In such instances, factors found to be associated with hospital deaths may relate to the capacity for survival up to the time of admission rather than to the genesis of a disorder.

Prevalence describes the amount of disorder existing in a population at a particular time regardless of time of onset. It therefore affords a useful measure of the current load of disorder to be provided for. However, prevalence compounds two measures: duration and frequency of occurrence (or incidence). As a result, the degree to which acute disorders of short duration—as compared to chronic disorders of long duration—will occur in a prevalence study can vary greatly, even when incidence rates are similar. Whereas chronic but generally nonlethal conditions such as peptic ulcer or psychoneurosis are likely to be found in any given set of prevalence statistics, serious but shortlived epidemics might not be detected at all unless histories of past illnesses are taken. Attacks of influenza, or deaths due to smog and even to heart disease, all take on an epidemic character, particularly in winter months and among old people.

From the distinctions made above between the demand for care and the full extent of ill health, and between incidence and prevalence, it follows that the precise numerators and denominators used in the calculation of rates affect the results. In incidence and prevalence rates the denominators—the average or midpoint population over a specified time period, or the population at one point in time respectively—are much the same. The crucial difference in the two types of rate resides in the numerator. The numerator is the outcome (or dependent variable) chosen as the index of ill health. This index can be one of the many described above, each of which will produce quite different rates for either incidence or prevalence.

We can illustrate the distinction between incidence and prevalence rates by looking at Down's syndrome. Many infants with Down's syndrome are born with anatomical defects and immunological deficiencies. Those most seriously affected tend to die in infancy or early childhood. Present day surgery can correct many of the anatomical defects, antibiotics reduce the risk of death from some recurrent infections, and immunization removes the danger of others, thereby greatly improving the chance of survival for affected infants. Thus, public health along with medical and surgical measures have increased the expectation of life for Down's syndrome infants. The greatest relative increase in survival has been under the age of 10; the chances of surviving until 10 have about doubled over the last 30 years.

There is an apparent paradox between the two measures of frequency discussed above, incidence at birth and prevalence at older ages. Although we have every reason to believe that incidence at birth is declining (in consequence of the decline in birth rates in older women who have the highest risk), prevalence at older ages is undoubtedly rising. Figures 2.1 and 2.2 illustrate the dynamics of these changes. Estimates of the number of affected infants have been made from the age-distribution of the childbearing population in England and Wales from 1920 to 1970. The figures incorporate available survey data but are essentially models.

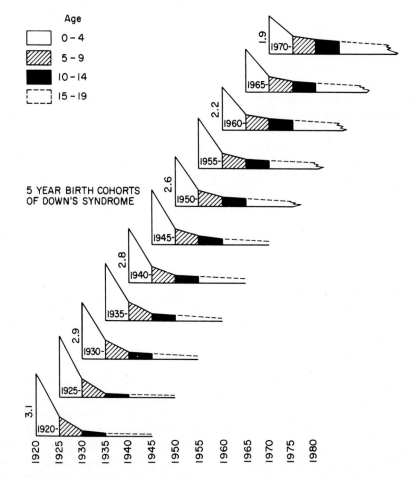

Figure 2.1 Successive five-year birth cohorts of Down's Syndrome from 1920 to 1970: Estimated incidence (per 1000) at birth and survival through ages 0–25 years. *Source:* Stein, Z. (1975). Strategies for the prevention of mental retardation, *Bull. N. Y. Acad. Med.*, 51, 130–142.

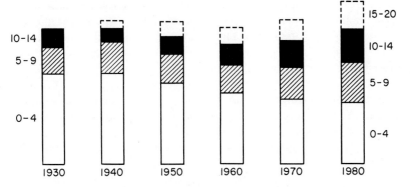

Figure 2.2 Estimated prevalence of Down's Syndrome in age-groups 0–4, 5–9, 10–14, 15–19 years for decennia 1930 to 1980. *Source:* Stein, Z. (1975). Strategies for the prevention of mental retardation, *Bull. N. Y. Acad. Med., 51,* 130–142.

Figure 2.1 shows the estimated numbers of births and their survival curves for successive five-year birth cohorts with Down's syndrome in this century. Although an estimated decline in incidence at birth took place, from 3.1 per 1000 in 1920 to 1.9 per 1000 in 1970, this decline was insufficient to balance the increase in prevalence at older ages owed to the increase in life expectancy at birth. The increasing accumulation of survivors brought about a corresponding rise in prevalence. This increase in prevalence, especially at older ages, is considerable in spite of the decrease in births. Clinical advances over the next decades are likely to improve further the chances of survival in Down's syndrome and prevalence at older ages can be expected to rise still more as a result.

Life-cycles and populations: age, time, and period

It is instructive to observe the influence of contrasting environments on the varying forms assumed by disease in the course of the life-cycle. The individual human organism, the phenotype, is a survivor of a process. In the course of this development, the expression of its genetic inheritance, the genotype, is modified, adapted, or impaired by wear and tear, and shaped by the acquisitions of experience. Some external sources of injury have immediate and observable effects on the organism, while others are embodied within it to produce long-lasting effects that are latent or deferred. For instance, infection by the tubercle bacillus produces, at each age, a constantly unfolding pathology. Pathogenesis begins with the "primary infection," dangerous to infants but otherwise seemingly benign until, after a variety of environmental assaults, the bacillus produces the acute cavitating fibrotic disease of older people. All the age-related effects are modified by the particular environmental experience of the individual. Within each individual, so to speak, is stored a memory both of genetic inheritance and of past experience.

When chronological age is used at any given time as an indicator of the outcome of this process of interaction between inheritance and experience, three dimensions of age as an attribute of individuals are involved. First, age is a description specific to the state of the individual at a particular point in time; it tells that he or she is young or old. Second, it is a statement of the duration of an individual's exposure to life experience; it quantifies the weathering caused by environment. Third, it is a mark of membership in a particular historical generation or birth cohort; age identifies the specific historical experience to which the individual was exposed. The nature and strength of the extraneous molding forces to which the individual has been subjected during aging can be inferred by comparing groups of people of the same age, each in the context of its special life experience and historical time.

Age as an attribute of populations is also complicated. The discrete individuals in a population are brought by the social structure into some sort of ordered relation with each other, to form social categories and groups. At a given point in time, any such population is young or old according to the distribution of age-groups within it. The age of a population is an outcome of the interplay of historical forces, a statement of the balance of fertility and mortality experience through time, and thereby an experience unique to each of the constituent generations.

The size and the composition of a closed population (i.e., one not subject to gains and losses by migration) are the outcome of an equation through time of rates of birth and death. Increase or decrease of a population depends on the difference between the two rates; likewise, the age and sex composition of the population depend on its history of fertility and mortality. High birth rates raise the proportion of the young; low birth rates, the proportion of older people. The overall birth rate itself depends on the age composition of the population, and on the rate of childbearing at each age. Similarly, the overall death rate is a function of the age-sex composition of the population and of the death rate at each age and for each sex. (*Birth rates*, like crude death rates, are usually stated per 1000 total population per year. The *fertility* of a population is usually stated as a rate per 1000 women of childbearing age, often 15 to 45 years.)

Mortality

The pattern of death is a useful starting point in the description and understanding of health conditions. The available data must be approached with caution, however, as crude indices rather than precise measures. Death certificates assign cause of death selected, at the best, by the subjective judgment of variously trained physicians; the certificates are coded by clerks using an unavoidably imperfect international classification of diseases; and most registration procedures lay down that in each case a single disease must be selected as the underlying cause of death, thus distorting reality, for where multiple diseases coexist and contribute to death, ordinarily only one is registered and analyzed as the cause.

Curves of mortality plotted by age have a characteristic shape (see Figure 2.3). Consistent features are the peaks among the newborn and the aged, and the higher rates for males than females throughout life. To take the United States in 1980 as an example, about one per cent of the population died each year, but this is the average of rates as low as .03 per cent in the age-group 5 to 14 years, and above 15 per cent

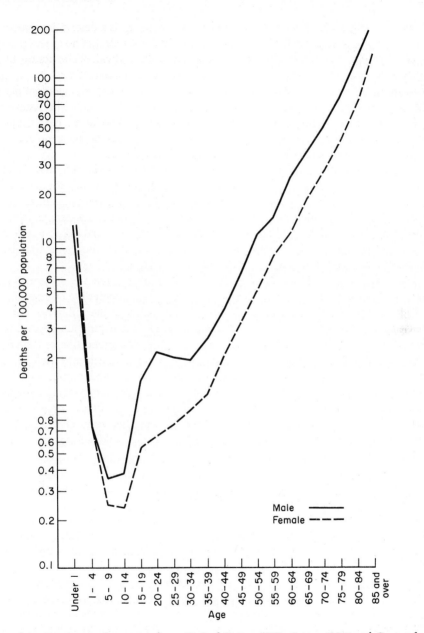

Figure 2.3 Death rates by age and sex, United States, 1980. *Source:* National Center for Health Statistics (1983). Advance Report of Final Mortality Statistics, 1980, *Month. Vit. Stat. Rep.*, vol. 32, No. 4, Supplement, p. 10.

at ages over 85 years. The death rate falls sharply from the high rates of the first years of life, and especially in the first month of life during which about three-quarters of first-year deaths occur, to reach its lowest point at puberty. The death rate then tends to rise exponentially, that is, the rate rises by the same *proportion* in each successive age-group. In 1980, at age 35 to 39 years the rate was 1.8 per 1000 persons; for each successive decade of age the rate more than doubled to reach 10.8 per 1000 at 55 to 59 years, 24.6 per 1000 at 65 to 69 years, and 54.9 per 1000 at 75 to 79 years. The overall age-adjusted male death rate (7.7 per 1000) was 80 per cent higher than the female rate (4.3 per 1000); in the age-group 15 to 29, it was almost three times as high as the female rate (1, 2, 3).

Populations can be thought of as collections of individuals who survive a process of selection; they are forged by the interaction of constitution and environment over time. A common method of analyzing the effect of exposure to environment on life and health is to examine age-specific period rates of relevant phenomena, that is, their frequency in successive age-groups at a defined period in time. The shape of the curve plotted by age reveals whether a phenomenon is characteristic of any particular age-group at that time and place; it shows whether the phenomenon varies in frequency as a function of age, which can be thought of as a measure of duration of exposure to the life situation as well as a measure of an intrinsic aging process. The constrasts revealed among populations by cross-sectional comparisons between different places at the same time, and by historical comparisons of the same place at different times, point to the influence of environmental and social conditions, provided the populations themselves can be taken to be comparable.

Statistical manipulations are commonly applied to data of this type to facilitate their interpretation. *Age and sex adjustment* aim to improve the comparability of different populations. Since, as we shall see, age and sex are powerful determinants of mortality and morbidity, and populations may differ markedly from one another in these respects, naked comparisons can be grossly misleading. Thus *the standardized death rate* tries to make comparable the crude or overall death rates of populations by correcting for age and sex differences in the populations. The standardized death rate is obtained by calculating the death rates per 1000 in the population being studied, for each sex- and age-group (i.e., age-specific death rates). The number of deaths expected in each sex- and age-group of a standard population, if these rates prevailed, is then calculated. The deaths in all the sex- and age-groups are then added, and an age- and sex-adjusted rate is thus obtained for the total population.

A standardized rate does more than improve the comparability of population measures; it also provides a summary statistic by which to make ready comparison. Thus it circumvents the laborious process of comparing each specific sex- and age-group, although not without loss of information.

Expectation of life is another summary statistic of this kind, but precisely the obverse of standardized mortality. The *expectation of life* at a particular age is the average number of years a population would be expected to survive beyond that age, if the population experienced the mortality rates for a given calendar year. At birth it is the expected average survival period of the population born in that year, calculated from the mortality rates in each age-group of the whole population for that year. Thus a *current life table* is constructed that provides a useful summary of potential survival. It is an arbitrary and erroneous assumption, if a useful one for comparative purposes, that the population will experience the mortality of a given year throughout life.

Period and cohort analysis

Comparisons over time within societies present problems that differ from those of simultaneous comparisons across societies and populations. In the modern world, economic and social forces induce continued rapid change in the configuration of society, including health and disease. Change in disease usually implies change in its causes. Hence for the epidemiologist in particular historical analyses of the health disorders of populations are a stock in trade. Any valid analysis of health patterns over time must therefore find means of taking account of the changes in society.

In the design of studies of *time-trends*, control of the components of the time variable presents special problems. People exposed to a particular historical period share the common experience of that period. Hence a typical approach to the study of time-trends and their causes is to compare the frequencies of health disorders at successive time periods separated by fixed intervals such as quinquennia or decennia. This is the method of *period analysis*. The comparisons made are between rates of a particular manifestation in the several age- and sex-groups of the population at each time period; they are viewed in cross section at successive points over the years under study.

In this way, period analysis relates health phenomena prevailing at given periods to the environment prevailing at those periods; each period, in effect, stands for a given environment. The causal assumption is of a current environment producing a *concurrent effect*. With an influenza epidemic, where the virus spreads rapidly and runs its course in a single winter season, the assumption is sound. In other circumstances, the assumption of concurrent effect can lead to gross error in interpreting time-trends. This applies to both the supposed causes and the outcomes being studied.

The error arises especially with chronic conditions, for instance, peptic ulcer, chronic renal disease, hypertension, and cigarette smoking. Each of these conditions has been interpreted as rising in frequency at a time when more appropriate analysis showed them to be declining. The error is rooted in the long *latent interval* that may occur between the operation of a cause and the manifestation of its effects in the form of chronic disease, and in the changes in trends that often supervene during such a latent interval. In period analysis latent intervals are necessarily ignored, since effects are treated as if they were concurrent with the environment of the period by which they were induced; it is assumed that they are immediately expressed in response to the enviroment of the period, among the assembly of age-groups as they exist at the point of analysis.

At any point in time, however, the consecutive age-groups then existing constitute an array of successive generations. Each of these generations has been exposed to an unique historical environment that coincides, not with the period under analysis, but with its life-span. Thus, period analysis cannot take into account that variation in phenomena arising from the different environments to which each age-group in the population was exposed as society changed during the time preceding the observation.

These historical differences between generations, or *generation effects,* are better approached by *cohort analysis.* Cohort analysis can be seen as an elaboration of the cohort study design applied to the study of time-trends. In the cohort design the study population is selected according to exposure to a hypothetical cause and observed thereafter for effects of exposure. In cohort analysis, the experience of a succession of generations, or cohorts, is traced over their life course (4).

Cohort analysis is accomplished by a simple device. The population is defined not at the point of occurrence of the events or outcomes under examination (for instance, date of death), but at the point of entry into the relevant period of experience leading to the event (for instance, date of birth or date of entry into an institution). To accomplish the transformation into birth cohorts, one need know only two facts—age at the time of the event and the date of the event—in order to derive the third fact of date of entry to the cohort. A birth cohort thus includes all those within a population who were born at the same time and who age together.

At any given period, the general population comprises the succession of survivors from each cohort, each of whom contributes a different age-group in the total array. Differences in population structure between periods follow from the combination of cohorts peculiar to each period. These combinations, and the size and demographic attributes of each cohort included, are determined by the differing rates of accessions through births and immigration, and of losses through deaths and emigration. The demographic structure that characterizes each period, in terms of age, sex, and social position, is a statement of the balance of fertility, mortality, and migration through time of all the cohorts combined.

Cohort analysis has converse limitations in the appropriate analysis of period effects. Any given calendar date or time period, as a variable applied to individuals, has three distinct dimensions. The date specifies an environment at a point in time; it denotes an historical experience unique for each generation; and it is a measure of the duration of exposure to life experience from conception up to that date. One of these three dimensions must be left uncontrolled by either period or cohort analysis. Period analysis examines the joint and separate effects of current experience, defined by the date of events observed, and age. But period analysis does not capture the effects of the experience of generations. Cohort analysis examines the joint and separate effects of generation experience defined by the date of birth or entry to the cohort, and age. But cohort analysis does not capture the effects of given periods.

The structural ties between the three variables—age, period, and cohort—have made quantification of their relative and joint effects difficult (5). Thus for the most part the method has been a graphic one in which interpretation has been founded on inspection. More recently a number of multivariate analytic approaches have been developed (6) that enable age, period, and cohort effects to be quantified given certain assumptions.

Cohort analysis can be used to reveal the effect of those differences in early life experiences that persist through time to manifest themselves only at later ages. One example addressed the idea of racial or social degeneration, with which many nine-teenth-century thinkers were obsessed, each rationalizing the idea in a different way. Karl Pearson, a social Darwinist and eugenicist, believed that the decline in infant mortality that began in England and Europe at the turn of the century was the herald of racial degeneration; the weak as well as the strong now survived to flout natural selection, and in their adult years they could only add to the general debility of the population (7). These fears were put to rest by one of the first cohort analyses to be applied to a health problem: Kermack, McKendrick, and McKinley in 1934 analyzed British and Swedish mortality trends. They showed quite clearly that as the infant mortality of each successive birth cohort declined, so equally regularly the age-specific mortality of each of these cohorts at successive ages declined. Figures 2.4 and 2.5 illustrate their analyses for Britain (8).

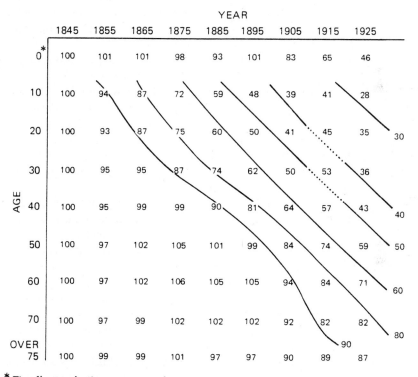

*The figures in the zero row refer to deaths under one year per 1000 births.

Figure 2.4 Age-specific mortality (around each central year of death at 10-year intervals and for 75 years and over) for England and Wales, 1845–1925. Birth cohorts indicated by free-hand diagonal lines. *Source:* Taken from Kermack, W.O., McKendrick, A.G., and McKinley, P.L. (1934). Death-rates in Great Britain and Sweden: Some regularities and their significance, *Lancet, 1,* 698–703; as cited by Susser, M. (1981). Environment and biology in aging: Some epidemiological notions, in McGaugh, J.L., and Kiesler, S.B., eds., *Aging: Biology and Behavior,* New York, 77–96.

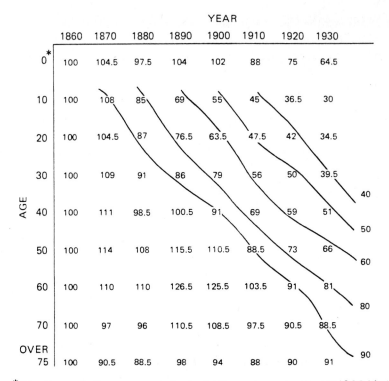

*The figures in the zero row refer to deaths under one year per 1000 births.

Figure 2.5 Age-specific mortality (around each central year of death at 10-year intervals and for 75 years and over) for Scotland, 1860–1930. Birth cohorts indicated by free-hand diagonal lines. *Source:* Taken from Kermack, W.O., McKendrick, A.G., and McKinley, P.L. (1934). Death-rates in Great Britain and Sweden: Some reqularities and their significance, *Lancet, 1,* 698–703; as cited by Susser, M. (1981). Environment and biology in aging: Some epidemiological notions, in McGaugh, J.L., and Kiesler, S.B., eds., *Aging: Biology and Behavior,* New York, 77–96.

In another example Wade Hampton Frost, in a classic paper published posthumously in 1939, demonstrated that the pattern of deaths from tuberculosis was consistent with a cause operating from early childhood. This cause was inferred from the distinctive pattern of mortality risk that was carried through life by each generation (9). Figures 2.6a and b are an updated version of Frost's analysis. Period analysis of trends in death rates in Massachusetts from 1880 to 1930 had revealed puzzling shifts, from one period to another, in age-peaks of deaths from the disease. Figure 2.6a shows, in the cross-section contours at successive dates, the gradual disappearance of an age-peak among young adults, together with a shift toward a pronounced peak in older age groups. Cohort analysis revealed a different age distribution. The death rates were consistent between successive generations, with each generation also maintaining a consistent position relative to the others from early childhood on. Figure 2.6b shows these features, with a consistent age-peak in the mid-twenties.

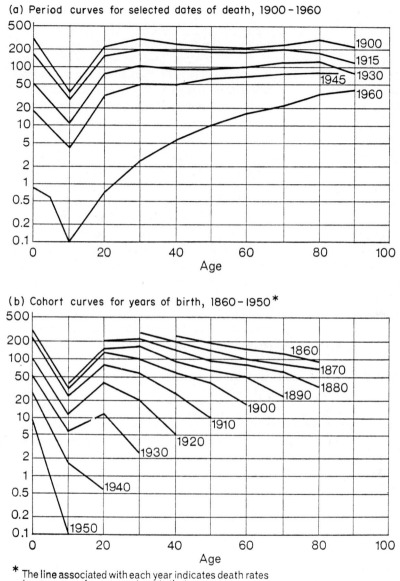

(a) Period curves for selected dates of death, 1900-1960

Age

(b) Cohort curves for years of birth, 1860-1950*

Age

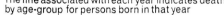

* The line associated with each year indicates death rates
by age-group for persons born in that year

Figure 2.6 Death rates for tuberculosis, by age, United States, 1900–1960 (per 100,000 population). *Source:* Doege, T.C. (1965). Tuberculosis mortality in the United States, 1900–1960, *J. Amer. Med. Ass.,* 192, 1045–48; as cited by Susser, M.W. (1969). Aging and the field of public health, in Riley, M.W., Riley, J.W., and Johnson, M.E., eds. *Aging and Society,* Vol. II, Russell Sage Foundation, New York, p. 141.

The shifts in age-peaks in the period analysis could best be explained as an artifact of the underlying assumptions of the period analysis. The apparent susceptibility acquired by the older age-groups in the more recent periods, suggested by period analysis, could be reinterpreted from the cohort analysis as the residuum of the high risk experienced by earlier generations. These findings gave new significance to the seemingly benign primary tuberculosis infection of early childhood. The primary condition was now confirmed as the forerunner of the fatal adult forms.° The target of primary prevention, which seeks to forestall the onset of a health disorder, in consequence had to shift from adults to the young.

The dimensions of age are a function of the dimensions of time. This example from Frost makes plain the value of cohort analysis for controlling age factors as well as time factors. Any age distribution of a condition within a population can be a consequence of aging processes of individuals, whether these are intrinsic, or caused by the increasing duration of exposure to the wear and tear of life as time passes, or to forces specific to the environments particular to some times at some places.

With any condition that is affecting later generations (cohorts) differently from earlier ones—either because of changes in cohort characteristics or in the life circumstances in which the cohorts were born—cohort analysis will reveal an association with age quite different from that shown by the more usual period analysis. If, for example, a condition begins to rise in incidence among new cohorts of later birthdate, then in a period analysis the rise will be reflected by the appearance of high frequency peaks in the newly affected younger age-groups, but without raising the rates among the old.

Figure 2.7 shows death rates from lung cancer over the period 1914 to 1961, and illustrates just such a case of a disease that is increasing and affecting cohorts of more recent birthdate with ever greater frequency (10). Mortality from the disease is rising rapidly and the curve for every birth cohort shows deaths rising regularly with age (continuous lines in the figure). By contrast, the curves for each date or period (broken lines in the figure) suggest that, after a peak around 70 years of age, the oldest age groups have relatively lower rates of lung cancer. Thus, the cross-sectional data of the period analysis create the impression that the oldest individuals have become less susceptible; but this impression rests on the incorrect assumption that the age-groups at each date of death, having had the same duration of exposure to life, have had equivalent experience.

Alternatively, if a condition begins to decline in incidence among new cohorts of later birthdate, then the decline will be reflected in the cross-section age curves of a period analysis by lowered rates among the young, but not necessarily among the old. These relationships are illustrated in the period analysis of tuberculosis, a declining disease, in Figure 2.6a and b. The higher rates among the older age-groups represented earlier cohorts that continue to manifest a residual mortality caused by their

---

° Years elapsed, however, before Frost's result was thoroughly incorporated into clinical thinking. It has since been argued that the differences between the causes of early- and late-onset tuberculosis are so great as to warrant classifying them as two different diseases.

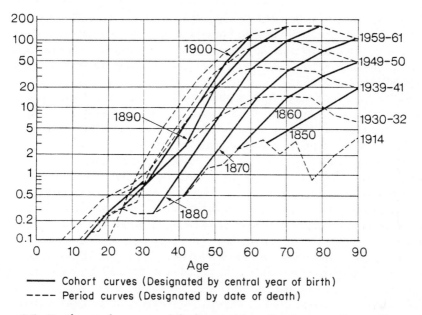

Cohort curves (Designated by central year of birth)
---- Period curves (Designated by date of death)

Figure 2.7 Death rates for cancer of the lung and bronchus, by age, white males, United States, 1914–1961 (rate per 100,000 males). *Source:* adapted from Case, R.A.M. (1956). Cohort analysis of mortality rates as an historical or narrative technique, *Brit. J. Prev. Soc. Med.*, *10*, 159–71; as cited by Susser, M.W. (1969). Aging and the field of public health, in Riley, M.W., Riley, J.W., and Johnson, M.E., eds. *Aging and Society*, Vol. II, Russell Sage Foundation, New York, p. 140.

experience in earlier years; the younger age-groups represent later cohorts that have escaped that experience and its effects on mortality.

Thus, cohort analysis of trends in the occurrence of disease is more discriminating than period or cross-section analysis in unravelling age and generation effects. Cohort analysis helps to sort out the component of life experience due to membership in particular cohorts from the component of intrinisic age changes as well as from that of concurrent period effects. For instance, cross-sectional studies of measured intelligence at different ages have shown a decline in measured intelligence among elderly persons, especially those in occupations that made few intellectual demands. Longitudinal studies of cohorts of old people, however, do not support the implication of steady intellectual deterioration among them; the apparent deterioration shown in cross-sectional analysis is almost certainly a result of successively less education among the older generations than among the younger generations that followed them.

Suicide rates among white males in the United States illustrate an instance of a cause of death that, though associated with age, has shown relative stability through time with little change in frequency between cohorts. In such a case, a cohort analysis is no more informative than a cross-section analysis; both will reflect the absence of secular change. In the short run, suicide rates are sensitive to current social forces, and thus illustrate the special utility of cross-sectional period analysis for phenomena affected by conditions associated with the time of observation (rather than with the time of birth). It can readily be seen from the cross-section age curves in Figure 2.8, for example, that regardless of age men showed a rise in the incidence of suicide after 1929 at the depth of the Great Depression, and a fall with the engagement of the Second World War (11).

Death rates among males from peptic ulcer in England and Wales illustrate the age patterns of a disease that first waxed and has since begun to wane (12). As this condition wanes, it too is now affecting later (i.e., younger) cohorts with decreasing frequency. At first sight, the trends of gastric and duodenal ulcer mortality are confusing in the extreme, as shown for male deaths in Figure 2.9a and b. The trends appear to show a rise in death rates among the old during the past 50 years, but a fall among the young. While biological and social phenomena are notorious for their irregularity as compared with the lesser vagaries of the physical world, the variability exhibited in these data is too great to make biological sense. The data begin to do so only when it is recognized that the diverging fan shape of these cross-section age curves for gastric and duodenal ulcer is characteristic of a condition that has both risen and fallen in frequency during the period of study (see Figure 2.10 a and b).

When these same data are converted to cohort graphs, as in Figure 2.11, the regularity of the age association of the disease becomes evident. In order to avoid overlapping contours in these graphs, it is necessary to plot mortality for each age separately. The mortality of each birth cohort at different ages is represented vertically, upward from one age contour to the next, while the differences in mortality at each

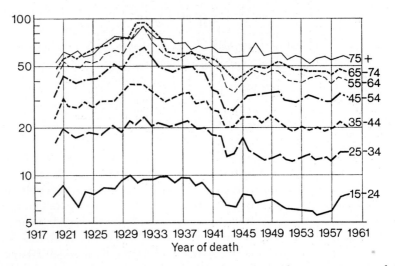

Figure 2.8 Suicide death rates by age, period curves for each age-group, United States, 1921–1964 (rates per 100,000 white males). *Source:* MacMahon, B., Johnson, S., and Pugh, T.F. (1963). Relation of suicide rates to social conditions, *Publ. Hlth Rep. (Wash.), 78*, 285–93; as cited by Susser, M. W. (1969). Aging and the field of public health, in Riley, M. W., Riley, J. W., and Johnson, M. E., eds. *Aging and Society,* Vol. II, Russell Sage Foundation, New York, p. 146.

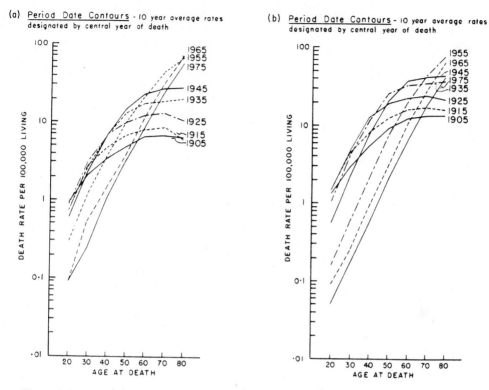

Figure 2.9 Period date contours for (a) duodenal and (b) gastric ulcer in males. Ten-year average rates designated by central year of death. *Source:* Susser, M. (1982). Period effects, generation effects, and age effects in peptic ulcer mortality, *J. Chron. Dis.*, 35, pp. 31, 33.

age among successive cohorts are represented horizontally, along each contour. With impressive regularity and regardless of age, the death rates rise for each of the cohorts born from the mid-nineteenth century until the last decade of that century; for all the more recent cohorts, rates decline. Mortality of each generation from gastric ulcer increases to a maximum for those born in 1885–1889, and from duodenal ulcer for those born in 1890–1894, and then as steadily declines for successive generations. The apparent divergence in the rates of peptic ulcer in different age-groups through time is again an artifact of statistical and graphic representation.

In keeping with this waxing and waning, the maximum incidence of other manifestations of peptic ulcer might be expected to have shifted to older age-groups, as the generations of the most affected men grew older, and their ranks were not reinforced by younger generations with similar high frequencies of the disease. This does indeed turn out to be the pattern for perforated ulcers. These complications have lately occurred on average at least ten years later in life than a generation ago. Mortality also behaves in accord with this expectation; it is rising at ages over 65, that is, in the most affected generations, and declining in the younger age-groups who succeed them.

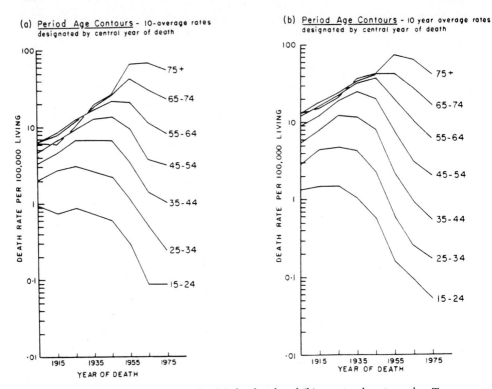

Figure 2.10 Period age contours for (a) duodenal and (b) gastric ulcer in males. Ten-year average rates designated by central year of death. *Source:* Susser, M. (1982). Period effects, generation effects, and age effects in peptic ulcer mortality, *J. Chron. Dis.*, 35, pp. 31, 33.

Where, as with peptic ulcer, cohort analysis indicates a generation effect by manifesting a constant frequency pattern across the age-groups of each cohort and a changing pattern between successive cohorts, the field of investigation can often be narrowed. Many factors may be seen to be incompatible with the generation effect. Particular treatments or fashions in diagnosis that affect all age-groups in the same way at the same time, for instance, can be excluded as the causes of a generation effect. With peptic ulcer, the decline in the disease first demonstrated by cohort analyses could not be attributed to improvements in surgery that had been introduced after the Second World War, because the distribution of the disease among age- and social-class groups was incompatible with the distribution of treatments in age-groups. A similar argument applied to the effects of diagnostic fashion.

This excursus on methods does not pretend to cover the necessary territory for the application of the social sciences to medicine. Nor does it aim to penetrate the thickets of obscurity with which social scientists must contend or, it must be allowed, with which they sometimes veil underlying incoherence. Our selectivity is deliberate. Since the available texts are in no need of duplication, we have treated only some special and even elementary topics that are often scanted.

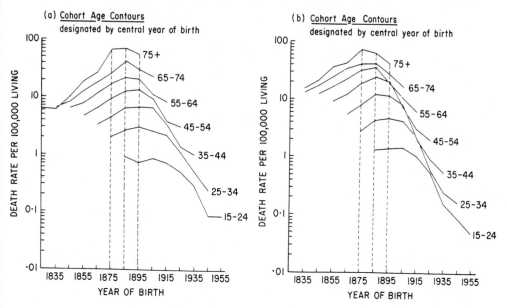

Figure 2.11 Cohort age contours for (a) duodenal and (b) gastric ulcer in males. Ten-year average rats designated by central year of death. *Source:* Susser, M. (1982). Period effects, generation effects, and age effects in peptic ulcer mortality, *J. Chron. Dis.*, 35, pp. 31, 33.

References

1. **National Center for Health Statistics** (1982). *Monthly Vital Statistics Report 32*, 4.
2. **Central Statistical Office** (1982). *Annual Abstract of Statistics*, H.M.S.O., London.
3. **U.S. Dept. of Health and Human Services** (1982). *Health, United States, 1982*, DHHS Pub. No. (PHS) 83-1232, Hyattsville, Maryland.
4. **Andvord, K. F.** (1930). What can we learn by studying tuberculosis by generations? *Norsk Mag Loegevidensk, 91*, 642–660.
   Springett, V. M. (1950). Comparative study of tuberculosis in mortality rates, *J. Hyg.* (Lond.) *46*, 361–395.
   Case, R. A. M. (1956). Cohort analysis of mortality rates as an historical or narrative technique, *Brit. J. Prev. Soc. Med., 10*, 159–171.
   MacMahon, B., and **Terry, W. D.** (1958). Application of cohort analysis to the study of time trends in neoplastic disease, *J. Chron. Dis., 7*, 24–35.
5. **Mason, K. O., Mason, W. M., Winsborough, H. H.,** and **Poole, W. K.** (1973). Some methodological issues in cohort analysis of archival data, *Amer. Sociol. Rev., 38*, 242–258.
   Glenn, N. D. (1976). Cohort analysts' futile quest: Statistical attempts to separate age, period and cohort effects, *Amer. Sociol. Rev., 41*, 900–904.
   Knoke, D. and **Hout, M.** (1976). Reply to Glenn, *Amer. Sociol. Rev. 41*, 905–908.
   Mason, W. M., Mason, K. O., and **Winsborough, H. H.** (1976). Reply to Glenn, *Amer. Sociol. Rev., 41*, 904–905.

Goldstein, H. (1979). Age, period and cohort effects—a confounded confusion, *Bull. App. Stat.*, 6, 19–24.

6. Greenberg, B. G., Wright, J. J., and Sheps, C. G. (1950). A technique for analysing some factors affecting the incidence of syphilis, *J. Amer. Stat. Assoc.*, 45, 373–399.

Walter, S. D., Miller, C. T., and Lee, J. A. H. (1976). The use of age-specific mean cohort slopes in the analysis of epidemiological incidence and mortality data, *J. Roy. Stat. Soc. A*, *139*, part 2, 227–245.

Barrett, J. C. (1978). The redundant factor method and bladder cancer mortality, *J. Epidem. and Comm. Health*, *32*, 314–316.

Osmond, C., and Gardner, M. J. (1982). Age, period and cohort models appied to cancer mortlaity rates, *Statistics in Med.*, *1*, 245–259

7. Morel, B. A. (1857). *Traite des degenerescences physiques, intellectuelles, et morales de l'espece humaine*, Paris.

Lombroso, C. (1911). *Crime: Its Causes and Remedies*, Boston.

Semmel, B. (1958). Karl Pearson, Socialist and Darwinist, *Brit. J. Sociol.*, *9*, 111–125.

McKenzie, D. (1983). *British Statistics 1865-1930*, Edinburgh.

8. Kermack, W. O., McKendrick, A. G., and McKinlay, P. L. (1934). Death rates in Great Britain: Some general regularities and their significance, *Lancet*, *i*, 698–703.

Kermack, W. O. McKendrick, A. G., and McKinlay, P. L. (1934). Death rates in Great Britain and Sweden: Expression of specific mortality rates as products of two factors, and some consequences thereof, *J. Hyg.*, *34*, 433–457.

9. Frost, W. H. (1939). The age selection of mortality from tuberculosis in successive decades, *Am. J. Hyg.*, *30*, 91–96.

10. MacMahon, B., Pugh, T. F., and Ipsen, J. (1960). *Epidemiological Methods*, Boston.

United States Public Health Service (1964). *Smoking and Health*, Publication No. 1103, Government Printing Office, Washington, D.C.

11. MacMahon, B., Johnson, S., and Pugh, T. F. (1963). Relation of suicide rates to social conditions, *Publ. Hlth. Rep.* (Wash.), *78*, 285–293.

12. Susser, M. and Stein, Z. (1962). Civilization and peptic ulcer, *Lancet*, *i*, 115–119.

Susser, M. (1982). Period effects, generation effects, and age effects in peptic ulcer mortality. *J. Chron. Dis.*, *35*, 29–40.

3

Health and disease
in the world economy

The health of any people—be they hunter-gatherers in the mountains of New Guinea, primitive agriculturalists along the Amazon, peasants in highland Chiapas, or assembly-line workers in Detroit—is bound up with their means of livelihood. An understanding of health and nutrition, it follows, requires a grasp of a broad economic front. General economic relations as well as local economic activity affect livelihoods and occupations. In the contemporary world, local economies are seldom isolated. They need to be seen within a larger context that is ultimately linked with a global system of production and exchange.

This is not to say that economic and productive activities rigidly determine the nature of social systems and cultures, but rather that they impose pressures and set limits on the possibilities of variation. Contemporary societies range in their economic and productive activities from simple food-gathering, through hunting, fishing, and subsistence agriculture, to mass production by processes of increasing complexity. In their social and political systems and in such cultural characteristics as language, customs, and values, these societies display a remarkable diversity. The diversity is striking even between societies with comparable economic and productive activities (1).

In every society systems of law, customs, moral imperatives, and institutions mold the personalities and aspirations of successive generations; in this sense people may be said to be the victims of their social relationships. Custom is not king, however, even in the simplest and most conservative society; in their unceasing interaction with their social heritage, people in every society continually accept and reject, rebel and reform, and thereby help to change the social system.

The comparative study of societies and human relationships is the means whereby sociologists attempt to achieve an understanding of the regularities in social and cultural phenomena and the reasons for their variation (2). In every society certain behaviors are repeated over and over again; there is an organized, formal, and regular means of achieving certain goals. These patterns of behavior, when thoroughly established, are termed *institutions*, and are represented by specific *associations*, so that universally there exists, for example, the institution of the family, represented by many individual families that are associations. Similarly, there are the institutions of religion, government, and war, all of which have their characteristic associations in churches, different forms of government, and armies; thus the Roman Catholic Church and the U.S. Army are associations. Organization of the associations that comprise social institutions may be formal—that is, governed by explicit rules and law— or informal, and guided by custom and convention.

Institutions determine normal social interaction, and by studying them a comparative analysis of social organization can be made and regularity and variation in patterns of behavior detected. At any point in time, small-scale subsistence societies may be compared with complex industrial ones; over time, the development of any given society may be shown through an analysis of its institutions at different historical periods. Medicine, the set of beliefs and practices that constitute the established procedures for dealing with disorders of health, is one such institution. Equally, the health of communities, as measured by morbidity and mortality which are the objects of medical attention, sheds light on the nature of society.

Economic development and underdevelopment

Between 1500 and 1800 a global economy emerged, dominated by Europe, that integrated diverse regions, economies, and societies into a network of production, exchange, and consumption. The unfolding of this system brought about the most fundamental transformation of the material conditions of life in human history. So massive was this change that it may be said to have divided pre-industrial from industrial eras, and traditional from modern societies (3). Of particular concern to us is how the arrangement of economic relations, activities, and social structures within this system shaped, and continues to shape, the conditions of health and disease in all economies, rich or poor, developed or underdeveloped, capitalist or socialist.

In this chapter we shall discuss the origins of the modern world economy, summarize the history of its expansion over the centuries, and examine its development and its consequences for health. This is done by comparative analysis under four sets of conditions. Two expositions that illustrate differences *between* societies at different stages of development are supplemented by two expositions that illustrate differences *within* societies. Thus we examine different societies in two sections that compare the conditions of the contemporary industrial nations of Great Britain and the United States, on the one hand, with those of contemporary underdeveloped countries on the other. In a third section, we examine a single contemporary society in a case study of South Africa, which exhibits features of both modern and traditional economies. The fourth and final section, which describes changes over time within Great Britain and the United States, aims to illustrate the dynamic historical aspect of development and its impact on health.

European economic growth was contingent in part on the subjugation of vast areas of the world through trade and conquest. Europe imposed a system of unequal economic interchanges between "advanced" and "backward" areas through which it exploited the material and human resources of the globe. Theories of the development of the modern world economy identify a system with three interacting zones—core, periphery, and semi-periphery—whose functions and dynamism shifted over time (4).

Initially, Northwestern Europe was the dominant or *core zone*. Composed of strong centralized states, Northwestern Europe was the first region to import agricultural products on a large affordable scale, diversify its own agriculture, increase its crop yields, and begin industrial production (specifically, textiles, shipbuilding, metal wares). Here too were located the centers of long-distance trade, credit, and exchange. The new European nation-states soon became managerial in form, highly bureaucratized and militaristic as the demands of politics and economics converged. Wage-labor replaced a manor-bound peasantry as the preferred labor system and at the same time the skill levels of the work force advanced.

The role of the *peripheral zone* between 1500 and 1800 was to supply raw materials to the core area for exchanges within Europe and between Europe and Asia. Later these areas also began to provide markets for the core's finished products. Composed of colonies, foreign dominated states, and the feudal regimes of Russia and Poland, these areas had specialized export economies: South America and Mexico were vast mining camps providing gold and silver for European coinage; the American and Caribbean basin plantations provided sugar and distilled spirits for the European diet and cotton for textile factories; Poland and Russia provided grains for the industrializing and urbanizing centers of Northwestern Europe, and timber for the fleets of England and the Dutch Republic; Africa provided slaves for the American plantations. The labor systems of serfdom, forced cash-cropping, and slavery sustained the system.

The *semi-peripheral zone* was an intermediate region that reflected the interests and institutions of both core and periphery. The advanced sectors of the semi-periphery were comprised mainly of Mediterranean states. Formerly a thriving commercial center in the Ancient and Renaissance worlds, the Mediterranean was displaced from the center of world economic activity. After 1600 the known world around it expanded, and the Atlantic-based economies expanded in turn. In its new position, it produced luxury commodities, conducted extensive credit and money transactions—as in the financing of the Portuguese and Spanish explorations of Africa and the New World—and maintained centers of learning. Coexisting with these advanced sectors was an underdeveloped sector that sustained large agrarian, pastoral, and nomadic populations into the contemporary twentieth century. These populations were linked to ossified systems of land tenure (embodied in the *latifundia*) and highly localized hinterland economies (5).

The Industrial Revolution (1750–1900) signified three conjoint occurrences within a larger process of change in the world economy. The first was accelerated and sustained growth in food and agricultural production and in human populations. The second was rapid advance in technology. The third was unprecedented social change (6). "Industrial revolution" is particularly associated with Great Britain, the first nation to industrialize (7). Because of its primacy and early dominance of world economic transactions, Britain exerted a powerful influence on world development. The overall structure of the world economy, however, had been established long before Britain's ascendancy as an industrial power, and has shown great resiliency in the face of extraordinary economic development and political change. Technical advances, political upheavals, the depletion of resources, and social developments such as urbanization and mass migration have continually changed the configuration of the world system. Shifts in relative position have occurred over time as formerly marginal societies became major economic and political powers. At various times industrial ascendancy has shifted among other European powers such as Germany, non-European powers such as the United States and Japan, and even non-capitalist powers such as the Soviet Union. In the twentieth century the core countries have had a near monopoly of global economic and political strength as well as military control in the world. Throughout this history, the structured inequalities of exchange and development have persisted; the dynamic development of the core zone is predicated on the underdevelopment of the periphery.

After World War II the former colonies and economically dependent "backward" territories in Asia, Africa, the Middle East, and Latin America gained their political independence. The absorption or realignment of these new economies in the international market economy was complicated by two considerations. The first was the division of the world into hostile American and Soviet blocs, with each attempting to garner allies through economic aid or coercion. This conflict gave rise to the widely used idea of three distinctive economic worlds: the first, made up of the United States, Western Europe, and Japan; the second, made up of the Soviet Union and Eastern Europe; and the third world, made up of Latin America, Africa, the Middle East, and Asia, including the People's Republic of China. The second consideration was the legacy of colonialism. Foreign control, and the institutionalized inequalities of exchange and development it had imposed, continued to have strong influence on the social and economic relationships in these former colonial possessions (8).

In the transition from colonial status to political autonomy Third World nations inherited enormous problems of poverty, malnutrition, and hunger and experienced rapid population growth and urbanization. These were problems exacerbated where not initially created by colonial rule; they were not solely the consequences of poor natural endowments such as soil and climate, or deficient technology, or preliterate cultures that lacked the means for the acquisition and deployment of new knowledge. Many newly emergent problems were outgrowths of the structure of economic relations between core and periphery; these were inheritances of the colonialism that had fueled the growth of the modern world economy. Indeed, so too are the alternatives to colonialism of the post-colonial phase. The relative poverty or prosperity of the new states is refracted in social relationships and states of health (9).

Economic theory and practice are difficult to disentangle from political considerations and pressures. The new governments, influenced by European theories of economic and social development—both capitalist and socialist—sought to solve their human and economic problems through industrialization and modernization. For them the visibly prosperous "advanced nations" were the economic models to emulate: advanced nations enjoyed the benefits of technology, high standards of living, and low mortality and fertility rates.

In the strict sense, *underdevelopment* refers both to a historical dynamic of unequal growth and to a set of present circumstances. Underdeveloped nations are characterized by high rates of illiteracy and unemployment, low levels of skill, productivity, and technology, large food imports, dependency on foreign capital and a burden of debts, an economy dominated by the export of a few cash crops or minerals, and rigidly stratified social structure (10).

As former colonies were integrated into the global economy, existing social systems were transformed. Peasant, agricultural, and nomadic people were converted first into plantation workers, and then often into the labor force of industrializing urban centers. Indigenous control over the local economy proved to be largely illusory. Foreign powers not only decided what goods were to be exchanged, they also controlled markets, capital, credit, local elites, and the labor supply as well. The advanced European and non-European economies continued to dominate erstwhile colonies in the periphery for their own benefit (4,6,10).

The social and economic structures in underdeveloped nations are the outcome of diverse histories. Each has a unique experience of conquest, colonization, settlement, and ongoing social transformations; each has its own particular internal class frictions, political confrontations, and economic policies. Marked differences result between underdeveloped regions and nations, despite gross similarities in their overall position in the world economy. By the 1930s, for example, South America was more urbanized than Asia and Africa, and was better integrated into the world economy. This difference is partially explained by the fact that many of the nations of South America secured political independence from Spain and Portugal in the nineteenth century, while Asian states attained independence after 1945 (as resistance movements against the Japanese developed into liberation movements against European states), and Europe's African colonies and territories achieved self-government only in the 1960s and 1970s (8).

The transition from colonial possession to autonomous state, while ending direct political control from foreign states, did not necessarily end the economic dependency and exploitation that characterized the colonial system. The persistence of economic dependency, described by some as neocolonialism, engendered common problems for most if not all the emergent nations, many of which became virtual "client-states." Diversified local economies have often all but disappeared. Many underdeveloped economies are industrial or agricultural monocultures, dependent on a single mineral or crop for export and foreign trade. They tend to receive low prices for their exports, pay low wages for their labor, and provide markets for finished consumer goods produced elsewhere.

In the 1970s, however, in the absence of state regulation, powerful trade unions, and active environmental groups, some underdeveloped countries became repositories for industries too hazardous or costly to operate in developed countries. While the infusion of Western resources seems to have brought a few Third World states (such as South Korea and Taiwan) to the threshold of self-sustaining growth, most are still characterized by relations of dependency with the developed world. Exceptions must be made. Thus the ancient Chinese state is *sui generis*, and the unprecedented cartel formed by Third World oil-producing countries exercised immense influence on the developed world during the 1970s.

Within Third World countries, westernized modernist groups favoring urbaniza-

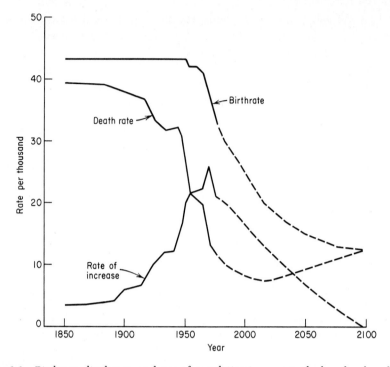

Figure 3.1   Birthrate, death rate, and rate of population increase in the less-developed countries, 1850–2100. *Source:* Coale, A. J. (1983). Recent trends in fertility in less-developed countries, *Science, 221,* 828–32.

tion and industrialization are often in political conflict with traditionalist groups representing the surviving peasant economy. Furthermore, the rapid rate of growth of predominantly young populations since 1940 has been a feature of the developing world—although there are early signs of a slowing rate (see Figure 3.1). While the rate of growth in the most advanced nations has slowed down and their populations have aged, Third World populations have nearly tripled. Three billion people live in less developed countries; one billion live in the developed countries. In 1981, the World Bank estimated that nearly 800 million people in the developing world lived in absolute poverty (11).

   In order to understand the effects on health and survival of the interdependencies and disparities of the components of the world economic system, one must relate and contrast states of development and of health. These contrasts can be derived from contemporaneous societies at different levels of development. They can be derived also from the historical evolution of single societies from one developmental level to another.

Developed economies

For epidemiological purposes one of the major differences between the developed and underdeveloped worlds is the availability of information in the form of *vital and health statistics.* These regularly updated records provide information about births and deaths, marriages and divorces, illness and health care, and health resources and facilities. Such data enable detailed pictures of the state of health and disease to be drawn. Our depiction of the general health conditions in the developed world will rely primarily on the experience of the United States and Britain (see Tables 3.1 and 3.2 for mortality rates).

A sufficiency of food is one foundation for high survival rates in the developed world. In 1980, the average daily intake in the United States was 3520 calories. Consumption of high-class protein in the form of animal protein like milk, meat, eggs, and fish is common. For the developed world as a whole daily average intake is high. Malnutrition caused by lack of food is uncommon. Although pockets of undernourishment persist, malnutrition seldom contributes directly to death although, especially among children, it may undermine immunity and sap resistance to infection (12).

The epidemic infections, and other acute infections that caused many deaths in the past, have yielded first to public health advances in environmental sanitation, and to improvements in host resistance that accompanied an enhanced food supply; only later did infections yield to advances in medical science in prevention and cure. Understanding of the nature of disease and the dynamics of its spread has been applied through sanitation, housing, general education, health care (first through immunization, later through chemotherapy and antibiotics), and legislation on all these matters. Because of such advances in industrial societies, a large proportion of those born survive to become adults and old people—a fact that necessarily raises the amount of chronic noninfectious disease, because of its intimate association with age. The risks of chronic disease are added to by the modes of life engendered by industrial societies. Their systems of production, the goods they afford, and kinds of consumption they encourage foster sedentary habits, overfeeding, and obesity, and add physical and chemical pollutants to the environment. Their characteristic patterns of social relations and behavior carry their own particular toll (see Chapter 4).

Mortality

Mortality at birth and in the first month of life, while higher than in later childhood, is low in comparison with underdeveloped societies. Such early deaths are usefully described as *perinatal:* this rate combines *stillbirths* (fetal deaths after 20 or 28 weeks of gestation according to definition) with *early neonatal* deaths (in the first week or month of life according to definition) and is stated per 1000 total births, live or dead. *Neonatal* deaths (through the first month of life) are often associated with low birthweight, prematurity and its related respiratory and metabolic dysfunctions, and with congenital malformations. As midwifery becomes more efficient, neonatal deaths are associated in declining degree with birth injuries and infections (see Table 3.3).

The prime persisting causes of death of the newborn are largely unknown. The association of perinatal and neonatal mortality with birthweight is extremely close; birthweight can account for more than 90 per cent of the variation in perinatal mortality. Prematurity accounts for a small proportion of deaths over and above birthweight, and it exerts its main effect through the low birthweight that is its conse-

Table 3.1 Percentages of deaths attributed to each of the 10 leading causes of death in each age-group: United States, 1980

Cause of death[a]	All ages	<1	1–4	5–14	15–24	25–34	35–44	45–54	55–64	65–74	75–84	85+
Heart Disease	38.2	1.8	4.1	.3	2.5	6.1	19.6	30.8	36.7	40.7	44.7	48.7
Malignant Neoplasms	20.9	.25	7.0	14.0	5.5	10.1	21.3	30.8	32.4	27.3	18.7	9.8
Cerebrovascular disease	8.6	.3	.7	.89	.85	1.9	3.7	4.3	4.8	7.3	11.8	14.3
Accidents	5.3	2.6	40.5	48.9	53.5	34.2	16.4	6.7	3.2	4.3	3.4	1.7
Chronic obstructive pulmonary diseases	2.8	.13	.6	.8	.28	.4	.7	1.7	3.2	2.2	2.0	1.4
Pneumonia and influenza	2.7	2.2	3.3	1.8	.7	1.1	1.5	1.3	1.4	1.9	.03	5.5
Diabetes mellitus	1.8	.009	.15	.35	.26	1.1	1.5	1.6	2.0	1.4	.46	1.2
Chronic liver disease and cirrhosis	1.5	.07	.15	.10	.25	2.6	6.0	5.2	3.1	2.0	1.8	1.8
Atherosclerosis	1.5	.004	0	0	0	.02	.08	.2	.4	.8	1.9	4.1
Suicide	1.4	0	0	1.3	10.7	11.8	6.7	2.7	1.9	.6	.3	.12

[a]As specified in the International Classification of Diseases (ICD).

Source: Adapted from National Center for Health Statistics, (1983) *Monthly Vital Statistics Report, 32, 4,* Suppl.

Table 3.2   Rates in 1980 for 10 leading causes of death in successive age-groups: (a) United States, (b) England and Wales

Under 1 Year			
United States		**England and Wales**	
Cause of death	Rate per 100,000	Cause of death	Rate per 100,000
All causes	1288.3	All causes	1203.7
1. Congenital anomalies	260.9	1. Certain conditions originating in the perinatal period	475.0
2. Accidents	33.0	2. Congenital anomalies	322.1
3. Pneumonia or influenza	28.6	3. Pneumonia and influenza	69.8
4. Diseases of the heart	22.8	4. Accidents	25.1
5. Septicemia	6.8	5. Chronic obstructive pulmonary disease	18.3
6. Nephritis	6.4	6. Other diseases of the nervous system	11.6
7. Homicide	5.9	7. Diseases of the heart	11.1
8. Cerebrovascular disease	4.4	8. Other diseases of the digestive system	5.6
9. Malignant neoplasms	3.2	9. Malignant neoplasms	4.0
10. Chronic obstructive pulmonary disease	1.6	10. Phlebitis	.6
1–4 Years			
All causes	63.9	All causes	51.1
1. Accidents	25.9	1. Accidents	11.8
2. Congenital anomalies	8.0	2. Congenital anomalies	9.7
3. Malignant neoplasms	4.5	3. Malignant neoplasms	5.5
4. Disease of the heart	2.6	4. Pnuemonia and influenza	3.5
5. Homicide	2.5	5. Other diseases of the nervous system	2.6
6. Pneumonia or influenza	2.1	6. Chronic obstructive pulmonary disease	1.5
7. Certain conditions originating in the perinatal period	.7	7. Diseases of the heart	1.3
8. Septicemia	.6	8. Other diseases of the digestive system	1.2
9. Cerebrovascular disease	.5	9. Cerebrovascular disease	.3
10. Chronic obstructive pulmonary disease	.4	10. Certain conditions originating in the perinatal period	.3
5–14 Years			
All causes	30.6	All causes	24.4
1. Accidents	15.0	1. Accidents	7.7
2. Malignant neoplasms	4.3	2. Malignant neoplasms	4.8
3. Congenital anomalies	1.6	3. Congenital anomalies	2.5
4. Homicide	1.2	4. Pneumonia and influenza	1.3
5. Diseases of the heart	.9	5. Other diseases of the nervous system	1.2
6. Pneumonia or influenza	.6	6. Diseases of the heart	0.8

Table 3.2   Continued

5–14 Years			
United States		**England and Wales**	
Cause of death	Rate per 100,000	Cause of death	Rate per 100,000
7. Suicide	.4	7. Chronic obstructive pulmonary disease	0.6
8. Cerebrovascular disease	.2	8. Cerebrovascular disease	.3
9. Chronic obstructive pulmonary disease	.2	9. Other diseases of the digestive system	0.2
10. Diabetes mellitus	.1	10. Diabetes mellitus	0.2
15–24 Years			
All causes	115.4	All causes	61.9
1. Accidents	61.7	1. Malignant neoplasms	7.0
2. Homicide	15.6	2. Suicide	4.7
3. Suicide	12.3	3. Accidents	3.0
4. Malignant neoplasms	6.3	4. Diseases of the heart	2.3
5. Diseases of the heart	2.9	5. Pneumonia and influenza	1.5
6. Pneumonia and influenza	1.8	6. Other diseases of the nervous system	1.4
7. Congenital anomalies	1.4	7. Cerebrovascular disease	1.2
8. Chronic and obstructive pulmonary diseases	.3	8. Chronic obstructive pulmonary disease	1.2
9. Diabetes mellitus	.3	9. Mental disorders	0.7
10. Nephritis	.3	10. Diabetes mellitus	.4
25–34 Years			
All causes	135.5	All causes	72.4
1. Accidents	46.3	1. Accidents	17.0
2. Homicide	19.6	2. Malignant neoplasms	16.0
3. Suicide	16.0	3. Suicide	8.7
4. Malignant neoplasms	13.7	4. Diseases of the heart	7.0
5. Diseases of the heart	8.3	5. Cerebrovascular disease	3.1
6. Chronic liver disease and cirrhosis	3.5	6. Pneumonia and influenza	2.0
7. Cerebrovascular disease	2.6	7. Congenital anomalies	1.2
8. Pneumonia and influenza	1.5	8. Other diseases of the nervous system	1.1
9. Diabetes mellitus	1.5	9. Certain conditions originating in the perinatal period	1.1
10. Congenital anomalies	1.3	10. Other diseases of the digestive system	.9
35–44 Years			
All causes	227.9	All causes	161.8
1. Malignant neoplasms	48.6	1. Malignant neoplasms	51.7
2. Diseases of the heart	44.6	2. Diseases of the heart	40.1
3. Accidents	37.3	3. Accidents	15.2

Table 3.2   Continued

35–44 Years			
United States		England and Wales	
Cause of death	Rate per 100,000	Cause of death	Rate per 100,000
4. Suicide	15.4	4. Suicide	11.8
5. Homicide	15.1	5. Cerebrovascular disease	9.1
6. Chronic liver disease and cirrhosis	13.6	6. Pneumonia and influenza	3.8
7. Cerebrovascular disease	8.5	7. Chronic obstructive pulmonary disease	3.4
8. Diabetes mellitus	3.5	8. Other diseases of the digestive system	2.3
9. Pneumonia or influenza	3.5	9. Congenital anomalies	1.7
10. Chronic obstructive pulmonary disease	1.6	10. Diabetes mellitus	1.5

45–54 Years			
All causes	584.0	All causes	512.3
1. Diseases of the heart	180.2	1. Diseases of the heart	183.0
2. Malignant neoplasms	180.0	2. Malignant neoplasms	182.7
3. Accidents	39.0	3. Cerebrovascular disease	32.4
4. Chronic liver disease and cirrhosis	30.9	4. Accidents	18.4
5. Cerebrovascular disease	25.2	5. Chronic obstructive pulmonary disease	17.0
6. Suicide	15.9	6. Suicide	13.2
7. Homicide	11.1	7. Pneumonia and influenza	11.3
8. Chronic obstructive pulmonary disease	9.8	8. Chronic liver disease and cirrhosis	6.6
9. Diabetes mellitus	9.6	9. Diabetes mellitus	4.4
10. Pneumonia and influenza	6.4	10. Other diseases of the nervous system	3.8

55–64 Years			
All causes	1346.3	All causes	1382.4
1. Diseases of the heart	494.1	1. Diseases of the heart	540.2
2. Malignant neoplasms	436.1	2. Malignant neoplasms	481.7
3. Cerebrovascular disease	65.2	3. Cerebrovascular disease	97.5
4. Chronic obstructive pulmonary disease	42.7	4. Chronic obstructive pulmonary disease	65.7
5. Accidents	42.6	5. Pneumonia and influenza	41.0
6. Chronic liver disease and cirrhosis	41.6	6. Accidents	24.7
7. Diabetes mellitus	26.7	7. Arterial disease (embolism, thrombosis, etc.)	17.8
8. Pneumonia and influenza	18.6	8. Other diseases of the digestive system	15.0

Table 3.2 Continued

55–64 Years			
United States		England and Wales	
Cause of death	Rate per 100,000	Cause of death	Rate per 100,000
9. Suicide	15.9	9. Suicide	14.7
10. Nephritis	9.0	10. Diabetes mellitus	10.7
65–74 Years			
All causes	2994.9	All causes	3432.3
1. Diseases of the heart	1218.0	1. Diseases of the heart	1357.6
2. Malignant neoplasms	817.9	2. Malignant neoplasms	958.0
3. Cerebrovascular disease	219.5	3. Cerebrovascular disease	378.2
4. Chronic obstructive pulmonary disease	129.1	4. Chronic obstructive pulmonary disease	199.5
5. Diabetes mellitus	64.9	5. Pneumonia and influenza	192.5
6. Accidents	57.7	6. Arterial disease (embolism, thrombosis, etc.)	63.8
7. Pneumonia and influenza	55.6	7. Other diseases of the digestive system	41.4
8. Chronic liver disease and cirrhosis	43.1	8. Accidents	41.0
9. Nephritis	24.6	9. Diabetes mellitus	32.2
10. Atherosclerosis	23.6	10. Phlebitis	26.6
75–84		75+ Years	
All causes	6692.6	All causes	10252.0
1. Diseases of the heart	2993.1	1. Diseases of the heart	3740.1
2. Malignant neoplasms	1232.2	2. Cerebrovascular disease	1633.4
3. Cerebrovascular disease	788.6	3. Malignant neoplasms	1536.9
4. Chronic obstructive pulmonary disease	224.4	4. Pneumonia and influenza	1469.0
5. Pneumonia and influenza	220.0	5. Chronic obstructive pulmonary disease	487.8
6. Diabetes mellitus	131.1	6. Atherosclerosis	249.9
7. Atherosclerosis	125.5	7. Accidents	156.6
8. Accidents	120.3	8. Arterial disease (embolism, thrombosis, etc.)	153.7
9. Nephritis	67.8	9. Other diseases of the digestive system	139.7
10. Septicemia	35.5	10. Ulcer of the stomach	88.7

Sources: Adapted from National Center for Health Statistics (1983) *Monthly Vital Statistics Report, 32*, 4, Suppl., and World Health Organization (1983) *World Health Statistics Annual,* Geneva.

Table 3.3 Infant mortality rate by age and for 10 selected causes of death: United States, 1981

Age and cause of death	Rate per 1000 live births
Total, under 1 year	11.7
Under 28 days	7.8
28 days to 11 months	3.9
Certain gastrointestinal diseases	.08
Pneumonia and influenza	.2
Congenital anomalies	2.4
Disorders relating to short gestation and unspecified low birthweight	1.03
Birth Trauma	.2
Intrauterine hypoxia and birth asphyxia	.4
Respiratory distress syndrome	1.2
Other conditions originating in the perinatal period	2.9
Sudden infant death syndrome	1.4
All other causes	1.9

Source: National Center for Health Statistics (1982), *Monthly Statistics Report, 30,* 13.

quence (see Figure 3.2). Both premature delivery and low birthweight are frequent where social conditions are poor (13). Congenital malformations are sometimes caused by antenatal virus infections, drugs, irradiation, and a rising proportion of genetic disorders. Cigarette smoking during pregnancy, and probably alcohol consumption as well, reduce birthweight and thereby add to the risks of infant death. Many other environmental factors are under investigation, although few have been firmly established as causes of newborn death. Today the infections most dangerous to the newborn child no longer arise from poor hygiene in the home. They are usually viruses, or staphylococci and Gram-negative organisms that, because of their resistance to antibiotics, flourish in the hospital ward. For these organisms effective drugs have proved difficult to find. For several causes of newborn death, however, the same strong relationship with birthweight holds irrespective of the specific cause (see Figure 3.3).

In the post-neonatal period the sudden infant death syndrome, the causes of which remain obscure, has become the predominant cause of death, with a peak at 3 to 5 months of age (14). In part, the prominence of sudden infant death is the residuum of the elimination of causes of death among children in the remainder of the first year of life that were common and more subject to control than those that cause death among the newborn. Many deaths during this post-neonatal period follow infection, especially respiratory infection. Cigarette smoking in mothers, and probably air pollution as well, contribute both to respiratory infection and to sudden infant death syndrome. Overall, however, infant death rates have diminished rapidly. In 1980 in England and Wales the infant mortality rate had fallen to 11.8 per 1000 live births and in the United States to 12.6 (15,16). The decline occurred in the absence of much change in birthweight, and the cause must probably be sought in perinatal factors including newborn medical care (see Figure 3.4).

In the later years of childhood deaths become fewer, although accidents begin to

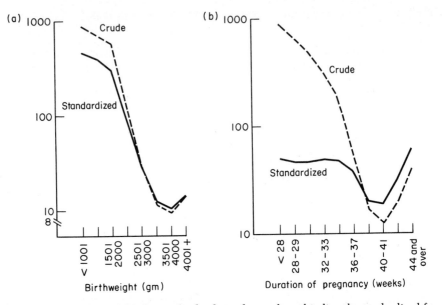

Figure 3.2 (A) Perinatal death rates by *birthweight*: crude and indirectly standardized for *duration of pregnancy*; (B) Perinatal death rates by *duration of pregnancy*: crude and indirectly standardized for *birthweight*. British Perinatal Survey, 1958. *Source:* Susser, M., Marolla, F. A., and Fleiss, J. (1972). Birth weight, fetal age and perinatal mortality, *Amer. J. Epi.*, 197–204.

take a rising toll, first within the home and then outside it. In the United States in 1979 accidents accounted for 41 per cent of all deaths in the 1 to 4 year age-group (although the mortality rate has been declining through time) (17). Because of the marked decline in deaths from infections, especially influenza and pneumonia, congenital malformations and malignant neoplasms have come to account for relatively

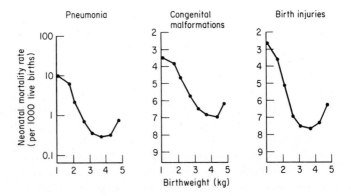

Figure 3.3 Birthweight-specific neonatal mortality curves for three specific causes of death, United States, whites, 1960. *Source:* Wilcox, A. J., and Russell, I. T. (1983). Birthweight and perinatal mortality: II. On weight-specific mortality, *Internat. J. Epi.*, 12, 319–25.

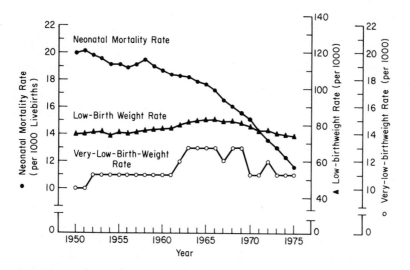

Figure 3.4 Neonatal mortality, low birthweight, and very low birthweight in the United States, 1950–1975: rate per 1000 live births. *Source:* Lee, K., Paneth, N., Gartner, L., Pearlman, M., Gruss, L. (1980). *Amer. J. Pub. Hlth., 70,* 15–21.

more deaths, although they too are declining in frequency as causes of death. At the same time deaths associated with congenital malformations and other handicaps have been deferred from infancy to later ages.

In the 5 to 14 year age-group in the United States school age children die from accidents (1.5 per 1000) more often than from diseases; in England and Wales, accidents account for about a third of all deaths in this age group. The high proportions are again relative, and reflect the decline of other causes of death (primarily infections). Death rates are lowest at pubescence, when human beings reach a peak of hardiness and vitality.

After puberty the death rate rises slowly. Tuberculosis, like other infections, has long been displaced as a main cause of death. This one-time intractable, chronic, and fatal disease no longer maintains an important position, and persists largely in limited but persistent foci—for instance, among old men in "skid row" and lodging houses, and among migrant laborers in overcrowded dwellings. For youths especially, accidents on the roads and violence of various kinds have replaced the social diseases of poverty among the leading causes of death. Accidents and violent death in general are intimately linked with the customary behavior of young men and the related values, social priorities, and technical innovations of industrialized societies. The high death toll of motor vehicle accidents associated with the drinking of alcohol illustrates the point. Violent and accidental deaths largely accounted for the 3:1 ratio of male to female mortality in the United States for ages 15 to 24 in 1980. In 1980 in the United States deaths from accidents, homicides, and suicides together amounted to nearly 80 per cent of the total in this same age-group (17).

For the age-group 25 to 34 years in both England and the United States accidents, and especially motor vehicle accidents, remain the leading cause of death. In the United States, accidents are followed by homicide and suicide, which still account for over a quarter of the deaths in the age-group. In England and Wales, accidents are followed closely by malignant neoplasms and distantly by suicide and diseases of the heart.

Later in life, chronic noninfectious disease becomes prominent and the death rate rises steeply. In middle-age both in the United States and in Britain cardiovascular disease is the leading cause of death. In the latter years, malignant neoplasms compete for dominance with cardiovascular diseases. In the age-group 35 to 64 years in the United States, heart disease accounts for a third and cancer for a little less than a third of all deaths; in England and Wales, the comparable proportions are 37 per cent and 35 per cent, respectively. Cerebrovascular disease (mainly stroke) also grows steadily in frequency with age (although arterial diseases of the brain, in common with those of the heart, have declined significantly over the past decade and more).

Beginning in middle age, women suffer a progressively heavier toll from both breast cancer and cancer of the genital organs. At these ages deaths from diabetes are prominent; rates have increased, deferred from younger ages by effective treatment in the same fashion as those from congenital malformations and severe mental subnormality among children. During the 1960s and into the 1980s, in both the United States and Britain, diabetes appears among the ten leading causes of death in males and females beginning in the 5 to 14 age group (17,18). In the United States, too, deaths from cirrhosis of the liver have increased, to make it one of the ten leading causes in general and one of the six leading causes for ages 25 to 64. Alcohol abuse and hepatitis are the chief known factors in cirrhosis, and the rise in mortality has occurred in the face of better control of hepatitis. Deaths from cirrhosis have recently increased in Britain as well, but the problem is much less severe than in the United States. This difference between the two countries could be due in part to the stiffer tax policies and closer regulation of the hours during which drinking establishments may be open in Britain. The regulation of alcohol use, as with prohibition in the United States, correlates strongly with death rates from cirrhosis (19).

In late middle age and among the old, the number of deaths from chronic disease of the lung (lung cancer, chronic bronchitis, and emphysema) becomes notable, especially among men. These respiratory conditions burden cigarette-smoking cultures and urban societies. Smoking is the major cause of these two respiratory problems. An urban factor is almost certainly pollution of the air by industrial and domestic wastes (20). Chronic bronchitis (or emphysema) has long been known as the "English disease," but this can no longer be so easily claimed. Since particulate pollution from coal was controlled in England by the Clean Air Act of 1956, this disease is a less obvious affliction, although it still accounts for 13 per cent of all deaths at ages over 54.

Among the elderly in the United States in 1980 heart disease, cancer, and stroke accounted for 75 per cent of all deaths; influenza, pneumonia, and diabetes together accounted for 5 per cent. All these causes, excepting cancer, are in decline. One way of gauging the number of untimely deaths that continue to occur is to estimate those that are preventable in the light of current medical knowledge. In the United States, such "sentinel deaths" would include those from tuberculosis, throat and lung cancer, myeloid luekemia, chronic bronchitis, and emphysema, and, among age-groups younger than 50, influenza and pneumonia. By this measure a 1976 estimate suggests that 12.9 per cent of all deaths might have been preventable (21). This figure does not include an uncertain number of deaths related to occupational hazards.

Morbidity

Measures of sickness rather than death bring to view a somewhat different configuration of diseases. Many diseases do not have an issue in death, and mortality rates cannot show the impact of acute minor ailments such as upper respiratory and gastrointestinal infections, which are the commonest of all causes of sickness. Nor can they reflect acute or chronic psychiatric disorders of the nonorganic type, and other nonfatal chronic diseases, for instance, skin diseases and osteoarthritis.

Moreover, in those chronic diseases that are sometimes fatal, a highly selected aspect of the disease is likely to be represented in the death rates. Peptic ulcer is an example. It appears as a cause of death largely because of the complications of acute perforation and hemorrhage, but these definitive events are not representative of all ulcers; the risk of their occurrence is not the same for all age- and sex-groups and for all types of ulcer. Complications occur in more patients with gastric than with duodenal ulcers, in more men who have ulcers than women and in more old people than young. Those patients with peptic ulcers who have undergone operations or have complications have been found to have a higher proportion of nonsecretors of blood group substance than others; those who bleed have a higher proportion of blood group O. The statistics relating to hospital admissions or surgery for peptic ulcer will reflect these characteristics as well as the distribution of the disorder in the general population (22).

Morbidity rates therefore modify the spectrum of disease disclosed by mortality rates. (The index of morbidity used will in part determine the spectrum, as discussed in Chapter 2.) Morbidity rates also vary with the source of the statistics, depending on whether the population studied includes all those at risk, or only those who come into the purview of professional medical care. Many illnesses are never reported to medical services. Some diseases have long latent periods before being expressed in symptoms; even then people who become aware of symptoms may not complain about them; and those who do seek treatment for their complaints may defer medical consultation until they have exhausted the resources of family, neighbors, wise old women, and the pharmacist on the corner. Finally, the availability and type of medical services determines their use. Thus, expressed demand for medical services is an outcome both of the chain of referrals that follows on perceived illness, and of the perceived supply. Diabetes goes unrecognized as often as it is recognized; undiagnosed mental disorders are common sources of distress; anemias in women of reproductive age seldom produce distinctive symptoms and often remain silent; hypertension and glaucoma pose latent unknown threats to the health of many persons past middle age (23).

Surveys of populations can reveal some of these hidden disorders, although often with loss of diagnostic precision, and not without many difficulties that are inherent in surveys of prevalence (24). Since 1957, the National Health Survey of the United States Public Health Service has provided some of the most representative and extensive information through its continuing Health Interview Survey. The interview obtains reports of illnesses suffered from representative national samples of households. Diagnosis is sharply limited by dependence on respondents' information and memory, however, and recall of the events of illness has proved to be somewhat selective. A smaller proportion of such stigmatized events as admissions to mental hospitals was reported than of more neutral events, and likewise underreporting increased as events receded into the past.

In part to correct such deficiencies, the Health Examination Survey, initiated in 1959, administers a thorough physical examination and selected clinical and laboratory tests to samples of the population (usually about 6000 persons) intended to be representative. Naturally, a relatively small sample cannot represent in any force many subgroups of the national population. Population surveys, in turn, are supplemented by review of hospital records. This allows national estimates of disease prevalence to be made. Table 3.4 shows the characteristic increase with age both in admission and length of stay in acute hospitals in the United States in 1980. In Britain the best current information is to be had from the National Health Services Hospital In Patient Inquiry and from the Morbidity Series of the Office of Population Censuses and Surveys (25).

In childhood the bulk of illnesses are acute infections and exanthemata (17,26). Respiratory disease accounts for by far the most hospital admissions—28 per cent under age 15 in the United States in 1980. The incidence of such exanthemata as measles and rubella, once taken to be the inevitable price of childhood, has been sharply reduced by vaccination. (Indeed, measles has been all but eliminated in the United States.) Measles vaccination prevents the occasionally severe consequences of the disease in sickness and complications for the child itself; rubella vaccination of school children in the United States and adolescent girls in Britain aims to protect, not the vaccinated, but fetuses in the first trimester of gestation from the congenital malformations caused by rubella transmitted from the mother in utero.

Table 3.4 Discharges from short stay hospitals per 1000 population by age-group and sex: United States, 1980

Age-group	Males	Females	Total
<15	78.9	64.3	71.8
15–44	92.7	207.6[a]	151.3
45–64	196.9	195.1	196.0
65+	427.4	384.7	405.2

[a] Much of the female excess in this age-group is accounted for by obstetric care for childbirth.

Source: Adapted from National Center for Health Statistics (1983). Inpatient utilization of short stay hospitals by diagnosis: United States, 1980, *Vital and Health Statistics*, Series 13, Number 74.

The incidence of acute illness declines rapidly in adolescence, and then more gradually in old age. Of these acute episodes, around 70 per cent were presumed owed to infection, and about 17 per cent to injuries. In the United States in 1981, each school child between 6 and 16 lost on average 4.9 school days because of acute illness. Each employed person lost 4.9 workdays, and each person suffered 19.1 days of restricted activity and 6.9 days of bed disability (15,27,28).

Diseases of all kinds have become steadily less important among children; the everyday concerns in their primary medical care are now problems of growth, development, and psychological and social adjustment. Diptheria and whooping cough yielded to vaccines before poliomyelitis, and long before measles, rubella, and mumps. Measles outbreaks tend to occur only in communities with low vaccination rates and living in poor circumstances or at much older ages, as in university students who were never vaccinated or when immunity is waning. In the United States, the disease is on the verge of elimination as a regularly recurring epidemic. Even the rising incidence of venereal diseases among adolescents represents primarily a problem of social and sexual behavior; one can include as a facet of the same problem the sexually transmitted microorganisms resistant to antibiotic treatment, either because resistant strains of bacteria have emerged or because the herpes or other viruses are involved. Even the prevalence of physical handicaps caused by chronic disorders seems to have diminished. This is less likely to be true for developmental conditions like cerebral palsy, epilepsy, and severe mental subnormality, although the evidence is not conclusive. Down's syndrome frequency as described in Chapter 2 is illustrative. In these conditions, incidence is probably on the decline, but to produce a decline in prevalence requires that incidence must fall enough to balance the increment from increased survival among the births at high risk, for instance, those of very low birthweight or the congenitally deformed (29).

Adult chronic illness increases with age and markedly at middle age. Indeed, the amount of chronic illness provides a measure of the process of aging. Because prevalence compounds frequency and duration, the contrast in the age distributions of acute and chronic illness is even more marked than with incidence. As an analysis of some years ago in Figures 3.5 and 3.6 shows, in incidence chronic disabling illnesses exceeded acute disorders only over the age of 75 years; but in prevalence they were about equal from adolescence to 40 years of age, and above that age chronic illnesses exceeded acute by a progressively larger margin. Many patients with chronic disorders are ambulatory, so that the load of care is borne largely by general practice and outpatient services rather than by hospital wards (25).

In 1967, one out of five persons below the age of 17 years, and four out of five above the age of 65, had chronic disorders as defined by the United States Health Interview Survey. In the United States in 1981, it was estimated that one in seven persons experienced a limitation of activities because of chronic conditions (see Figure 3.7). As expected, restriction of activity increased with age, from 3.8 per cent for those under 17 years of age, to 45.7 per cent or more than tenfold for those 65 years of age and over (15,30). Heart disease was by far the most frequent cause of restricted activity in persons 45 years and older.

The rates reported by the Health Interview Survey tend to be underestimated. The

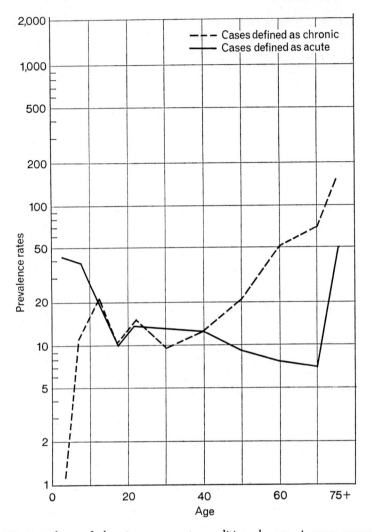

Figure 3.5 Prevalence of chronic versus acute conditions, by age. Average annual prevalence of disabling cases per 1000 population, 1938–1943. *Source:* Collins, S. D., et al. (1961). Age incidence of specific causes of illness found in monthly canvasses of families, *Publ. Hlth Rep.* (Wash.), *66*, 1227–45 (adapted); based on sample of Eastern Health District of Baltimore; as cited by Susser, M. W. (1969). Aging and the field of public health, in *Aging and Society*, Vol. II, eds. Riley, M. W., Riley, J. W., and Johnson, M. E., Russell Sage Foundation, New York, p. 124.

surveys exclude a concentration of persons with chronic disorders resident in institutions. In the United States in 1981 people in institutions comprised almost 1 per cent of the total population. Today, 85 per cent of the residents of nursing homes are over 75 years old. Most are women, and most suffer from multiple chronic diseases and impairments and significant functional disability. About 20 per cent of those who

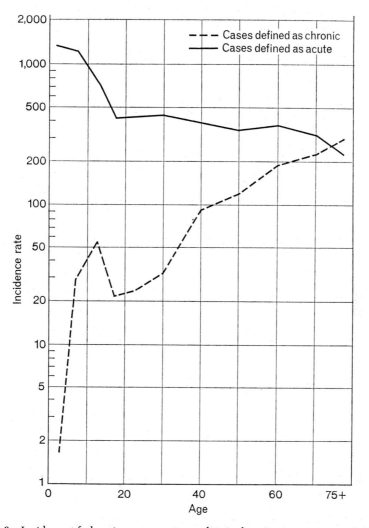

Figure 3.6 Incidence of chronic versus acute conditions, by age. Average annual incidence of episodes of disabling illness per 1000 population, 1938–1943. *Source:* Collins, S. D., et al. (1961). Age incidence of specific causes of illness found in monthly canvasses of families, *Publ. Hlth Rep.* (Wash.), *66*, 1227–45 (adapted); based on sample of Eastern Health District of Baltimore; as cited by Susser, M. W. (1969). Aging and the field of public health, in *Aging and Society*, Vol. II, eds. Riley, M. W., Riley, J. W., and Johnson, M. E., Russell Sage Foundation, New York, p. 125.

dwell in institutions live in mental hospitals; the rest live in nursing homes, long-term facilities, and correctional institutions (31).

At this point it must be noted that useful generalization about the impact of disease at different ages is limited by marked variations in the distribution of specific diseases by sex, social class, and ethnic group; by heterogeneity in the causes of similar disa-

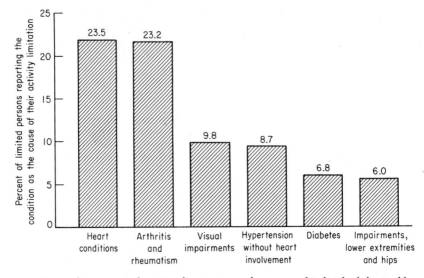

Figure 3.7   Leading causes of activity limitation, and per cent of individuals limited by each cause, at ages 65 years and over, United States. *Source:* Adapted from National Center for Health Statistics (1974), *Vital and Health Statistics*, Series 10, No. 111.

bilities; as well as by imprecision in the description and reporting of severity. Table 3.5 shows sex differences by age-group for leading causes of admissions to acute hospitals in the United States in 1980; these rates for diagnosis at discharge approximate measures of incidence of severe disease, although they include repeat admissions, that is, the data are based on episodes and not on persons. In general, males have a slight advantage over females in morbidity rates for both acute and chronic illness, in contrast to their marked disadvantage in death rates. Among acute conditions, males report notably higher rates only for injuries and the childhood diseases.

Females have distinctly higher rates of chronic conditions, and this can be demonstrated for a number of diagnoses—such as respiratory disorders, hypertension, and diabetes—as well as for chronic disability in general. (It is a matter of debate whether these higher rates are a matter of biological sex, of the social environment of women, or of the sickness behavior expected of women—issues to be discussed in later chapters.) In the case of mental disorder younger men in their twenties and thirties are the main victims of the onset of schizophrenia, and young women in their thirties of the onset of depressive illnesses, whereas both disorders persist and become prevalent among older people of both sexes. Coronary heart disease, peptic ulcer, alcohol dependency, and (in Britain) bronchitis are diseases that are concentrated among middle-aged and old men, and they make a large contribution to the load of chronic sickness. Rheumatoid arthritis, diabetes, and iron deficiency anemias (related to the loss of blood with the menstrual cycle and with gynecological disorders) are forms of chronic sickness concentrated among middle-aged women of the lower social classes. In the United States, hypertension is much more common among black people than white, and especially among black women. In all age groups, reported disability from sick-

Table 3.5   Diagnosis (first listed) per 1000 discharged from short-stay hospitals by age and sex: United States, 1980

Diagnostic category	Male	Female
A. *Under 15 years of age*		
Viral diseases	1.9	1.7
Otitis media and eustachian tube disorders	4.5	3.2
Diseases of the respiratory system:		
Acute respiratory infections	5.9	4.6
Chronic disease of tonsils and adenoids	5.4	6.4
Pneumonia, all forms	5.2	3.6
Asthma	3.0	1.8
Diseases of the digestive system		
Inguinal hernia	3.0	0.6
Regional enteritis and idiopathic proctocolitis and other noninfectious gastroenteritis and colitis	4.1	3.7
Congenital anomalies	4.0	3.2
Fractures, all sites	3.7	2.4
Intracranial injury (excluding concussion with skull fractures)	1.9	1.1
B. *15–44 years of age*		
Neoplasms:		
Malignant neoplasms	1.4	2.1
Benign neoplasms, carcinoma-in-situ and neoplasms of uncertain behavior	0.7	4.8
Mental disorders:		
Psychosis	3.1	2.4
Anxiety states and other neuroses and personality disorders	1.5	2.6
Alcohol dependence syndrome	3.6	1.0
Heart disease	3.0	1.7
Regional enteritis and idiopathic proctocolitis and other noninfectious gastroenteritis and colitis	1.5	2.3
Inflammatory disease of female pelvic organs	. . .	5.1
Disorders of menstruation and other abnormal vaginal bleeding	. . .	6.6
Pregnancy with abortive outcome	. . .	9.9
Females with delivery	. . .	70.9
Intervertebral disc disorders	2.4	1.5
Fractures, all sites	6.3	2.3
Lacerations and open wounds	3.5	0.8
Persons admitted for sterilization	0.2	4.7
C. *45–64 Years of Age*		
Neoplasms:		
Malignant neoplasms	14.5	16.7
Benign neoplasm, carcinoma-in-situ, and neoplasms of uncertain behavior	2.4	6.7
Diabetes mellitus	4.6	6.4
Alcohol dependence syndrome	6.4	1.5
Heart disease	34.0	17.9
Acute myocardial infarction	6.1	1.8
Coronary atherosclerosis	6.3	2.5
Other chronic ischemic heart disease	7.8	2.5
Cerebrovascular disease	4.7	3.4
Diseases of the digestive system:		
Gastric, duodenal, and other and unspecified peptic ulcer	4.2	3.5
Inguinal hernia	7.0	0.5
Cholelithiasis	2.4	4.7

Table 3.5.   Continued

Diagnostic category	Male	Female
C. *45–64 Years of Age*		
Neoplasms:		
Intervertebral disc disorders	3.7	2.9
Fractures, all sites	4.1	4.6
D. *65 Years and over*		
Malignant neoplasms	48.0	30.4
Malignant neoplasms of large intestine and rectum	5.5	4.7
Malignant neoplasms of trachea, bronchus, and lung	10.7	2.4
Diabetes mellitus	7.7	11.5
Heart disease	81.5	69.3
Acute myocardial infarction	12.4	8.0
Coronary atherosclerosis	15.3	13.9
Cardiac dysrhythmias	10.1	8.7
Congestive heart failure	13.6	13.2
Cerebrovascular disease	25.4	23.1
Pneumonia, all forms	15.6	10.4
Diverticula of intestine	3.2	6.0
Cholelithiasis	4.5	6.5
Hyperplasia of prostrate	18.8	. . .
Rheumatoid arthritis and allied disorders	3.8	7.4
Fractures of neck and femur	3.9	9.9
Other Fractures	4.1	10.6

Source: Adapted from the National Center for Health Statistics (1983). Inpatient utilization of short stay hospital by diagnosis: United States, 1980, *Vital and Health Statistics*, series 13, Number 74.

ness observes a strict socioeconomic gradient; those families with lower income report a progressively greater amount of restricted activity, confinement to bed, and work loss. The permutations of disease and its consequences according to personal attributes, environmental variables, and social position are endless. They do not call for further elaboration here, since they are the substance of this book.

Underdeveloped economies

Underdeveloped economies have patterns of health and disease quite different from those of developed economies. The contrasts between them are a legacy, on the one side, of unequal economic development on a global scale, and on the other of economic and institutional disparities distinctly local in origin. In the developed world many deaths are the result of chronic diseases whose causes are not clear and which we cannot yet prevent. In the underdeveloped world most deaths are the result of acute and chronic diseases that medicine and public health know how to control. The fact that such diseases flourish in the face of this knowledge can be ascribed to the weakness and poverty of the economy, of education, of government, and administration. The conjuncture of sporadic disasters like war, crop failure, and famine with ineffective institutions adds to the toll.

Indicies of morbidity and mortality in the developing world necessarily present a restricted view of health conditions. Impoverished societies maintain impoverished data systems. Thus there are serious shortcomings in the registration of vital events. Many deaths go unrecorded, and for many that are recorded, causes of death are unidentified or misclassified. Statistics are frequently drawn only from urban areas, thereby excluding or underrepresenting rural areas. In short, unreliable health statistics exist for 75 per cent of the world's population (32). In spite of these limitations, we can sketch the conditions of health and disease in the developing world by drawing on a variety of sources (18,33).

Population structure

The populations of less developed countries are relatively young. There is a high birthrate, and therefore many children; but there is also an excessive death rate among children, and in many places 50 per cent may not survive to the age of fifteen, or even to the age of five. Nearly one-half of all reported deaths in less developed countries occur in children under the age of five. Mortality rates for infants and young children in less developed countries tend to be 10 to 20 times higher than in developed countries. The result is gross disparity in life expectancies (see Table 3.6).

In the harshest environments, the survivors of the hazards of early life tend to die off at a high and even rate throughout the rest of life. Statistically, this model of mortality resembles some nonhuman phenomena, for instance, the experience of robins in the wild (34), or even the random destruction of annealed glasses in a restaurant; at each successive age the survivors run the same high risk of death, quite unlike the age-related increase in risk that characterizes the senescent populations of developed societies. Contrast, for example, the survival curve for British India in 1921–1930, as shown in Figure 3.8, with the curves for other populations at other times. In harsh conditions, after high mortality in the first years of life, there is no *modal* or most common age at death (35). Less-developed countries therefore lack this characteristic feature of developed countries, with its accompanying health pattern of an aging population—although, of course, some hardy individuals in less-developed countries do survive into old age. Only when more favorable social and economic circumstances reduce the rate of death in childhood does the vulnerability of older age-groups emerge. An increasing probability of death as people grow older becomes evident and a modal age at death tends to appear which, in any society, is thus an expression of the level of economic development.

Mortality

The stillbirth (or fetal death) rate is high. This is defined as the number of infants born dead after reaching a viable stage of gestation (sometimes taken as 20 weeks and sometimes 28) for every 1000 total births, alive and dead. Many infants are born dead from preventable causes. Ignorance of the principles of hygiene and vulnerability to infection combines with the mother's unremitting work throughout pregnancy and the deficiencies in her nutrition, a combination that in all likelihood leads to prematurity and low birthweight and a high risk of infant death. The single largest known

Table 3.6 Life expectancy at birth in various countries: national averages

Age	Country
76	Iceland, Japan
75	Denmark, Netherlands, Norway, Sweden, Switzerland
74	Australia, Canada, France, Greece, United States
73	Belgium, Bulgaria, Cuba, Finland, Ireland, Italy, New Zealand, Spain, United Kingdom, West Germany
72	Austria, Cyprus, East Germany, Israel, Poland, Singapore
71	Czechoslovakia, Fiji, Hungary, Luxembourg, Malta, Portugal, Romania, Taiwan, Uruguay
70	Albania, Argentina, Barbados, Costa Rica, Jamaica, Panama, Trinidad and Tobago, USSR, Yugoslavia
69	Guyana, Kuwait
67	Venezuela
66	Bahrain, Brunei, Chile, Lebanon, Sri Lanka
65	Mexico, Paraguay, South Korea, Syria
64	China, Malaysia, Mauritius, North Korea
63	Brazil, Mongolia, Philippines, Vietnam
62	Colombia, El Salvador, Thailand, Turkey, United Arab Emirates
61	WORLD AVERAGE Dominican Republic, Ecuador
60	Jordan, South Africa
59	Guatemala
58	Honduras, Iran, Peru, Tunisia
57	Qatar
56	Algeria, Libya, Nicaragua
55	Egypt, Iraq, Kenya, Morocco
54	Saudi Arabia, Zimbabwe
53	Burma
52	India, Tanzania, Uganda
51	Haiti, Namibia, Pakistan
50	Bolivia, Indonesia, Lesotho, Liberia, Papua New Guinea
49	Ghana
48	Botswana, Nigeria, Zambia
47	Oman
46	Bangladesh, Benin, Cameroon, Congo, Equatorial Guinea, Ivory Coast Madagascar, Malawi, Mozambique, Rwanda, Sierra Leone, Sudan, Swaziland, Togo, Zaire
45	Yemen People's Democratic Republic
44	Central African Republic, Gabon, Guinea, Nepal
43	Laos, Somalia
42	Burundi, Mali, Mauritania, Niger, Senegal, Yemen Arab Republic
41	Angola, Chad, Gambia, Upper Volta
40	Afghanistan, Cambodia, Ethiopia

Source: Sivard, R. L. (1983). *World Military and Social Expenditures*, Washington, D.C., p. 22.

factor in low birthweight in the Third World is almost certainly malarial infection of the placenta; this contrasts with the developed world where it is undoubtedly maternal smoking (36). Deaths are also caused by ill-advised, if traditional, forms of intervention. In obstetric medicine the dangers of inappropriate interference in parturition slowly came to be understood, and they are emphasized by adverse outcomes of the customary conduct of labor in some peasant societies.

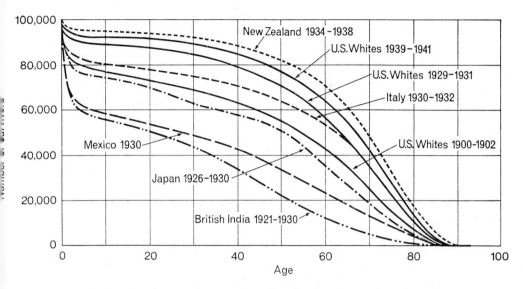

Figure 3.8 Survival under varied environmental conditions. Estimated number of survivors, at 10-year age intervals, of 100,000 male births. *Source:* Comfort, A. (1956). The biology of aging, *Lancet, 2,* 772–78; from life tables for selected countries, after Greville, 1946; as cited by Susser, M. W. (1969). Aging and the field of public health, in *Aging and Society,* Vol. II, eds. Riley, M. W., Riley, J. W., and Johnson, M. E., Russell Sage Foundation, New York, p. 131.

Traditional practices are no less important as an unwitting cause of infant loss after birth. While smallpox was still rife, health campaigns to vaccinate during an epidemic often failed where custom proscribed variolation of children with the exudate of the lesions of smallpox victims, or where spirits were thought to demand appeasement, because the people saw these campaigns as the intrusion of uncomprehending authorities. Among people in a changing environment, where they are deprived of customary foods, or where dietary restrictions and usages from the past persist for lack of other means or new knowledge, infants may be deprived of nutrients essential to growth and survival (37).

Mortality for the first year of life is relatively higher even than the stillbirth rate, and reflects the great vulnerability of infants to environmental forces. Infant mortality rates properly enumerated on a national level may range between 100 and 300; that is, 100 to 300 deaths occur in the first year of life for every 1000 live births in the same year. On a regional, or local level, the rates are often higher still. Many of these deaths are the result of nutritional disorders and infections and, again in contrast with developed countries, congenital malformations cause a tiny proportion of infant deaths. Diet is often markedly inadequate, so that undernutrition and malnutrition are widespread and the daily food intake of the adult population is likely to be 2000 calories or less. United Nations estimates suggest that 29 per cent of the population of the Far East suffer from malnutrition, 28 per cent in Africa, 16 per cent in the Near East, and 15 per cent in Latin America (37).

Lack of animal protein has been considered to be the single deficiency of most consequence, and its effects appear in such conditions as kwashiorkor in children who are artificially fed or who are fed at the breast into childhood with inadequate supplements. Deficiency of calories—simply insufficient food—is now seen to entail equal consequences. Malnutrition also contributes largely to childhood deaths from infection, principally gastrointestinal and respiratory infections. Wasted children are little able to resist measles and pneumonia in the colder months, or gastroenteritis in the summer. Epidemics of measles in the winter and diarrhea in the summer literally decimate the children of some peasant communities (38). Depressed mental performance accompanies the malnourished state; the production of permanent deficits requires the cooperating causes of social and intellectual deprivation and poverty (39).

After the first years of life the overall death rate declines, but nutrition and infection retain their importance. Epidemic killing diseases like typhoid, typhus, cholera, and plague flourish where water is impure, food contaminated, and rodent and insect vectors are uncontrolled. These diseases account for a good proportion of deaths, and the endemic killers like malaria, tuberculosis, and syphilis for even more. In a study in the Punjab, India, infectious diseases contributed 52 per cent of adult mortality. Tuberculosis was found to be the single most important cause of death, followed by heart disease and cancer. In Latin America 40 per cent of all deaths were attributed to infectious diseases; deaths from circulatory diseases accounted for only 20 per cent (40). A complex of ecological factors determines the spread and degree of each.

Enteric infections are borne by food, water, and flies. These involve a constant and repetitive cycle between human host and microorganism of fecal contamination and oral ingestion. All infections that take the enteric route flourish where clean water, effective sanitation, and strict hygiene in food handling and other matters are lacking. Thus bacterial diseases like typhoid and other salmonella organisms, dysentery and cholera, and viral diseases like infectious hepatitis and poliomyelitis are common causes of morbidity and mortality, and great havoc results from infantile gastroenteritis—although all these are eminently preventable. Heavy infestations by intestinal worms are common.

Airborne infections too account for much morbidity. They spread easily and rapidly in the conditions characteristic of poor, rapidly urbanized societies with overcrowding, intimate social contact among large numbers and large proportions of susceptible young. Thus heavy contributors to child morbidity as well as mortality are such preventable epidemic diseases as measles, whooping cough, diphtheria, various meningitides, and the somewhat less lethal chicken pox. The pneumonias too are responsible for much disease in both children and adults. In ill-ventilated tribal huts in highland areas, the smoke from indoor wood fires adds to the burden of respiratory disease. The airborne spread of tuberculosis, a preventable but continuing scourge of less-developed countries, makes it a familial disease; the bovine form, spread by contaminated milk, has a more sporadic distribution consistent with the mode of spread.

Vector-borne disease is markedly more common in developing than in developed countries. The snails that carry schistosomiasis, the fleas that carry plague, the mosquitoes that carry malaria, dengue fever, and yellow fever, and the lice that carry typhus readily find ecological niches no longer available in most developed countries.

Accidental deaths are fewer and of different types from those in industrial societies almost by definition, for the factories, machinery, and vehicles characteristic of industrial countries are scarce in underdeveloped countries. Where machines exist, injuries and fatalities take a high toll for want of safety regulations. Accidents are related to primary production in agriculture or mining, to exposure to the elements, and on occasion to wild animals and reptiles.

Chronic diseases of the various systems of the body are not uncommon as causes of death in less developed countries but they are not ranked in the same order of precedence as in developed countries. Although heart diseases attain importance in adults, and include rheumatic and hypertensive heart disease as they do in industrial societies, coronary disease is uncommon in many less developed societies, and in Africa especially; on the other hand, obscure cardiomyopathies may cause up to a third of all heart disease (41).

Survival and mortality in chronic disease have been little studied in Third World populations. Prevalence of equivalent but treatable disorders such as diabetes, hypertension, and others is assuredly lower in less developed than in developed countries for lack of medical care. On the whole, deaths from chronic noninfectious disease make up a minor proportion of the total because of the small size of the aged population. Many cancers are of less importance, of different type, and more evenly distributed throughout the age-groups. Only some of these variations are determined by the age- and sex-structure of the population. Carcinoma of the liver, rare in industrial societies, is one of the commonest cancers in the developing world—whether in the Far East or among blacks in southern Africa—and it often occurs in the young and middle aged. The hepatitis B virus, highly prevalent in the poor conditions of underdeveloped economies, is now known to carry a high risk for this cancer (42). Other factors, the aflatoxin that contaminates certain crops, and malnutrition, may also contribute. Burkitt's lymphoma, hardly seen in Europe and America, is the commonest malignant tumor among central African children. In central Africa, it has a geographical distribution related to the altitudes and temperatures at which malaria occurs, and it clusters locally, suggestive of infection carried by an insect vector. The Epstein-Barr virus is a microorganism frequently associated with the tumor. Thus the likely complex of causes leading to Burkitt's lymphoma includes acquired malaria together with susceptibility to the virus because of an immune deficiency (43). The Kaposi tumor (rare in the developed world except together with the newly emerging immune deficiencies among persons exposed to drastic chemotherapy for malignant disease and promiscuous homosexual men in the United States—the AIDS syndrome) is not uncommon in southern and central Africa. Variations in cancers of these kinds, that can be attributed to the features of the locale rather than to the age, sex, and genetic make-up of the population, are central to the hypotheses of recent decades that the causes of a large proportion of cancers reside in the environment (44).

Relative to men, overall mortality among women is higher than in developed countries. Women in many tribal or peasant societies are expected not only to bear and rear children through their whole reproductive period, but also to work in the fields. A woman with child continues her work throughout pregnancy. Children are valued, for the more hands there are to work, the more food people are likely to have. Thus women in societies dependent on subsistence agriculture are exposed to the risks of frequent pregnancies, and at the same time are exposed no less than men to the hazards of work and weather. Their problems increase as availability of land decreases and subsistence agriculture is replaced by large-scale farming, leading to displacement, migration, and disruption of roles. The emphasis laid on fertility in these societies is such that in many of them barrenness of the wife is a ground for the husband to seek divorce; in some, barren women become concubines or prostitutes, and their social standing is low. Hence anxiety about sterility and childbirth is common, and may form the focus of conversion hysterias such as those reported in Zulu women in the rural areas of Natal (45,46).

Women's experience of disease and death is therefore closely linked to their social and economic position. The risk of cancer of the neck of the womb (cervix uteri) for instance, which occurs at relatively young ages, is increased with coitus and marriage at early ages, and the available data for peasant societies show it to be the most frequent malignant neoplasm of women. On the other hand, in comparison with the developed world the risk of cancers of the body of the womb (corpus uteri) and of the breast is reduced, for these occur most often in relatively infertile older women. Breast cancer risk is reduced also by the infrequency of late first pregnancies, which raise the risk.

Morbidity

Morbidity in developing countries differs no less markedly than mortality from that in industrial societies and, like mortality, is dominated by nutritional disorders and infections. In British and American hospitals it is possible for conditions like pellagra to present a rare diagnostic problem, and for the less obvious guises of infection, like acute arthritis of the hip, to elude diagnosis. Cases of this type are routine in many African hospitals south of the Sahara, whereas collagen diseases and blood dyscrasias are less often seen or recognized, and tend to present difficulties in diagnosis. Even such everyday conditions in the hospitals of the developed world as ischemic heart disease, peptic ulcer and diabetes, disorders of the thyroid, and multiple sclerosis are rarely reported in Africa, excepting a few major cities, whether or not they occur.

The assumption that a particular disease does not occur in societies is often doubtful, and creates difficulties of comparison. The ways in which patients come to enter the overcrowded hospitals and clinics secludes many from professional view. Among those who are seen, lack of technical facilities and staff, and barriers of language and culture between patients and health professionals, can all obstruct accurate observation. Physicians are conditioned by training and attitude to make some diagnoses before others. In Uganda, where few peptic ulcers had been discovered in the past, either clinically or through complications, a special prospective necropsy study of the tribal prevalence of ulcer revealed rates in African males reaching 15 per cent. Ten years before, the same investigator had found, in a retrospective study of hospital records, the very low rate of three incidental cases in 1020 necropsies, some 50 times less than in the later population survey. The point is further illustrated by a study of the records of a large hospital for Africans in Durban where amebiasis is rife. Twelve of 27 patients with peptic ulcer presented with epigastric pain, and before the diagnosis was made seven of these had had a full course of antiamebic treatment, therapy that was not without dangers (47).

The recognition of sickness and the recording of deaths and their causes therefore present in themselves a significant contrast between industrial and underdeveloped countries. Industrial countries have comprehensive systems of registration of vital statistics, as well as censuses at regular intervals, which provide the numerators and denominators respectively for the calculation of a number of standard rates. Underdeveloped countries do not have the administrative resources for collecting the statistics necessary for exact comparison with industrial societies. As noted above, mortality statistics for these countries are usually based on incomplete registration and inaccurate counts of population. Morbidity statistics are difficult to collect even in industrial countries, and ordinarily require special investigations to establish accurate rates.

The data on which we have based our conclusions about underdeveloped economies are therefore derived from sources that include special local surveys and sample areas. The differences between developed and underdeveloped economies are so gross, however, as to leave no real doubts about the major contrasts in mortality and morbidity. In developed economies the main part of the residue of preventable deaths not prevented will yield in the main to socially induced changes in individual behavior. In underdeveloped economies, direct control of the physical environment alone— hygiene, sanitation, and nutrition—can prevent the main part of preventable disease. This is not to say that custom, politics, and socially induced individual behavior are unimportant in such societies.

In underdeveloped economies when the death rate is controlled by any means, the population expands at a rapid rate because the same means do not automatically control births. Fertility continues at the same high level as before. As the chance of survival rises, so does a larger proportion of girls reach reproductive age. Once the population of fertile women grows, the birthrate—with the total population as denominator—can rise even though the (age-specific) fertility rate remains stable at the maximum for given conditions.

If the resulting increase in numbers is not foreseen, as in Mauritius in the 1950s, population may outrun slender economic resources. Reduced death rates readily follow as an unanticipated consequence of rising standards of living, housing, and nutrition, or as an intended consequence of sanitary and public health measures that can be effective without enlisting the active choices of individuals. Reduced fertility rates, however, can only follow from the individual choices and acts of mating couples. Their choices are likely to depend on their aspirations, and on their perception of how best to rear their families and achieve these aspirations. In peasant societies where the family remains the unit of production, children ensure both the strength of the family labor force and ultimately the support of the elders in old age. As a result, reductions in birth rate to balance a reduced death rate have usually been slow to materialize. The consequence is seen first in the so-called "population explosion" beginning in Europe in the eighteenth and nineteenth centuries, and then through the twentieth century spreading successively to Asia, South America, and Africa (48).

Coexisting patterns: a case study

Gross differences in patterns of health occur not only between developed and developing countries, but also within countries. The health problems of the rural poor, of marginal urban dwellers living in shantytowns, and of urban dwellers, for example, are seldom the same. Mortality rates in developing countries—unlike Europe in the nineteenth century—seem generally to be higher in rural than in urban areas (33). These health conditions of developing countries are far from static. The major adjustments in personal, familial, and communal life that must be made in adapting to the modernization and industrialization occurring in many developing countries have consequences for health.

Conversion from the traditional work of subsistence farming to landless labor in large-scale farming or to industrial labor often disrupts traditional social and family relationships. These transitions have been connected with a variety of disorders, such as hypertension, ischemic heart disease, peptic ulcer, diabetes, and appendicitis. A complex of causes is involved. Few can be exactly specified, although nutrition and psychosocial stressors are most often suspected.

By contrast, the incidence of disease caused by specific agents often has social origins. For example, the transformation of rural economies prompts rural exodus. Urban migration separates families and breaks up support networks, isolates men and women from families and segregates them, and in turn increases both alcohol abuse and its consequent disorders and extramarital sex and venereal diseases. Work scarcity and unemployment add to the problems. In 1981 (admittedly a time of economic recession), 40 per cent of the work force in developing market economies was underemployed. On the other hand, the expansion of large-scale farming and industrial activity brings hazards noted above such as machine-related accidents, toxic contamination from pesticides or refining activities, and the dust-related respiratory diseases of mining and textile industries. The absence of workers' unions, combined with the weakness of government administration, lead to unregulated economic exploitation. For example, in Brazil, the highest mortality rates appeared where economic growth was most rapid and the environmental safeguards least (32,49). Thus, changes in the nature, the frequency, and the distribution of many disorders of health accompanied the metamorphoses of peasant into industrial societies. Among indigenous populations in underdeveloped economies today, this process of change can be observed, almost as it happens, despite the lack of adequate statistics.

In this chapter so far, the connection between health and the economy has been sought in comparisons between underdeveloped and developed societies. In Britain and the United States health and disease patterns characteristic of both types of societies were separated in time, during which economic and social changes took place. Both patterns, however, may be found existing side by side, particularly in those tribal and peasant societies where an industrial economy has been superimposed and where, as a result, industrial and traditional societies coexist in a transitional phase. The Republic of South Africa is a country in this transitional phase, and there two distinct patterns of disease can be observed (45,50). In this segregated, castelike society, the distribution of resources is uniquely enforced through the laws of the country. Contrasts of quality on each side of the caste line are apparent in all aspects of life—in education, in occupations, in living places, in dwellings, and in economic resources and the ownership of land. Health serves as a paradigm for the whole.

In the generation following the Second World War especially, and for reasons embedded in the history of colonialism, imperialism, and world capitalism, an industrial economy was superimposed on the pre-existing indigenous economy of South Africa. Among blacks, this was a mixed subsistence economy, chiefly pastoral and partly horticultural, which had gradually been absorbed into the money economy. Among the Afrikaner trekkers who penetrated the interior from the Cape in the eighteenth and nineteenth centuries the same was true, although they had the advantages of literacy, guns, wheels, and horses. The advent of the British during the Napoleonic wars brought a new set of mercantile interests to bear. These interests became frankly imperial with the discovery of rich diamond and gold fields in the 1860s and 1870s, which brought a flood of immigrants. Increasingly acute struggles between Boer pastoralists and English-speaking immigrants backed by imperial Britain reached a climax in the three-year war at the turn of the century. A half century after the Union of South Africa was created as a British dominion in 1910, however, Afrikaner nationalists achieved political independence in the Republic of South Africa.

On coming to power in 1948, the Nationalist Party adopted *apartheid* as government policy. Although *apartheid* is the ideology of Afrikaner nationalists whose traditional background was pastoral and agricultural, Afrikaners now share economic power in finance and industry with English-speaking whites. Reciprocally, many English-speakers share the doctrines of Afrikaners about race, just as they share in the spoils of white political power. Blacks provide labor, but they are excluded from political power, economic power, and landownership, as well as being socially segregated (51). *Apartheid* and the health consequences that follow can thus be thought of as extreme phenomena of class, engrafted on a history successively of European colonization, imperialism, and internal colonialism. In any event, whether owed to class, caste, or ideology, the social structure is held in place by the laws of *apartheid*.

Today, white and black live together within the overarching industrial economy and share many reciprocal relationships but in fixed positions of superiority and inferiority. These relationships in no way override the social and economic segregation entrenched by law, nor the restrictions on the economic growth of tribal society into new forms. Thus the disparity between the two opposed ethnic groups has been sustained. White South Africans in the cities have enjoyed the amenities and the health of an affluent industrial economy. Black South Africans in the tribal areas have retained the customs and diseases of an impoverished indigenous economy while suffering the newly imported disorders of colonialism. Those black Africans who moved from the country to the cities have exhibited the intermediate patterns of early industrialization in subsistence societies.

Johannesburg, the largest southern African city, exemplifies this postwar era. Birth, death, and morbidity rates of the white population resident in a good suburb were similar—with significant exceptions discussed below—to those of the population in a "good" residential area in Britain or North America. Babies did not die from malnutrition, summer diarrhea, and dehydration, nor from the epidemic diseases of childhood. Syphilis was rare and tuberculosis occasional. Children were well fed and well grown. One such suburb is separated only by a main street from the Alexandra location° where in the 1950s one square mile was populated entirely by 80,000 black South Africans. In this area syphilis was widespread, tuberculosis rampant, and stab wounds and head injuries a commonplace. Each summer, 10 per cent of the infant population died from gastroenteritis. The average child was stunted; up to 40 per cent of preschool children might have stigmata of malnutrition (45). The same is still true (52).

The contrasting prevalence of disease that existed in adjacent neighborhoods can be explained only in terms of South Africa's history and the evolution of her economic and social system. Within a few decades, the rapid growth of industry had elevated the living standards of the politically dominant whites. At the same time, this economic growth undermined the subsistence economies of the indigenous black people, and revolutionized their traditional way of life. After white colonial settlement and conquest, little more than one-tenth of the land of South Africa (13 per cent in fact) was reserved for black Africans. The reserves—now designated "homelands"—soon became overcrowded and impoverished. Nutrition suffered as the food yield of shrinking tribal lands fell. The migrant labor system exposed the males to the hazards of the industrial and urban world, and undermined the traditional roles of family life. At any one time, not less than 50 to 70 per cent of the men might be absent, working for wages in the mines and factories of the towns and cities, or on the farms owned by the whites. Women remained to till the land and tend the cattle, to rear the children, and to care for the sick and old.

The large body of unskilled migrants to the cities has been the main labor force on which the viability of South African industry depends. The flow of migrants between the so-called homelands and the towns is controlled and directed by "pass laws," part of an overall system of "influx control" that prevents nonwhite settlement in white and particularly in urban areas—precisely those where the hope for economic development and employment lies. Pass laws are complemented by a "resettlement policy," a policy for the mass removal of nonwhite communities from areas designated for whites. The "homelands" thus continue to function, as the reserves always did, as a labor pool. In the money economy that has absorbed the tribal economy, unemployment, poverty and the necessity to earn cash for taxes ensure the supply of cheap, unskilled migratory labor.

Under this system, the majority of blacks in the cities are and remain transient residents by law. Even rigorous enforcement, however, could not prevail entirely over the economic necessities of both employers and workers so that by now large black populations have achieved permanent residence in the vast townships outside the major cities. Their conditions, standards of living, and education contrast sharply with those of the people excluded from such privileges.

Men in search of work have usually migrated alone to the towns, although many have been followed by wives and families to live in poverty and overcrowded slums.

°Locations are areas reserved by law or regulation for black settlement. They can, not inappropriately, be described as ghettos.

The social disturbance invariably generated by such conditions is reflected in high disease and crime rates. Temporary liaisons and casual sexuality became widespread, and in Johannesburg the illegitimacy rate has been reported to be 70 per cent. The effect of this social differentiation between blacks and whites appears in the epidemiology of such disorders as the venereal diseases (including cervical cancer), tuberculosis, infant deaths, and serious injuries.

Syphilis, probably first brought to South Africa by European immigrants, was rapidly disseminated. In the 1950s up to 20 per cent of apparently healthy African women seen in antenatal clinics had positive blood tests. Some of these results were false positives, but the high rate was also a consequence of the system of migratory labor, with its unbalanced sex ratio and unstable unions (53). Thus high rates persist in the rural hinterlands. Pulmonary tuberculosis, also probably introduced to South Africa by Europeans, was common. The prevalence of active disease was at least ten times as high among blacks as among whites. The spread of tuberculosis, like that of syphilis, was favored by the labor system, but in a different way. Black migrant workers who fell sick in the city carried the disease home to the rural areas. Even if treatment had been available to them—and in the gold mines, the major industry, it was not until recently—they could not remain in the city because, once sick, they lacked the support of wages or of social services. Malnutrition further diminished resistance to the disease; in crowded dwellings the infection passed rapidly from one person to another, and the countermeasures were usually not known or available to the victim.

In South Africa, no systematic morbidity data are available at national, provincial, or local levels, with the exception of certain notifiable infectious diseases and of occasional local sample surveys. Some mortality data are available. In these there are limitations with regard to blacks beyond the usual problems found with mortality as a health indicator. The number of deaths by cause, age, and sex is published by the Government Department of Statistics in two series. One series for whites, Asians, and coloureds covers the whole country. Another for blacks covers only recent years and selected (magisterial) districts, which comprise "approximately 3.4 million people" living in the main urban areas—less than 15 per cent of the black population. Census data giving age distributions for the needed denominators are not to be had for this selected population, but only for blacks resident in white urban areas. In rural areas, in which more than half the black population dwells, useful estimates of mortality rates cannot be made. Even infant mortality—in the underdeveloped world still the most important single comparative health index—is not universally available for blacks: birth statistics for blacks are not collected by the central government, and thus both the numerators and denominators for blacks are scanty and incomplete. In a few major cities, the medical officers of health have estimated infant mortality rates. Even these rates are subject to errors of uncertain direction because of the ambiguity in the resident status of a large part of the population who reside there illegally.

The available mortality statistics, to which we now turn, reflect in a variety of ways the impact of the South African socioeconomic and political structure on health. First, we compare the mortality of white South Africa with that of England or Wales. This cross-national comparison gains cogency from the common origin of the medical training, practice, and culture of the two countries during the past century: diagnostic and certification practices are highly comparable. (In the absence of necessary data, of course, national comparisons including all nonwhites cannot be made.)

It is at once evident that South African whites—who are found only in the upper economic strata of a wealthy country—have mortality rates less favorable than the overall rates of England and Wales (which reflect the entire range of social classes) (see Table 3.7). Yet it is more than a reasonable guess that the people of England and Wales as a whole are less well placed economically than white South Africans. The disadvantage of white South Africans in mortality rates points to a discrepancy between health status and economic status. Relative risks for particular causes of death suggest three kinds of reasons for this apparent paradox.

One set of diseases points to the impact of cultural and behavioral factors super-imposed on economic wealth. It is reasonable, if speculative, to suppose that these patterns relate to the personal freedom of a way of life shaped by a frontier-type existence of the past. The lack of constraints fostered in the gold boom towns is now shared by the descendants not only of the *uitlanders* of the gold rush, but also of the once pastoral and thoroughly Calvinist Afrikaners. All whites enjoy the rights and privileges that inhere in high castes and aristocracies. Transposed into a modern world of affluence and high technology, such privilege and power can have unwonted and unwanted consequences. Ways of life are surely reflected in automobile accidents, violent deaths and suicides, heart disease, and cirrhosis of the liver.

For motor vehicle accidents, the mortality risk for white South Africa, relative to England and Wales, for males is 3.5, and for females 3.7; at ages 35 to 44 years, the risks are 6.1 and 6.2 respectively. For suicides, the relative risk for males is 2.9 although for females it is only just over 1; between 15 and 24 years, the risk for males is 3.3, for females 1.9. For accidents, poisonings, and violence, the relative risk for males is 2.8, for females 1.8. For cirrhosis of the liver (to some degree at least a drink-ing disease), the relative risk for males is 4.3, for females 4.5. Although for cardio-vascular diseases the relative risk for males is 1.3 and for females 1.2, for the specific component of ischemic heart disease the risks—at ages 35 to 44 years 2.5 and 2.6 respectively—are the highest in the Western world. These risks one may plausibly relate to the common or garden-variety risk factors and venial sins of smoking, glut-

Table 3.7 Age-specific mortality rates (per 1000) and relative risks (RR) for whites in South Africa compared with England and Wales, 1970

	Age group (years)								
	Under 1	1–4	5–14	15–24	25–34	35–44	45–54	55–64	65–74
Males									
England & Wales	21.15	.79	.38	.94	.99	2.25	7.02	21.01	53.44
RR (South Africa)	1.2	1.6	1.6	2.4	2.3	2.2	1.7	1.3	1.1
Females									
England and Wales	16.19	.64	.26	.40	.60	1.69	4.32	10.24	27.79
RR (South Africa)	1.2	1.6	1.4	1.9	1.9	1.5	1.4	1.3	1.2

Source: Adapted from Wyndham, C. H. (1980). A comparison of the mortality rates of white South Africans with those of the population of England and Wales, *S. Afr. Med. J.*, 57, 729–41, in Susser, M., and Cherry, V. (1982). Health and health care under Apartheid, *J. Pub. Hlth Policy*, 3, 455–75.

tony, and sloth, although among Afrikaners familial hypercholesterolemia must also be considered (54).

A second set of diseases points directly to the structure of a caste society that juxtaposes gross disparities. For infectious and parasitic diseases, the risks of white South Africa, compared with England and Wales, are for males 2.5, and for females 3.0; among infants, the risk is 3.2. In this instance, it seems that the health of whites, in spite of their economic and social distance from blacks, is directly affected by contacts with them, even though almost all take place within limited and prescribed roles of superiority and subordination, masters and servants, employers and employees.

A third set of disorders, what are called "symptoms and ill-defined conditions," points to the entirely different issue of the distribution of medical care in urban and rural areas. Thus the much higher rate in South Africa than in England and Wales of this nebulous category, as well as of such disorders as "senility" (with relative risks for males of 5 and for females of 3) may indicate less sophisticated terminal care and diagnostic precision for the sizeable population of white rural dwellers with limited access to medical centers.

The single category listed in which white South Africa has lower rates than are found in England and Wales is diseases of the respiratory system, and in particular lung cancer. This difference might reside in the kinds and amounts of cigarettes smoked, or, alternatively, in weather and levels of air pollution. In fact, the difference is more a British than a South African peculiarity. Lung cancer rates in South African whites are very similar to the rates for United States whites and, indeed, so are the rates for most of the leading causes of cancer deaths (55).

The *estimated* population of South Africa at the 1980 census (56) stood at 23.77 million, stratified by race as follows:

Black	15.97 million
White	4.45
Coloured	2.5
Asian	0.79

These numbers exclude about 5 million blacks in the so-called "homelands." Thus blacks make up 67.2 per cent of the population in "white" South Africa, and whites 18.7 per cent. Since this racial stratification embodies social, economic, and political stratification it is a fundamental determinant of inequality in South Africa, in health as in any other matter. As will be shown in Chapter 6, social class has invariably been the most powerful social determinant of health patterns within developed countries. In the United States and Britain, for example, striking inequalities in the mortality and morbidity of higher and lower social classes remain. Even greater disparities reside in the rigid South African strata.

Precise comparisons of mortality across groups are hard to come by, however. Even within the better-documented white group, published indices besides location, age, and sex by which to stratify mortality statistics are not to be had. The absence of basic vital statistics and census data for blacks, as we have noted above, is itself a reflection of the body politic. This typical condition of an underdeveloped country is embedded in a social structure where the dominant minority lives under conditions typical of a developed country. The selected magisterial districts for which deaths are registered and published are much the better-off areas, placed where officials and resources are sufficient to engender recognition of the need for them.

The best available comparisons of mortality among the four race groups show rates for black and colored that are similar to each other (58). Both far exceed those of whites (see Figure 3.9). Asians hold an intermediate position, overall and for many specific causes of death, that mirrors their political and economic position in South African society. The dramatic contrasts in overall mortality are among infants, and among children aged 1 to 4 years.

Under age one the relative mortality for blacks compared with whites is sixfold, and for one to 4 years fourteen-fold. It is familiar public health lore that in harsh conditions infants are highly sensitive to poor hygiene and infections, and that weanlings, no longer protected against infectious diseases by maternal antibodies in breast milk, are especially vulnerable to malnutrition. Beyond early childhood, the relative mortality is much lower and gradually declines, from about three in the age group

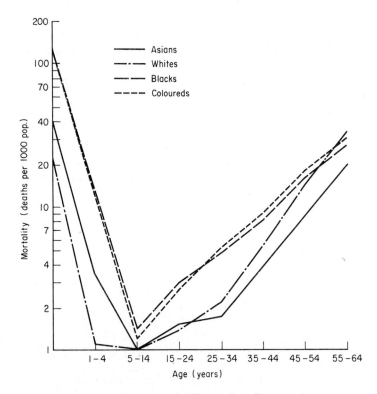

Figure 3.9 Age-specific mortality rates of different "race" groups for registration areas in South Africa in 1970. *Source:* Constructed from Wyndham C. H., and Irwig, L. J. (1979). A comparison of the mortality rates of various population groups in the Republic of South Africa, *S. Afr. Med. J.*, 55, 796–802; as cited by Susser, M. and Cherry, V.P. (1982). Health and health care under apartheid, *J. Pub. Hlth, Pol.*, 3, 455–75.

five to 14 years, to between two and three up to age 44, to less than two among survivors of 45 years and more. In the rural areas and the homelands, such knowledge as we have—from local studies and special surveys—points to an abysmal health pattern for blacks. In 1979 in certain rural areas, infant mortality was estimated to reach above 30 per cent (320 per 1000); overall, the minimum was thought to be above 20 per cent (220 per 1000) (56).

For coloured people, overall mortality rates up to age five are even worse than for the blacks in the selected registration districts. As to where the source of the blight might be, a study of coloured infant mortality in the city of Capetown is illustrative (58). The rates fell sharply over three decades from 149.6 per 1000 in 1941 to 25.9 per 1000 in 1977. The rates for the coloured people in South Africa as a whole, however, do not show this sharp decline, and the rate remains well over 100 per 1000. In Johannesburg, infant mortality rates for blacks also declined, from 232 in 1950 to 41.73 in 1977 (57)—again, far different from other areas of the country. The approximately sixfold fall in the mortality of the coloured infants in Capetown and black infants in Johannesburg shows what is self-evident. In the face of overcrowding, unemployment, and other adversities, it is quite feasible to reduce the inequalities in infant mortality that persist in the rest of South Africa. The improvement probably stems from a combination of higher living standards, better nutrition, and better access to and use of health services.

When one turns to consider specific *causes* of sickness and death it becomes plain that black and white live in different worlds. Whites, despite the differences noted above from Europeans in life-style and their vulnerability to infection across the color bar, die of European-type diseases; blacks and coloureds—so-called non-Europeans— die of Third World diseases. Diseases of the circulatory system and of neoplasms predominate among whites, childhood infections and malnutrition among nonwhites.

Table 3.8 selects from published data (58) specific causes of death, chiefly those with a relative risk (RR) for nonwhites of more than two. Fearsome mortality risks decimate blacks, for instance, gastroenteritis (RR 19.6), tuberculosis (RR 27), nutritional disorders (RR 62), and homicide (RR 20.7). For death from some chronic diseases too—as for hypertension and diabetes—blacks, like coloureds and Asians, are at a marked disadvantage (although Asians are at special risk from diabetes) (59). But for ischemic heart disease whites have a tenfold higher risk than blacks, for cancer of the lung twofold, and for suicide more than twofold (2.25).

To attribute the whole of this divergence to the political and economic structure of South African society is to make too sweeping and simple-minded a claim. Where constitution and culture diverge, the pattern of disease also diverges, an inescapable truth in South Africa (45,60). Both constitution and culture are shaping forces that exist in varying degree independently of political and economic structure (see Chapter 4). Here studies of morbidity illumine better than do those of mortality.

On the one hand, the frequency of hypertension in blacks is a likely reflection of the economic pressures underlying urban migration and acculturation (61). The frequencies of the leading cancers among blacks—for instance, the rising rates of lung cancer as cigarette smoking is diffused among urbanized blacks (55)—obviously reflect those pressures too. Rates of diabetes among blacks higher in the newer urban

Table 3.8   Relative mortality risks (age-adjusted) for Asians, Coloureds, and Blacks compared with whites for ICD groups and selected specific causes at ages 15–64: South Africa, 1970

Cause of death[a]	White rate per 1000	Relative risks		
		Asian	Colored	Black
Infective and Parasitic	7.0	5.2	15.8	14.9
Gastroenteritis	.8	5.2	12.5	19.6
Tuberculosis	2.9	7.6	31.2	27.0
Neoplasms	102.8	.7	1.4	1.0
Lung	20.2	.4	1.1	.5
Endocrine	6.1	6.6	2.6	2.9
Diabetes	5.0	7.4	2.1	2.1
Nutritional	.1	22.0	30.0	62.0
Circulatory	259.1	1.6	1.4	0.8
Hypertension	7.9	6.5	5.6	4.3
Ischemic Heart Disease	167.5	1.1	0.6	0.1
Respiratory	54.5	2.3	2.6	2.3
Pneumonias	21.0	2.6	3.5	3.9
Digestive	25.3	1.8	1.7	1.6
Symptoms and ill-defined	7.9	3.7	4.8	16.1
Accidents and Violence	101.6	.8	1.8	1.8
Suicide	18.1	.9	.4	.4
Homicide	3.4	2.3	14.4	20.7

[a] As specified in the International Classification of Diseases (ICD).

Source: Susser, M. and Cherry, V. (1982). Health and health care under Apartheid, *J. Pub. Hlth. Policy, 3*, 455–75.

than in traditional rural settings are presumably linked with a combination of economic and dietary changes. Overcrowding in black households in Soweto° is reflected in the unusually high rate of rheumatic heart disease among children—the result of recurrent untreated streptococcal infection of the respiratory tract (62).

On the other hand, several cancers can readily be linked with indigenous or long-standing cultural practices. The extremely high rate of esophageal cancer in the Transkei (63) is related to the smoking—in pipes or rolled cigarettes—of pipe tobacco, although rates in some large cities are also high and increasing (55). The high rates of cancer of the cervix and the low rates of cancer of the breast can both be connected with age at first coition and age at first pregnancy—behavior influenced by cultural tradition as well as by economic and demographic forces. Low rates of stomach cancer are perhaps related to diet; the notably low rates of colorectal cancer too might be related to diet, for instance, to high fiber content.

On the constitutional side, it might be argued, in whites both in the United States and South Africa mortality rates for cancers are remarkably similar; coloured rates

°Soweto is an acronym for the vast segregated area outside Johannesburg (the South West Township) with almost a million residents according to the census and probably twice that number in actuality (that is, including "illegal" residents).

for the most common cancers in some instances resemble those for United States blacks, in others those for South African blacks. Environment, however, is equally likely to produce these variations.

The connection with the sociopolitical structure is not in doubt for the diseases that create the sharpest contrasts in black and white sickness and health, namely, childhood infections superimposed on malnutrition, summer diarrhea in babies, parasitic and other infections. Even in a major city such as Durban, protein-energy malnutrition was recorded as present in from 32 to 51 per cent of pediatric admissions to the King Edward VIII Hospital from 1959 to 1975. In 1979, among 6765 pediatric admissions overt malnutrition was diagnosed in 41 per cent of cases, and was associated with 66 per cent of deaths. Where malnutrition was the primary diagnosis, as many as one-quarter died. In Soweto, Johannesburg, in 1978 23.6 per cent of pediatric admissions were for kwashiorkor or marasmus. Both the admission rate and the fatality rate of 7.1 per cent, it should be said, indicate distinct improvement over the past 25 years. In the population at large, especially in rural areas and "homelands," malnutrition is widespread. Among rural Asians in Natal, more than 60 per cent of children were reportedly malnourished. Among rural blacks in the Ciskei, about 50 per cent of the two- to three-year-olds were reportedly malnourished.

In the absence of detailed data and standard criteria, such reports can be challenged, but they surely reflect serious nutritional deprivation. A collation of reports both rural and urban from across the country shows substantial proportions of children, often a majority, below the third percentile for weight and height standards (64). The shortfall is not constitutional: in Johannesburg in the 1950s, the children of black women who were qualified nurses attained weights and heights much like those of higher class Americans of the same age (65). As noted above, in the major cities over the past few decades mortality trends have improved as overall economic productivity improved, without diminishing the relative deprivation of blacks. In the rural areas and "homelands," where documentation is even scarcer, scattered local reports do not suggest improvement and some suggest deterioration (66).

The South African case today has salience for public health theory. Edwin Chadwick wrote the *Report on Sanitary Conditions of the Labouring Population of Great Britain* in 1842 in part to bolster the utilitarian argument that disease caused poverty, and that the elimination of disease by sanitation would enrich the nation (67). The results in health and productivity of the sanitary revolution left little doubt that he was right. His thesis is illustrated afresh for blacks in South Africa by the positive health effects of introducing ideas of comprehensive hygiene into defined rural and urban populations without benefit of economic improvement (68).

In counterpoint, Friedrich Engels, in his *Condition of the Working Class in England in 1844*, argued the converse thesis that working-class poverty created by early industrial capitalism was itself a powerful cause of disease (69). That this is also true can be argued from improvements in health, especially those occurring without benefit of improved hygiene, that followed the reduction in the absolute level of poverty. In the major South African cities of Johannesburg and Capetown, nutrition and growth indices of black and coloured children respectively have all improved concurrently with wages, living standards, facilities, and in several instances without any known effective intervention to prevent or reduce disease. We noted above the substantial decline in infant mortality in the two cities for blacks and for coloureds, respectively. In Johannesburg there was also a relative narrowing of the gap between whites and blacks.

Engels had a still greater concern with the overriding thesis that the order of economic relations and the class relations they engender determine social relations, including health. Under *apartheid*, the sharp relief of the health contours holds despite the improvement over time in the large cities and the apparent narrowing of the gap between race groups. The configuration is the unequivocal mark of politically defined racial groups from which there is no legal or illegal escape.

Changes over time

Accelerating change in many domains typifies industrial societies. Just as the populations of industrial societies have not always had their present characteristics, so they have not always enjoyed a favorable experience of health and disease. In nineteenth century Britain, according to the earliest reliable statistics, the population age-structure, birth and death rates, and causes of death, resembled those now recorded in regions of the developing world. These similarities between pre-industrial Europe and the underdeveloped world of the present-day occur in the face of marked differences in ecology, economy, and historical circumstances. Economic development has created a new configuration of health and disease at the core of the world economy.

This does not imply that the means of "modernization" in Britain—rapid industrialization through technological innovation, land enclosures, urban migration, and the control of overseas markets and sources of raw materials—should or can be prescribed elsewhere. The underdevelopment of much of the rest of the globe was the counterpoint to the economic advance and the improvement in living conditions that can be documented in Britain from the latter part of the nineteenth century (70). Britain does, however, provide the most convenient example of changes over time in a developed country, for its national vital statistical system dates back to 1837 and uniquely included registration of causes of death almost from the beginning.° The changes can be discussed in terms of mortality, population structure, and morbidity.

Mortality

During the century 1851–1951, the rise in standard of living, together with parallel advances in sanitation, personal hygiene, and medical therapeutics, increased life expectancy at birth from 40 to 66 years for males, and from 42 to 71 for females. By 1978 life expectancy at birth in England and Wales was 70 years for males and 76.1 for females (16). Changes similar to these in Britain occurred in the indices of most

---

°William Farr, a founder of modern epidemiology, was appointed Compiler of Abstracts in the General Register Office in 1839; in this post he was responsible for the compilation of tables on the registration of births, deaths, and marriages, and he introduced a system of recording and classifying deaths at the outset of his 40-year career (71).

countries that underwent industrialization in the past century. For example, in the United States from 1900 to 1980, life expectancy at birth for males rose from 48 to 70.0 years, and for females from 51 to 77.5.

The chance of death fluctuates throughout an individual's life-cycle, and the main point of impact of the forces of mortality depends in large part on the social and economic circumstances of the population. As the standard of living rose during the past two centuries, the main point of impact shifted from the first five years of life to the first year, and finally to old age. A fall in death rates began in Britain probably about 200 years ago; this seems the most reasonable explanation, if not the only one, for the rise in population that also then began (72). Thus the Industrial Revolution can be said to have created its own internal labor force by increasing production, wages, consumption, and ultimately survival. The increased survival of the young into maturity led to a birthrate far in excess of the death rate, with a resulting rapid population growth.

After 1838, when reliable mortality statistics became available, the decline in deaths could be attributed to reductions in the toll of deaths from specific causes. Tuberculosis accounted for about half the decline up to the end of the nineteenth century, probably because of increased host resistance as more food was produced and diet improved. Typhus and typhoid fevers accounted for about one-fifth of the decline, and cholera, dysentery, and diarrhea for about one-tenth; their decline can safely be attributed to the clean water achieved by the closed-circuit sanitation systems introduced by Edwin Chadwick that separated water supplies and sewage disposal. Smallpox accounted for about one-twentieth of the decline, in the main because of vaccination, while scarlet fever accounted for one-fifth. The decline in scarlet fever is believed to be due to reduction in the virulence of the hemolytic streptococcus but, as with the other diseases, enhanced host resistance through improved diets probably played a role. The series of figures illustrating the historical course of major infectious diseases (see Figure 3.10) emphasizes the substantial effects of historical change alone on the death rate of each disease. In several instances, interventions by means of vaccines and chemotherapy of known efficacy produced effects scarcely perceptible in the grand sweep of declining mortality curves. That is, undirected economic, social, and political change outweighed directed technical advances.

In age-specific terms, the greatest single contribution to the improvement in death rates has been the fall in infant mortality. Because the deaths occur early in life, the decline of the infant mortality rate has a marked and disproportionate impact on estimates of expectations of life. This improvement came late in the cycle of change. Throughout nineteenth century Britain the rate had remained at about 150 per 1000 live births; at the turn of the century, it began to decline rapidly and reached 11.1 in 1982. In the United States similar declines have been observed. The total death rate in 1982 was less than one-third that of 1900; the infant mortality rate in 1981 (11.9) was about one-fifth of the 1935 rate of 55.7 (15). In the decade 1955–1964, however, the death rates tended to level off in all age-groups. A similar halt occurred in Britain and several other countries, but at a lower level than in the United States—good reason to believe that in the United States, at least, mortality could be further reduced. Since then, mortality rates among the newborn, among infants, and at later ages have resumed a steady decline.

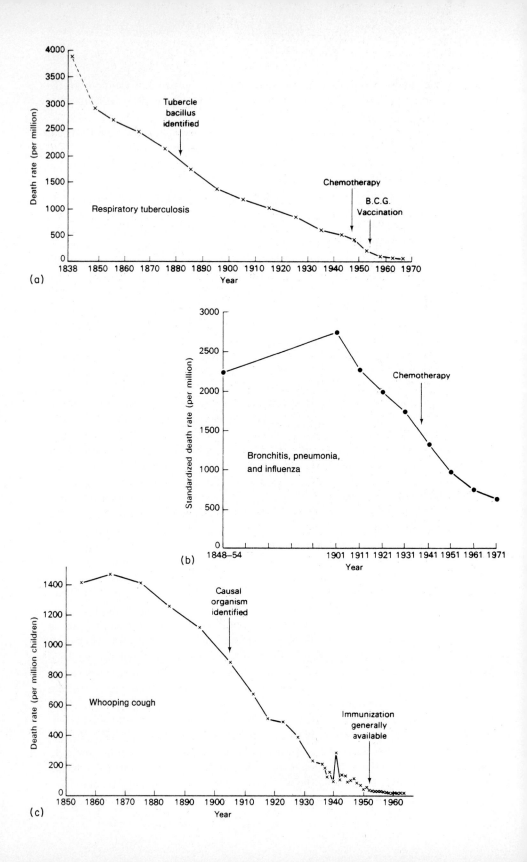

(a)

(b)

(c)

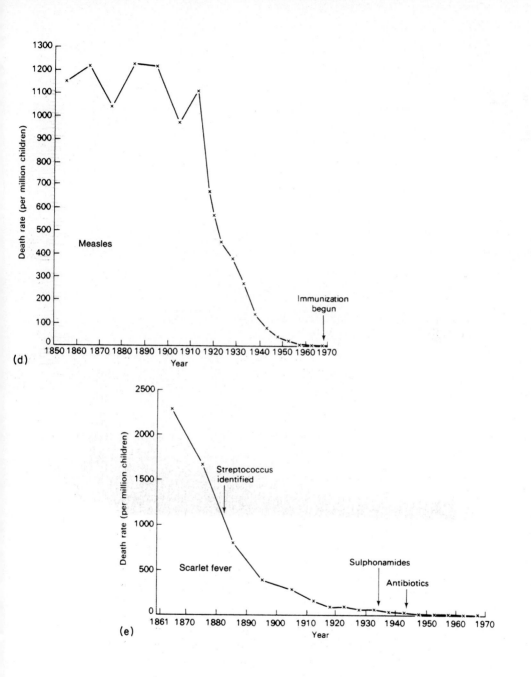

Figure 3.10 Death rates over time per million population, or per million children under 15, England and Wales, for major infectious diseases, indicating also the approximate point at which prophylaxis or effective treatment was deployed.

Source: McKeown, T. (1976). *The Modern Rise of Population*, London, pp. 93, 94, 96, 98, 99.

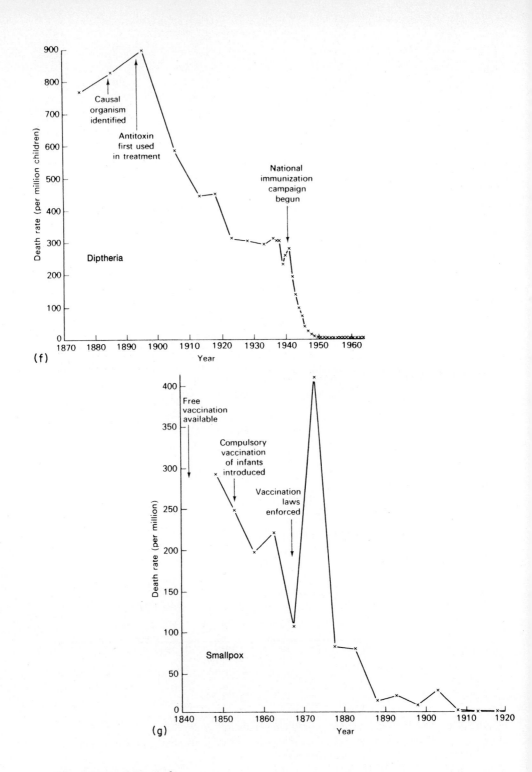

(f)

(g)

Figure 3.10 Continued

The impact of reduced infant mortality has not been uniform throughout the first year, and has been most striking after the neonatal period (see Chapter 6). Infancy is a stage of development highly sensitive to environmental influences so that, under severe conditions, most other causes of death are overshadowed by environmental causes. With the removal of this pressure, causes of death emerge that are less directly related to environmental stress. In infancy these residual causes are connected with gestation and birth, and the rise in their relative importance is reflected in the distribution of infant deaths by age. In the past, indeed as late as 1930 in the United States, fewer deaths occurred in the newborn period than in the remainder of the first year, whereas now most deaths occur among the newborn, and especially within the first hours and days. [*Neonatal death* is defined as occurring in the first 28 days of life, *early neonatal death* in the first seven days of life.] In Britain in 1980 the neonatal death rate was 7.7 per 1000 live births compared with only 4.4 in the 11 months of the post-neonatal period; in the United States in 1981, comparable figures were 7.8 and 3.9 respectively (15,16).

Neonatal mortality throughout the developed world has declined substantially in the past quarter century. In the United States in the years 1950–1965 neonatal mortality rate fell by 14 per cent (from 20.5 to 17.7 per 1000), but over the next decade dropped further to reach 7.8 per 1000 in 1981. In Britain a comparable decline occurred for the years 1961–1982: from 15.8 to 7.7 per 1000, better than 50 per cent. Analysis of United States trends indicates that the most significant factor in neonatal deaths—the distribution of low birthweight babies—showed little change during this period (see Figure 3.4). The improvement can in all probability, therefore, be attributed to enhanced chances of survival at each birthweight, and this, in turn, is likely to be the result of improved newborn care.

Sex ratio

Increasingly from birth onwards, vitality cannot be considered apart from social factors. These have a profound influence on the ratio of males to females in the total population. [The ratio may be stated as males per 100 females, a *masculinity ratio*, or as females per 100 males, a *femininity ratio*. Both ratios are used, sometimes in the same book or article, because of the convention of stating whichever ratio is greater than unity.] More males than females are born. In Britain, for instance, since 1870 the ratio of males to females at birth has fluctuated from 103 to 106. The sex ratio at conception is not known, although it may not be unity; in experiments, sperm bearing the male Y-chromosome are more efficient in penetrating ova in vitro. Moreover, the probability of a male conception seems to vary with the interval between ovulation and insemination. Thus one might surmise that at conception the excess of males to females is even greater than at birth, and that the excess is reduced by a greater loss of males from abortions during pregnancy and from stillbirths at parturition. Recent data support the expectation of a higher rate of spontaneous abortions among male conceptions (73).

Some authorities have speculated that even at this early stage the loss of males varies with the severity of the environment (74). In most animal species that have been studied, though not in all, males are more vulnerable and shortlived than females. This is true for human beings in the developed world in postnatal life at all ages. In the late 1970s in the United States, overall male mortality was 60 per cent higher than that of females. The high mortality of males could be related to their intrinsic constitutional vitality, to their behavior patterns, or to their exposure to environmental hazards. Sex differences in vitality is the most plausible explanation for the sex differences in prenatal growth rates, birthweight, and newborn mortality. Males grow more rapidly during gestation and are heavier at birth than females. Birthweight has a powerful effect on newborn mortality but despite the advantage of males in weight they are probably less "mature" and their perinatal mortality rates are higher; adjustment for weight-at-birth exaggerates the male disadvantage. While these differences are likely to be intrinsic to each sex, the balance of male and female sex hormones during gestation can influence not only postnatal somatic, sexual and physical development but behavior as well (75).

Later in life, the effect of sexual behavior on the health and survival of the sexes has been considered. In some species, for example, the joys and perils of mating have been found to shorten the life-span of males but in others to lengthen it (76). The question has been given due consideration in our own species as well, within a clinical tradition that dates back to the treatment of the aged and dying King David by having him cherished by young women. An early and unrefined analysis failed to settle the issue by comparing the mortality of celibate Roman Catholic priests with that of noncelibate Anglican clergy. A growing number of microorganisms are recognized as capable of being transmitted sexually but, in general, these have had a greater impact on morbidity and fertility than on mortality. Syphilis is an exception. It was an important cause of death from its rise at the end of the fifteenth century until its containment by chemotherapy and antibiotics in the twentieth. In the past two decades, changes in sexual mores have led again to a rapid rise in many venereal diseases, especially gonorrhea, nonspecific urinary tract infections, and herpes virus and not excepting syphilis. Men have suffered more frequently than women, an imbalance of which acquired immune deficiency syndrome (AIDS) is the newest manifestation. Probably at most times more men than women have been promiscuous, although the smaller number of promiscuous women will have had a higher average of sexual contacts.

For women, in the past the main consequence of mating for mortality has been the losses with childbearing. These losses have become minimal. We now find that sexual experience and reproduction relate not only to venereal diseases but to certain cancers in which there is a strong presumption of underlying sexually transmitted infections, in particular cervical cancer with herpes and human papilloma viruses. Patterns of sexual and reproductive behavior also relate, in the opposite direction, to hormone-dependent cancers of the female reproductive tract. That is, cancers of breast, body of the uterus, and ovaries are all associated with celibacy, late marriage, and low fertility. In breast cancer, an association with early menarche and late first pregnancy, and also the effect of hormones on the course of the established disease, strengthens the inference of hormone dependency (77).

Marked variations in sex ratios appear in different types of environmental circumstances, depending on conditions that act unequally against each sex (48). In India, for example, statistics have shown a preponderance of males in the population despite their constitutional vulnerability. The preponderance appears to have been maintained by the high death rate among women from very frequent maternities, as well as tuberculosis and other causes. It may also have been maintained by cultural practice, for females have less social significance than males, and it has been suggested that village headmen responsible for the census count frequently omitted female children from the enumeration.

In societies where environmental conditions are less severe, females outnumber males (78). In England and Wales, females have exceeded males in number for the past one hundred years, and this excess reached a maximum of 10 per cent after the First World War. The reversal from an excess of males at birth to an excess of females in later age-groups has tended over the years to occur at successively later ages. This shift is the result of the low absolute death rates for males up to these ages; more time is now needed before attrition among the excess of males existing at birth is enough to reverse the sex ratio. In less than a half century, the age at which an excess of females had first appeared has shifted from adolescence to 45 to 54 years, after which age the proportion of women increases in each successive age-group and into old age (see Table 3.9).

The female excess rests on different combinations of factors as one generation succeeds another. In Britain in the first half of the twentieth century, war fatalities and emigration affected men particularly. Later, middle-aged men were the chief victims of the epidemic smoking diseases and of the so-called diseases of civilization of the twentieth century (peptic ulcer, coronary heart disease, and lung cancer in particular). At the same time, women benefited most from declining mortality. The increase in expectation of life has been greatest among middle-aged women. Females already enjoyed lower mortality rates than males in the nineteenth century, except between the ages of 10 and 20, but they now have consistently lower mortality rates throughout life.

Table 3.9 Sex ratios (males per 100 females) in the U.S. population within age groups at variable intervals from 1950 and projected to 1980

Age and projection series	1950	1960	1970	1976	Projected 1980
Under 15 years	103.8	103.4	103.9	104.2	104.5
15 to 29 years	98.7	97.7	97.8	100.3	101.3
30 to 44 years	97.4	95.5	95.2	95.8	96.6
45 to 59 years	99.8	96.9	93.4	94.8	95.3
60 to 64 years	100.4	91.2	87.7	87.9	87.9
65 to 69 years	94.0	87.8	80.7	79.3	79.7
70 to 74 years	91.3	85.3	73.9	73.5	72.4
75 to 84 years	85.0	77.4	65.9	61.0	60.3
85 years and over	70.0	63.8	53.2	47.0	44.7

Source: U.S. Bureau of the Census, "Current Population Reports," series P-25, nos. 311, 519, 614, 643, and 704, as cited by Siegel, J. S. (1980). Recent and prospective demographic trends for the elderly population and some implications for health care, in *Epidemiology of Aging: Second Conference*, ed. Haynes, S. G. and Feinleib, M., U.S. Department of Health and Human Services, NIH Publ. No. 80-696, Bethesda, Maryland, p. 297.

The sharp increase in expectation of life of adult women during this century must be attributed in no small part to the remarkable reduction in childbearing over the last century. Of the women married in Britain during the decade 1870–1879, 61 per cent bore five or more children. In contrast, of the women married in Britain in 1971, fewer than 10 percent will bear four or more children. A typical Victorian mother would have spent the greater part of her married life in bearing and rearing children. Many contemporary mothers, having completed their families within less than ten years of marriage, have more than half their lives before them. These changes follow closely upon the altered economic and social position of women during the last century. Women have gained more control over their own fertility through the introduction of techniques of birth control that they manage themselves. They have attained equality before the law in most matters, and now command potential economic independence because of demand for their labor.

This is not to gainsay the continuing large proportion of morbidity and health service usage in women that is related to reproduction. Among women aged 15 to 44 years in the United States in 1980, deliveries accounted for almost a third of admissions to short-stay hospitals out of a total of 208 per 1000 population. And, on the contrary, tubal sterilization is being performed at a rate of 14 per 1000 annually (79). In this age-group, too, notable sex differences begin to emerge in benign neoplasms (females 0.7 vs. males 4.8 per 1000); in alcohol dependent syndromes (females 1 vs. males 3.6 per 1000); in heart disease (females 1.7 vs. males 3 per 1000); in fractures, lacerations, and wounds (females 3.1 vs. males 9.8 per 1000).

In contrast, high death rates among adult and middle-aged men have been maintained by greater exposure to such hazards as smoking, polluted air and cold weather, alcohol abuse, and accidents at work and on the roads. These compounded factors make a substantial contribution to male deaths from bronchitis and emphysema, bronchial cancer, and fatal injuries. To these must be added the large number of deaths from coronary heart disease, and a much smaller number from peptic ulcer, in both of which sex differences in smoking and in work-oriented behavior type play a part (see Chapter 6). In England and Wales in 1981 the death rate between 55 and 64 years among men (17.5 per 1000) was almost double that of women (9.3 per 1000). In the United States, the comparable rates in 1981 were virtually the same (17.8 vs. 9.4 per 1000). In 1980 in the United States male mortality for all ages was 9.6 per 1000 and female mortality 7.8 per 1000.

Male socialization and behavior patterns are reflected in these as well as in a number of other causes of death. Thus most of these sex differences are related to the fundamental divergence not only in the constitutions but in the life experiences of males and females. The contribution of life experience to the growing current disparity is suggested by the relative absence of notable sex disparities in the epidemics of the past, or in those that afflict contemporary peasant societies. In recent years women—and especially higher class and professional women—have begun, so to speak, to die like men. That is to say, they are acquiring more of the behavior and of the causes of death that have been typically male (80). As the impact of cigarette smoking among them is felt, their death rates from lung cancer and also from coronary heart disease have begun to rise. If the use of sex hormones for contraception and for menopausal symptoms has added to morbidity, this may well be balanced by a reduction in morbidity from other conditions and certainly from the pregnancies prevented. Oral contraceptives exacerbate the coronary disease risks from smoking. At the same time, oral contraceptive use appears in some instances to reduce mortality from cancer of the breast and ovary, in others to increase it. The precise effects, according to one group of investigators, seem to depend on the balance of estrogens and progestogens prescribed, and on the ages or stages of development of the reproductive cycle at which they are used. If a high progestogenic effect is introduced in very young or in menopausal women, the risk of breast cancer appears to be raised. Substitute estrogens, given for menopausal symptoms, in high doses multiplied the risks of cancer of the body of the uterus; this effect must be balanced by the decrease in fractures of the hip in older women because such treatment retards the erosion of bone by osteoporosis that many women suffer from middle life on (77, 81). These changes are far from righting the balance between male and female survival. Thus, while age-adjusted mortality for persons aged 65 years and over fell by 27 per cent from 1950 to 1979, the decline was twice as great for females as for males.

The consequences of sex disparity in deaths in industrial societies are more obvious than the causes. At current death rates in the United States, about one-third of men aged 20 can be expected to die before the age of 65, a loss to society of about one-tenth of the work potential of an age-cohort. A woman five years younger than her husband must face the prospect of an average of 11 years of widowhood; as a result, in 1980 there was a 73 per cent excess of women at ages 75 years and over.

Population

The changing sex ratio prevalent in the population at large, falling birth rates and death rates, and the increased expectation of life have brought about radical changes in the structure of populations (see Figure 3.11). In England and Wales, the rate of birth, which now fluctuates from 15 to 16 per 1000 of the total population, was twice as great throughout the nineteenth century; women who married in the period 1870–1879 bore an average of 5.8 children, whereas those who married in 1964 bore only 2.17. Family size is closely correlated with living standards and nutrition, and the sharp reduction in family size that followed the fall in the birthrate during the last century combined with the enhanced economic productivity of the enlarged working population in the new industrial system to raise living standards still further. Between 1871 and 1981, persons aged 65 years or more increased in the population from 5 per cent to 17 per cent, while those aged less than 15 years decreased from 36 per cent to 22 per cent. This reshuffling of age-groups represents a more than fivefold increase in the ratio of persons over the age of 65 to those under 15.

The proportion of productive workers has not fallen, however, and has actually been supplemented by the increase in the numbers of working women. Indeed, the main effect of the age changes has been to increase the relative numbers of the middle aged. Compared with the young, the expectation of life for those who reach old age has not been greatly extended, although the proportion of the old is so much larger. In general, the age-structure of the population in the United Kingdom has changed

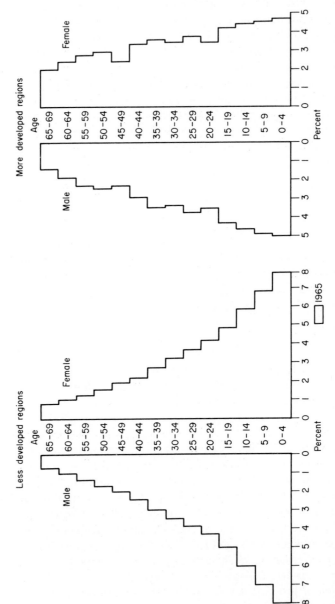

Figure 3.11 Sex- and age-structure of the population in less-developed and more-developed regions, 1965. *Source:* Adapted from United Nations Secretariat (1975) World and regional population prospects, in *Population Debate*, vol. 1, part II, United Nations, New York, p. 32.

over the last two centuries from that typical of a "traditional" society, in which the risk of death remains much the same throughout life, to that of an industrial society, with a "senescent" age curve showing a modal age at death beyond the sixties (see Figure 3.8) (35).

In the United States as in Europe, the population has grown rapidly, and exhibits similar changes in age-structure. Between 1900 and 1981, persons aged 65 years and more increased from 4.4 to 17 per cent, while those aged less than 20 decreased from 44.3 to 34.3 per cent, that is, a fivefold increase in the ratio of those over the age of 65 to those under 20. It is expected that over the next 30 years, the proportion of old people will rise by about 60 per cent compared to the 1970 population and the proportion of middle-age groups by roughly 100 per cent. This pattern has come about because sustained high birth rates in the postwar period, during a time of falling death rates, produced a large natural increase in population with a large proportion of young. These large postwar birth cohorts enlarge the current population of adults in successive age-groups as they age.

Demographic changes of this magnitude lead to fundamental changes in disease patterns, what has been described as an epidemiologic transition. In brief, many of the leading causes of death of 50 years ago are now insignificant, and have been replaced by the so-called "degenerative" diseases of senescence, chronic heart and lung disorders, long-latency cancers, and vehicular accidents (see Table 3.1).

Morbidity

Patterns of morbidity and the care of the sick, like those of mortality, reflect the demographic transformation of industrial societies, and the gathering pace of social change during the past two centuries. Patterns of thought reflect the change as well. The assumptions of society about disease change as profoundly, but less rapidly, than do the actual manifestations and social realities of disease. The lag between transformation and perception often obscures comprehension of these realities.

Most notably perhaps, with the passage of time the sphere of medical competence has been expanded (82). Sickness has come to embrace new classes of behavior. In the process, medicine has become in some degree an instrument of social control, drawing its authority from the supposedly value-free precinct of science. In the past half century such matters as neurosis, alcoholism, child behavior disorders, drug addiction, delinquency, violence, and even the youth revolt of the 1960s and urban militancy have been newly claimed as matters for medical concern. Proper objects of medical care now include healthy infants and schoolchildren, pregnant mothers, and business executives; all these are groups of people who may have no known illness, but who nevertheless qualify for periodic examinations meant to detect and prevent the progress of early deviations from health norms. Insofar as psychotherapy is classified as medical care, the boundaries are even wider. Within the specialty of public health, such personal behavior as smoking, modes of sexual intercourse, exercise, and diet earn increasing scrutiny as health hazards.

In order to accommodate changes in phenomena of disease and their perception, disorders can be classified under four headings (83):

1. Disappearing disorders
2. Residual disorders
3. Persisting disorders
4. Newer epidemic disorders

Disappearing disorders. Among disorders that were once commonplace in developed countries and have all but disappeared in their epidemic form during the past century are such conditions as chlorosis, conversion hysteria, and acute ulcers of the gastric cardia, all among young women. The specific causes of their disappearance remain unknown. We have already noted that rampant infection has been brought under control by social and medical advances. Improved nutrition enhanced the general resistance of populations to infection. Sanitation blocked the spread of endemic and epidemic enteric diseases. Immunization has eliminated smallpox, all but eliminated poliomyelitis and measles, and controlled diphtheria, whooping cough, tetanus, rubella, and mumps. Chemotherapy and antibiotics cured bacterial infections. Malaria, in developed countries, yielded to the ecological tactics of physical and chemical warfare against the mosquito vectors of the protozoa. [In underdeveloped regions, however, such tactics have suffered severe setbacks in recent times where the economic, political, and administrative resources to sustain anti-malaria campaigns are lacking; vector resistance to DDT and other poisons, as well as plasmodium resistance to antimalarial chemotherapy, is increasingly common (84).] Tuberculosis, like scarlet fever, began its decline long before the advent of specific antibacterial treatment, but the introduction in the late 1940s of specific antibiotics (streptomycin) and then chemotherapy undoubtedly accelerated its decline (see Figure 3.10a). Other viral disorders like hepatitis B can be controlled by immunization, and the new recombinant DNA technology being developed should help produce the vaccines to control many others. All that is needed with this class of disorders is to continue with time-tested methods based on sound epidemiological knowledge, while keeping a watch for recrudescence and for the unpredictable effects that changes in society and a changed ecological balance so often throw up.

Residual disorders. In these disorders something of the key contributory factors is known, but despite this knowledge society has failed to deal effectively with them. Residual disorders cluster in certain social groups and among special categories of people. Notable are the traditional venereal diseases (syphilis and gonorrhea); a good part of perinatal and infant mortality among the disadvantaged; and the diseases of tobacco and alcohol abuse. Lung cancer is an outstanding example, although because of its unabated frequency in older cohorts, and its accelerating rise among women, it still qualifies as a rising epidemic.

One reason for the persistence of residual disorders is the structured inequality combined with the political and administrative inertia of the contemporary metropolis. Delivery of many services often has been rendered ineffectual by the social and ecological stratification that segregates white and black, poor and rich, into ghettos and suburbs; and by a consequent inability to direct education and health services according to social need. Even where equal utilization of health services can be achieved, there is no guarantee that equalization in health status will follow. In the United States in the 1960s, as a result of the liberalized welfare measures of President Johnson's Great Society Programs, health coverage was extended to vast numbers of previously uninsured poor people. Improvement in mortality rates over the next decade, particularly neonatal mortality and maternal mortality, probably owed something to this expansion of care. Still, increased use of medical services by the poor has not closed the gap in health status between socially disadvantaged people and the better off. Whether measured by morbidity, mortality or disability, the gap actually widened during the period of expanding eligibility and access to services from 1964 to 1973 (85).

Educational deficiencies augment the disorders of health. These deficiencies stand as a bar to family planning, to the recognition of hazards to health, to the cultural control of risk-taking behavior, and to the efficient use of services to prevent or combat them. The social failure to control preventable diseases will persist so long as prevention depends on personal responses that the existing social structure and culture conspire to block. A primary task of public health is to discover and document these problems and to find ways through the blocks.

Persisting disorders. Many disorders that persist from the past have no ready solution. The vast bulk of mental illness, of cancers, and of cerebrovascular diseases fall under the head of persisting disorders. There are overlaps between the category of persisting disorders and the category of residua. Just as enteric infections yielded to sanitary methods on the erroneous assumptions of the miasma theory of disease°, so nonspecific action might diminish some of the persisting disorders. For instance, well-off and well-cared-for populations have low rates of low birthweight—and consequently of infant mortality—although the specific causal factors for low birthweight that have been eliminated among the well-off, and yet persist among the socially disadvantaged, have not been identified.

Mild mental retardation without brain damage has a distribution similar to low birthweight and infant mortality that has been attributed directly to social disadvantage. The condition has been thought to be in decline in some developed societies, and good evidence from Sweden suggests that it is indeed a disappearing disorder (86). By analogy low birthweight is likely to yield to the same favorable conditions as this form of mental retardation has been shown to do. Severe mental retardation, virtually all of which involves structural or metabolic brain disorder, is almost certainly decreasing in incidence, although the countervailing increase in survival has led to a rise in prevalence in many if not all its causal categories (see Chapter 2).

Mental disorder, too, taken as a global category, has a similar distribution to mild mental retardation and could be expected to respond to favorable conditions. Popular belief to the contrary, it does not qualify for the class of new epidemic disorders. Such data as are available for severe mental illness show no evidence of a rise in age-adjusted incidence. On the other hand, here too overall prevalence is likely to have

---

°The theory prevalent from the time of the "English Hippocrates" Thomas Sydenham, in the seventeenth century, that epidemic diseases were caused by the noxious effluvia or exhalations of foul places.

increased because of longer survival and the increasing proportion of elderly persons. Thus among people in their eighties, senile dementia has an incidence of perhaps five per cent per year, although the onset of the condition often presages a short remaining life-span. Yet with regard to adult psychological disorder in general over the whole adult age range, one of the few available longitudinal studies of a community sample—in which scales of mental impairment derived from symptom inventories were repeated after a 20-year interval—suggests a decline in frequency (87).

Most of the residual and persisting disorders are longer lasting than the disappearing disorders, many of which were either remitting or fatal. The changed balance between the incidence of these types of disorders has made for greater numbers of long-lasting disabilities and of survivors into later life. The result is a great increment of individuals who are dependent on others either because of illness or the infirmities of old age.

In response there has been a large increase in provision for the care and maintenance of dependent persons, both ambulatory and residential, though by no means a sufficient one. The burden of such provision, with its relatively small returns in improving the quality of life, highlights the issue of how to allocate scarce and costly resources, especially when the state formulates and bears the cost of such policy. Thus in the United States especially the politics of health care has been converted into the politics of costs; even the National Health Service in Britain has not been immune from this displacement.

The new balance of disease requires that the search for causes and for methods of primary prevention be intensified. At the same time the new balance demands examination of the means and agencies by which persons with chronic disorders can best be cared for, and by which the social disabilities of such disorders can be alleviated. The social stigma attached to dependency, and the seclusion from political and social power of dependent people, adds to the plight of the growing numbers of the elderly.

New epidemic disorders. The rise in the twentieth century of new, chronic, noninfectious but epidemic diseases such as lung cancer, coronary heart disease, and peptic ulcer is familiar knowledge. In 1980 in the United States, diseases of the circulatory system accounted for the largest proportion of all hospital discharges, and diseases of the digestive system for almost as many.

Yet the secular trends for many of these conditions have not continued in a simple upward linear curve. Like several diseases of the cardiovascular renal group, in the United States coronary heart disease mortality began to decline in the late 1960s; the rate fell by 36 per cent from 1968 to 1980. However, it remains a leading cause of death; in 1980, coronary heart disease comprised 28 per cent of all deaths, and 74 per cent of all cardiac deaths. In Britain too, coronary disease remains a leading cause of death. Although British rates have been lower than American, they have begun to converge (36 per cent of total deaths and 71 per cent of all cardiac deaths in 1980). In Britain, while the rate of increase has slowed, an absolute decline in rates has not yet appeared (88).

The halt and decline in mortality from coronary heart disease can be explained as in part the result of a reduction in incidence. The reduction in risk factors in the population—smoking, dietary cholesterol, the level of exercise, and hypertension—is sufficient to produce such a result. At the same time, improved medical care in acute episodes and the reduction of recurrent episodes by drug treatment and other regimens may also have contributed (89).

All these are plausible explanations. The decline in mortality from a number of other diseases, however, is not so simply explained. Over the past two decades mortality from hypertension and chronic kidney disease has seemed to decline spontaneously, that is, without any known effective intervention. The decline seems likely to continue. In the case of hypertension, although the advent of effective treatment in the early 1950s and its widespread distribution in the past decade must have contributed substantially to the control of the disorder, cohort analysis shows that the decline in mortality preceded the effective application of treatment (90). In the case of cerebrovascular disease and stroke, the decline in mortality relates to the decline in hypertension, which is a strong risk factor for stroke; it also relates to the decline in coronary artery disease, since some of the underlying factors related to arterial disease—such as smoking—are held in common. Chronic kidney disease too is a cause of hypertension; mortality from this condition, which on period analysis seemed to be on the rise, was shown by cohort analysis of British and American data to be in decline, much like that from hypertension. The decline affects both chronic nephritis and chronic renal infections (91). Chronic nephritis is held to be an autoimmune response to infection (like rheumatic fever, which among better-off people can be classed as a disappearing disorder). Its decline, as well as that of chronic kidney infections, is a part of the general decline of mortality from bacterial infections.

The waxing and waning of twentieth century epidemics of chronic diseases has been a complex process to decipher. In part, the time trends of diseases with long latent periods have been obscured by the conflation of period with generation effects, and also of incidence, prevalence, and mortality, which may go in contrary directions. Thus, the prevalence of diabetes is undoubtedly rising because of improved survival, but there is nothing to indicate rising incidence. In part, the complexity is social. Many of these diseases have moved vertically from one social class to another at the same time as they changed in frequency through time. Such changes point strongly to a source in the environment as the explanation for the behavior of these diseases. It is therefore entirely conceivable that a new "sanitary era" could remove noxious agents and control disease much as water and sewage systems and vaccination did in the nineteenth century.

A substantial proportion of all cancers—some authorities believe as much as 80 per cent—can be presumed to have an environmental origin. As we noted above, the presumption follows from the observed variation in cancer rates across circumstances and populations, on the premise that the lowest rates only might be regarded as intrinsic and unavoidable, and the surplus over and above these rates can be assigned to environmental sources. In some instances, the preventable cause is known and the remedy at hand. Among these, as we have noted, cigarette smoking and lung cancer is the most dramatic example. In a second instance, estrogens to treat menopausal and postmenopausal states underlay the rise in cancer of the body of the uterus. In others, a probable explanation is known: with malignant melanoma of the skin, increased exposure to sunlight at young ages is the probable explanation for its increasing incidence. In still others, supposed causes are no more than hypothesis, as for instance the role of carotene (precursor of Vitamin A) in a variety of cancers that maintain a steady or slowly rising incidence, for instance, cancers of the colon and pancreas, and perhaps in lung cancer also (44).

A substantial amount of preventable disorders in modern society can reasonably be labeled as "social pathology," that is, disorders that arise directly and obviously from failure to control distortions in the productive relations in society and the economic forces governed by those relations. Occupational hazards provide a simple example (92). In 1978, the rate of work-related fatalities was 8 per 100,000 workers. Many more suffer injury or contact-diseases of the skin at the workplace, and still more are likely to go unreported. The scale of cancers related to the physical environment of the workplace, while a matter of debate, at a national level is not negligible. Coronary heart disease too is possibly related to the psychosocial environment of the workplace, although more studies are needed to establish a firm causal association.

Technological development provides another set of examples, some simple and some not. Medicine itself engenders significant health hazards as the complement of its therapeutic powers, technical virtuosity, and organizational forms. Iatrogenesis—disease or impairment directly traceable to medical intervention—has reached frequencies high enough to be detected in population rates. In hospitals, nosocomial infections acquired by patients undergoing care for other disorders, complications caused by treatment, and accidents all contribute to the estimated one in fourteen hospital patients who suffers a compensable injury (93). The disorders of behavior and social function that arise with prolonged institutionalization among inmates of mental hospitals have long been recognized (94). Oral contraceptives prevent conception but, like the pregnancies they avert, they occasionally give rise to adverse consequences, as noted above; these include thrombosis of blood vessels, hypertension, and possibly cervical cancer and breast cancer (95). In some extreme opinions even smallpox vaccination entailed dangers that outweighed its benefits (96). Controversy about whether the approximately twofold raised risk of the rare encephalopathy following whooping cough vaccination outweighs its manifest benefits still rages (although there is little doubt that a rational decision favors the vaccine) (97).

Secondary effects on health have followed all the major technical revolutions of our time. Foreign substances like DDT, strontium-90, lead, mercury, and asbestos are known to lodge, far from inert, in the bodies of people and animals. High-speed transport has led not only to motor vehicle accidents and air pollution, but to the importation of such exotic diseases as plague and cholera into parts of the world usually free of them. In the developed world, communication through electronic media influences a wide range of behavior relevant to health. Much advertising must be considered harmful. People are encouraged or induced to use alcohol, cigarettes, and addictive drugs, and to adopt foods promoted for their commercial and not their nutritional value. All countries are beset by the multiple consequences of the smoking plague. Alcohol abuse too has multifarious consequences, with road accidents and cirrhosis of the liver among the more prominent. Cirrhosis is a disease that seems to be on the increase in the United States, but its fluctuations in frequency bear closely on the availability of alcohol in a given society or at a given time. In the developing world, mothers who give up breast feeding for the sake of desperately needed employment, and who substitute inadequate amounts of expensive advertised infant formula foods under conditions that make the sanitary preparation of the formula impossible (98), place their infants at risk of malnutrition, gastroenteritis, and death. At the same time, the purveying of knowledge about health directly has done much to promote healthier living.

The profound effects of previous development in industry and agriculture may be matched by the dislocations that follow automation. About health consequences, however, we have little notion. We understand somewhat better the consequences of atomic physics which, along with its benefits, added to nuclear irradiation and created the possibility of nuclear annihilation. Although the health hazards of irradiation are well established (99), the impact of the nuclear threat on emotions, individual behavior, and social relations has still to be studied. Moreover, atomic weapons have brought about quite another class of effects, namely, the domination of industrial societies by military priorities set above all others, including health. (For a comparison of the expenditures on military, social and health programs in 142 countries in 1980, see Tables 3.10 and 3.11.)

Table 3.10   Ranking of countries, military and social indicators

	Military						Economic-social standing[b]	GNP per capita	
	Public expenditures per capita		Public expenditures per soldier[a]		Public expenditures per sq. km.				
	Rank[f]	US$	Rank	US$	Rank	US$	Avg. Rank	Rank	US$
WORLD		122		22,032		4,123			2,619
Developed°		403		44,668		7,897			8,477
Developing		34		7,737		1,504			794
AMERICA									
North America		590		69,834		7,688			11,233
United States°	8	632	8	70,231	26	15,377	9	16	11,347
Canada°	26	195	10	59,519	90	471	11	19	10,159
Latin America		25		7,514		451			2,172
Argentina	61	58	56	11,629	84	588	37	37	4,361
Barbados	71	36	70	9,000	19	22,500	33	48	3,301
Bolivia	84	19	111	4,417	123	96	84	76	1,071
Brazil	97	13	95	5,678	113	182	62	57	2,002
Chile	36	132	40	16,545	64	1,923	49	51	2,506
Colombia	102	12	109	4,576	104	265	68	70	1,251
Costa Rica	—	—		—		—	52	58	1,923
Cuba	40	114	99	5,340	34	9,565	35	60	1,864
Dominican Rep.	84	19	94	5,684	60	2,204	69	72	1,175
Ecuador	75	26	100	5,333	81	732	63	66	1,358
El Salvador	104	11	76	7,714	55	2,571	88	92	725
Guatemala	94	14	87	6,313	76	927	86	75	1,096
Guyana	78	24	120	2,857	124	93	69	95	680
Haiti	126	4	121	2,750	79	786	119	124	266
Honduras	102	12	113	4,091	93	402	94	96	633

Table 3.10   Continued

	Military Public expenditures per capita		Military Public expenditures per soldier[a]		Military Public expenditures per sq. km.		Economic-social standing[b]	GNP per capita	
	Rank[i]	US$	Rank	US$	Rank	US$	Avg. Rank	Rank	US$
Jamaica	111	9	104	5,000	67	1,818	56	77	1,069
Mexico	104	11	81	7,065	95	383	60	50	2,590
Nicargua	73	28	47	14,000	86	538	81	87	837
Panama	111	9	128	1,636	106	237	48	61	1,666
Paraguay	81	21	112	4,313	116	170	66	67	1,346
Peru	75	26	106	4,760	98	356	73	78	1,056
Trinidad & Tobago	94	14	42	16,000	50	3,200	44	32	5,268
Uruguay	49	90	72	8,667	70	1,477	41	46	3,398
Venezuela	66	46	37	18,875	78	828	50	43	3,726
EUROPE									
NATO Europe		330		38,921		37,292			8,939
Belgium°	16	402	19	44,989	5	127,710	9	13	12,023
Denmark°	20	314	16	46,000	14	37,442	3	10	12,504
France°	9	492	13	53,467	13	48,384	4	12	12,156
Germany, West°	14	434	12	54,018	7	107,382	6	8	13,399
Greece	24	236	51	12,522	25	17,265	32	36	4,384
Iceland°		—		—		—	5	14	12,009
Italy°	28	171	30	26,224	16	31,887	21	27	7,012
Luxembourg°	33	143	14	52,000	24	17,333	15	5	14,297
Netherlands°	17	373	17	45,887	4	128,707	13	15	11,399
Norway°	15	409	18	45,135	44	5,154	2	9	13,357
Portugal	51	87	44	14,400	35	9,391	39	52	2,393
Turkey	62	55	110	4,450	49	3,230	80	68	1,327
United Kingdom°	11	478	5	81,386	6	109,738	14	22	9,213
ALL NATO (inc. US & Canada)		443		52,355		11,538			9,937
Warsaw Pact		391		30,793		6,271			4,614
Bulgaria°	35	133	74	7,919	31	10,631	31	39	4,219
Czechoslovakia°	27	180	45	14,103	21	21,484	27	28	5,821
Germany, East°	18	360	23	37,160	9	55,741	19	21	7,226
Hungary°	44	103	53	11,828	29	11,828	28	40	4,200
Poland°	38	121	49	13,522	27	13,738	34	41	3,929
Romania°	60	61	77	7,337	42	5,672	35	42	3,851
USSR°	10	490	26	35,490	41	5,803	25	34	4,564
Other Europe		157		17,503		8,267			6,822
Albania	57	71	108	4,634	39	6,552	56	83	898
Austria°	39	118	38	17,860	31	10,631	17	17	10,508
Finland°	29	170	34	20,325	58	2,412	8	18	10,333
Ireland°	51	87	36	19,733	46	4,229	22	33	5,074
Malta	88	16	90	6,000	23	20,000	42	45	3,406
Spain	43	107	55	11,708	38	7,929	28	30	5,550
Sweden°	12	459	11	57,848	36	8,484	1	7	13,962
Switzerland°	19	331	3	117,389	12	51,537	12	4	16,188
Yugoslavia	41	113	67	9,534	33	9,832	46	49	2,651

Table 3.10 Continued

	Military						Economic-social standing[b]	GNP per capita	
	Public expenditures per capita		Public expenditures per soldier[a]		Public expenditures per sq. km.				
	Rank[i]	US$	Rank	US$	Rank	US$	Avg. Rank	Rank	US$
ASIA									
Middle East		313		27,323		6,508			2,925
Bahrain	13	454	7	78,500	3	261,667	38	24	8,474
Cyprus	65	49	116	3,444	48	3,444	42	44	3,496
Egypt[h]	67	44	103	5,063	66	1,856	93	99	600
Iran	37	126	33	20,413	52	2,973	71	55	2,160
Iraq	25	206	59	11,194	40	6,228	58	48	2,791
Israel°	4	1,470	22	38,818	2	314,238	23	29	5,635
Jordan	32	144	83	6,701	45	4,582	73	73	1,154
Kuwait	7	693	6	79,250	11	52,833	17	3	24,434
Lebanon	45	101	58	11,609	17	26,700	47		na
Oman	5	1,012	4	84,786	43	5,599	71	31	5,365
Qatar	1	2,540	2	120,400	10	54,727	30	1	28,034
Saudi Arabia	2	1,862	1	373,191	37	8,158	54	11	12,484
Syria	21	256	69	9,093	28	12,189	75	63	1,481
United Arab Emirates	3	1,734	9	68,320	22	20,333	24	2	27,975
Yemen, Arab Rep.	56	72	52	12,063	63	1,979	124	100	578
Yemen, People's Dem. Rep.	58	65	102	5,167	96	372	111	106	423
South Asia		7		3,559		1,183			226
Afghanistan	124	5	124	2,000	121	123	137	127	240
Bangladesh	132	2	123	2,167	75	1,083	136	138	129
India	117	6	114	4,032	71	1,354	117	128	230
Nepal	134	1	131	1,000	119	156	138	137	135
Pakistan	91	15	119	2,895	69	1,581	123	121	292
Sri Lanka	130	3	112	2,733	83	621	82	123	279
Far East		34		6,363		3,237			1,063
Brunei	6	714	20	44,000	20	22,000	25	6	14,162
Burma	117	6	130	1,172	100	301	113	134	171
Cambodia		na		—		—	134		na
China	73	28	88	6,292	53	2,918	91	120	298
Indonesia	91	15	65	9,657	74	1,153	105	105	460
Japan°	53	85	21	41,079	18	26,613	20	23	8,975
Korea, North	55	73	126	1,917	30	10,744	76	74	1,151
Korea, South	48	91	91	5,995	15	36,765	65	65	1,388
Laos		na		—		—	122	140	87
Malaysia	46	97	32	20,636	47	4,127	61	62	1,623
Mongolia	42	108	86	6,429	122	115	54	86	854
Philippines	97	13	96	5,602	61	2,110	79	91	728
Singapore	23	245	46	14,095	1	986,667	45	35	4,422
Taiwan	31	149	89	6,071	8	83,094	51	54	2,255
Thailand	75	26	93	5,368	58	2,412	85	94	691
Vietnam	87	17	133	875	54	2,727	103	135	161
OCEANIA		194		46,449		490			8,102
Australia°	22	249	15	51,338	89	474	7	21	9,943
Fiji	88	16	62	10,000	85	556	53	59	1,875
New Zealand°	34	142	28	33,846	68	1,636	15	25	7,727
Papua New Guinea	97	13	64	9,750	126	84	98	88	811

Table 3.10 Continued

| | Military | | | | | | Economic-social standing[b] | GNP | |
| | Public expenditures per capita | | Public expenditures per soldier[a] | | Public expenditures per sq. km. | | | per capita | |
	Rank[i]	US$	Rank	US$	Rank	US$	Avg. Rank	Rank	US$
AFRICA		26		9,449		410			827
Algeria	69	37	82	6,980	101	296	77	56	2,091
Angola	—	—				—	97	82	902
Benin	117	6	60	11,000	111	195	125	117	322
Botswana	69	37	41	16,500	128	55	87	84	886
Burundi	115	8	92	5,833	72	1,250	135	131	210
Cameroon	109	10	54	11,714	115	173	101	90	743
Central African Rep.	117	6	85	6,500	131	21	126	115	333
Chad	124	5	78	7,333	133	17	142	139	113
Congo	68	39	61	10,167	114	178	89	80	1,014
Equatorial Guinea	78	24	129	1,200	108	214	114	98	608
Ethiopia	91	15	125	1,943	97	366	141	136	137
Gabon	47	93	24	37,000	103	276	59	38	4,279
Gambia	—	—		—		—	121	112	384
Ghana	126	4	117	2,941	109	209	112	114	359
Guinea	132	2	131	1,000	129	37	132	118	315
Ivory Coast	88	16	31	20,833	94	388	96	71	1,235
Kenya	86	18	35	20,000	88	515	98	109	412
Lesotho	—	—		—		—	95	102	505
Liberia	94	14	101	5,200	107	234	108	101	515
Libya	30	167	68	9,491	102	286	40	20	10,119
Madagascar	104	11	79	7,231	118	160	106	113	366
Malawi	111	9	48	13,750	91	466	127	126	248
Mali	117	6	75	7,800	130	31	139	133	196
Mauritania	82	20	115	3,750	132	29	128	108	414
Mauritius	117	6		na	51	3,000	67	81	1,011
Morocco	63	53	66	9,655	56	2,506	102	85	872
Mozambique	97	13	84	6,667	110	200	115	110	394
Namibia	—	—		—		—	90	64	1,443
Niger	130	3	73	8,500	134	13	131	116	325
Nigeria	72	30	43	15,671	57	2,476	104	79	1,035
Rwanda	126	4	97	5,550	77	846	128	128	226
Senegal	104	11	80	7,111	99	327	119	103	471
Sierra Leone	126	4	107	4,667	112	194	130	119	306
Somalia	82	20	127	1,694	117	165	133	122	283
South Africa	54	81	29	26,977	65	1,900	64	53	2,387
Sudan	104	11	117	2,941	127	80	116	107	418
Swaziland	80	22	50	13,000	80	765	83	89	786
Tanzania	97	13	105	4,808	104	265	110	125	264
Togo	111	9	93	5,750	92	404	107	111	388
Tunisia	64	52	57	11,621	62	2,055	77	69	1,301
Uganda	109	10	39	17,857	87	530	109	104	468
Upper Volta	117	6	71	8,750	120	128	139	130	221
Zaire	116	7	62	10,000	125	85	118	132	201
Zambia	50	89	25	36,857	82	685	100	97	609
Zimbabwe	59	63	27	34,143	73	1,223	92	93	718

Table 3.10 Continued

	Education									
	Public expenditures per capita		School-age population per teacher[c]		% School-age population in school		% Women in total university enrollment		Literacy rate[d]	
	Rank	US$	Rank	Number	Rank	Number	Rank	%	Rank	%
WORLD		130		45		54		40		70
Developed*		448		25		69		44		99
Developing		31		54		51		34		59
AMERICA										
North America		591		22		84		49		99
United States*	16	571	7	22	1	85	12	49	1	99
Canada*	8	784	17	24	8	72	12	49	22	98
Latin America		75		45		58		37		80
Argentina	40	157	28	28	48	61	32	42	34	93
Barbados	30	233	21	26	5	76	52	39	22	98
Bolivia	79	38	45	36	81	55	76	30	78	63
Brazil	69	63	63	45	87	53	55	38	62	76
Chile	50	113	57	43	8	72	45	40	37	92
Colombia	91	24	72	49	73	57	55	38	46	86
Costa Rica	47	117	67	46	81	55	55	38	34	93
Cuba	39	162	10	23	24	68	20	46	27	95
Dominican Rep.	91	24	96	72	66	58	40	41	64	74
Ecuador	76	49	69	47	53	60	62	36	57	81
El Salvador	84	29	113	97	99	47	86	27	74	65
Guatemala	95	21	112	95	120	33	86	27	90	50
Guyana	72	59	54	42	48	61	82	29	39	90
Haiti	130	4	118	114	119	34	82	29	118	29
Honduras	97	20	101	76	98	48	59	37	81	60
Jamaica	63	76	63	45	31	66	26	44	40	89
Mexico	60	78	63	45	20	69	76	30	55	83
Nicaragua	86	26	95	68	85	54	66	35	71	66
Panama	59	87	48	38	24	68	5	54	49	85
Paraguay	102	18	62	44	87	53	28	43	46	86
Peru	99	19	78	54	31	66	70	32	58	80
Trinidad & Tobago	38	170	76	51	81	55	62	36	27	95
Uruguay	60	78	42	35	60	59	6	53	31	94
Venezuela	33	188	57	43	73	57	45	40	56	82
EUROPE										
NATO Europe		458		27		63		40		94
Belgium*	9	732	17	24	42	63	59	37	1	99
Denmark*	6	868	3	19	16	70	32	42	1	99
France*	13	599	10	23	24	68	12	49	1	99
Germany, West*	12	616	21	26	34	65	62	36	1	99
Greece	54	101	40	34	24	68	40	41	42	88
Iceland*	19	500	7	22	8	72	66	35	1	99
Italy*	27	321	10	23	60	59	32	42	27	95
Luxembourg*	5	920	17	24	66	58	32	42	22	98
Netherlands*	4	947	35	31	43	62	76	30	1	99
Norway*	2	1,197	5	20	16	70	45	40	1	99
Portugal	56	91	31	30	8	72	20	46	58	80
Turkey	81	35	85	56	99	47	86	27	74	65
United Kingdom*	20	494	10	23	4	77	59	37	1	99

Table 3.10   Continued

	Education									
	Public expenditures per capita		School-age population per teacher[c]		% School-age population in school		% Women in total university enrollment		Literacy rate[d]	
	Rank	US$	Rank	Number	Rank	Number	Rank	%	Rank	%
ALL NATO (incl. US & Canada)		516		25		72		46		96
Warsaw Pact		214		28		59		49		99
Bulgaria*	36	176	36	32	73	57	6	53	31	94
Czechoslovakia*	35	182	42	35	60	59	40	41	1	99
Germany, East*	28	304	42	35	43	62	17	47	1	99
Hungary*	32	201	21	26	60	59	17	47	1	99
Poland*	41	135	47	37	81	55	9	50	1	99
Romania*	47	117	37	33	43	62	28	43	22	98
USSR*	31	231	21	26	60	59	9	50	1	99
Other Europe		353		30		64		40		93
Albania		na	45	36	48	61	26	44	65	72
Austria*	17	561	10	23	77	56	52	39	1	99
Finland*	15	585	21	26	53	60	12	49	1	99
Ireland*	25	359	29	29	13	71	28	43	22	98
Malta	55	99	21	26	13	71	93	26	49	85
Spain	47	117	37	33	20	69	52	39	34	93
Sweden*	1	1,350	1	18	34	65	40	41	1	99
Switzerland*	7	831	50	39	48	61	70	32	1	99
Yugoslavia	45	124	37	33	53	60	45	40	44	87
ASIA										
Middle East		156		49		53		32		48
Bahrain	29	249	29	29	38	64	8	52	107	40
Cyprus	46	122	31	30	53	60	40	41	49	85
Egypt[h]	89	25	91	62	99	47	75	31	90	50
Iran	34	183	76	51	66	58	70	32	99	47
Iraq	58	89	52	41	13	71	70	32	103	43
Israel*	21	467	7	22	38	64	20	46	42	88
Jordan	67	69	70	48	77	56	45	40	84	58
Kuwait	10	707	6	21	29	67	3	57	78	63
Lebanon		na	10	23	34	65	62	36	62	76
Oman	44	125	80	55	121	32	124	15	90	50
Qatar	3	1,156	20	25	24	68	2	64	126	20
Saudi Arabia	11	680	57	43	112	39	86	27	123	25
Syria	64	73	54	42	53	60	93	26	87	55
United Arab Emirates	23	400	1	18	20	69	20	46	86	56
Yemen, Arab Rep.	99	19	135	189	132	22	130	12	139	9
Yemen, People's Dem. Rep.	102	18	100	74	105	42	76	30	120	27
South Asia		6		85		38		27		39
Afghanistan	126	5	129	153	134	20	118	17	126	20
Bangladesh	134	2	121	121	122	30	116	18	106	41
India	121	7	104	79	108	41	86	27	107	40
Nepal	134	2	120	120	122	30	106	20	131	19
Pakistan	126	5	125	127	125	29	86	27	117	32
Sri Lanka	118	8	54	42	38	64	32	42	49	85

Table 3.10 Continued

						Education				
	Public expenditures per capita		School-age population per teacher[c]		% School-age population in school		% Women in total university enrollment		Literacy rate[d]	
	Rank	US$	Rank	Number	Rank	Number	Rank	%	Rank	%
Far East		57		43		59		32		72
Brunei	26	341	31	30	16	70	9	50	77	64
Burma	131	3	123	123	108	41	12	49	71	66
Cambodia	na		115	99	131	23	112	19	98	48
China	104	17	51	40	60	59	76	30	71	66
Indonesia	116	10	72	49	77	56	93	26	70	67
Japan°	18	524	31	30	6	73	103	23	1	99
Korea, North	77	39	98	73	38	64		na	49	85
Korea, South	74	56	93	64	20	69	104	22	31	94
Laos	na		94	67	105	42	93	26	102	44
Malaysia	53	102	70	48	53	60	68	34	65	72
Mongolia	71	60	63	45	48	61	1	71	27	95
Philippines	115	11	80	55	66	58	4	55	40	89
Singapore	42	133	67	46	73	57	28	43	37	92
Taiwan	62	77	57	43	53	60	45	40	49	85
Thailand	94	23	57	43	93	50	32	42	46	56
Vietnam	122	6	78	54	43	62	70	32	44	87
OCEANIA		476		28		66		45		92
Australia°	14	597	10	23	6	73	25	45	1	99
Fiji	56	91	48	38	8	72	84	28	60	79
New Zealand°	22	409	21	26	3	79	32	42	1	99
Papua New Guinea	79	38	116	102	122	30	131	11	104	42
AFRICA		39		80		44		22		38
Algeria	37	171	86	58	77	56	100	24	104	42
Angola	86	26	90	60	93	50	32	42	136	15
Benin	109	13	126	132	116	35	116	18	119	28
Botswana	68	68	80	55	66	58	45	40	107	40
Burundi	122	6	138	249	140	12	106	20	120	27
Cameroon	86	26	110	88	87	53	124	15	90	50
Central African Rep.	112	12	130	165	116	35	128	13	114	33
Chad	131	3	140	313	137	18	136	5	134	18
Congo	66	70	74	50	93	50	126	14	80	62
Equatorial Guinea	na		124	126	110	40		na	126	20
Ethiopia	131	3	139	271	132	22	126	14	141	7
Gabon	43	131	74	50	16	70	98	25	81	60
Gambia	106	14	98	73	129	24		na	126	20
Ghana	118	8	80	55	104	44	128	13	107	40
Guinea	109	13	132	180	135	19	134	10	131	19
Ivory Coast	51	104	109	86	105	42	112	19	111	35
Kenya	89	25	80	55	29	67	106	20	99	47
Lesotho	109	13	103	77	66	58	17	47	68	69
Liberia	82	33	101	76	114	37	84	28	123	25
Libya	24	399	3	19	2	83	100	24	84	58
Madagascar	106	14	114	98	93	50	68	34	90	50
Malawi	126	5	133	181	116	35	104	22	114	33
Mali	117	9	137	232	139	15	134	10	138	10
Mauritania	95	21	136	202	137	18		na	135	17
Mauritius	70	62	40	34	43	62	121	16	60	79

Table 3.10   Continued

	Education									
	Public expenditures per capita		School-age population per teacher[c]		% School-age population in school		% Women in total university enrollment		Literacy rate[d]	
	Rank	US$	Rank	Number	Rank	Number	Rank	%	Rank	%
Morocco	75	53	104	79	114	37	98	25	122	26
Mozambique	134	2	131	178	112	39	20	46	114	33
Namibia	na	na	86	58	93	50		na	90	50
Niger	106	14	141	335	140	12	106	20	137	10
Nigeria	77	39	89	59	85	54	121	16	113	34
Rwanda	122	6	128	150	110	40	131	11°	90	50
Senegal	99	19	127	138	129	24	112	19	131	19
Sierra Leone	112	12	118	114	128	26	121	16	126	20
Somalia	126	5	133	181	135	19	131	11	142	6
South Africa	52	103	86	58	66	58	100	24	74	65
Sudan	97	20	117	109	126	27	93	26	125	22
Swaziland	73	57	52	41	31	66	55	38	101	45
Tanzania	105	15	104	79	90	52	106	20	67	70
Togo	91	24	108	82	34	65	118	17	111	35
Tunisia	64	73	91	62	90	52	76	30	97	49
Uganda	118	8	122	122	126	27	112	19	89	52
Upper Volta	122	6	142	504	142	9	106	20	139	9
Zaire	112	12	96	72	99	47	136	5	88	54
Zambia	85	28	107	81	90	52	118	17	81	60
Zimbabwe	83	31	110	88	103	46	86	27	68	69

	Health									
	Public expenditures per capita		Population per physician		Population per hospital bed		Infant mortality rate[e]		Life expectancy[f]	
	Rank	US$	Number	Rank	Rank	Number	Rank	Rate	Rank	Years
WORLD		100		1,125		272		87		61
Developed°		381		416		100		20		73
Developing		12		2,310		580		96		58
AMERICA										
North America		446		550		163		13		74
United States°	13	439	26	550	34	171	19	13	8	74
Canada°	10	515	26	550	24	112	10	11	8	74
Latin America		27		1,210		341		69		64
Argentina	65	22	16	470	39	195	56	45	38	70
Barbados	35	120	51	1,240	26	117	38	27	38	70
Bolivia	82	11	56	1,510	77	448	117	131	98	50
Brazil	55	32	50	1,150	48	250	75	77	63	63
Chile	48	58	58	1,620	55	289	49	38	50	66
Colombia	72	16	68	2,000	92	586	69	64	67	62
Costa Rica	62	25	55	1,500	61	318	35	24	38	70
Cuba	50	50	32	640	43	221	30	19	13	73
Dominican Rep.	65	22	77	2,620	76	432	70	68	72	61
Ecuador	72	16	57	1,600	83	491	77	82	72	61
El Salvador	79	12	81	3,160	93	590	59	53	67	62
Guatemala	72	16	76	2,540	90	535	73	72	76	59
Guyana	71	17	91	5,840	40	202	55	44	47	69
Haiti	120	2	92	5,990	129	1,361	101	115	95	51
Honduras	82	11	83	3,180	107	757	81	90	77	58

Table 3.10 Continued

	Public expenditures per capita		Population per physician		Population per hospital bed		Infant mortality rate[e]		Life expectancy[f]	
	Rank	US$	Number	Rank	Rank	Number	Rank	Rate	Rank	Years
Jamaica	57	27	78	2,880	56	293	25	16	38	70
Mexico	82	11	66	1,840	117	887	67	60	55	65
Nicaragua	53	37	70	2,060	80	482	81	90	82	56
Panama	43	84	49	1,130	51	264	43	34	38	70
Paraguay	102	5	64	1,800	104	691	57	47	55	65
Peru	87	9	53	1,470	91	543	80	88	77	58
Trinidad & Tobago	36	116	53	1,470	50	260	37	26	38	70
Uruguay	53	37	20	510	46	248	51	40	29	71
Venezuela	40	97	48	1,090	67	364	54	42	49	67
EUROPE										
NATO Europe		516		518		110		46		72
Belguim°	11	481	5	400	22	106	10	11	13	73
Denmark°	4	826	15	460	28	122	3	8	3	75
France°	7	743	29	590	8	82	9	10	8	74
Germany, West°	2	884	12	440	11	87	19	13	13	73
Greece	32	132	8	410	32	160	29	18	8	74
Iceland°	5	768	16	470	1	61	3	8	1	76
Italy°	16	418	2	340	20	101	22	14	13	73
Luxembourg°	29	154	36	730	10	84	14	12	29	71
Netherlands°	6	758	16	470	5	80	7	9	3	75
Norway°	3	881	20	510	3	67	3	8	3	75
Portugal	44	77	22	520	38	187	46	35	29	71
Turkey	79	12	59	1,690	79	481	109	123	67	62
United Kingdom°	12	443	31	620	27	121	14	12	13	73
ALL NATO (incl. US & Canada)		486		531		128		31		73
Warsaw Pact		132		310		88		32		70
Bulgaria°	42	85	8	410	14	90	31	20	13	73
Czechoslovakia°	26	176	3	360	5	80	27	17	29	71
Germany, East°	19	341	19	490	17	94	14	12	23	72
Hungary°	34	127	5	400	23	109	34	23	29	71
Poland°	27	164	22	520	29	133	33	21	23	72
Romania°	30	149	34	680	25	113	39	39	29	71
USSR°	37	113	1	270	8	82	47	36	38	70
Other Europe		332		490		124		19		72
Albania	59	26	41	890	30	154	58	48	38	70
Austria°	9	589	5	400	14	90	22	14	23	72
Finland°	17	410	25	530	2	64	3	8	13	73
Ireland°	21	293	39	790	21	103	14	12	13	73
Malta	38	104	42	910	19	98	25	16	29	71
Spain	24	189	10	420	37	182	10	11	13	73
Sweden°	1	1,035	13	450	4	68	1	7	3	75
Switzerland°	8	720	10	420	12	88	7	9	3	75
Yugoslavia	31	138	35	690	33	167	41	33	38	70
ASIA										
Middle East		35		1,350		578		99		57
Bahrain	25	188	44	950	58	312	59	53	50	66
Cyprus	47	60	47	1,080	36	180	27	17	23	72
Egypt[h]	94	7	45	970	85	498	90	103	85	55
Iran	51	39	75	2,470	109	777	96	108	77	58
Iraq	65	22	63	1,790	89	534	76	78	85	55

Table 3.10 Continued

	Public expenditures per capita		Population per physician		Population per hospital bed		Infant mortality rate[e]		Life expectancy[f]	
	Rank	US$	Number	Rank	Rank	Number	Rank	Rate	Rank	Years
Israel[*]	28	157	4	380	53	285	22	14	23	72
Jordan	57	27	65	1,820	124	1,175	71	69	74	60
Kuwait	20	297	29	590	45	241	50	39	47	69
Lebanon	78	13	22	520	49	253	53	41	50	66
Oman	41	91	60	1,730	84	492	114	128	107	47
Qatar		na	52	1,270	69	376	59	53	81	57
Saudi Arabia	39	103	61	1,740	102	675	100	114	89	54
Syria	102	5	74	2,270	116	883	68	62	55	65
United Arab Emirates	22	289	40	880	63	339	59	53	67	62
Yemen, Arab Rep.	94	7	99	7,620	132	1,684	137	170	130	42
Yemen, People's Dem. Rep.	120	2	97	7,430	98	661	124	146	123	45
South Asia		2		3,330		1,415		126		51
Afghanistan	129	1	113	13,860	138	3,309	140	205	140	40
Bangladesh	137	0.5	107	9,780	139	4,602	120	136	108	46
India	120	2	80	2,910	127	1,312	109	123	92	52
Nepal	129	1	129	30,780	140	5,865	131	150	124	44
Pakistan	129	1	85	3,630	134	1,844	112	126	95	51
Sri Lanka	97	6	95	7,220	64	343	51	40	50	66
Far East		35		2,180		392		59		62
Brunei	23	195	71	2,200	59	314	31	20	50	66
Burma	120	2	89	4,810	125	1,196	89	101	91	53
Cambodia		na		na	121	951	142	212	140	40
China	97	6	73	2,250	86	506	66	56	59	64
Indonesia	113	3	110	11,630	133	1,782	84	93	98	50
Japan[*]	18	394	38	770	12	88	1	7	1	76
Korea, North	113	3		na	113	832	43	34	59	64
Korea, South	113	3	62	1,750	96	608	43	34	55	65
Laos	129	1	121	17,290	122	1,022	115	129	128	43
Malaysia	59	26	87	4,000	70	383	42	31	59	64
Mongolia	79	12	13	450	16	92	63	55	63	63
Philippines	108	4	79	2,900	87	527	63	55	63	63
Singapore	46	66	46	1,050	46	248	14	12	23	72
Taiwan	48	58	42	910		na	35	24	29	71
Thailand	102	5	94	6,940	100	665	63	55	67	62
Vietnam	129	1	88	4,330	52	270	81	90	63	63
OCEANIA		359		680		94		43		70
Australia[*]	14	428	28	560	5	80	10	11	8	74
Fiji	51	39	72	2,230	66	355	48	37	29	71
New Zealand[*]	15	423	32	640	17	94	19	13	13	73
Papua New Guinea	62	25	118	15,580	44	236	93	104	98	50
AFRICA		8		7,960		554		122		49
Algeria	68	21	84	3,620	71	387	105	118	82	56
Angola	87	9	117	15,510	62	327	133	154	136	41
Benin	102	5	120	16,980	117	887	131	150	108	46
Botswana	69	20	101	8,100	75	420	78	83	104	48
Burundi	120	2	134	42,040	114	834	107	122	130	42
Cameroon	97	6	114	14,300	68	371	97	109	108	46
Central African Rep.	102	5	127	23,380	97	642	129	149	124	44
Chad	129	1	136	49,070	127	1,312	129	149	136	41
Congo	59	26	90	5,170	42	213	116	130	108	46
Equatorial Guinea		na	133	41,670	73	404	122	143	108	46

Table 3.10 Continued

	Health									
	Public expenditures per capita		Population per physician		Population per hospital bed		Infant mortality rate[e]		Life expectancy[f]	
	Rank	US$	Number	Rank	Rank	Number	Rank	Rate	Rank	Years
Ethiopia	120	2	139	69,600	137	2,672	127	147	140	40
Gabon	45	68	82	3,170	35	174	104	117	124	44
Gambia	91	8	103	8,950	110	804	139	198	136	41
Ghana	113	3	100	7,730	103	690	90	103	103	49
Guinea	113	3	137	50,140	94	592	136	165	124	44
Ivory Coast	72	16	119	16,110	111	810	113	127	108	46
Kenya	87	9	104	9,130	95	593	79	87	85	55
Lesotho	108	4	111	13,390	82	488	101	115	98	50
Liberia	91	8	105	9,490	106	742	133	154	98	50
Libya	32	132	37	740	41	206	87	100	82	56
Madagascar	91	8	108	9,960	74	412	72	71	108	46
Malawi	108	4	138	50,180	88	539	121	142	108	46
Mali	120	2	128	26,190	135	1,884	133	154	130	42
Mauritania	97	6	115	15,020	136	2,653	122	143	130	42
Mauritius	64	24	67	1,900	60	317	41	33	59	64
Morocco	85	10	109	9,980	112	812	95	107	85	55
Mozambique		na	131	39,170	120	918	101	115	108	46
Namibia		na		na		na	106	120	95	51
Niger	113	3	132	39,490	131	1,641	124	146	130	42
Nigeria	94	7	106	9,590	126	1,251	118	135	104	48
Rwanda	120	2	130	31,180	101	670	107	122	108	46
Senegal	97	6	112	13,730	119	902	127	147	130	42
Sierra Leone	108	4	123	18,050	115	872	138	180	108	46
Somalia	113	3	122	17,970	108	772	124	146	128	43
South Africa	85	10	68	2,000	31	155	85	96	74	60
Sudan	129	1	102	8,650	123	1,115	111	124	108	46
Swaziland	70	19	96	7,240	57	302	118	135	108	46
Tanzania	102	5	125	20,690	80	482	90	103	92	52
Togo	87	9	124	18,560	105	729	97	109	108	46
Tunisia	56	30	86	3,760	78	464	87	100	77	58
Uganda	108	4	126	23,280	99	662	86	97	92	52
Upper Volta	120	2	135	48,330	130	1,599	141	211	136	41
Zaire	129	1	116	15,060	65	352	99	112	108	46
Zambia	76	15	98	7,500	54	288	94	106	104	48
Zimbabwe	77	14	93	6,580	72	388	74	74	89	54

	Nutrition				Water	
	Calorie supply per capita[g]		Protein supply per capita[h]		% Population with safe water	
	Rank	Number	Rank	Grams	Rank	%
WORLD		2,614		69		57
Developed°		3,426		99		94
Developing		2,360		60		44
AMERICA						
North America		3,625		106		99
United States°	5	3,652	6	107	5	99
Canada°	24	3,358	20	98	5	99
Latin America		2,591		66		61
Argentina	22	3,386	3	112	61	60
Barbados	34	3,054	37	85	1	100

Table 3.10   Continued

	Nutrition				Water	
	Calorie supply per capita[g]		Protein supply per capita[h]		% Population with safe water	
	Rank	Number	Rank	Grams	Rank	%
Bolivia	113	2,086	104	53	88	39
Brazil	67	2,517	84	59	58	63
Chile	54	2,738	53	75	46	76
Colombia	76	2,417	100	55	55	64
Costa Rica	64	2,635	80	61	39	81
Cuba	55	2,717	61	71	59	62
Dominican Rep.	105	2,133	119	47	65	57
Ecuador	112	2,092	112	49	71	51
El Salvador	102	2,163	88	58	77	48
Guatemala	114	2,064	95	56	85	42
Guyana	70	2,483	84	59	23	93
Haiti	128	1,882	125	44	119	12
Honduras	100	2,175	108	52	66	55
Jamaica	66	2,570	77	63	37	82
Mexico	52	2,803	58	72	63	59
Nicaragua	90	2,284	72	65	79	46
Panama	87	2,290	95	56	36	83
Paraguay	43	2,902	44	81	96	28
Peru	101	2,166	95	56	74	49
Trinidad & Tobago	58	2,702	53	75	27	89
Uruguay	47	2,868	36	87	42	78
Venezuela	62	2,649	61	71	39	81
EUROPE						
NATO Europe		3,410		95		92
Belgium°	1	3,938	7	105	27	89
Denmark°	15	3,502	18	99	5	99
France°	23	3,381	7	105	16	97
Germany, West°	10	3,537	31	90	5	99
Greece	8	3,629	5	108	16	97
Iceland°	37	3,013	1	119	5	99
Italy°	6	3,643	11	104	33	86
Luxembourg°	1	3,938	7	105	13	98
Netherlands°	17	3,490	32	88	16	97
Norway°	27	32,88	25	95	13	98
Portugal	30	3,196	37	85	25	92
Turkey	39	2,965	42	83	51	69
United Kingdom°	26	3,315	30	91	5	99
ALL NATO						
(incl. US & Canada)		3,503		100		95
Warsaw Pact		3,434		100		64
Bulgaria°	7	3,638	12	102		na
Czechoslovakia°	18	3,472	18	99	42	78
Germany, East°	4	3,746	12	102	37	82
Hungary°	11	3,533	26	94	83	44
Poland°	9	3,545	7	105	66	55
Romania°	20	3,396	22	97		na
USSR°	21	3,389	17	100		na

Table 3.10   Continued

	Nutrition				Water	
	Calorie supply per capita[g]		Protein supply per capita[h]		% Population with safe water	
	Rank	Number	Rank	Grams	Rank	%
Other Europe		3,380		96		77
Albania	50	2,837	42	83		na
Austria°	16	3,495	32	88	30	88
Finland°	32	3,127	26	94	34	84
Ireland°	3	3,764	4	109	48	73
Malta	35	3,046	28	92	1	100
Spain	25	3,333	22	97	42	78
Sweden°	31	3,157	28	92	5	99
Switzerland°	13	3,525	32	88	21	96
Yugoslavia	12	3,528	15	101	64	58
ASIA						
Middle East		2,838		75		68
Bahrain		na		na	1	100
Cyprus	29	3,199	24	96	22	95
Egypt[h]	40	2,950	50	77	34	84
Iran	42	2,912	52	76	71	51
Iraq	63	2,642	69	67	56	76
Israel°	36	3,045	12	102	5	99
Jordan	78	2,397	80	61	54	66
Kuwait		na		na	27	89
Lebanon	69	2,496	72	65	26	91
Oman		na		na	70	52
Qatar		na		na	16	97
Saudi Arabia	44	2,889	46	79	55	64
Syria	48	2,863	48	78	50	71
United Arab Emirates		na		na	30	88
Yemen, Arab Rep.	91	2,272	64	70	128	4
Yemen, People's Dem. Rep.	111	2,103	104	53	92	37
South Asia		2,015		49		41
Afghanistan	132	1,833	91	57	123	10
Bangladesh	129	1,877	130	41	53	68
India	121	1,998	115	48	87	41
Nepal	125	1,914	122	46	121	11
Pakistan	85	2,300	82	60	95	29
Sri Lanka	92	2,251	125	44	106	22
Far East		2,472		64		48
Brunei	59	2,664	46	79	49	72
Burma	88	2,286	84	59	102	23
Cambodia	134	1,795	129	42	81	45
China	72	2,472	72	65		na
Indonesia	86	2,296	119	47	107	19
Japan°	46	2,883	32	88	13	98
Korea, North	38	2,972	39	84		na
Korea, South	41	2,926	48	78	41	79
Laos	131	1,856	111	50	77	48
Malaysia	61	2,650	84	59	55	64
Mongolia	56	2,711	15	101		na
Philippines	82	2,315	108	52	66	55
Singapore	33	3,094	44	81	1	100
Taiwan		na		na		na

Table 3.10   Continued

	Nutrition				Water	
	Calorie supply per capita[g]		Protein supply per capita[h]		% Population with safe water	
	Rank	Number	Rank	Grams	Rank	%
Thailand	84	2,301	115	48	102	23
Vietnam	117	2,029	112	49	100	24
OCEANIA		3,111		93		84
Australia°	28	3,202	20	98	16	97
Fiji	45	2,885	68	68	51	69
New Zealand°	14	3,511	2	116	23	93
Papua New Guinea	88	2,286	119	47	113	16
AFRICA		2,249		56		32
Algeria	77	2,406	78	62	42	78
Angola	108	2,110	130	71	110	17
Benin	83	2,310	104	53	110	17
Botswana	99	2,181	58	72	81	45
Burundi	104	2,152	91	57		na
Cameroon	73	2,451	82	60	74	49
Central African Rep.	103	2,161	128	43	108	18
Chad	133	1,808	88	58	98	26
Congo	98	2,200	130	41	117	13
Equatorial Guinea		na		na		na
Ethiopia	135	1,729	88	58	117	13
Gabon	49	2,844	50	77	129	1
Gambia	93	2,250	100	55	119	12
Ghana	120	2,016	125	44	73	50
Guinea	124	1,934	130	41	123	10
Ivory Coast	65	2,623	95	56	115	14
Kenya	115	2,055	91	57	100	24
Lesotho	74	2,442	56	73	102	23
Liberia	71	2,474	115	48	123	10
Libya	19	3,418	39	84	32	87
Madagascar	75	2,436	91	57	98	26
Malawi	95	2,219	69	67	83	44
Mali	122	1,996	100	55	102	23
Mauritania	116	2,051	64	70	110	17
Mauritius	57	2,703	78	62	61	60
°Morocco	60	2,651	64	70	69	53
Mozambique	127	1,891	134	33	127	7
Namibia	94	2,224	39	84		na
Niger	96	2,217	69	67	74	49
Nigeria	81	2,337	104	53	96	28
Rwanda	97	2,201	95	56	90	38
Senegal	79	2,389	61	71	94	35
Sierra Leone	109	2,106	124	45	126	9
Somalia	107	2,131	58	72	90	38
South Africa	51	2,826	55	74		na
Sudan	80	2,371	64	70	79	46
Swaziland	68	2,499	75	64	92	37
Tanzania	118	2,028	115	48	88	39
Togo	109	2,106	122	46	121	11
Tunisia	53	2,751	56	73	59	62

Table 3.10 Continued

	Nutrition				Water	
	Calorie supply per capita[g]		Protein supply per capita[h]		% Population with safe water	
	Rank	Number	Rank	Grams	Rank	%
Uganda	130	1,862	112	49	113	16
Upper Volta	119	2,018	75	64	115	14
Zaire	105	2,133	134	33	108	18
Zambia	123	1,992	100	55	85	42
Zimbabwe	126	1,911	110	51		na

* Developed country

—none or negligible   na Not available

[a]"Soldier" represents all members of the armed forces.

[b]Represents average of ranks for GNP per capita, education, and health.

[c]Ages 5–19.

[d]Represents % of adult population (over 15) able to read and write.

[e]Deaths under one year per 1,000 live births.

[f]Expectation of life at birth.

[g]Represents supply of food available per day per capita, in calories, and grams of protein.

[h]Egypt is shown in the political grouping of Middle East rather than in Africa.

[i]RANK shows the standing of the country among those in the table. The rank order number is repeated if more than one country has the same figure.

Source: Sivard, R. (1983) World Military and Social Expenditures, Washington, D.C., pp. 36–41.

Table 3.11 Military and social trends: world, developed, and developing countries, 1960, 1970, 1980, 1981

	1960	1970	1980	1981
Military Expenditures				
billion US $				
World	100	183	543	595
Developed	90	156	426	465
Developing	10	27	117	130
% of GNP				
World	6.9	5.8	4.6	4.9
Developed	7.5	6.0	4.6	5.1
Developing	4.1	4.9	4.3	4.5
per capita, US $				
World	33	50	122	131
Developed	103	160	403	437
Developing	5	10	34	37
Arms Exports				
billion US $				
World	na	5.8	26.1	na
Developed	na	5.6	24.4	na
Developing	na	.2	1.7	na

Table 3.11   Continued

	1960	1970	1980	1981
Arms Imports				
billion US $				
World	na	5.8	26.1	na
Developed	na	2.1	6.6	na
Developing	na	3.9	19.5	na
Foreign Economic Aid				
billion US $				
World	5.2	8.3	38.8	35.8
Developed	5.0	7.6	29.4	27.8
Developing	.2	.7	9.4	8.0
GNP				
billion US $				
World	1,441	3,161	11,666	12,070
Developed	1,195	2,612	8,958	9,193
Developing	246	549	2,708	2,877
GNP per capita				
US $				
World	473	855	2,619	2,657
Developed	1,365	2,674	8,477	8,642
Developing	114	202	794	827
Population				
millions				
World	3,046	3,697	4,463	4,542
Developed	876	977	1,057	1,064
Developing	2,170	2,720	3,406	3,478
Armed Forces				
thousands				
World	18,550	21,484	24,642	25,311
Developed	9,851	10,146	9,538	9,581
Developing	8,699	11,338	15,104	15,730
Physicians				
thousands				
World	1,668	2,317	3,946	na
Developed	1,226	1,658	2,482	na
Developing	442	659	1,464	na
Teachers				
thousands				
World	14,526	22,129	32,142	32,860
Developed	6,580	8,823	9,960	9,960
Developing	7,946	13,306	22,182	22,900

Source: Adapted from Sivard, R. (1983) *World Military and Social Expenditures,* Washington, D.C., p. 32.

The growth of this technological economy, with its large-scale organizations in complex societies, has given a new momentum to social and spatial mobility at all levels, and has altered the forms of social relations in general. Again, the social, the psychological and somatic results are probably extensive, but they are still to be identified. The major task in relation to such consequences is to try and recognize their appearance and their scale, and then to set about their control.

References

1. **Hobhouse, L. T., Wheeler, G. C.,** and **Ginsberg, M.** (1915). *The Material Culture and Social Institutions of the Simpler Peoples,* London.
   Forde, C. D. (1934). *Habitat, Economy, and Society, London.*
   Childe, V. G. (1951). *Social Evolution,* London.
   Firth, R. (1951). *Elements of Social Organization,* London.
   Epstein, A. L., ed. (1967). *The Craft of Social Anthropology,* London.
2. **Radcliffe-Brown, A. R.** (1958). *Method in Social Anthropology,* ed. Srinivas, M. N., Chicago.
   Geertz, C. (1973). *The Interpretation of Cultures,* New York.
3. **Dobb, M.** (1946). *Studies in Economic Development,* Cambridge.
   Braudel, F. (1981). *The Structure of Everyday Life,* New York.
   Wolf, E. (1982). *Europe and the People Without History,* Berkeley.
   Braudel, F. (1983). *The Wheels of Commerce,* New York.
4. **Wallerstein, I.** (1974). *The Modern World System,* New York.
5. **DeVries, J.** (1976). *The Economy of Europe in an Age of Crisis, 1600–1750,* Cambridge.
6. **Landes, D. S.** (1969). *The Unbound Prometheus,* Cambridge.
   Hobsbawm, E. J. (1975). *The Age of Capital,* New York.
7. **Hobsbawm, E. J.** (1968). *Industry and Empire,* London.
   Dean, P. (1969). *The First Industrial Revolution,* Cambridge.
8. **Amin, S.** (1974). *Accumulation on a World Scale,* London.
   Wallerstein, I. (1979). *The Capitalist World Economy,* Cambridge.
   Murdoch, W. (1980). *The Poverty of Nations,* Baltimore.
   Barnet, R. (1983). *The Alliance,* New York.
9. **Hughes, C. C.** and **Hunter, J. M.** (1971). Disease and development in Africa, in *The Social Organization of Health,* ed. Dreitzel, H.-P., New York, pp. 150–214.
   Gereff, G. (1983). *The Pharmaceutical Industry and Dependency in the Third World,* Princeton, N.J.
10. **Frank, A. G.** (1969). The development of underdevelopment, in Frank, A. G., *Underdevelopment or Revolution,* New York.
    Payer, C. (1975). *The Debt Trap: The IMF and the Third World,* New York.
    Duncan, K. and **Rutledge, I.,** eds. (1977). *Land and Labor in Latin America,* Cambridge.
    Rodney, W. (1982). *How Europe Underdeveloped Africa,* rev. ed., Cambridge, Mass.
    Becker, D. G. (1984). *The New Bourgeoisie and The Limits of Dependency,* Princeton, N.J.
11. **World Bank** (1980). *World Development Report,* Washington, D.C.
    World Bank (1981). *World Development Report,* Washington, D.C.
12. **Chandra, R. K.** and **Newberne, P. M.** (1977). *Nutrition, Immunity and Infection,* New York.

Morley, D. C. and **Woodland, M.** (1980). *See How They Grow: Monitoring Child Growth for Appropriate Health Care in Developing Countries,* Oxford.

13. **Susser, M., Marolla, F.,** and **Fleiss, J.** (1972). Birthweight, Fetal age and perinatal mortality, *Amer. J. Epi., 96,* 197–204.

    Wilcox, A. J. and **Russell, I. T.** (1983). Birthweight and perinatal mortality: I. On the frequency distribution, and II. On weight-specific mortality, *Int. J. Epidem., 12,* 314–25.

    Barron, S. L., and **Thomson, A. M.** (1983). *Obstetrical Epidemiology,* New York.

    Mammelle, N., Laumon, B., and **Lazar, P.** (1984) Prematurity and occupational activity during pregnancy, *Amer. J. Epi., 119,* 309–22.

14. **Shannon, D. C.** and **Kelly, D. H.** (1982). SIDS and near-SIDS, Part I, *New Eng. J. Med., 306,* 959–65; 1022–28.

15. **National Center for Health Statistics** (1984). *Mon. Vit. Stat. Rep., 33,* 3, Suppl.

16. **Central Statistical Office** (1982). *Annual Abstract of Statistics,* H.M.S.O., London.

17. **United States Department of Health and Human Services** (1982). *Health, United States, 1982,* Hyattsville, Maryland.

18. **World Health Organization** (1982). *World Health Statistics Annual,* Geneva.

19. **Terris, M.** (1967). Epidemiology of cirrhosis of the liver: National mortality data, *Amer. J. Pub. Health, 57,* 2076–88.

20. **Martin, A. E.** (1964). Mortality and morbidity statistics and air pollution, *Proc. R. Soc. Med., 57,* 969–75.

    Reid, D., Anderson, D. O., Ferris, B. G., and **Fletcher, C. M.** (1964). An Anglo-American comparison of the prevalence of bronchitis, *Brit. Med. J., 2,* 1487–91.

    Stocks, P. (1967). Lung cancer and bronchitis in relation to cigarette smoking and fuel consumption in 20 countries, *Brit. J. Prev. Soc. Med., 21,* 181–85.

    Anderson, D. O. (1967). The effects of air contamination on health; Parts I–III, *Canad. Med. Ass. J., 97,* 528–36, 585–93, 802–6.

    Ferris, B. G. (1968). Epidemiological studies on air pollution and health, *Arch. Environm. Hlth., 16,* 541–55.

    United States Environmental Protection Agency (1982). Epidemiological studies on the effects of particulate matter and sulfur oxides on human health, p. 14-1–14-141, in *Air Quality Criteria for Particulate Matter and Sulfur Oxides,* Vol. III, EPA-600 8-82-029c, Research Triangle Park, North Carolina.

21. **Rutstein, D. D., Berenberg, W., Chalmers, T. C., Child, C. G., Fishman, A. P.,** and **Perrin, E. B.** (1976). Measuring the quality of medical care, a clinical method, *N. Engl. J. Med., 294,* 582–89.

22. **Susser, M. W.** (1967). Causes of peptic ulcer: A selective epidemiological review, *J. Chron. Dis., 20,* 435–56.

23. **Last, J. M.** (1963). The iceberg—completing the clinical picture—in general practice, *Lancet, 2,* 28–31.

    Logan, R. F. L. (1964). Studies in the spectrum of medical care, in *Problems and Progress in Medical Care,* ed. McLachlan, G., London.

    Elwood, P. C., Waters, W. E., Green, W. J., and **Wood, M. M.** (1967). Evaluation of a screening survey for anaemia in adult non-pregnant women, *Brit. Med. J., 1,* 714–17.

    Morris, J. N. (1975). *Uses of Epidemiology,* 3rd ed., Edinburgh.

24. **Susser, M. W.** (1968). *Community Psychiatry: Epidemiologic and Social Themes,* New York, pp. 205–77.

    MacMahon, B., and **Pugh, T. F.** (1970). *Epidemiology: Principles and Methods,* Boston.

25. **Office of Population Censuses and Surveys,** *Hospital In Patient Inquiry,* Morbidity Series MB4, H.M.S.O., London.

Office of Population Censuses and Surveys (1978). Morbidity Statistics from general practice 1971–72. Second National Study, *Studies on Medical and Subject Population,* No. 36, H.M.S.O., London.

See the **National Center for Health Statistics:**

Series 10. Data from the Health Interview Survey.

Series 11. Data from the Health Examination Survey and the Health and Nutrition Examination Survey (HANES).

Series 13. Data on Health Resources Utilization.

Series 22. Data from the National Natality and Mortality Surveys.

Centers for Disease Control. *Morbidity and Mortality Weekly Report,* Washington, D.C.

26. **Collins, S. D.** (1951). Age incidence of specific causes of illness found in monthly canvases of families, *Publ. Hlth. Rep.* (Wash.), *86,* 1227–43.

Douglas, J. W. B., and **Blomfield, J. M.** (1958). *Children Under Five,* London.

Miller, F. J. W., Court, S. D. M., Walton, W. S., and **Knox, E. G.** (1968). *Growing up in Newcastle upon Tyne,* London.

Danner, C. C., Korns, R. F., and **Schuman, L. M.** (1968). *Infectious Disease,* Vital and Health Statistics Monographs, American Public Health Association, Cambridge, Mass.

27. **National Center for Health Statistics** (1975). Acute Conditions: Incidence and associated disability, United States, July 1973–June 1974, *Vital and Health Statistics,* Series 10, Number 102.

National Center for Health Statistics (1983). Disability Days: United States, 1980, *Vital and Health Statistics,* Series 10, Number 143.

28. **National Center for Health Statistics** (1982). Current Estimates from the National Health Interview Survey, *Vital and Health Statistics,* Series 10, Number 141.

29. **Paneth, N., Kiely, J., Stein, Z.,** and **Susser, M. W.** (1981). Cerebral palsy and newborn care. III: Estimated prevalence rates of cerebral palsy under differing rates of mortality and impairment of low-birthweight infants, *Develop. Med. Child. Neurol., 23,* 801–17.

30. **Colvez, A.,** and **Blanchet, M.** (1981). Disability trends in the United States Population, 1966–1976: Analysis of reported cases, *Amer. J. Publ. Hlth., 71,* 464–71.

31. **U.S. Department of Commerce and Bureau of the Census** (1983). *Statistical Abstract of the United States, 1982–3,* Washington, D.C.

Vladeck, B. C. (1982). Nursing Homes, in *Handbook of Health, Health Care and the Health Professions,* ed., Mechanic, D., 352–65, New York.

32. **Edge, P. G.** (1947). *Vital Statistics and Public Health Work in the Tropics.* London.

Kuczynski, R. R. (1949). *Demographic Survey of the British Colonial Empire,* Vol. II, London.

Sabben-Clare, E. E., Bradley, D. J., and **Kirkwood, K.** (1980). *Health in Tropical Africa during the Colonial Period,* Oxford.

Escudero, J. C. (1980). On lies and health statistics: Some Latin American examples, *Int. J. Health Services, 10,* 421–34.

Evans, J. R., Hall, K. L., and **Warford, J.** (1981) Health care in the developing world: Problems of scarcity and choice (Shattuck Lecture), *New Eng. J. Med., 305,* 1117–27.

33. **Puffer, R. R.,** and **Serrano, C. V.** (1973). *Patterns of Mortality in Childhood,* Pan America Health Organization, Scientific Publication No. 262, Washington, D.C.

World Health Organization (1975). *The Population Debate: Dimensions and Perspec-*

tives: Papers of the World Population Conference, 1974, Bucharest, 573–97, United Nations, New York.

World Health Organization (1975). Mortality and morbidity trends, 1969–72, *WHO Chronicle, 29,* 377–86.

World Health Organization (1982). *Levels and Trends of Mortality since 1950: A joint study by the United Nations and the World Health Organization,* United Nations, New York.

United Nations (1982). *Demographic Annual,* 34th edition, New York.

34. Lack, D. (1954). *The Natural Regulation of Animal Numbers,* Oxford.

35. Comfort, A. (1956). The biology of ageing, *Lancet, ii,* 772–78.

36. McGregor, I. A., Wilson, E., and Billewicz, W. Z. (1983). Malaria infection of the placenta in The Gambia, West Africa; its incidence and relationship to stillbirth, birthweight and placental weight, *Trans. R. Trop. Med Hyg., 77,* 223–44.

   Stein, Z., and Susser, M. (1984). Intrauterine growth retardation: Epidemiological issues and public health significance, *Seminars in Perinatology, 8,* 5–14.

37. Williams, C. D. (1933). A nutritional disease of childhood associated with a maize diet, *Arch. Dis. Childh. 8,* 423–33.

   Brock, J. F., and Autret, M. (1952). *Kwashiorkor in Africa,* W.H.O., Geneva.

   Scrimshaw, N. S., Taylor, C. E., and Gordon, J. E. (1968). *Interactions of Nutrition,* WHO Monograph Series, No. 57, Geneva.

   Olson, R. E., ed. (1975). *Protein-Calorie Malnutrition,* New York.

   Alderman, M. H., Wise, P. H., Ferguson, R. P., Laverde, H. T., and D'Soua, A. (1978). Reduction of young child malnutrition and mortality in rural Jamaica, *Trop. Ped. Environ. Child Hlth., 24,* 7–11.

   Escudero, J. C. (1978). The magnitude of malnutrition in Latin America, *Int. J. Hlth. Serv., 8,* 465–90.

   World Health Organization (1980). *Sixth Report on the World Health Situation, 1973–1977,* Geneva.

   LePage, P., Munyakazi, C., and Hennart, P. (1981). Breastfeeding and hospital mortality in children in Rwanda, *Lancet, ii,* 409–11.

   Beaton, G. H. and Ghassemi, P. D. (1982). Supplementary feeding programs for young children in developing countries, *Amer. J. Clin. Nutr., 35,* 864–916.

38. LePage, P., and DeMol, P. (1979). Measles mortality in Rwanda, *Lancet, ii,* 1133–34.

   Aaby, P., Bukh, J., Lisse, I. M., and Smits, A. J. (1983). Measles mortality, state of nutrition and family structure: A community study from Guinea-Bissau, *J. Infect. Dis, 147,* 693–701.

39. Susser, M. W. (1980). Prenatal nutrition, birthweight, and psychological development: An overview of experiments and quasi-experiments in the past decade, *Amer. J. Clin. Nut., 34,* 784–803.

40. Gordon, J. E., Singh, S., and Wyon, J. B. (1965). Causes of death at different ages, by sex and by season in rural population of Punjab, *Ind. J. Med. Res., 53,* 911.

   Laurell, A. C. (1981). Mortality and working conditions in agriculture in underdeveloped countries, *Int. J. Health Serv., 11,* 13–20.

41. Gillanders, A. D. (1951). Nutritional heart disease, *Brit. Heart J., 13,* 177–96.

   Davies, J. N. P., and Ball, J. D. (1955). The pathology of endomyocardial fibrosis in Uganda, *Brit. Heart J., 17,* 337–59.

   Grusin, H. (1957). Acute reversible heart failure in Africans, *Circulation, 16,* 27–35.

Schwartz, M. B., Schamroth, L., and Seftel, H. C. (1958). The pattern of heart disease in the urbanised (Johannesburg) African, *Med. Proc.*, 4, 275–35.

Seftel, H. C., and Susser, M. W. (1961). Maternity and myocardial failure in African women, *Brit. Heart J.*, 232, 43–52.

Shaper, A. G., Kaplan, M. H., Mody, N. J., and McIntyre, P. A. (1968). Malarial antibodies and auto-antibodies to heart and other tissues in the immigrant and indigenous peoples in Uganda, *Lancet, i*, 1342–46.

42. Berman, C. (1951), *Primary Carcinoma of the Liver: A Study in Incidence, Clinical Manifestations, Pathology and Aetiology*, London.

Higginson, J., and Oettle, A. G. (1957). The incidence of liver cancer in South Africa, *Acta Un. Int. Cancer*, 13, 602–5.

Szmuness, W. (1978). Hepatocellar carcinoma and the hepatitis B virus: Evidence for a causal association, *Prog. Med. Virol.*, 24, 40–69.

43. Roulet, F. C., ed. (1964). *Lymphoreticular Tumours in Africa*, International Union Against Cancer, Monograph Series 3, Basel.

Burkitt, D., and Wright, P. (1966). Geographical and tribal distribution of African lymphoma in Uganda, *Brit. Med. J.*, 1, 569–73.

Pike, M. C., Williams, E. M., and Wright, B. (1967). Burkitt's tumour in the West Nile district of Uganda, 1961–65, *Brit. Med. J.*, 1, 395–99.

Burkitt, D. (1983). The discovery of Burkitt's lymphoma, *Cancer*, 51, 1777–86.

44. Doll, R., and Peto, R. (1981). *The Causes of Cancer*, Oxford.

45. Susser, M. (1957). African Township: A sociomedical study, *Medical World*, 86, 385–400.

46. Loudon, J. B. (1959). Psychogenic disorder and social conflict among the Zulu, in *Culture and Mental Health*, ed. Opler, M. K., New York.

47. Susser, M. W. (1967). Causes of peptic ulcer. A selective epidemiologic review, *J. Chron. Dis.*, 20, 435–56.

48. Titmuss, R. M., Abel-Smith, B., assisted by Lynes, T. (1961). *Social Policies and Population Growth in Mauritius*, London.

George, S. (1977). *How the Other Half Dies: The Real Reasons for World Hunger*, Montclair, N.J.

Chossudovsky, M. (1983). Underdevelopment and the political economy of malnutrition and ill health, *Int. J. of Health Services*, 13, 69–87.

Ross, J., ed. (1982). *International Encyclopedia of Population*, Vols. I and II, New York and London.

Coale, A. (1983). Recent trends in fertility in less developed countries, *Science*, 221, 828–32.

49. Davis, S. H. (1977). *Victims of the Miracle*, London.

Doyal, L., and Pennel, I. (1979). *The Political Economy of Health*, London.

50. Susser, M., and Cherry V. (1982). Health and health care under Apartheid, *J. Pub. Hlth Policy*, 3, 455–75.

Susser, M. (1983). Apartheid and the causes of death: Disentangling ideology and laws from class and race (A commentary), *Amer. J. Pub. Hlth.*, 73, 581–83.

51. Wilson, M., and Thompson, L. (1969). *Oxford History of South Africa*, London.

Fredrikson, G. M. (1981). *White Supremacy: A Comparative Study in American and South African History*, New York.

52. Robins-Browne, R. M. (1984). Seasonal and racial incidence of infantile gastroenteritis in South Africa, *Amer. J. Epi.*, 119, 350–55.

53. **Kark, S. L.** (1949). The social pathology of syphilis in Africans, *S. Afr. Med. J.*, 23, 77–84.

54. **Wyndham, C. H.** (1978). Ischaemic heart disease mortality rates in white South Africans compared with other populations, *S. Afr. Med. J.*, 54, 595–601.
    Seftel, H. C., Baker, S. G., Sandler, M. P., Forman, M. B., Joffe, B. I., Mendelsohn, D., Jenkins, T., and Mieny, C. (1980). A host of hypercholesterolaemic homozygotes in South Africa, *Brit. Med. J.*, 281, 633–36.

55. **Shonland, M. and Bradshaw, E.** (1968). Cancer in the Natal African and Indian, *Ind. J. Canc.*, 3, 304–16.
    Shonland, M., Bradshaw, E. (1969). Some observations on cancer of the uterine cervix in Africans and Indians of Natal, *S. Afr. J. Med. Sci.*, 34, 61–71.
    Bradshaw, E., and Harington, J. S. (1981). The cancer problem among Blacks: South Africa, in *Cancer Among Black Populations*, eds. Mettlin, C., Curtis, N., and Murphy, G., New York.

56. **Gordon, L.,** ed. (1980). *Survey of Race Relations in South Africa 1979*, South African Institute of Race Relations, Johannesburg.
    Gordon, L., ed. (1981). *Survey of Race Relations in South Africa 1980*, South African Institute of Race Relations, Johannesburg.

57. **Stein, H.** (1982). *The Sick Black Child*, Johannesburg.

58. **Wyndham, C. H., and Irwig, L. J.** (1979). A comparison of the mortality rates of various population groups in the Republic of South Africa, *S. Afr. Med. J.*, 55, 796–806.
    Wyndham, C. H. (1980). A comparision of the mortality rates of white South Africans with those of the population of England and Wales, *S. Afr. Med. J.*, 57, 729-41
    Wyndham, C. H. (1981). The loss from premature deaths of economically active manpower in the various populations of the RSA. Part I: Leading causes of death; health strategies for reducing mortality, *S. Afr. Med. J.*, 60, 411–19.

59. **Seftel, H. C., and Schultz, E.** (1961). Diabetes mellitus in the urbanized Johannesburg African, *S. Afr. Med. J.*, 35, 66–71.
    Campbell, G. D. (1963). Diabetes in Asians and Africans in and around Durban, *S. Afr. Med. J.*, 37, 1195–1208.

60. **Cassel, J.** (1955). A comprehensive health program among South African Zulus, in *Health, Culture and Community*, ed. Paul, B. D., New York, pp. 15–42.
    Steuart, G. W., and Kark, S. L., eds. (1962). *A Practice of Social Medicine*, Edinburgh.

61. **Scotch, N. A., and Geiger, M. S.** (1963). The epidemiology of essential hypertension. II. Psychologic and sociocultural factors in etiology, *J. Chron. Dis.*, 16, 1183–1213.
    Henry, J. P., and Cassel, J. (1969). Psychosocial factors in essential hypertension: Recent epidemiological and animal experimental evidence, *Am. J. Epidem.*, 90, 171–200.
    Seedat, Y. K., Seedat, M. A., and Hackland, D. B. T. (1982). Prevalence of hypertension in the urban and rural Zulu, *J. Epidem. Comm. Hlth.*, 36, 256–61.

62. **MacLaren, M. J.** (1975). Epidemiology of rheumatic heart disease in Black school-going children in Soweto, *Brit. Med. J.*, 23, 474–78.

63. **Burrell, R. J. W.** (1957). Oesophageal cancer in the Bantu, *S. Afr. Med. J.*, 31, 401–9.

64. **Moosa, A. and Coovadia, H. M.** (1981). The problem of malnutrition in South Africa, *S. Afr. Med. J.*, 59, 888–89.

65. **Kahn, E. and Freedman, M. L.** (1959). The physical development of a privileged group of African children, *S. Afr. Med. J.*, 33, 934–36.

66. **Wilson, F., and Westcott, G.** (1980). *Economics of Health in South Africa*, Vols. I and II., Capetown.

67. **Chadwick, E.** (1842). *Report on Sanitary Conditions of the Labouring Population of Great Britain*, H.M.S.O., London.
68. **Kark, S. L.,** and **Cassel, J.** (1952). The Pholela Health Center: A progress report, *S. Afr. Med. J.*, *26*, 101–4, 132–36.
    Kark, S. L., and **Steuart, G. W.** (1957). Health education and neighborhood family practice, *Health Educ. J.*, *15*, 131–39.
69. **Engels, F.** (1887). *The Condition of the Working Class in England in 1844*, English translation by J. W. Lovell Company, New York.
70. **Pollard, S.** (1981). *Peaceful Conquest: The Industrialization of Europe, 1760–1970*, Oxford.
71. **New York Academy of Medicine** (1975; originally published 1885). *Vital Statistics: A Memorial Volume of Selections from the Reports and Writings of William Farr*, edited for the Sanitary Institute of Great Britain by Noel A. Humphreys, with an Introduction by M. Susser and A. Adelstein, No. 46, History of Medicine Series, Metuchen, N.J.
72. **McKeown, T.** (1976). *The Modern Rise of Population*, London.
73. **Hassold, T., Quillen, S. D.,** and **Yamane, J. A.** (1983). Sex ratio in spontaneous abortions, *Ann. Hum. Genet.*, *47*, 39–47.
74. **Crew, F. A. E.** (1948). *Measurements of the Public Health*, Edinburgh.
    Martin, W. S. (1948). The sex ratio, *Med. Offr.*, *79*, 153–56.
75. **Erhardt, A.** (1981). Effects of prenatal sex hormones on gender related behavior, *Science*, *211*, 1312–18.
76. **Hamilton, J. B.** (1948). The role of testicular secretions as indicated by the effects of castration in man and by studies of pathological conditions and the short life span associated with maleness, *Recent Prog. Hormone Res.*, *3*, 257–322.
77. **Kelsey, J. L.** (1979). A review of the epidemiology of human breast cancer, *Epidemiol. Rev.*, *1*, 74–109.
    MacMahon, B. (1979). Oestrogens in the genesis of endometrial and breast cancer, *INSERM*, *83*, 81–92.
78. **Wiehl, D.** (1938). Sex differences in mortality in the United States, *Milbank mem. Fd. Quart.*, *16*, 145–55.
    Yerushalmy, J. (1943). Age-sex composition of the population resulting from natality and mortality conditions, *Milbank mem. Fd. Quart.*, *21*, 37–63.
    Enterline, P. E. (1961). Causes of death responsible for recent increases in sex mortality differentials in the United States, *Milbank mem. Fd. Quart.*, *39*, 312–28.
79. **National Center for Health Statistics** (1983). Inpatient Utilization of Short Stay Hospitals by Diagnosis, United States 1980, *Vital and Health Statistics*, Series 13, Number 74.
80. **Waldron, I.** (1978). The coronary prone behavior pattern, blood pressure, employment and socio-economic status in women, *J. Psychosom. Res.*, *22*, 79–87.
81. **Vessey, M., Doll, R., Peto, R., Johnson, B.,** and **Wiggins, P.** (1976). Long-Term Follow-Up Study of Women Using Different Methods of Contraception—An Interim Report, *J. Biosocial Sci.*, *8*, 373–427.
    Palesch, Y. Y., Brody, J. A., and **White, A.** (1980). Risks and benefits of the decline in oestrogen use by postmenopausal women, *J. Chron. Exp. Geron.*, *2*, 65–77.
    The Centers for Disease Control (1983). Long term oral contraceptive use and the risk of breast cancer: The Centers for Disease Control Steroid Hormone Study, *J. Amer. Med. Assoc.*, *249*, 1591–95.
    Kampert, J. B., Wood, D. A., and **Paffenbarger, R. S.** (1983). Oral contraceptives and breast disease, in *Breast Carcinoma: Current Diagnosis and Treatment*, ed. Feig, P., New York, pp. 597–607.

Pike, M. C., Henderson, B. E., Krailo, M. D., Duke, A., and Roy, S. (1983). Breast cancer in young women and use of oral contraceptives: Possible modifying effect of formulation and age at use, *Lancet, ii*, 930–34.

Vessey, M. P., Lawless, M., McPherson, K., and Yeates, D. (1983). Neoplasia of the cervix uteri and contraception—A possible adverse effect of the pill, *Lancet, ii*, 934–38.

Rosenberg, L., Miller, D. R., Kaufman, D. W., Helmrich, S. P., Stolley, P. D., Schottenfeld, D., and Shapiro, S. (1984). Breast cancer and contraceptive use, *Amer. J. Epi.,* *119*, 167–76.

82. Susser, M. (1974). Ethical components in the definition of health, *Int. J. Hlth. Serv., 43*, 539–548.

Starr, P. (1982). *The Social Transformation of American Medicine*, New York.

83. Susser, M. (1971). The public health and social change: Implications for professional education in public health in the United States, *Int. J. Hlth. Serv.*, 1, 60–70.

84. Chapin, G. and Wasserstrom, R. (1981). Agricultural production and malarial resurgence in Central America and India, *Nature, 293*, 181–85.

Peters, W. (1982). Anti-malarial drug resistance: An increasing problem, *Brit. Med. Bull.,* *38*, 187–92.

Peters, W. (1982). Editorial: Chemotherapy of malaria in mouse and man, *Lancet, i*, 318–20.

85. Havighurst, C. C., and Weistart, J. C. (1972). *Health Care*, Dobbs Ferry, N.Y.

Somers, A. R., and Somers, H. M. (1977). *Health and Health Care Policies in Perspective*, Germantown, Md.

Wilson, R. W., and White, E. L. (1977). Changes in morbidity, disability and utilization differentials between the poor and the nonpoor: Data from the Health Interview Survey: 1964 and 1973, *Medical Care, 15*, 636–46.

Davis, K., and Schoen, C. (1978). *Health and the War on Poverty: A Ten Year Appraisal*, Washington, D.C.

86. Stein, Z., and Susser, M. (1970). Mutability of intelligence and epidemiology of mild mental retardation, *Rev. Ed. Res., 40*, 29–67.

Hagberg, B., Hagberg, G., Lewerth, A. and Lindberg, U. (1981). Mild mental retardation of Swedish school children, I. Prevalence, *Acta Pediatr. Scand., 70*, 441–44.

87. Srole, L. and Fischer, A. (1980). The Midtown Manhattan longitudinal study vs "The Mental Paradise Lost" doctrine, *Arch. Gen. Psychiat., 37*, 209–21.

88. Marmot, M. G., Adelstein, A. M., Robinson, N., and Rose, G. A. (1978). Changing social class distribution of heart disease, *Brit. Med. J., 2*, 1109–12.

Office of Population Censuses and Surveys (1981). *Mortality Statistics*, Series DH, No. 2, H.M.S.O., London.

89. Alderman, M. H. (1980). The epidemiology of hypertension: Etiology, natural history, and the impact of therapy, *Cardiovascular Reviews and Reports, 1*, 509–19.

Gillum, R. F., Folsom, A., Luepker, R. V., Jacobs, D. R., Jr., Kottke, T. E., Gomez-Maria, O., Prineas, R. J., Taylor, H. L., and Blackburn, H. (1983). Sudden death from acute myocardial infarction in a metropolitan area, 1970–80: The Minnesota Heart Survey, *New Eng. J. Med., 309*, 1353–57.

90. Krueger, D. E., Williams, J. L., and Paffenbarger, R. S. (1967). Trends in death rates from cerebrovascular disease in Memphis, Tennessee, 1920–60, *J. Chron. Dis., 20*, 129–37.

91. Hansen, H., and Susser, M. (1971). Historic trends in deaths from chronic kidney disease in the United States and Britain, *Amer. J. Epi., 93*, 413–22.

92. **U.S. Department of Labor** (1980). *Occupational Injuries and Illnesses in 1978: Summary*, Report 586, Washington, D.C.

U.S. Department of Health, Education and Welfare (1978). *Estimates of the Fraction of Cancer in the United States Related to Occupational Factors*, National Institute for Occupational Safety and Health, Bethesda, Maryland.

Centers for Disease Control (1983). Leading work-related diseases and injuries—United States, *Morbidity and Mortality Weekly Report, 32*, 24–6; 189–91.

93. **U.S Department of Health, Education, and Welfare** (1973). *Report of the Secretary's Commission on Medical Malpractice*, 2 vols., Washington, D.C

Freeman, J., and McGowan, J. E., Jr. (1981). Day-specific incidence of nosocomial infection estimated from a prevalence survey. *Amer. J. Epidem., 114*, 888–901.

Eickhoff, T. C. (1982). Nosocomial infections—1981, *J. Am. Geriatr. Soc., 30*, 326–28.

94. **Barton, R. W. A. G.** (1959). *Institutional Neurosis*, Bristol.

Wing, J. K. and Brown, G. W. (1970). *Institutionalism and Schizophrenia*, Cambridge.

95. **Newton, M. A., Sealey, J. E., Ledingham, J. G., and Laragh, J. M.** (1968). High blood pressure and oral contraceptives, *Amer. J. Obstet. Gynec., 101*, 1037–45.

Vessey, M. P., and Doll, R. (1968). Investigation of relation between use of oral contraceptives and thromboembolic disease, *Brit. Med. J., 2*, 199–205.

Sloane, D., and Shapiro, S. (1969). Computer analysis of epidemiologic data on effect of drugs on hospital patients, *Pub. Hlth. Rep., 84*, 39–52.

96. **Kempe, C. H.** (1960). Studies on smallpox and complications of smallpox vaccination, *Pediatrics, 26*, 176–89.

Dixon, C. W. (1962). *Smallpox*, London.

Dick, G. W. A. (1962). Prevention of virus diseases in the community, *Brit. Med. J., 2*, 1275–80.

97. **Broome, C. V., and Fraser, D. W.** (1981). Pertussis in the United States, 1979: A look at vaccine efficacy, *J. Infect. Dis., 144*, 187–90.

Stewart, G. T. (1981). Whooping cough in relation to other childhood infections in 1977–79 in the United Kingdom, *J. Epidemiol. Comm. Hlth., 35*, 139–45.

Miller, D. L., Alderslade, R., and Ross, E. M. (1982). Whooping cough and whooping cough vaccine: The risks and benefits debate, *Epidemiologic Reviews, 4*, 1–24.

98. **Jelliffe, D. B.** (1972). Commerciogenic malnutrition? *Nutrition Reviews, 30*, 199–205.

Manderson, L. (1982). Bottle feeding and ideology in colonial Malaya: The production of change, *Int. J. Hlth. Serv., 12*, 597–616.

99. **Committee for the Compilation of Materials on Damage Caused by the Atomic Bombs in Hiroshima and Nagasaki** (1981). *Hiroshima and Nagasaki, The Physical, Medical and Social Effects of the Atomic Bombings*, New York.

4

Culture and health

To be sick is to be placed in a situation that is defined by the social interaction of the patient with family, friends, employers, and caretaking agents. The sick person, as Henry Sigerist pointed out long ago, has a special position, a social role with implicit rules and privileges (1). Sickness is synonymous neither with illness nor with disease, although it usually includes both. *Illness* can be defined as a state of psychic awareness of disordered function, and *disease* as an underlying state of physiological or psychological dysfunction (see Chapter 1). The crucial distinction from sickness is that both illness and disease affect the individual organism and are confined within it, whereas *sickness* refers to a state of social dysfunction that affects the individual's relation with others. States of affliction do not go unattended in human communities. Societies have devised supports—symbolic and material—that aid their members in the pain, grief, rage, and confusion of periodic crises, and mediate the meaning and impact of affliction. Illness is one such crisis. Once a person becomes aware of illness, the forms of social relations peculiar to a given society set the conditions in which sick privileges are conferred.

All social life is a process, a sequence of interactions between human beings in time. The effects of the actions of individuals on one another, and of their joint actions, are so complex that their relationships must be arbitrarily isolated into social units if they are to be comprehended and studied. "Societies" are the most comprehensive of these social units (2). The !Kung San of the Kalahari Desert and the citizens of Great Britain form two distinct societies in this sense; each group has its own particular social and cultural characteristics and occupies a defined territory. These conditions are not the only ones by which to define a society, however. Until 1966 when Botswana won independence, the !Kung San and the British were both under the jurisdiction of the same state and could have been considered members of the same society if one regarded the Commonwealth as a society. Conversely, the present-day hunting and gathering society of the nomadic !Kung San can be usefully distinguished from the

132

settled, pastoral life of their compatriots in eastern Botswana. In the same way, gypsies in Europe can be said to form a society, as can other social and ethnic groups within particular countries whose members regard themselves, and are regarded by others, as distinct and separate.

Although the term "society" is used imprecisely and its meaning depends on context, for practical purposes *society* may be defined as the system of social relationships that characterizes some particular aggregate of individuals who are dependent upon one another for survival and procreation, and who as a group enjoy some measure of political independence. A system of social relationships has a perceptible degree of regularity and permanence, and is typically described in terms of its constituent institutions and associations. While the structure of society—say, its division into social classes—may constrain behavior, this structure is not simply an impersonal force acting on passive groups of individuals or families. Rather, society is an elaborate web of interaction, joint action, and conflict, regulated by law and custom, and based to some degree on a common set of values (3).

If society is considered as a system of social relationships, then the *culture* of a society is the system of values and meanings in terms of which social behavior takes place (4). Behavior is here taken to include all the activities of an individual, whether physical or mental, overt or hidden. Culture is, at the same time, preeminently symbolic in nature, a body of tradition borne, enacted and shared by members of a society and transmitted from one generation to the next. It includes norms, values, knowledge, and beliefs that serve as standards of behavior and that define a way of life peculiar to that society or a segment of it. How people interpret and respond to the mundane, including disease and illness, is thus an expression of culture. In general, then, culture constitutes a set of selected adaptations that sustain a society in a specific environment (see Chapter 1) and endow the members of society with a particular definition of reality and a sense of what may be rightly expected of others. Culture forges our identities as social beings (5).

So thoroughgoing is this initiation that culture becomes, in effect, "second nature" for its members. All children must be taught to walk and to speak, but the manner in which this is done and the language children learn are fixed by the society in which they are born. The process of socialization is universal, but the method of teaching and the content of what is taught vary from one society to another, and the variations are innumerable. Every individual in a society learns how to express needs and feelings in a way that other members of society can understand and accept. At the same time, individuals learn to interpret the behavior of others towards themselves.

The system of social relationships we call a society persists as a stable structure beyond the life-span of individuals. The elementary family of two generations, for instance, may be seen as a structure of relationships through which the behavior appropriate to husband and wife, and parents and children, is transmitted to successive generations of individuals. Although the actual behavior of members of elementary families, that is, the content of their relationships, varies between one society and another, or between families in the same society, this behavior is never completely arbitrary, nor simply the outcome of mutual affection or a clash of wills. The existence of certain rights and obligations and of the emotional ties that characterize family relationships (the love of a mother for her child, for example) are common to human-kind everywhere. Wide variations exist, however, in the ties that are recognized, in the manner in which these are expressed, and in the sanctions imposed on individuals who break the legal or customary rules that regulate these relationships (6).

Every society, therefore, may be said to have its own particular system of social relationships and its own distinctive culture, within which a range of allowable customary behavior may be discerned. In medical practice, the influence of culture and social organization is detectable in even such basic decisions as whether a severely deformed newborn is considered alive or whether death has occurred in victims of trauma (7). In this chapter, we shall take as one theme the influence of culture on behavior in general, and on sickness behavior specifically. A second theme will be the influence of culture on communication, in particular between doctors and patients, and between health professionals and communities. Finally, we shall examine the influence of culture on health and disease, on modes of adaptation, and on mental states.

Culture and behavior

Culture, genes, and behavior

The rich diversity of societies and cultures was often ascribed in the past to racial differences between human beings; this belief is still sufficiently widespread to be a potent social and political force in many societies. The notion of "race" is problematic; race cannot be simply defined as a discrete entity. People vary in such obvious physical matters as skin color, hair form, and head shape as well as in less obvious characteristics such as susceptibility to disease. The frequency of certain genes varies between populations, although few if any genes are confined to a single race. The more distant populations are from each other the more distinct are their characteristics, but the extremes are connected by intervening populations with intermediate characteristics.

The human species thus shows genetic diversity. A species that is genetically uniform is more limited in the range of habitats it can exploit than one that shows individual variation within populations; a species differentiated into subspecies or races is capable of occupying a wider territory than a species consisting of only a single race; and a species that can alter its genetic constitution when the environment changes is more likely to endure than less flexible species. Geographical race, therefore, is best thought of as a statistical notion describing population types, not individuals. Within societies, recognition of racial diversity varies greatly. North Americans, for example, typically distinguish three or four categories, whereas Brazilians can identify three or four hundred (8).

The genetic diversity expressed in individual variation within populations, and in the racial variation between populations, has furnished the means for the unique biological adaptation of *Homo sapiens sapiens*. Human control of the environment through intellect and social organization, flowing from and overtaking this process of adaptation, has furnished the means for further human evolution. If any relation exists between racial characteristics and the variant forms of society it is an obscure one. The same physical type can live in societies of every description. People of Mongoloid stock, for instance, live in societies that range from simple nomadic tribes of Siberia to the elaborate civilization of China. On the other hand, a diversity of racial types adapt themselves successfully to the industrial societies of Europe and America. Race cannot be regarded as the cause of a particular form of social organization or culture; races have no culture (9).

Race is only one type of genetic configuration among many that sociobiological theorists advance as a source of cultural variation. Nature and culture interact intimately and continuously to produce the evolutionary process. It has been plausibly argued, for example, that the neocortex evolved in prehistory out of the reciprocal interaction of the use of tools, the demands that use placed on the brain, and the minimum of social organization and culture engendered thereby (10). But the precise nature of the linkage between nature and culture remains much in dispute. An extreme version of sociobiology holds that genes are the key to human nature and behavior. Cultural beliefs, practices and values are to be explained by the manner in which they favor the propagation of selected, kin-based genes. Residual phenomena, those which resist such a functional explanation, are thought to be few and relatively insignificant, and may then be relegated to the cultural sphere (11).

One need not deny human biology to deny primacy to such sociobiological interpretations. Comparisons between human and other species are hazardous and, indeed, inadequate where they impinge on speech, learning, and the use of technology in human societies. Thus sociobiologists are often reduced to describing animal societies in terms of analogies and metaphors drawn from human cultures. Altruism, applied to the behavior of ants, can be no more than a human metaphor. In general, sociobiological explanations of society lack parsimony; to hypothesize underlying genes in order to account for social phenomena that are readily intelligible on cultural grounds alone is redundant. Language is a system of signifying, and of conferring meaning and value, as well as a means of conveying information. Even if the process of acquiring language should prove to be genetically based, once acquired it transforms learning, individual behavior, and society. The diversity of cultures and their histories emphasizes the plasticity rather than the rigidity of our genetic heritage. In practice, for example, the complex tangle of kinship bonds and the rights and obligations these entail render futile any attempt to describe them as a means to enhance the survival chances of a given set of genes (12).

Although genetic legacies may create dispositions and impose constraints, the outcome in human behavior rests on the interplay of natural endowment with specific context. One may leave open the question of the degree to which such endowment operates. Cultural evolution takes place in untried situations that call forth novel responses from groups whose biological substrate is shared more than it differs. Genes certainly confer special attributes on individuals, including mental and artistic abilities, which in a given environment are uniquely elicited and expressed. Whether genes confer special attributes on populations that are uniquely elicited and expressed in culture is a hypothesis that can be argued, but without obvious profit to social analysis (13) (see Chapter 9).

The responses of adults to social situations, which include medical situations, are influenced by the manner in which they were reared and educated and by the mode of life peculiar to their society, and do not correspond with intrinsic racial characteristics. In New Guinea, for example, two peoples of the same racial stock, the Mundugamor and the Arapesh, lived near each other, but behaved quite differently (14). Mundugamor adults of both sexes were aggressively "masculine" in their behavior. Love-making was conducted like a prize-fight, and biting and scratching were common elements in foreplay. The women were said to have an active dislike of childbearing and rarely demonstrated overt affection for their children. Mothers suckled their children while standing, and pushed them away from the breast as soon as they appeared in the least satisfied. The Arapesh presented a marked contrast. Both sexes were timid and gentle, and Arapesh men habitually nursed and fondled children. Their behavior generally would have been considered effeminate by European standards. Children were allowed a protracted period of dependency, few demands were made on them, and interest was focused on feeding and the mouth. Despite the carping of some critics about the subjectivism of these early observations, variability in the typical sex-role behavior of males and females of the same stock is a well-established cultural phenomenon.

Because everyone tends to judge the behavior of others by his or her own standards, there are many mistaken beliefs about racial characteristics. Some people believe that American Indians have no sense of humor because they rarely laugh aloud in public, while others believe that tribal Africans feel no pain because they do not weep or cry out when injured. All people feel and think, but the manner in which they express even the deepest and most universal emotions is culturally determined. Because the Gahuku of highland New Guinea have no word for "love" in their language does not mean that they lack affection or fail to express it, or that enduring bonds between the sexes are not formed (15). Similarly, the threshold for perceiving a painful stimulus does not vary much in humans, although tolerance for pain and ways of expressing it do, sometimes in systematic fashion across cultures (16). Our clinical observation in South Africa suggested that black industrial workers reacted differently from white and Coloured to the shock of mutilation, as in cases of hand and upper-limb injuries sustained in industrial accidents (17). Blacks did not commonly show the marked vasomotor and nervous response of pallor, nausea, tachycardia, tremor, weakness, fall in blood pressure, and fainting seen in white and Coloured.

It seems likely that the reactions of these black urban workers to mutilation were related to general attitudes towards pain and injury acquired in the tribal societies from which many of them came. In the same way, an African woman's response to the lower abdominal pain of acute gonococcal salpingitis may seem exaggerated to European doctors, but it is of a piece with anxieties about sterility and the womb in tribal societies where barrenness is treated almost as an offence. In childbirth the same woman will be stoical.

Reactions to disease and pain are thus bound up with whole systems of beliefs, values, and modes of expression that influence people to respond distinctively when exposed to similar situations. In the Second World War troops of contrasting culture campaigning in the same conditions displayed contrasting sickness behavior. In the jungles of Arakan, Indian soldiers had lower rates of mental breakdown than their

British counterparts and their distress was not evoked by the same things. Hand-to-hand fighting, killing, and capture troubled the Indians less than the British; loss of face, physical ailments, and hospital care troubled them more (18).

Values, closed systems of thought, and sickness behavior

The incursion of social science into the health field has made familiar the notion that values—criteria by which people judge the moral worth or virtue of conduct—are determinants of the health behavior of health professionals as well as patients. Values are neither uniformly applied nor universally accepted, but vary across communities and social classes. Karl Marx and Emile Durkheim among others taught us that the relativity of morals and values derives from the structure of societies and the position accorded different social groups. Plato discussed this question in Book III of *The Republic:*

> ... Aesculapius was aware that, in all well-regulated communities, each has work assigned to him in the state which he must needs do, and that no one has leisure to spend his life as an invalid in the doctor's hands: a fact which we perceive in the case of the laboring populations, but which with ludicrous inconsistency we fail to detect in the case of those who are rich and happy.
>
> When a carpenter is ill, he expects to receive a draught from his doctor that will expel the disease by vomiting or purging, or else to get rid of it by cauterizing, or a surgical operation; but if any one were to prescribe for him a long course of diet, and to order bandages for his head, with other treatment to correspond, he would soon tell such a medical advisor that he had no time to be ill, and hint that it was not worth his while to live in this way, devoting his mind to his malady, and neglecting his proper occupation: and then, wishing his physician a good morning, he would enter upon his usual course of life, and either regain his health and live in the performance of his business; or, should his constitution prove unable to bear up, death puts an end to his troubles. Yes, and for a man in that station of life, this is thought the proper use to make of medical assistance. ...

Values denote not so much properties or traits as they do dispositions to act in certain ways under certain conditions. They exist not merely in the mind of the actor but are embedded in social practices themselves. Values have their underlying causes in economic and class interests, in political and social power, and in the culture created by the historical evolution of societies. Context plays a crucial role in determining which of the available value systems will be activated and how (19).

The clinical encounter is one context in which values are exercised. Doctors and patients, even when reared in the same society, can have widely divergent cultural values and responses, and each is likely to interpret the other's behavior in terms of his or her own values and beliefs. Even when divergence is recognized, either may ascribe distasteful behavior in the other to moral turpitude, stupidity, or to some other personal, genetic, or racial weakness. In American teaching hospitals and medical schools, hostile attitudes of teachers and students towards "crocks" (non-fee-paying charity patients with ill-defined multiple disorders in addition to their poverty) have been several times documented (20). An extreme example often occurs when a doctor from a Western culture is confronted with witchcraft beliefs in African patients.

Most Westerners would accept that the "cause" of tuberculosis is the tubercle bacillus. But an African tribesman may not accept this explanation, and may refuse to follow the treatment prescribed, because he believes that witchcraft is the important "cause" of his illness. He may accept the existence of bacilli shown under a microscope, and yet reject this as the sole cause of his illness. For him the presence of these bacilli does not explain why they happen to be active now, when before they did not harm him, nor why they are in his own lungs, and not in those of someone else. While he may not deny that the bacilli harm him, the tribesman attributes the coincidence of his illness at that particular time not to change in himself, nor predisposition, nor excessive exposure as we might do, but to supernatural forces operated by a witch who hates him.

Witchcraft is therefore a theory of multiple causality, and also a system of beliefs that explains *why* an event occurs, and not only *how* it occurs. (The example also shows that modern technical "hows" need not conflict with traditional "whys"; neat accommodations between the two systems of causality can be found in a number of preliterate societies (21).) Although theories of multiple causality are fashionable among epidemiologists of today, this rival mode of thinking appears unreasonable to most Westerners because they do not accept the existence of supernatural agencies, at least not in the form of witchcraft.

A classic analysis of the system of witchcraft beliefs held by the Azande tribe, an African people, showed that their mode of thought is less illogical than at first appears (22). If an Azande man stubs his toe against a tree stump while walking along a path, and the wound subsequently festers and troubles him, he puts this down to witchcraft. He does not exclude the immediate cause of his injury, the knock against the tree stump. He reflects that on other walks along this path he did not stub his toe and, if he did, the wound did not turn septic. He reasons then that the significant cooperating cause is not his own carelessness, but the malice of a witch, probably someone among his neighbors who bears him a grudge, and that he did not see this particular stump on this particular occasion because, for a moment, witchcraft blinded him. Witchcraft is called on to explain the singularity of experience, why one event or its consequences should differ from other similar events.

This mode of reasoning is a closed system of thought, in that given the initial premise it cannot readily be denied. In the absence of competing belief systems that are as strongly rooted in the texture of a culture, it provides a logical explanation by interrelating otherwise haphazard and meaningless events. Witchcraft is therefore used only to explain events and behavior that lack manifest motive. It cannot make a person lie, or steal, or commit adultery or assault, nor can it excuse failure in achievement if a person is stupid, clumsy, or careless. As a mode of reasoning for contingencies, witchcraft does not displace common sense, but fills the gaps and addresses the questions unexplained by common sense. Like religious systems of belief everywhere, witchcraft seeks to go behind appearances, to relate the seemingly unrelated, to account for the anomalous and to render the inexplicable intelligible within a coherent order of ideas (23).

Africans are not exceptional in seeking an answer to the profound human question of why events occur (24). Some people believe in the Will of God, others in Luck or Fate or Destiny, and others are content with materialist determinism or the theory of probability. This variability appears in the responses of persons in our society to such misfortune as sickness, or bereavement, or the birth of a handicapped child. On these occasions, as in Camus' *The Plague*, some turn to the consolation of religion, others forswear a belief in a god who could so harm them.

In contemporary Western society all these beliefs are found together; many religious, philosophical, and psychological systems, as well as some political systems, also use logical constructs to explain the totality of events in terms traceable to premises that are articles of faith. The universality of such systems and their imperviousness to skepticism derive from the sense of purpose and reassurance they provide for human beings confronted with the mysteries of existence. These coherent bodies of beliefs and values enable people to respond to misfortune, or moral transgression, or unhappiness, or to take some action when they are caught up in conflict.

The unarticulated hallmarks of witchcraft belief and thought—internal consistency, resistance to change, ability to absorb seemingly anomalous information, and absence of skepticism—are common to many of the closed systems of belief and thought current in industrial societies. Indeed, studies in the history and philosophy of Western science have revealed parallels in the tenacity with which scientific theories have been held in the face of evidence they cannot accommodate. Society plays a role in shaping both the old and the new ideas as well as what is relevant research, although the precise nature of social influence remains much in dispute (25).

Different systems of belief and opposed values lead to social conflict. Legal systems conflict with medical ones in their reluctance to allow medical and psychological explanations to diminish individual responsibility for crime or sin (26). Medical explanations of criminal behavior sometimes go contrary to the values enshrined in the legal code. In this code, the limits of individual responsibility for crimes committed by mentally disordered persons are closely defined. The law depends on continuity and precedents from the past. By contrast, the shifting ground of advancing medical knowledge and opinion threatens the permanence of the legal and penal code, because medical definitions of responsibility shift accordingly. In addition, the clinical approach denies the applicability of a law to every case.

To put this in another way, a conflict exists between the medical view that a criminal may be sick and need medical treatment, and the legal view that a criminal must be held responsible for his antisocial acts and should be punished. In English law a striking example was to be found, prior to the Suicide Act of 1961, in the treatment of persons who attempted suicide. Many were brought before the courts. Male homosexuals, too, were imprisoned whether or not psychiatrists held them to be sick men. (The American Psychiatric Association deleted homosexuality as a category of mental disorder from its diagnostic manual in 1973.) The greatest controversy, however, is provoked by the sociopath or psychopathic criminal because judgments of his clinical status are often uncertain, and depend in part on the antisocial behavior for which the courts would punish him.

The legal system and the system of medical care provide alternative and sometimes competing mechanisms for dealing with the social strains of deviance (27). Among the questions raised by the family planning and women's rights movements, for instance, the demand for legalizing abortion posed an acute challenge for obstetrics. The medical monopoly over this procedure was acquired in the 19th century, wrested in competition from the unsafe hands of untrained midwives. The consequent illegality of induced abortion except for specified indications eliminated it as a means of fertility control. As a result, safe abortion was denied to any women who insisted upon it. Gradually the refusal of obstetricians to perform abortions was eroded by humanist pressures. The discovery of teratogens like rubella and thalidomide helped in the erosion, but most of all the infiltration of issues of the mother's mental health undermined the established position. Finally, what had become an acute political and moral issue was depoliticized in Britain, by making the right to abortion a matter of medical judgment. Later, in the United States, it was made an individual woman's legal right. The ruling of the Supreme Court that accomplished this shift in the United States was instructive. The justices provided various legal grounds for abortion, including particularly the health of the mother. At the same time, they extended the definition of maternal health to defuse many questions of values. Included under the definition of health effects were such circumstances as the "stigma of unwed motherhood" and "the distress for all concerned associated with the unwanted child" (28).

The hundred years from the mid-nineteenth to the mid-twentieth century saw the rise of large medical institutions commited to the custodial care of patients suffering from mental illness and mental subnormality. For patients suffering from disorders such as the organic psychoses and severe mental deficiency, these institutions provided a substitute for the home and the social and nursing care that indigent families were unable to provide. But for sociopaths (i.e., psychopaths, so-called high-grade mental defectives, "moral imbeciles," narcotic addicts), and for some patients with functional psychoses, these institutions provided a means of constraining and disciplining individuals whose behavior, while it could not be termed criminal, deviated from standards acceptable to the values of the community. Admissions to institutions of persons with mild mental retardation commonly resulted from a combination of deviant behavior and homelessness (29). In the late nineteenth century custody became a prominent social function of medicine, in part by the default of social support for the masses of migrants to the cities, in part because the domain of medicine had been enlarged to encompass and treat a wider range of social disorders. A conflict was thus established between professional values of treatment and cure and managerial functions of detention and control.

The conflict is not easily resolved, since medicine has a social duty that it cannot escape. The actual functions of medicine in society extend beyond its avowed function. In industrial societies this avowed function is at the organic level, to cure and prevent disease. But it is quite evident that medicine has an additional function at the personal level. This is to reassure and to allay anxiety in individuals, whether healthy or diseased, who in their distress turn to the doctor; nearly half of patient visits in the United States were found to be for complaints with no readily ascertainable organic basis (30). Work at the personal rather than the organic level is the standby of the doctor in prescientific societies; in the idiom introduced earlier and in marked contrast to much of modern medicine, traditional healers treat illness—persons in felt distress—rather than disease, and their credits in this area balance their debits with organic disease (31).

Medicine has a third function at the social level. This is the function that brings medicine into the area of social control. Sickness for which a person demands or accepts medical care is a deviation from the norms for the everyday performance of social roles. All societies have social mechanisms to deal with the strains and conflicts that deviance of any kind inevitably creates (32). In many traditional societies, healers go beyond the diagnosis and treatment of individual ailments; they also use the occasion of illness to search for the presence of unresolved conflicts in the patient's social circle that both may have caused the trouble and could impair recovery. Techniques of cure, in turn, may have the intended effect of reordering the social context—relatives may be enlisted in healing ceremonies and allegiances reaffirmed in a social catharsis. Sickness, that is, is made to signify the presence of underlying social disorder of which one person's symptoms are but the surface evidence (33).

The power wielded by authorized healers is universally recognized. In preliterate societies, the sick may be treated by traditional doctors or by priests or lay healers. In industrial societies, the sick are dealt with by vast and growing systems of medical care. Here is a paradox. This modern burgeoning of medicine has gained its strength from an armamentarium of technical facilities and treatments, and these are controlled by ever-narrowing specialties based on discrete organ systems or on particular technical expertise. Yet, at the same time, the bounds of medical competence have been extended, and medicine deals increasingly with personal and social problems. Its implicit function is to adjust the capacities of individuals to the complicated behavior demanded of them by their society (34).

This appears in the common dilemma that faces doctors in issuing a certificate of sickness to cover a patient's absence from work. Practitioners in Britain often receive requests for such certificates from patients who have no detectable disease, frequently for short absences and sometimes for longer ones (35). Individual deviance is inevitable, and in this instance dysfunction—whether for manifest illness or not—is connected with an economic and social system that requires a strict and time-bound conformity in work from most people, in return for which they gain regular employment and financial security.

The problem for doctors lies in the conflict between the responsibilities incurred through their contract with the state, which imposes on them a duty to certify accurately that sickness was a cause of absence, and their professional obligation to their patients, which requires that they should maintain strict confidence and do their best to help the sick. This conflict in medical practice is reported to have been acute in the Soviet Union at the time when the state placed a heavy responsibility upon the doctors to maintain the labor force at work (36). In Britain and the United States, it is equally a conflict for industrial medical officers who accept similar responsibilities and duties from the firms that employ them, as well as for physicians in the employ of the armed services (37). Doctors may find themselves pressed to accommodate their professional values, their concepts of health, and their criteria of what constitutes sickness to the demands of employers and patients. In Britain, when welfare supports were complemented by full employment opportunities, the practitioner resolved the conflicts of sickness certification by establishing a norm of compromise in responding to patient requests. In some countries where the worker is heavily dependent on keeping his job, it is not unknown for cash bribes to resolve the conflicts.

The functions of medicine in social control were of special concern to the early sociologists of medicine, such as Talcott Parsons. From the perspective of maintaining a given social order, the sick-role was seen as a unique means of containing and neutralizing potential threats. In exchange for strict adherence to a regimen of care, the patient is offered conditional exemption from customary responsibilities. One effect of the act of diagnosis is to remove responsibility for illness from the individual and to attribute it instead to forces outside individual control (1,38). The resultant dependence of the sick on the nonsick prevents coalitions of the dissatisfied from forming and confines the attention of the sick to the task of getting better. Implied in the notion of sickness as deviance is the proposition that sickness is a kind of refusal. To fall sick is to withdraw from the demands of everyday life. "Taking a sick day," for example, legitimizes what may be a needed respite from a demanding job. For Parsons, sickness is both an expression of real suffering and a protest against the conditions that require such suffering.

In summary, medicine as a social institution is empowered both to treat disease, a technical function, and to validate the felt distress of illness in terms of sickness, a social function (39). In the latter function, medicine reflects the interests of the wider society in which it is embedded. Medicine treats not only disease but also the uncertainty, frustration, or anger that illness may occasion, and the social dislocations of sickness. The fact that the "why?" of affliction is not well tended to in developed societies does not mean that the question ceases to be asked. In birth and death, and in the pain and dysfunction of disease, medicine performs—simply by virtue of the circumstances of its practice—what in traditional societies was the priestly function of enabling people to cope with human trials (31).

Communication between doctors and patients

Members of industrial societies differ in race, sex, age, occupation, status, and a host of other personal and social characteristics. Many of them may be members of localized groups with such distinct patterns of speech, habits, values, and standards that they may be distinguished as a subculture within society. The accidents of geography, history, and economic development tend to produce these distinctive local groups in large-scale societies: within Britain people may be Welsh or Scots, Lancastrians or Yorkshiremen, Londoners or Mancunians, although they are all British. In South Africa there are Afrikaners, Zulus, Indians, and so on. In the United States a multitude of subgroups exists: they are defined by region, as between North and South, East and West; by color, as between whites, blacks, and Native Americans; by ethnicity, as between Hispanics, Irish, Italians, and many others; by religion, as between Protestants, Catholics, Jews, and the many cohesive sects like the Hutterites, the Amish, and the Hasidim. Thus, the national and regional groups are marked by particular clusters of occupations, customs, dialects, religious beliefs, and idiosyncratic modes of behavior that distinguish them clearly from one another, although all are united within the same economic, social, and political framework.

In addition to these distinctions, persons of different occupation and upbringing in industrial societies have specific cultural characteristics related to their social class position. In the United States as in Britain, members of the "upper classes" differ in occupation and recreation, modes of speech, social conventions, and system of values from members of the "lower classes." These forms of social behavior and modes of social interaction are the source of subjective feelings of social class and class loyalties (40). People can be observed to categorize others favorably as "people like us," or pejoratively as "them," and to adjust their behavior accordingly. National, regional, and class characteristics influence diffuse personal relations generally as well as the more particular choice of spouses, friends, and neighbors. The behavior of individuals in industrial societies is therefore complex and variable, and their values often conflict.

Doctors and individuals. These conflicts are important in the practice of medicine, particularly in the matter of communication between doctors and patients. Communication is not merely, or solely, a matter of language: both acts and words may be given different interpretations by different people. In an Israeli study, patients were asked, before seeing the doctor and again afterward, whether they considered they had a dangerous or a minor illness; the doctors were asked to make a similar rating (41). Forty per cent of those patients rated by the doctor as having minor illness had thought, before seeing the doctor, that their condition was serious. The doctors rated less than 10 per cent of the patients' conditions as serious. After seeing the doctor, 10 of the 40 per cent no longer thought their condition serious but the original number was exactly retained by the substitution of others who had come to think their illness serious. In the patients' perception of their illnesses, hardly any shift could be attributed to the consultation. Although the doctors did in fact succeed in communicating instructions about treatment that were understood by their patients, they had not succeeded in communicating either reassurance or information about disease.

All doctors have been harassed at one time or another by the apparent illogicality of some patients, who appear to hold ignorant and mistaken beliefs concerning the nature of their troubles. Most have been frustrated as well by patients who fail to comply with prescribed treatment regimens. But consideration of the patients' beliefs in terms of their social background and the peculiar circumstances of the clinical encounter may show that there is reason in the "illogicality" or "noncompliance." Failure to communicate, to understand, or to follow through may result from a clash in cultural views, views that produce different expectations, different agendas, and, consequently, different criteria for what constitutes a satisfactory doctor-patient transaction.

Studies of doctor-patient interaction have revealed just how discordant this clash of perspectives can be and how it may impair and even defeat the original purpose of the visit. Doctor and patient come to the encounter each burdened by a distinct set of questions, propelled by different motives, and ready to proceed along lines of inquiry that need not coincide. For a doctor working in a clinic, "seeing" the next patient is routine, part of workaday reality; it is an occasion for the presentation of a problem, elicitation of the information needed to assess it, and determination of an appropriate course of action. Rarely is it something out of the ordinary. The physician's foremost objective is a practical one: to fashion the information gleaned from the patient into a pattern which can then be compared with textbook descriptions of disease types or past clinical experience, and from which prognosis and treatment follow.

For the patient, the circumstances of the encounter are strikingly different. Illness interrupts daily life in ways that range from minor irritation to crippling pain or disability. Almost by definition, a visit to the doctor is out of the ordinary, accompanied by uncertainty, anxiety, and dependency. At the extreme, it is occasioned by a crisis thought to be life threatening. The doctor is there to diagnose and treat; the patient is there to seek understanding, reassurance, and help.

Given the divergent agendas of the two parties to the encounter some degree of confusion is inevitable. Regular compliance with medical prescription is not to be expected (42). Should a doctor make a diagnosis of tuberculosis, for example, a situation fertile for misunderstanding and discord is created. The doctor will understand that the patient has a serious and possibly long-lasting disease, although nowadays a cure can be expected in a few months. The physician no longer fears later complications, nor subsequently imposes restrictions on the patient's habits other than those of moderate living. In accord with cultural precept, the patient may view the matter otherwise. Tuberculosis may conjure up the specter of "galloping consumption"; it may be regarded as a sentence of death, a curse on one's family, a punishment for sin. Some people, English and American, attach a stigma to the disease, and consider the whole family of a patient as contaminated and dangerous, an attitude that often extends to cancer patients as well (43). In another example, for a middle-aged man, in for a routine physical, to be told that he has "essential hypertension" of unknown origin, and that he will have to restrict his salt intake and avoid stressful situations where possible, and faithfully take a lifelong medication which may produce impotence and dizziness as side effects, and for all this to happen when he came in for the examination feeling fine, is for him to contract an illness where before he had only an undetected and asymptomatic disease.

Under the terms and conditions of the clinical encounter, moreover, it is the doctor's agenda that takes priority. In the language of medical practice, patients—and especially "problem patients"—are "managed." From recordings of actual doctor-patient interactions, it is possible to construct a set of implicit rules that govern the behavior of both parties in the encounter. Doctors tend to control not only the terms, but also the content and duration of the exchange. They may explain the workings of disease in the technical language of their profession, to the bewilderment of their patients. Many patients do not feel at liberty to question or to counter the doctor's pronouncements, or to interpose unanswered queries of their own. One study of 800 mothers consulting pediatricians about their children's ailments, for example, found that nearly half the mothers left the doctor's office without a clear understanding of what was wrong with their child. Some 300 mothers felt that they somehow bore responsibility for their child's illness; over a quarter had not voiced their gravest worry, either because they were blocked from doing so or felt it to be inappropriate (44).

In general, patients tend to be passive, undemanding, and obedient. Silence on the patient's part, mistaken by the doctor for concurrence, may mask simple confusion. A mother who nods agreeably at a doctor's suggestion of dietary changes may yet fail to comply with the diet and in the eyes of the physician "sabotages" the treatment, never having understood the need for it in the first place. The asymmetry of the exchange can be redressed when the rules of the clinical encounter are no longer in force. When recounting a visit to the doctor to friends, patients frequently portray themselves as much more active, assertive, and controlling than they were in fact during the consultation (45).

The clinical encounter is embedded within a wider array of social relationships and cultural practices. In the colonial situation of North Africa, for example, compliance with prescribed treatment was hampered by the distortions of the white doctor–black patient relationship (46). In the United States, power relations in the society at large infiltrate in various ways the clinical situation, as when a black, lower-classs woman is treated by a white, upper-class physician (47). Discrepancies are intensified by the vulnerability and dependency that the patient role entails.

Cultural influences operate at a number of levels and through various channels. Belief systems, modes of perception, and labeling practices,° as well as the values attached to suffering and impairment, all influence the experience and expression of illness. In effect, people learn to be ill in culturally sanctioned ways, just as they must learn to court, to grieve, or to celebrate. The health problems that people perceive, the gravity imputed to certain symptoms or disease labels, how and where help is sought, are all affected. How one comprehends and responds to a bout of illness, accordingly, will be influenced by the heterogeneities of culture associated with social class, ethnic background, education, occupation, and religious affiliation (50).

Cultural discrepancies between doctors and patients, and between types of patients, can be found in any stratified society. In New York City, no less than elsewhere, ethnic groups have orientations to disease and the use of medical services that vary in the degree that they are based in folklore or science. One study of whites, Puerto Ricans, and blacks showed that the greater the cohesion and exclusiveness of the ethnic group and the stronger its ties with family and friends, the more people were oriented to folk medicine, skeptical of medical care, and ready to look to their own social group for comfort in illness (51). Conversely, in Salt Lake City, an ethnically homogeneous community well integrated into mainstream American culture, no association was found between tight social ties and distrust of modern medicine (52).

Our examples illustrate how failures in communication residing in the undiscerned incongruence of subcultures and the inherent inequalities of the clinical situation may affect the manner of treatment, and limit the use of facilities and the acceptance of treatment. An estimated 70 to 90 per cent of all illness episodes are handled outside the formal system of medical care (53). Some women, even when in danger of their lives, refuse to enter maternity hospitals. Again, maternity and child welfare services are used least by those who are usually considered to need them most (54). People

---

°"Labeling" results when a diagnosis assigned to an individual carries implications of a stigmatized identity that override the other status attributes of the individual. The initial use of the term was with reference to mental illness (48); another application has been to mental retardation (49).

with symptoms of such critical disorders as malignant new growths delay in seeking treatment, and find psychological mechanisms to deny the existence of the condition even when they have been carefully told of it (55).

Health professionals and communities. Failures of communication at the community level occur for many reasons. Sometimes the values propounded ignore the exigencies of livelihood. An example is provided by a nutrition program in rural Colombia (56). A careful study of nutritional status, food purchasing and consumption, and crop yields documented the existence of protein deficiency. The research team concluded that to correct this protein deficiency, the community need only withhold 7 per cent of its soya crop from the market for home consumption. Such advice had little chance of acceptance in the face of the objective circumstances: 30 per cent of the people were landless and an additional 50 per cent owned too little for subsistence; the cooperative arrangements of the community economy had long since withered in the face of wage labor; and the costs of foregoing cash income from the crop were imminent and immediate, while the gains in stature and weight were deferred and not self-evident.

More subtle problems arise when the values propounded are at odds with the nonexplicit value system of a community. Such a conflict was illustrated by an attempt at mental health education in Canada. A great many people fear psychiatric treatment—although less so than in the past—and even some general practitioners have been reluctant to suggest this form of treatment for their patients. Many persons confronted with mental disorder tend to judge and to act by standards remote from those accepted by science and medicine. To overcome these difficulties in the way of bringing people early into treatment in the community, a psychiatric team devised a mental health education program and tested it in a small town (57). They took such precautions as enlisting the support of local organizations and talking to the leaders of the community. They tested people to discern their attitudes towards mental illness, and repeated these tests at the end of a six-month campaign to evaluate its effect. During the campaign they publicized a set of propositions throughout the community which they hoped would lead to the social acceptance of mentally ill persons, and thereby block popular misconceptions that drove patients into hospitals.

These propositions were: first, that the range of normal behavior is wider than is ordinarily believed; second, that abnormal behavior does not simply happen but has a cause, and therefore can be understood and often cured; and third, that abnormality and normality are not distinct but shade into one another in a continuum. The townspeople not only accepted the first proposition but went beyond the psychiatrists in the range of behavior they regarded as "normal." They accepted the second proposition too, and could be persuaded that mental illness was curable. But the third proposition, which blurred the line between normal and abnormal, provoked anxiety and hostility, and by the end of the campaign people had begun to boycott the psychiatrists' meetings, film shows, and other activities. Finally the team secretary, a local person and a supporter of the campaign, was herself admitted to the hospital in an acute anxiety state.

The psychiatrists explained this reaction as follows. People feared mental illness and were made anxious by it. They would rather ignore than confront it. Hence, they tolerated unusual behavior without attributing it to mental illness. But when, finally, an individual had exhausted tolerance, people at once wished him or her packed off to the hospital and segregated as a danger to the community. Admission to the hospital identified the sick person as different; it was the dividing line between sanity and insanity.

The third proposition attacked this attitude of the community: if people admitted that abnormality was merely one end of a continuum, then a sick person might not be "different" from themselves, and segregation was not an obvious answer to the problem. This logic created a threat to their system of values, as well as to their sense of security, for it implied that anyone could become "different"—that is, insane. Attitudes toward the mental hospital were ambivalent, because although admission was felt to place the indelible stigma of insanity on the patient, people wished to believe that a hospital could cure, and that they were consigning the sick person to a good place. The ambivalence had its source in the definition of "insanity" as "sickness." The discomfort of two values in conflict caused people to reject the theories of the psychiatrists.

Other interpretations could be put on this result. To health educators, as to most doctors, optimism and the conviction that professional knowledge is superior to lay beliefs are necessary to effective practice. Faith and conviction sometimes lie close to a didactic approach that evokes hostility and blocks understanding in controversial matters. As this experiment illustrated, what is controversial for a given group is specific to its system of values, and can only be discovered by studying these values.

Values are always at work in the behavior of individuals, and dissimilar values may induce courses of action that are directly opposed, even when motives are similar. Dissimilar values confuse understanding between individuals in many social situations, and all medical situations are social situations. Doctors need to be aware of the social determinants of their own practices and attitudes (58). Cultural values cannot be neglected in clinical assessments by doctors of their individual patients, for these have helped to shape the personality and capacities of both parties, and to determine their customary beliefs and behavior.

The use of services involves transactions between users and dispensers. To ensure effective use, both sides of the transaction need to be considered. Health and medical activities rely for their effect on the transmission of messages about health to patients and communities. Responses can be seen as a sequence of perceptions, first about illness, second about action against illness (59). Whether a person allows symptoms to rise above the threshold of complaint depends on the ways in which that person perceives illness and is moved to act about it as well as on relevant social relations and situations (50,60).

To begin with, the perception of a health condition has two phases: a person may or may not interpret a condition as illness, and if one perceives it as illness, one may or may not perceive oneself as being susceptible to the illness and threatened by it. For instance, in Britain smokers with morning cough and sputum, and in Egypt fellaheen (peasants) with blood in the urine from schistosome parasite infection in the bladder, may share their disorders with a majority of their age and sex peers, and often they either do not consider themselves to be ill at all, or regard these potentially serious symptoms as trivial. The effect of the perception of a threat to health has been demonstrated in studies, among others, of health care in children. In a school health program parents who considered their children unusually susceptible to illness were more likely to carry out the instructions given (61). In a prophylactic program against the recurrence of rheumatic fever, those whose children had had rheumatic fever and who believed they would suffer a recurrence took fuller part (62). Within a single industrial society, as in the United States, education is a critical variable in the amount and the kind of information that can be taken to underlie shared cultural perceptions of the threat posed by illness (63).

In the literate society of the United States, however, psychological readiness to seek care contributes but a small part of the variance that exists in the actual use of services. The second part of the sequence of perceptions leading to the use of health services—perception of the action to be taken—contributes more. This part of the sequence also has two phases: first, once a person has perceived a condition as an illness threatening health, he or she must recognize avenues of action to deal with it; second, he or she must see those avenues of action as appropriate, helpful, and preferable to the threat of illness. People classify illness within rubrics of the common lore of their culture; among the most educated the classification will be the closest to that of contemporary medicine.

The class to which the illness is assigned is a guide to what help it is appropriate to seek. In South Asia, for example, a peasant can turn for aid to herbalists, snakebite specialists, diviners, and the vaidyas and hakims trained in the ancient ways of Indian folk medicine. In the previous chapter we noted that a similar array of treatment agencies is available to, and used by, the migrant workers in the growing towns of South Africa. In these circumstances, native informants tend to report that mental illness and chronic vague disorders are often assigned to folk treatment, and injury or severe illness with well-defined symptoms to "scientific" treatment. They also report resorting to the alternative agency in the event of the failure of the first to deal adequately with the presented problem. In actual practice, however, multiple therapeutic use is the rule, often owing to the divergent preferences of various members of the extended family network. In industrial societies, too, exchanges of patients, often unwitting, occur between "respectable" and "fringe" practitioners (64).

A limiting condition in the use of services is their accessibility, a term which takes in costs, availability and visibility. In a national survey in the United States, among people who recognized that they had personal problems, knowledge about services and their accessibility influenced use more than did the psychological factors of the perception and interpretation of the nature of their problems (65). Use of such services depends upon the participation of the agency as well as of the patient, and health agencies may not appear as blandly neutral or as welcoming to patients as they feel themselves to be (66). Burdensome costs, confusion and inefficiency in the delivery of care, and uncomprehending behavior on the part of providers all play a role in the willingness of community members to make use of health care facilities (66). Clinics may be seen as hostile by some patients, and among those who make little use of services feelings of rejection are common. Studies within hospitals in England and the United States give clues to the objective basis for such unlooked-for reactions (67). Explanations of illness given by staff are tailored to the patient's education and social class. Those who seem to know less receive less. Thus clinical interaction is partly a function of the social distance between the patient and the source of care.

To modify the structure and culture of institutions is likely to prove easier than to modify the cultural attitudes of social groups. Indeed, experiment shows that the behavior of staff toward patients can be changed. In the emergency clinic of a Boston hospital a new policy prescribed prompt and detailed personal attention for alochol- ics, long a category of patients considered untreatable, with avoidance of undue wait- ing and cursory contact. A spectacular rise in the return rate of these patients resulted. Staff action modified the response of the alcoholic patients, and in turn these responses modified staff attitudes to alcoholics (68).

Culture and health disorders

In the annals of medical investigation, the solution to problems has often emerged only as the role of some cultural practice has been suspected and traced. A dramatic example is the story of kuru, a fatal neurological disorder. In 1953, in a highland New Guinea hamlet, an Australian government patrol observed a small girl "shivering vio- lently . . . her head jerking spasmodically from side to side." Her kinspeople saw her as a victim of sorcery, and considered death imminent. The log of this patrol provides the first official description of the disease.

By 1957, epidemiological studies had established that kuru was confined to the Fore (a slash-and-burn agricultural group) and those neighbors with whom they intermar- ried, that it ran in families, and that it attacked women and children primarily (69). The original impression of Western clinicians that it was a form of hysteria culturally induced through fear of sorcery had to be discarded in the face of the gross damage to the central nervous system of its victims. Clinically, kuru progresses from a first stage of subtle difficulties of motor coordination which might be apparent only to the victim, through a second stage with spasms, trembling, emotional lability, and loco- motor difficulty, until in a third and final stage there is total disability with shaking, incoordination, difficulty in swallowing, and inability even to sit up. Death usually follows within a year of onset (70). For Fore males, it was estimated, not less than one in five could expect to contract the disease. For Fore females nine out of ten could expect to succumb to kuru before completing their childbearing years (71).

The pattern of familial aggregation and high incidence in a small interrelated pop- ulation at once provided the basis for a genetic hypothesis. For such a hypothesis to explain a common disorder, the disease must have been present for generations. Native informants were certain that kuru first made its appearance well within the memory of elder tribesmen, however, not more than 40 years before. They were able, too, to trace the progress of the disease from community to community after its arrival from the north. But Fore seeking work out of their home territory had not carried kuru with them. It was slowly realized that the familial distribution fitted no regular

Mendelian pattern; kuru was a disease of women and children of either sex, but adult males were seldom affected.

Fore culture was marked by a sharp segregation of the lives of men and women. Men resided communally in separate dwellings, spending their days together disputing or hunting small game. Women resided with their children and their pigs, and performed most of the agricultural work. Men had first claim on high-quality protein sources, wild and domestic pig especially. Wild game had become scarce with the depletion of the forest reserves, and Fore women and children (and a few older men) had adopted the practice, early in this century, of cooking and eating flesh of deceased kin, not excluding those who had died from kuru. By 1962, a similarity between the pattern of cannibalism and the epidemiological profile of kuru was noted. The preparation and distribution of the cannibalized flesh was a matter for female kin and children, an assignment of rights and duties that could account for the imperfect mimicry of a genetic disorder. Still, no alternative mode of transmission had been identified.

The resolution came in 1966, when after a three-year wait, kuru was shown to have been transmitted from affected human brains to the chimpanzee (72). In 1959, striking similarities had been remarked in the pathologies of kuru and scrapie, a neural degenerative disease of sheep. Scrapie was known to be an infectious disorder, transmissible by inoculation, but only after remarkably long incubation periods of up to several years. Kuru, like scrapie, indeed turned out to be a "slow virus" infection.

The picture, allowing for expected differences in individual susceptibility, now appears complete. Water boils at a lower temperature at the high altitudes of the New Guinea highlands; cooking infected flesh under such conditions would not inactivate the virus. The mode of transmission was probably through cuts in the skin, rather than through ingestion. In the late 1950s, the Australian government had suppressed cannibalism. Consistent with a break in the chain of transmission, the distribution of the disease changed. In the early 1960s, the childhood cases all but disappeared, and throughout the 1960s and 1970s annual incidence continued to decline. By May of 1978, the youngest case of kuru was over 20 years old. New cases showed a more balanced sex ratio, such as would be anticipated after long incubation in victims infected in childhood, when both boys and girls partook of cooked flesh (73,74).

To this day the Fore believe kuru to be the work of sorcerers in their midst. Cultural beliefs about the origins of illness express fundamental notions about the nature of reality as well, and are not dislodged by the mere presence of a suspect—and, not obviously superior—competitor (74). Alert cultural observation has led, in the case of kuru, to the discovery of a new class of infective processes of far-reaching significance. In this respect, it is but the latest of several discoveries in which cultural observation had a signal role.

Examples which show how the customs of a people affect their physical health are legion. It is scarcely surprising that tetanus neonatorum is common among those African peoples who apply a herbalist's mixture containing powdered dung to the cut cord of each newborn baby, or where tetanus spores shed by domestic animals lie thick about the huts with their caked dung floors (75). Nor is it surprising that the men of the Karamajong tribe of East Africa, whose diet includes a daily pint of blood drawn from the jugular veins of their cattle, should be better nourished, with higher red cell counts, than men of neighboring tribes who do not have this custom (76).

Distinctive cultures create distinctive patterns of health and disease, even within the confines of a single town. In Durban, for instance, Africans and Indians lived side by side, strikingly unlike in their habits and customs (77); the stillbirth and infant mortality rates for each ethnic group were also strikingly unlike. These health indices were studied in detail in four separate neighborhoods: in an African slum and an Indian one, and in an African housing project and an Indian one (78). Both ethnic groups therefore lived under comparable conditions, divided between neighborhoods of slum housing and good housing, each with a different array of the material and biological factors known to influence rates for stillbirth and infant mortality.

Africans in both housing project and slum had higher income and less overcrowding than Indians in either. African mothers had had more formal education than Indian mothers, they were younger, had borne fewer children, and had made more use of the antenatal and midwifery services. African babies in Durban also tend to be heavier than Indian babies. In these respects the African mothers had an advantage over the Indian mothers, for older mothers are known to lose more babies at birth than young mothers, mothers of high parity lose more than those of lower parity, and light babies are at higher risk of death than heavier ones (below an optimum weight) (79). In addition, in a situation of this kind, the use of maternity services reduces the risk of perinatal infant deaths (80). Indian mothers were favored only by smaller rates of first births and of illegitimacy, both of which carry a higher risk. Although the Indian mothers had a lower rate of positive blood tests for syphilis, this advantage was reduced because the African mothers made more use of facilities for treatment.

The Indian mothers had a clear disadvantage in this array of factors, but they nevertheless had consistently lower rates for stillbirth and for infant mortality, particularly neonatal mortality, than the African mothers in either housing estate or slum (See Figure 4.1). Although racial factors may contribute to these results, their distinctive culture assisted Indian mothers in adapting to poor conditions. Traditional methods of confinement, infant feeding, and child care derived from the villages and cities of India seemed to be better suited to urban life in South African than practices derived from tribal life in Africa.

There are innumerable variations in the prevalence of disease between ethnic and cultural groups. Carcinoma of the esophagus, for instance, is frequent in black South Africans (81), and in the town of East London cases were clustered within certain parts of the "location," the dwelling area to which they were confined (82). The focus in each cluster appeared to be a *shebeen*, a place in which illicit liquor or *skokiaan* could be bought by black people, who were forbidden by law to purchase alcohol. The shebeen functioned as a social center in much the same way as an English "pub" or European cafe, although somewhat modified by constant liability to police raids. To avoid police trouble, the "shebeen queen" sought two properties for her ideal brew: the effects should be rapid and produced at a gulp, and they should keep the customers quiet. Hence she laced the *skokiaan* with bizarre ingredients, among which

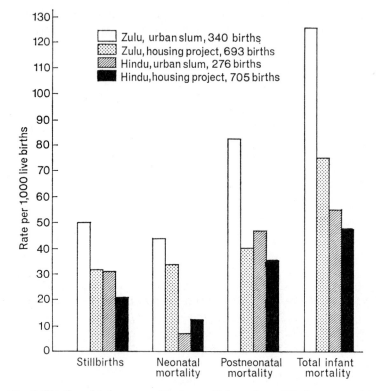

Figure 4.1 Stillbirth and infant mortality in two Zulu and two Hindu communities, Natal, South Africa, 1943–1951. *Source:* Constructed from Kark, S. L., and Chesler, J. (1956). Survival in infancy: A comparative study of stillbirths and infant mortality in certain Zulu and Hindu communities in Natal, *S. Afr. J. Lab. Clin. Med.*, 2, 134–59.

carbide had a high place because of its anesthetic effects. In East London the illicit liquor was brewed in drums that had once contained such carcinogens as petroleum and asphalt.

Personal behavior

The upsurge of the new discipline of public health and preventive medicine in the nineteenth century emphasized control of the physical environment, of water, sewage, food, housing, and workshops. The role of personal practices in everyday life was recognized later, and child welfare and maternity clinics were set up to attack "ignorance," to eradicate practices inimical to health, and to encourage those that promote it (83). The apparently simple task of gaining acceptance for even such public health measures as vaccines, however, proved to be a complex one of changing behavior, a task that still vexes practitioners today (84). Habits that affect health, in childbearing and midwifery, in nutrition and in daily living, are not merely the negative result of ignorance among people who know no better. They are often intrinsic elements in a way of life, customs that have adaptive value and symbolic significance.

Cervical cancer. Cancer of the neck of the womb is one of the two commonest cancers among women. Its incidence varies with social and cultural factors (see Table 4.1). Thus, in industrial societies it accounts for fewer deaths than cancer of the breast, while in the conditions of black people in southern Africa it accounts for more. It is now certain that some factor connected with sexual intercourse enhances the risk of this cancer. The unfolding epidemiology of this condition illuminates the conclusion.

Opportunities for sexual intercourse or for celibacy, and the conditions of hygiene in which they occur, depend on social and cultural factors; this is true not only for premarital and extramarital intercourse, but for marital intercourse too (85). In Britain, age at marriage has been young and fertility high among the lower social classes (86). Mortality and morbidity from cervical cancer have been consistent with the sexual activity to be inferred from these facts (87). The disease is most frequent among fertile married women, particularly those who have borne large families. Married women who have not borne children are less susceptible, which suggests that the physical trauma or the metabolic changes of childbirth may also be related to it. This cannot be the only factor, however, because deaths from this cancer among single women are only about half as many as among infertile married women, and hardly occur at all among nuns. Sexual intercourse probably underlies the apparent effect of childbearing, for the most fertile women marry younger, and consequently have histories of intercourse beginning at an earlier age and of longer duration than the infertile. When age and parity have been controlled, the effect of parity has usually been reduced to insignificance. A large proportion of women with the disease have married before the age of 20 (88).

This hypothesis, that some factor connected with sexual intercourse enhances the risk of the disease, gained early support from the high rate among prostitutes; in an early Danish study, prostitution was four times as common among women with cancer of the cervix as among controls of similar age and social background without the

Table 4.1 Cervical cancer risks reported in various studies

Low risk	High risk
Moslem	Inmates of a women's prison
Jewish	Prostitutes
Amish	Veneral disease clinic patients
Seventh-Day Adventist	American Negro
Irish-American Immigrants	Puerto Rican
Italian-American Immigrants	Mexican Immigrants
Churchgoers (Protestant and Catholic)	Non-churchgoers (Protestant and Catholic)
High social class	Low social class
Rich	Poor
Rural	Urban

Source: Adapted from Martin, C. E. (1967) Marital and coital factors in cervical cancer, *Amer. J. Publ. Hlth.*, 57, 803–814.

disease (89). The question of sexual activity has been further explored at the individual level. With a high degree of consistency, women with cervical cancer have experienced sexual congress earlier in life, and with a greater number of male partners both in and out of marriage, than their controls. These results gain strength from the similar results of a study of American Jewish women, in whom the disease is relatively uncommon. The husbands of affected women, too, tend to have had more sexual partners than the husbands of controls (90) (see Table 4.2).

Cervical cancer has also been associated with methods of contraception; it occurs less frequently with obstructive methods. This points to a role for hygiene. Contraceptive methods have had a distinctive social distribution during this century; different methods have been in vogue among different classes and cultures, changing with time, and shifting from one group to another, most often from the higher to the lower classes (91). The introduction of oral contraceptives, because they may both alter sexual behavior and dispense with any need for obstructive contraceptives, may have complicated effects on the social distribution of cervical cancer. For at this point in time it seems reasonable to characterize cervical cancer as a venereal disease whose spread is facilitated by promiscuous sexual contact (see Table 4.3). The hunt is on for a likely virus that males might transmit from one woman to another. The herpes virus and more recently the human papilloma (wart) virus have already been indicted, although a causal relationship is far from being proved.

Tobacco smoking. The emerging picture of cervical cancer brings an intimate matter of personal life into the orbit of public health concern. Tobacco smoking is by now a notorious and more visible example of personal behavior that is of public health concern. Woven into the daily social intercourse of many contemporary societies, smoking is much more than a simple personal habit from which people will abstain when

Table 4.2   Factors differentiating cases and controls in a sample of Jewish women with diagnosed cervical cancer

	Per cent with factor	
Coital factor	Cases N = 40	Controls N = 36
Coitus with two or more partners[a]	42.5	16.7
Induced abortion[a]	42.5	16.7
First coitus before 20[a]	52.5	30.6
Extramarital coitus of either spouse[a]	27.5	8.3
Extramarital coitus of husband[a]	25.0	2.8
First coitus with non-Jew[a]	17.5	0.0
Any coitus with non-Jew[a]	22.5	5.6
Married to uncircumcised non-Jew[a]	12.5	0.0
Foreign born	32.5	19.4
Marriage dissolved	37.5	19.4

[a]Significant at 5 per cent level of probability.

Source: Adapted from Martin, C. E. (1967) Marital and coital factors in cervical cancer, *Amer. J. Publ. Hlth.*, 57, 803–814.

Table 4.3 Relative risks of cervical abnormalities[a] according to age at first intercourse and number of sexual partners

Age at first intercourse (years)	Number of sexual partners				χ_1^2 for linear trend (row)
	0–1	2	3–5	6+	
21+ or never	1·00 (18)[b]	2·42 (6)	7·09 (11)	6·44 (4)	4·50[c]
19–20	0·81 (9)	1·93 (6)	15·04 (14)	12·89 (6)	5·76[c]
17–18	1·40 (10)	5·09 (15)	5·98 (26)	10·03 (14)	3·98[c]
<17	1·55 (6)	1·90 (5)	8·83 (26)	7·52 (14)	3·51[c]
χ_1^2 for linear trend	−1·01	−0·36	0·11	0·14	

[a]Cervical dysplasia or carcinoma *in situ.*

[b]The numbers of women with cervical abnormalities in each category are shown in parentheses. All risks are relative to women with one or no sexual partners, and whose age at first intercourse was 21 years or more.

[c]$P < 0·001.$

Source: Harris, R. W. C., Brinton, L. A., Cowdell, R. H., Skegg, D. C. G., Smith, P. G., Vessey, M. P., and Doll, R. (1980) Characteristics of women with dysplasia or carcinoma *in situ* of the cervix uteri, *Br. J. Concer, 42,* 362.

they are told of the danger associated with it. This danger is now known to be considerable; smokers have an appreciably (70 per cent) greater overall chance of death than nonsmokers. Cigarette smoking is associated not only with cancer of the lung (squamous epithelioma of the bronchus), but also with cancers of the larynx, oral cavity, esophagus, urinary bladder, kidney, pancreas, and uterine cervix. Smoking now ranks as one of the three chief risk factors for heart attacks and its presence potentiates the effect of other risk factors as well. Smokers report being sick more often than do nonsmokers and, clinically, the habit is associated with bronchitis, the flaring-up of tuberculosis, and the failure of peptic ulcer to heal. In addition, pregnant women who smoke tend to have smaller babies, suffer greater perinatal losses, and have more miscarriages (92). Smoking is surely a causal factor in many of these disorders; in others the predisposition to smoke and to the disease may both occur in individuals of a particular type of constitution or experience.

Virtually beyond doubt, the statistical association between cigarette smoking and squamous cell carcinoma of the bronchus is a causal one (see Table 4.4). This disease, like the cigarette-smoking habit, has rapidly increased in incidence and caused one death in eight among men aged 45 to 54 years in Britain in 1975; in the United States heavy smokers run a relative risk more than 20 times as high as nonsmokers. Tobacco smoke contains carcinogens and these reach the bronchial epithelium (93). Smoking exerts a number of independent noxious effects, for instance, by direct irritation of the respiratory and alimentary tracts, and through physiological and biochemical mechanisms on the blood vessels.

In those cases where predisposition to the disease and to smoking could occur together, the causal role of smoking is difficult to establish. Differences in temperament have been shown to exist between smokers and nonsmokers, and a study of twins also provided some evidence for a common constitutional factor in smokers (94). Thus, psychological and even genetic factors may play a part in the smoking habit,

Table 4.4 Comparison of mortality rates for smokers and nonsmokers by age and sex; based on data from U.S. veterans study and Hammond study

Study population, sex, and measure of mortality	35–44 years	45–54 years	55–64 years	65–74 years	75–84 years
U.S. Veterans: men					
Mortality ratio[a]	1.83	1.76	1.72	1.67	1.36
Excess deaths as percentage of total[b]	33	43	21	17	8
Hammond: men					
Mortality ratio[a]	1.89	2.28	1.83	1.51	1.23
Excess deaths as percentage of total[b]	33	38	25	13	4
Hammond: women					
Mortality ratio[a]	1.12	1.26	1.20	1.17	0.99
Excess deaths as percentage of total[b]	5	9	4	2	—

[a]Mortality ratios—death rate for current cigarette smokers divided by death rate for those who never smoked regularly.

[b]Excess deaths among current cigarette smokers (i.e., additional deaths that occurred among current cigarette smokers per year above those which would have occurred if smokers had the same death rates as those who never smoked regularly). This is expressed as a percentage of all deaths occurring in that age–sex group.

Source: Adapted from *The Health Consequences of Smoking, A Public Health Service Review* (1967), U. S. Department of Health, Education, and Welfare, Washington, D.C., p. 13.

but social and cultural causes overshadow individual predisposition. A study of a cohort of Harvard University students 30 years ago showed that social background was significant in their smoking habits (95). The nonsmokers tended to come from middle-class or lower-middle-class families and were moving upward in the social scale. They came mostly from families who were strict Protestants imbued with "work morality." The smokers tended to come from families whose social position was already secure, and they had entered the university from upper-class schools.

In industrial societies cigarette smoking, the most dangerous form of smoking, now shows a strong inverse relation to class position, having its highest prevalence among men of the lower social classes. The habit first took hold at the turn of the century among upper-class men, and then among lower-class men. The trenches of the First World War produced the first cohort of teenaged smokers. Later, in the twenties, at the time of the movement toward social as well as legal sex equality, "emancipated" upper-class women began to smoke cigarettes. In recent years the habit has been taking greater hold among lower-class women, at a time when at last men of the most highly educated classes are beginning to smoke less (96).

Although historical data on smoking among children are meager, recent studies show it also to be most prevalent among lower-class children and among those with the poorest educational attainments. The prevalence of smoking among children is related to smoking both among parents and older sibs, and among their friendship groups (97). Smoking is thus displaying a pattern common to the transmission of many forms of behavior among children as they grow into social beings by acquiring the mores, the habits, and the knowledge of their culture. The adoption of a habit that is forbidden is, on the one hand, prematurely to preempt the privileges of adults in an attempt to establish independence and personal identity, and, on the other, to emulate and identify with the model provided by parents. Lately in the United States, it seems that prevalence in children may be following the trend toward decline found among adults.

Eradication of this danger to health has proved to be no simple matter. In Edinburgh in the 1950s an antismoking campaign found three out of four men, and three out of eight women, to be habitual smokers. A major health education campaign directed against smoking used a battery of publicity and educational techniques for a period of six months, and its effects were then measured. This campaign not only failed to bring about a decrease in smoking, as might be expected in an attempt to deal with an addiction in so short a period, but it failed even to change attitudes toward smoking (98). Two major health reports each undersigned by experts of the highest prestige—namely that of the Royal College of Physicians of London, and that of the Surgeon General of the United States Public Health Service—merely caused sales of cigarettes to falter for some months before the upward trend was resumed. More than five years later signs of a halt were only beginning to be discovered, spreading first from physicians to men of other professions (99).

The difficulty in preventing smoking underlines the strength of the social and psychological factors which maintain the habit, of the commercial forces that exploit them, and of the other private and public economic interests that collude with those forces. The various studies show that an apparently simple habit such a smoking is related to a wide variety of diseases, and that prevention is difficult because in addition to the problems of the psychology and physiology of addiction, the habit is interwoven with the web of culture, social relations, and the economy.

The failures of short-term health education campaigns to induce population changes in smoking have sapped the morale of health educators, and contributed much to a sense of ineffectiveness in preventive programs. Nevertheless, close analysis of the distribution of smoking through time among different social groups—defined by sex, age, and social class—shows that the habit is distinctly on the decline, and that this decline tends to have been earliest and sharpest among those who adopted the habit first, that is, upper-class men. Just as the adoption of the habit spread to lower-class men, then to upper-class women, then lower-class women, so it seems the quitting of the habit is likely to go.

The phenomenon we are witnessing is best described as a *social movement*. A social movement expresses socially shared demands for social change in an aspect of the social order. Such movements may work in a directed manner through formal associations, structured groups with identified leaders and specific programs, of which the public health movement is one. Simultaneously or alternatively they may work in an undirected manner through loose social groups and informal interaction. Social movements reject prevailing values, adopt and promote another set of values, and strive for converts. They attempt to implement their policies both through public policy and through private persuasion. Value changes brought about in this way are at the root of the changes we now observe in health behavior.

Infant feeding. Some psychologists have interpreted tobacco smoking as an adult substitute for the comfort of suckling at the maternal breast. The Harvard study of smoking mentioned above provides some basis for this association, if the doubtful accuracy of retrospective histories of breast feeding is passed over. The men who found it easiest to give up smoking were those who had been longest at the breast. Later research continues to explore impulses related to oral craving (100). The nub of these hypotheses is that infant feeding experiences influence the development of an individual's personality, an idea that gained wide currency from the work of Freud. At the turn of this century he described his concept of the oral component of the libido, essentially an inborn drive to secure oral gratification; he considered that the strength of this drive was influenced by infant experience at the breast (101). A later discovery of an association between thumb sucking in children and a lack of opportunity to suck at the breast in infancy suggested that thumb sucking, and perhaps other behavior, was a response to frustration of the oral drive (102). The manner, duration, and time of weaning in different societies and groups have been studied in pursuit of this idea. Weaning seems to produce varying degrees of emotional upset in infants, but with no consistent pattern to validate the hypothesis (103).

This hypothesis is difficult to substantiate because of the lack of objective measures of personality standardized for different cultures, and because of the penumbra of maternal attitudes and family values associated with any particular mode of infant feeding. In other words, a whole culture is involved. It must be admitted that within a single culture also the more objective and systematic attempts to connect patterns of infant rearing with adult personality traits have often failed (104). There can be little doubt, however, that in many societies feeding methods are crucial to the health and survival of infants (105). Although in industrial societies gross failures of infant feeding that result in deficiency diseases or deaths are uncommon, more subtle metabolic disturbances may ensue.

In underdeveloped societies all health workers are confronted by the crucial role of feeding practices in infant growth and development. The problems begin before birth, during gestation. In some tribal and peasant cultures, from the Arctic to Africa, custom and taboo restrict the food intake of pregnant women, often of vital foods. The pregnant Zulu bride, for instance, may not partake of milk in the patrilocal kraal where she must live with her husband and his family, and eggs too are frowned on since they are thought to make women licentious (106). The effects of these restrictions are problematical, but quite possibly serious. After birth, the infant usually draws adequate sustenance, attested by growth curves that match those of European infants for the first six months of life. But it is usually held that the infant must be protected from possible dangers inherent in adult foods, and until weaned he or she will be fed only on bland foods of low nutrient value. Hence growth curves fall off after the first six months of life, and the failure of breast feeding, or even weaning, can lead to the catastrophe of protein-calorie malnutrition syndromes, including marasmus and kwashiorkor (107).

Even in the big cities of industrial societies, like New York and Glasgow, elements common to the life-styles of the poor in other societies have been described among migrants and in the most deprived social strata. In these cities, too, inadequate feeding of the children of working mothers has its outcome in failure to thrive, iron deficiency anemias, and deficiency diseases like rickets.

Feeding practices vary between societies and between racial and socioeconomic groups in the same society (108). European and African, upper class and lower class, do not use the same methods. In Scotland, three-quarters of a sample of young mothers had given up breast feeding at three months (109), whereas in South Africa only one-tenth of African mothers had done so (110). Only about two-thirds of the Scottish mothers had an adequate milk supply, whereas most African mothers might be expected to have sufficient milk. As noted previously, growth in breast-fed African babies in the first six months of life compares favorably with European norms, although thereafter African babies show the effects of deficient supplementary diet (111). The advanced motor behavior of African babies, noted by a number of observers, could contribute to more efficient suckling, for the effective sucking-power of an infant seems to be correlated with its milk-getting capacity and its general vitality (112).

The distinctiveness of breast-feeding practices is illustrated in comments made by some black women about the practices of white mothers in South Africa, and reflects the values implicit in the role of mother in two cultures within the same society (110):

"It is not true to say that European mothers, or most of them, have not sufficient breast milk, or that it dries up because they want it to do so. They feed their babies according to fixed times, and breasts normally do not work according to the clock. Since they force the breasts to work at the time they want them to, they meet such results as milk drying off or decreasing until they say they cannot feed their babies because they have no milk. . . ."

"The Europeans feed by the clock with intentions not mainly to nurse, but to keep themselves up with daily enjoyments, which otherwise would be denied them if they had to feed their babies each time they wanted the breast. . . ."

"It is also a shame amongst many European mothers to feed in public, even in the presence of another female. One mother for whom I worked, when she had to breast feed, would close the door, draw the curtains, sit down comfortably, taking time before she started feeding. If anybody came into the house she would attend to the guest. That baby was not properly fed; it did not have what it should have because she was ashamed of feeding it in the presence of people. A woman's pride lies in the successful nursing she has given."

Distinctions also occur among people in the same society but of different social class or ethnic group, or race. In the postwar period, women of the upper classes in Britain and the United States tended to breast-feed babies more often and for longer periods than women in the lower classes (108). While women of all social classes experienced the same difficulties in breast feeding, upper-class women were less easily discouraged than lower-class women. In a Scottish survey, mothers of all social classes experienced mastitis and sore nipples but these did not prevent women from the professional and technical classes from continuing to suckle, whereas three-quarters of the fishwives with these conditions gave up breast feeding. A high success rate in breast feeding was associated with favorable attitudes toward it, and such attitudes were commoner among the women of the professional classes. The investigators in Scotland concluded that the mother who chooses to breast-feed in contemporary urban society often

accepts a heavy load of discomfort and disability, and this arises less from psychological factors than from her way of life. Most working-class women preferred bottle
feeding, and many gave up breast feeding despite the strongest medical advice. This
is, in part, a further instance of two sets of values in conflict. People of the social class
to which doctor, nurse, and health visitor usually belong place a high value on breast
feeding, and tend to recommend it, often on "scientific" grounds. On the other hand,
given the exigencies of the daily life found in modern cities, working women will
often need to resort to bottle feeding.

Breast feeding customs also change with time and with altered social conditions.
An Englishman traveling in France just before the French Revolution noted that the
most fashionable women, influenced he thought by Rousseau, had become ashamed
of not nursing their own children. Leo Tolstoy held a similar and characteristically
strong view, and projected some of his own conflicts with his wife in the matter of
breast feeding onto Natasha in *War and Peace* (113). In contemporary industrial societies (see Figure 4.2), the rate of breast feeding, having declined for several decades,
is on the rise again (114). In Natal, it was found that the rate for Zulu women who
had migrated to the towns was less than for those still living in the country. At six
months, no less than 97 per cent of rural mothers were breast feeding, as compared
with 82 per cent of urban mothers.

The illustrative material set out here about sex behavior, smoking habits, and
infant-feeding practices is sufficient to indicate the never-ending interplay of health
with the personal behavior customary in various cultures. We turn now to a further

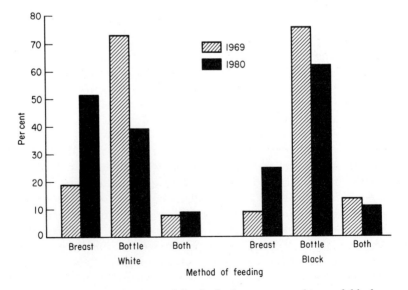

Figure 4.2 Percentages of breast and bottle feeding among white and black women—
United States, 1969 and 1980. *Source:* National Natality Survey of the National Center for
Health Statistics (1984). *Morbidity and Mortality Weekly Report*, Vol. 33, No. 11, p. 153.

aspect of culture as it relates to health; its effect on personality, psychological adaptation, and "stress" disorders.

Culture, personality, and health disorders

The previous pages referred to the intricate connections of infant feeding practices with health. Cultural variations in feeding practices have repercussions that must be looked for in both physical and mental health, because infant feeding belongs to the class of basic physiological activities that are also basic social activities. By such social mechanisms immature individuals are transformed into conscious members of society. The precise manner in which each generation transmits its cultural heritage to its successor is a field of study that concerns both sociology and psychology. Many studies of personality have attempted to analyze individual psychology in terms of variant cultures. Qualities on which one society places a high value, these studies show, another often ignores or deprecates (115). What Western diagnosticians would consider pathological behavior may be highly valued and culturally enfranchised in some societies. Among Eskimos, Washo, Iroquois and Apache Indians, and the Zinacantecan people of northern Mexico, for example, personality traits and behavior patterns which Westerners associate with mental illness are channeled into the role of the priest-healer or shaman. Such societies, it should be added, do not fail to distinguish betwen true shamans and "crazy people" (116). The social advantage and recognition accorded such behavioral traits in a culture could give them a selective advantage, or elicit the traits where they are latent, and so shape the personalities of the members of a culture. One school of personality theorists has held that the molding of the structure of adult personality is founded on methods of childrearing. Freud's many fertile inferences—made however from intensive retrospective observations of adult patients—provided the theoretical basis: personality differences, not only between individuals of the same stock, but also between groups of different stock, could be explained by infant experience at the mother's breast, in weaning, in toilet training, and so on.

The guiding hand of Freud is also apparent in many of the field studies of personality development carried out by anthropologists in this century. Early investigators tended to assume an isomorphism of culture and personality; culture was viewed as "personality writ large," or alternatively, personality was viewed as a microcosm of the culture as a whole. Descriptions of "national character" done in this spirit were popular in the period around the Second World War. These were weak observations and bold inferences from which to derive "modal" personality types. Later work has aimed rather to describe the range of personality types in a given culture (117).

If we use the term *socialization* to signify the universal process by which the norms, values, beliefs, and behavioral patterns of a society are transmitted from generation to generation, then the term *enculturation* may be used to describe the particular way in which this process occurs in a specific society. The different styles of caretaking that Japanese and American mothers practice, for example, are congruent with the ways in which adults in each of these cultures treat the very young, the very old, and the disabled. Japanese mothers were more inclined to soothe and quiet their babies, while in the United States activity and vocal responsiveness were encouraged. That the differences are culturally induced and not genetic is seen from the similarity of Japanese-American mothers' handling of their infants to that of their American counterparts (118).

Numerous studies attest to the importance of childrearing practices in enculturation, in the development both of personality traits and of skills. Children raised in extended families have been found to show more spontaneous altruism than those raised in nuclear families (119). The accelerated sensorimotor development observed in African infants has been attributed to the fact that their mothers handle their newborn babies much more freely than European mothers handle theirs, although constitutional differences appear to play a part (120).

Likewise, what appear to be cognitive deficits in members of preliterate societies—when measured by Western test scales—may be the result of patterned differences in modes of perception and thinking common to such societies. Both cultural and physical environmental factors may be at work. As the witchcraft example cited earlier shows, deviations from familiar modes of causal reasoning cannot be considered abnormal in cultures which allow for magical influences on the normal course of events. Similarly, the poor performance of West African children on a geometric task involving the manipulation of patterned blocks is owed to their lack of familiarity with techniques of graphic representation rather than to any innate defect in spatial perception; they readily learn the task if properly trained. People who live in environments dominated by right-angular forms—such as building corners, intersecting streets, and rectangular houses—have been found to be more susceptible to certain optical illusions than those who do not (121). The possible variations are endless, given the plasticity of the human nervous system and the array of environmental and cultural situations it has adapted to.

With regard to personality, however, both the adequacy of the observations in terms of objectivity, validity, and reliability, and the existence of a statistical association of given traits of personality with particular childrearing experiences, have been disputed (104). Yet these hypotheses, which have so exercised the imagination of this century, cannot altogether be put aside. Behaviorist as well as psychoanalytic theory opened a gateway to the understanding of personality in general, and of the manner in which social forces can mold personality in individuals.

Two American theorists of socialization, Cooley and Mead, who dealt with the development of self-consciousness, grounded their theories in a different set of concepts. Each took a sociological view of socialization. Cooley claimed that self-consciousness can only arise in society, and cannot be distinguished from social consciousness (122). In other words, the manner in which an individual conceives of him or herself as appearing to someone else is an essential element in one's own conception of oneself. This is Cooley's idea of the "looking-glass" conception of the self, and he considered that self-consciousness in a child does not appear until two years of age, in conjunction with consciousness of others outside oneself. The role of other people in the development of self-consciousness was again emphasized by Mead (123). For him, the genesis of the self lay in learning the meaning of our own gestures and emotions through the responses of others. People meet and interact with many others and this could imply a whole series of different selves. Mead postulated that we lump all these others into one entity, the "generalized other," which incorporates the social group of which we are members. We make a continuous response to the "generalized other" and hence the self is continuous or consolidated. Mead further distinguished between the "I" and the "me," that is, between the subjective "I" as initiator of thought and action, and the objective "me," the consequence of responses to the attitudes and behavior of others, the "generalized other." The "I" and "me" are social products because they reflect the values and world views of the community. This "dramaturgic" conception of the self has since been applied in studies of everyday social interaction, of the culture of "total institutions" (such as asylums), and of the evolution of deviant identities (124).

The social character of even so individual a matter as personal identity is strikingly apparent when the typical Western notion of a self bounded by the skin of the body is contrasted with corresponding notions of selfhood in such traditional communities as Java, Bali, and Morocco (125). These notions seem to conform better with the social dramaturgy of Mead and Cooley than with the individualism of much Western psychology. In Java, the self is seen as the outcome of a constant interplay between inner feeling, which is described as "coarse," and the strict rule of etiquette. In Bali, individual identity seems to merge with successive social roles through which the individual's life-cycle is articulated with the ongoing drama of community life. In Morocco, personal affiliations (with family and place of origin) are defined so flexibly, according to the requirements of specific social situations, that the self becomes virtually an *ad hoc* product of the moment.

To summarize the discussion thus far: society provides a culture pervaded by expressive symbols, faiths, and emotional attitudes; it provides a structure of social relations that rests on the distinctive positions and statuses accorded individuals of different sex, age, power, and prestige; and it provides a value system with moral and legal sanctions. At the same time these elements of society are learned and internalized by individuals. This cycle of successive social transmission and individual internalization produces a self-perpetuating system of belief and behavior, and a recognizable patterning of the personalities within each culture (126).

Personality, through its network of psychic pathways tied in with the body's nervous and metabolic pathways, can be taken to modulate the individual's physiological reactivity to the environment. Culture in turn, through its influence on the formation of personality, thus finds an indirect route to influence overt organic responses and disease, in particular so-called psychosomatic and stress diseases. Indeed, the Hippocratic concept of humors can be seen as a precursor of one formulation of the psychogenic theory of disease. The postulate is that certain combinations of humors or constitutions—or in today's jargon, certain personalities—predispose to certain kinds of disease. A variety of pathogenic mechanisms has been advanced to link the personality type with the disease. Inherent susceptibility is one such mechanism. Another would be characteristic psychodynamic processes, set in train by symbolic repetition of childhood events, that issue in physiological responses so excessive, or prolonged, or inappropriate, as to be converted into pathological responses (127,128). The pathology attributed to such processes has been both physical and mental, for example on the one side peptic ulcer and ulcerative colitis, and on the other conversion hysteria and obsessional neuroses.

It must be admitted that since the time of the Hippocratic works the scientific substantiation of these hypotheses has made slow progress. One of the better-documented diseases studied in this light is peptic ulcer. The part of affect in peptic ulcer and its complications has been suggested by a number of observations (129). For example, objective social events with emotional connotations have been found to precede the onset of symptoms and of the complications of perforation and hemorrhage, and as with the bombing of Britain during the Second World War, to accompany peaks in the incidence of perforations and deaths.

Physiological experiment indicates how external factors that produce emotion may find a pathway to the gut. The notable effect of emotion on the function of the stomach has long been known and elaborated (130). Conflicts and provocations produce hypermotility and hypersecretion in some people, and at the same time a lower pain threshold and fragility of the mucosa. Such hyperfunction of the stomach is characteristic in duodenal ulcer; a high level of acid is one of its more constant physiological accompaniments. During periods of personal conflict hyperfunction can also be accompanied by a rise in blood and urine levels of pepsinogen, an enzyme secreted by the stomach and capable of digesting protein, including that of the intestinal wall (131).

Harmful emotional responses may thus be a contributory cause of peptic ulcers, although experiment has so far failed to produce persisting effects that could maintain chronic ulceration, and all these signs regress when the emotional provocation is removed. If these harmful emotions are of a specific type, they may be nourished by particular personalities (132) and therefore by families enmeshed in a certain social structure or pattern of relationships. In coronary heart disease, for instance, recent studies have made a good case for the existence of two different personality types, one at high and one at low risk of being affected (see Chapter 6).

To continue with peptic ulcers, the central conflict of the "peptic ulcer personality" is seen in one hypothesis as the struggle between feeling dependent on parents on the one hand, and striving for adult independence on the other (133). Many studies in this field have been poorly designed and their results conflicting. An early controlled study revealed no differences between ulcer patients and other hospital patients in such informative family characteristics as the size of family and its composition and social class, nor in such personal experiences as educational level, childhood illness, or early separation from parents (134).

A few careful studies have been more successful in relating psychological attributes to peptic ulcers. For instance, some studies have tested psychological predictions against physiological markers related to gastric hypersecretion. A battery of psychological tests showed that among men inducted into the U.S. Army those with duodenal ulcer more often exhibited unresolved conflicts about emotional dependence. Subsequently the test battery was able to discriminate between duodenal ulcer patients and controls, and was correlated with the level of urinary catecholamines, particularly a low noradrenaline level (135).

In London, an attempt was made to elucidate subtle and dynamic elements of relations in a study of the families of 32 young men with duodenal ulcer, compared with controls selected from a general practice. A pattern consistent with the hypothesis of emotional dependency was found (136). As compared with the parents of controls, the mothers of ulcer patients appeared to be more dominating and ambitious for their children, and their fathers weaker, passive and unassertive. The young men themselves were reported to be psychologically dependent on their mothers, while at the same time nursing deep inward feelings of resentment and hostility towards them. One group of patients' families did not show this distinctive pattern, but these all had a family history of ulcer. A familial incidence of ulcer has been demonstrated several times (137). It therefore seemed not unlikely that some ulcers were influenced more by inheritance, and others more by the emotions generated by typical family situations. These stresses might not have their origin in personality so much as in external forces that impinge directly on the personality.

Culture and indices of "stress"

The concept of *stress* was used by Hans Selye to reclassify a number of disorders which he believed, on the basis of animal experiments, might share a common pathogenesis in the hyperfunction of the adrenal cortex (138). Other writers have elaborated psychogenic theories around this concept (139). The word "stress" has led to semantic confusion; it has described both stimuli in the environment and responses in the organism to those stimuli. Selye named the stimuli "stressors," the immediate responses "stress," and the chronic adaptations, "strains." In this text we follow a similar usage.

Research of varying quality through the 1950s supported common observation in human beings that stressors can provoke immediate psychic and somatic reactions (140). They can also provoke, in animals, chronic somatic reactions, and simulate natural disease process. When we turn to such reactions in humans, theory outruns the data to be garnered from experiment. Observations are taken from the course and treatment of such disorders as asthma, warts, eczema, urticaria and other skin reactions, colitis, menstrual syndromes, and abdominal pain in children; they are also taken from the psychological states that coexist with these somatic states and from histories of stressful experience that preceded their onset. The results are far from precise or even consistent. Mental disorders do not yield much firm evidence either, particularly because the definition of a case is so difficult; it follows that the definition of the effect of stressors is also difficult (141).

Nonetheless, evidence is slowly building up, both that accumulation of stressors has an impact and that mental symptoms vary with life situations that generate different strains (142). Blood-pressure levels, for instance, have been found sensitive: in working men who anticipated the shutdown of their factories and the loss of jobs, pressures were raised, and high levels persisted as long as the men had not obtained new jobs (143). In this longitudinal study, other physiological indices also fluctuated according to the men's social situation: serum uric acid levels were high during the phase of anticipation, and fell sharply when new jobs were obtained; serum cholesterol levels rose only when unemployment followed, but also fell when jobs were obtained (144).

The nature of the conflicts that an individual faces, as well as the degree of resulting stress and strain, may be expected to vary from one culture to another. A wide range of stressors can be related plausibly to particular social situations, and cross-cultural surveys have been made of a variety of indicators—alcohol abuse, mental disorder, homicide, and suicide—in attempts to do so. The data from which cross-cultural studies can be made are imprecise, and do not lead to firm conclusions. Even in industrial societies sickness statistics are difficult to collect and not always reliable, and they cannot easily be compared with the statistics from simpler societies. The documentation of customary patterns of behavior is still more difficult, although these data for some small-scale preliterate societies are perhaps more extensive and easier to handle than those for complex industrial societies (145).

Various indices have been used to compare the elements of strain in societies. *Suicide* is one of these indices, and suicide rates have been intensively studied ever since the pioneering work of Morselli and particularly of Durkheim at the turn of the century (146,147,148). Durkheim postulated three forms of suicide: *altruistic, egoistic, and anomic.*° The altruistic suicide of certain cultures is not socially disapproved, but rather in the nature of a duty. The distinction between egoistic and anomic suicide is fine and of doubtful validity, and both can be subsumed under the head of *anomie.* Anomie is a state of confusion, inchoate values, and loss of cohesion in *social groups.* The impact of such situations on the mental state of *individuals*, it is held, gives rise to uneasiness, a sense of separation and isolation, frustration, powerlessness, and apathy. This subjective state in individuals is variously described as *anomie* (149) or *alienation* (150).

The state of anomie can arise from a conflict of values and ways of life between cultural groups in the same society, as among immigrants and their hosts; or from the deterioration of systems of values in one society; or where the social structure prevents achievement of approved goals. Anomie is therefore found where the cultural norms and goals which impel people to behave in certain ways are disjoined from their capacity to act in accord with them: for instance, when men *en masse* are unable to find work, or when immigrant groups in a new society are discriminated against or are otherwise unable to adjust to social and cultural demands. The anomie hypothesis predicts that suicides should increase with the rapid growth of industrial cities peopled by immigrants who are physically isolated from their original homes, and culturally isolated from the dense mass of people who surround them in their new society.

Although Durkheim's statistical techniques were primitive by modern standards, his sociological and epidemiological analysis is a classic of its kind, and the evidence he presented is impressive (151). He searched the official statistics of Western Europe for associations between suicide rates and such factors as religion, occupation, marital status, and economic cycles. He found a high rate of suicide in Protestant countries,

---

°A fourth type, *fatalistic* suicide, was for Durkheim an anomaly: "the suicide deriving from excessive regulation, that of persons with futures pitilessly blocked and passions violently checked by oppressive discipline" (148). He considered it too rare in his time to warrant more than a footnote.

a low rate in Roman Catholic countries, and a moderate rate in countries with mixed populations of Catholics and Protestants.

These results have been criticized, but Durkheim put this relationship beyond chance by the epidemiological method of replication, which helped to show that it was independent of the many other associated differences between Catholic and Protestant countries. To do this he tested the relationship within countries by breaking down the figures for groups and regions. In Switzerland the relationships with predominant religious persuasion held for each language group, in Prussia and Bavaria for each province, and in all for 17 essentially independent comparisons.

It must be allowed that unavoidable flaws existed in the sources of the data. Regardless of how refined Durkheim's definition of suicide was, he was still faced with an insurmountable problem in investigating its causes: there was no guarantee that the statistics he used were based on a similar understanding, on the part of those who collected and recorded them, of what suicide was, and of what would count as an instance of it. For many reasons, a large proportion of suicides, in an estimated range from 25 to 40 per cent, go unreported (152). In fact, when it is a private event, only a suicide note, a history of previous attempts, or a record of psychotherapy for depression will in any way guarantee that a suicide will be officially labeled as such.

There are practical reasons for underreporting—loss of insurance benefits, for example. Other reasons are social: suicide is often purposely misdiagnosed and erroneously recorded by physicians and public officials who may attempt to protect members of their practice or constituency from public shame. Still other reasons are cultural. To take an often-cited example, a suicide in an Irish Catholic community is quite likely to be labeled as "death by misadventure," particularly if the death certificate is signed by the family physician. The official Irish suicide rate is suspiciously low—1.8/100,000 compared with 22/100,000 in Sweden or 11/100,000 in the United States (153). More generally, the power to control public access to and classification of private events rises with social status and thus throws a possible skew into official statistics. In the United States, for example, attempted suicide by upper-class individuals seen by private practitioners is less likely to show up in case registries than attempted suicide by working-class people seen in hospital emergency rooms (154).

However, results both from Durkheim's analysis and others are consistent with the hypothesis that an individual's participation in the life and work of a society bears on the suicide rates of its members. Thus, suicide rates decline in times of war, when national sentiment brings social cohesion, and they rise with economic depression and unemployment (155). In urban areas with ecological features suggestive of anomie— single-person households, the unmarried, the old—more than an average number of suicides occur. Rates are high among the old, among whom alienation can be the outcome of the process of aging and retirement, and among the mentally ill, alienated not only by their state of mind, but by inhospitable living conditions and social rejection as well (156). Rates are high among the single and the childless, who lack domestic support, and among the divorced and the widowed who have lost it, and for widows especially in the period after bereavement (157). Among minority groups such as Chicanos, Native Americans, and blacks in the in the United States, the male age-group from 15 to 24 years especially experiences very high unemployment rates and exhibits many signs of social alienation, and over the past 30 years they have also exhibited steadily rising suicide rates (158,159).

Suicide always has a social connotation. In some societies the individual may be so closely integrated that a higher value is placed on the persistence of core values than on one's own life, and suicide may reflect this altruism, as in the *seppuku* of Japanese warriors, or in the now rare *suttee* of Hindu widows. In other societies, suicide may be the final sanction that an individual can use to influence the behavior of others. For example, the Mambwe people in Africa believed that the spirit of a suicide is able to punish those of his kin who have done him an injury or disservice; one chief hanged himself in order to punish a headman and villagers who against his will had given shelter to a runaway wife when she refused to return to him. The supernatural sanctions were feared and respected, and the village subsequently disintegrated (160). A suicide rate is clearly not a simple index. It points to complicated social and cultural processes and beliefs in which the behavior of the living can be influenced by the dead. Abundant case histories confirm this generalization for industrial as well as peasant societies.

Suicide has been interpreted psychologically as the ultimate expression of aggression turned in upon the self, and in-turned aggression may be the product of a strict moral upbringing which emphasizes conscience and reinforces feelings of guilt and depression; suicide is the ever-present danger in depressive states (161). Durkheim conceived the possibility that within a single society suicide and homicide were competing forms of aggression and self-destruction. Thus, depending on culture and mores, social forces conducive to suicide in some societies may lead to homicide in others. If a warlike Crow Indian became depressed, he would chant the songs and wear the garb that marked him as a "Crazy Dog," pledged to die fighting the enemy within the season. His will to self-destruction was thus achieved through homicide, a means acceptable to his society and akin to that sometimes suspected by psychologists in the bravado of racing drivers or fighter pilots. In Britain one-third of all homicides are said to be followed by suicide (162). Durkheim showed that the proposition that suicide and homicide are competing causes of death could hold only for some societies, for the two causes of death did not occur consistently in inverse ratio.

If the sensitivity of suicide to environmental factors makes it an apt case for epidemiological analysis, its complexity makes it a difficult one. In the first place, suicide, along with many other forms of self-destruction, is under certain circumstances a rational act. It is also an act of unusual opacity: often private, sometimes bungled, occasionally not meant at all, and always subject to a variety of interpretations as to its true cause. Moreover, the meaning of the act in any given instance is seldom self-evident to anyone, not excepting the actor (163). Indeed, there is no such thing as *the* suicide act. There are, instead, many species of acts. In the absence of a working typology, the catalogue of suicides remains as ill-defined as the eighteenth-century notion of fevers.

Mental disorders, of all health disorders, seem likeliest to be sensitive to the cultural environment. In some African tribes, conversion hysterias have been found to be common among adult women, whereas in some African towns adolescent schoolgirls most often manifested the symptoms (164). In Britain, however, conversion hysterias were common in the First World War, and uncommon a generation later in the Second World War.

These disparities in prevalence could reflect the degree of strain in each social and cultural situation. Before the conclusion can be accepted, it is necessary to ensure that the disparities in prevalence cannot be attributed to imperfections in measurement, data sources, and reporting (165), nor to social selection in the populations observed which could cause a clustering or a deficiency of the condition, nor to genetic variation with such disorders as alcoholism and the functional psychoses (depression and schizophronia) that have a genetic component. Given these safeguards, other cultural hypotheses remain to be ruled out. Thus, the social approval given to the expression of symptoms varies, as noted above in the case of the election of shamans in certain cultures. Tolerance of particular forms of behavior is not the same between societies, and at different times in the same society. A hypothesis of this type has been advanced to explain a decline in neuroses reported in a British factory population over a period of time, and accompanied by an apparently compensatory rise in gastric disorders. The hypothesis in essence postulates competing guises for an underlying stress that is bound to be manifest in some form (166).

Certainly, the content and expression of mental illness can be determined by culture (167). Every society makes distinctive demands upon its members and encourages some forms of behavior while it restricts others. Schizophrenia occurs everywhere. In the underdeveloped world, however, where chronic sick roles (see Chapter 7) are not encouraged and there is no dearth of useful work even for the impaired, the course of recovery from schizophrenia appears to compare favorably with that characteristic of the disorder in the developed world. The delusions and the catatonic states that occur in schizophrenia also have a cultural content. Technology accounts for some of the obvious differences. Delusions of thought control by radio waves can only occur in societies familiar with such devices. Cultural belief systems also play a part. In Brazil catatonia in middle-class Bahian patients who share Western ideas assumed the classical form with physical immobility and complete withdrawal from human relationships. They directed their paranoid anxieties and hostility toward other persons. But some lower-class Bahian catatonics whose beliefs were less rationalistic were able to continue with human relationships of a sort; mutism, stupor, and negativism were rare, and they were able to enter into social relations with others. These lower-class patients displaced their hostility on to spirits and supernatural agencies.

In Britain the content of schizophrenic delusions has been found to vary by sex and by social background. Women for example, had more sexual delusions than men, especially of sexual assaults and pregnancy. Those schizophrenics who showed a trend toward grandiose delusions came mainly from the higher social classes, or from among the educated, or were the eldest in families. Those who showed a trend, less marked, toward delusions of inferiority came mainly from the lower social classes, or from the less well educated, or were the youngest in their families. Elements of the actual social positions of these patients seemed to be incorporated in their delusions (168).

In the United States schizophrenic male patients of Irish and Italian descent presented contrasting sets of symptoms. The Irish suffered more from alcoholism, from preoccupations with sin and guilt, and from fixed delusions. The Italians showed markedly more overt homosexuality, behavior disorders, and hostility toward authority. These contrasts were attributed to the influence of their social and cultural backgrounds; a parallel study of Irish and Italians in New York had enabled the researchers to predict some of these responses. Irish families were often dominated by mothers, with the fathers shadowy and their sons "forever boys and burdens," anxious, sexually repressed, and with a gift for fantasy rather than for action. Italian families were dominated by fathers, and sanctioned the free expression by their sons of emotion, physical aggression, and sexuality (169). Immigrant Jews in America were reported to resort more often than other immigrants to psychiatric and psychological treatment, while Irish immigrants had a high degree of alcoholism (170). A number of other comparative studies point to variation in the content and expression of mental illness with social and cultural differences (171).

No firm conclusions can be drawn about the general or specific stressors of a culture causing mental illness, or any other manifestation taken as an index, because of the dearth of adequate comparative material. Although much work has gone into criteria for diagnoses and nomenclature (172), methods of selecting populations and case-finding vary; indeed, the recognition of psychiatric disorder is itself culturally determined. This lack of comparability has to some degree invalidated even the best surveys of the prevalence of mental disorders. One team of researchers applied the same case-finding technique developed for a prevalence survey in Nova Scotia to a survey among the Yoruba in Nigeria (173). The overall prevalence of mental impairment was remarkably similar in these two populations. However, both the definition of mental impairment and the measures of prevalence can be criticized, and even if the variation had been great, there is no assurance that the responses to the same questions of Acadians and Yoruba had the same significance for mental impairment.° Indeed, studies among whites, blacks and Puerto Ricans living side by side in New York suggest that the responses of different ethnic groups cannot be accorded the same significance (142).

Comparative problems are fewer with different cultural groups living in the same country and using the same language. A study of the Hutterites, an Anabaptist sect in North America, did suggest that their social cohesion and Puritan values influenced the prevalence and the types of mental illness among them. The Old Order of Pennsylvania Amish are another exclusive religious group like the Hutterites, and they separate themselves from many of the material goods and technical advances—including the use of electricity—of the world that surrounds them. The distribution of mental disorder among them has unusual features, some of which can be attributed to this distinctive culture. Among more than 12,000 people, a survey discovered no drug abuse, alcoholism, or sociopathy. *Major depressive disorder*—unipolar and

---

°For instance, the positive responses of the Yoruba to many questions probably had a basis in their high frequency of somatic disorders.

bipolar—was the predominant form, and accounted for 71 per cent of the 112 cases reported in the five-year period 1976–80. Another remarkable feature of these depressive disorders was their equal frequency among men and women in contrast with the higher frequencies among woman consistently found elsewhere. The finding suggests either that Amish women have relatively more support and less stress than women elsewhere, or that in other social groups much depression among males masquerades as alcoholism and sociopathy. In either case, the Amish culture would account for the unusual equal sex ratio (174).

The examples of this chapter show that the frequency and form of disorders as well as the way people respond to them have a cultural dimension. While we have drawn here on cross-cultural studies to illustrate patterns of health and personality, the concept is one that is relevant to the diversity of industrial society. These patterns vary not only between societies, but within the social groups of a single society. Within industrial societies social class is the most cogent of the divisions that reveal such differentiation, and we turn now to that topic.

References

1. **Sigerist, H. E.** (1929). Die Sonderstellung des Kranken. *Kyklos*, 2, 11–20, reprinted as Sigerist, H. E. (1960). The special position of the sick, in *The Sociology of Medicine*, ed. Roemer, M. I., New York.
2. **Firth, R.** (1951). *Elements of Social Organization*, London.
   Schapera, I. (1956). *Government and Politics in Tribal Societies*. London.
3. **Ogburn, W. F.,** and **Minkoff, M. F.** (1947). *A Handbook of Sociology*, London.
   Nadel, S. F. (1951). *The Foundation of Social Anthropology*, London.
   Radcliffe-Brown, A. R. (1952). *Structure and Function in Primitive Society*, London.
   Emmet, D. (1958). *Function, Purpose, and Powers*, London.
   Williams, R. (1958). *Culture and Society*, New York.
   Harris, M. (1968). *The Rise of Anthropological Theory*, New York.
   Murphy, R. (1979). *An Overture to Social Anthropology*, Englewood Cliffs, N.J.
4. **Linton, R.** (1936). *The Study of Man*, New York.
   Lynd, R. S. (1939). *Knowledge for What?*, Princeton, N.J.
   Kroeber, A. L. (1952). *The Nature of Culture*, Chicago.
   White, L. A. (1959). *The Evolution of Culture*, New York.
   Goodenough, W. H. (1971). *Culture, Language, and Society*, Reading, Mass.
   Leach, E. R. (1976). *Culture and Communication*, Cambridge.
5. **Kaplan, D.,** and **Manners, R. A.** (1972). *Culture Theory*, Englewood Cliffs, N.J.
   Geertz, C. (1973). *The Interpretation of Cultures*, New York.
   Sahlins, M. (1977). *Culture and Practical Reason*, Chicago.
6. **Fox, R.** (1967). *Kinship and Marriage: An Anthropological Perspective*, Harmondsworth.
   Lévi-Strauss, C. (1971). The family, in *Man, Culture, and Society*, ed. Shapiro, H. L., New York, pp. 333–357.
7. **Sudnow, D.** (1967). *Passing On: The Social Organization of Dying*, Englewood Cliffs, N.J.
   Kovit, L. (1978). Babies as social products: The social determinants of classification, *Social Science and Medicine*, 12, 347–351.

8. **Dobzhansky, T.** (1959). *Evolution, Genetics and Man*, New York.
   Harris, M. (1970). Referential ambiguity in the calculus of Brazilian racial identity, *Southwestern J. Anthropology, 26*, 1–14.
9. **Klineberg, O.** (1935). *Race Differences*, New York.
   Hooton, E. A. (1947). *Up from the Ape*, New York.
   Boas, F. (1948). *Race, Language and Culture*, New York.
   Park, R. E. (1950). *Race and Culture*, Glencoe, Ill.
   Bibby, C. (1960). Race prejudice and education, *U.N.E.S.C.O. Courier, 13*, 6–12.
   Montagu, A. M. F. (1974). *Man's Most Dangerous Myth: The Fallacy of Race*, 5th ed., New York.
10. **Washburn, S. L.** (1959). Speculations on the interrelations of tools and biological evolution, in *The Evolution of Man's Capacity for Culture*, ed. Spuhler, J. M., Detroit, pp. 21–31.
    Wallace, A. F. C. (1961). *Culture and Personality*, New York.
    Geertz, C. (1962). The growth of culture and the evolution of mind, in *Theories of the Mind*, ed. Scher, J., New York, pp. 713–740.
11. **Wilson, E. O.** (1975). *Sociobiology: The New Synthesis*, Cambridge, Mass.
    Dawkins, R. (1976). *The Selfish Gene*, New York.
    Lumsden, C. J., and **Wilson, E. O.** (1981). *Genes, Mind and Culture: The Coevolutionary Process*, Cambridge, Mass.
12. **Lewontin, R. C.** (1976). The fallacy of biological determinism, *The Sciences, 16*, 6–10.
    Sahlins, M. (1976). *The Use and Abuse of Biology*, Ann Arbor.
    Washburn, S. L. (1978). Animal behavior and social anthropology, *Society, 15*, 35–41.
13. **Holtzman, E.** (1977). The sociobiology controversy, *Int. J. Hlth. Serv., 7*, 515–527.
    Kreniske, J. (1985). *Sociobiology, The Runcible Science*, Unpublished Ph. D. Dissertation, Columbia Univ., New York.
    Caplan, A., ed. (1979). *The Sociobiology Debate*, New York.
14. **Mead, M.** (1935). *Sex and Temperament in Three Primitive Societies*, London.
15. **Read, K. E.** (1965). *The High Valley*, New York.
16. **Wolff, H. G.** (1958). Disease and patterns of behaviour, in *Patients, Physicians and Illness*, ed. Jaco, E. G., Glencoe, Ill.
    Wolff, B. B., and **Langley, S.** (1968). Cultural factors and the responses to pain, *American Anthropologist, 70*, 494–501.
    Clark, W. C., and **Clark, S. B.** (1980). Pain response in Nepalese porters, *Science, 209*, 410–412.
17. **Morgan, G. D.** (1959). Traumatic fore-quarter avulsion, *Brit. Med. J., 1*, 511.
18. **Williams, A. M.** (1950). A psychiatric study of Indian soldiers in the Arakan, *Brit. J. Med. Psych., 23*, 130–81.
19. **Taylor, C.** (1971). Interpretation and the sciences of man, *Review of Metaphysics, 25*, 3–51.
    Rock, P. (1974). The sociology of deviancy and conceptions of moral order, *Brit. J. Criminology, 14*, 139–149.
    Wolf, E. (1974). *Anthropology*, New York.
20. **Merton, R. K., Reader, G. G.**, and **Kendall, P. L.**, eds. (1957). *The Student Physician: Introductory Studies on the Sociology of Medical Education*, Cambridge, Mass.
    Hammond, K. R., and **Kern, R.** (1959). *Teaching Comprehensive Medical Care*, Cambridge, Mass.
    Duff, R. S., and **Hollingshead, A. B.** (1968). *Sickness and Society*, New York.

21. **Geertz, C.** (1960). *The Religion of Java*, Glencoe, Ill.
   Goody, J. (1962). *Death, Property and the Ancestors: A Study of the Mortuary Customs of the Lodagaa of West Africa*, Stanford.
   Murphy, J. (1964). Psychotherapeutic aspects of shamanism on St. Lawrence Island, in *Magic, Faith and Healing*, ed. Kiev, A., New York, pp. 53–83.
   Imperato, P. J., and **Traore, D.** (1968). Traditional beliefs about smallpox and its treatment in the Republic of Mali, *J. Trop. Med. Hyg.*, 71, 224–28.
   Smith, M. E. (1972). Folk medicine among the Sicilian-Americans of Buffalo, New York, *Urban Anthropology*, 1, 87–106.
   Fabrega, H. J. (1974). *Disease and Social Behavior*, Cambridge, Mass.
   Janzen, J. (1978). *The Quest for Therapy in Lower Zaire*, Berkeley.
22. **Evans-Pritchard, E. E.** (1937). *Witchcraft, Oracles and Magic among the Azande*, London.
   Gluckman, M. (1944). The logic of African science and witchcraft: An appreciation of Evans-Pritchard's *Witchcraft, Oracles and Magic Among the Azande of the Sudan*, *Human Problems in British Central Africa*, 1, 61–71.
   Forde, C. D., ed. (1954). *African Worlds*, London.
   Gluckman, M. (1955). *Custom and Conflict in Africa*, Oxford.
23. **Horton, R.** (1967). African traditional thought and Western science, *Africa*, 37, 50–60.
   Rappaport, R. A. (1979). *Ecology, Meaning and Religion*, Richmond, Calif.
   Morley, P., and **Wallis, R.,** eds. (1979). *Culture and Curing: Anthropological Perspectives on Traditional Medical Beliefs and Practice*, Pittsburgh.
24. **Weber, M.** (1946; first pub. 1915). Religious rejections of the world and their directions, in *From Max Weber: Essays in Sociology*, ed. Gerth, H. H., and Mills, C. W., pp. 323–359.
   Lienhardt, G. (1961). *Divinity and Experience: The Religion of the Dinka*, London.
   Geertz, C. (1966). Religion as a cultural system in *Anthropological Approaches to the Study of Religion*, ed. Banton, M., London, pp. 1–46.
25. **Fleck, L.** (1979; first pub. 1935). *Genesis and Development of a Scientific Fact*, ed. Trenn, T. J., and Merton, R. K., Chicago.
   Harris, E. (1970). *Hypothesis and Perception: The Roots of Scientific Method*, Atlantic Highlands, N.J.
   Kuhn, T. (1970). *The Structure of Scientific Revolutions*, 2nd ed., Chicago.
   Lakatos, I., and **Musgrave, A. E.,** eds. (1970). *Criticism and the Growth of Knowledge*, Cambridge.
   Feyerabend, P. (1975). *Against Method*, London.
   Laudan, L. (1977). *Progress and Its Problems: Towards a Theory of Scientific Growth*, Berkeley.
   Harris, M. (1979). *Cultural Materialism: The Struggle for a Science of Culture*, New York.
26. **St. John-Stevas, N.** (1951). *Life, Death and the Law*, London.
   Lewis, A. (1953). Health as a social concept, *Brit. J. Sociol.*, 4, 109–24.
   Wootton, B. (1959). *Social Science and Social Pathology*, London.
   Szasz, T. S. (1961). *The Myth of Mental Illness: Foundations of a Theory of Personal Conduct*, New York.
   Sedgwick, P. (1973). Mental illness is illness, *Salmagundi*, 20, 196–224.
   Foucault, M. (1967). *Mental Illness and Psychology*, New York.
27. **Rieff, P.** (1968). *The Triumph of the Therapeutic*, New York.

Pitts, J. R. (1968). Social control: The concept, *International Encyclopedia of Social Sciences*, ed. Sills, D. L., vol. 14, pp. 381–396.

Kittrie, N. (1973). *The Right to Be Different*, Baltimore.

Spitzer, S., and Scull, A. T. (1977). Social control in historical perspective: From private to public responses to crime, in *Corrections and Punishment*, ed. Greenberg, D. F., Beverley Hills, Calif., pp. 265–286.

Arney, W. R., and Bergen, B. J. (1984). *Medicine and the Management of Living*, Chicago.

28. Fox, R. (1977). The medicalization and demedicalization of American society, in *Doing Better and Feeling Worse, Health in the United States*, ed. Knowles, J. H., New York.

Illsley, R. (1980). *Professional or Public Health? Sociology in Health and Medicine*, London.

29. Stein, Z. A., and Susser, M. W. (1960). The families of dull children: A classification for predicting careers, *Brit. J. Prev. Soc. Med.*, 14, 83–8.

Saenger, G. (1960). *Factors Influencing the Institutionalization of Mentally Retarded Individuals in New York City*, A Report to the New York State Interdepartmental Health Resources Board, New York.

30. Balint, M. (1957). *The Doctor, His Patient and the Illness*, London.

Stoeckle, J., Zola, I. K., and Davidson, G. (1964). The quantity and significance of psychological distress in medical patients, *J. Chron. Dis.*, 17, 959–970.

31. Frank, J. (1961). *Persuasion and Healing*, Baltimore.

Illich, I. (1976). *Medical Nemesis: The Expropriation of Health*, New York.

Eisenberg, L. (1977). Disease and illness: Distinctions between professional and popular ideas of sickness, *Culture, Medicine and Psychiatry*, 1, 9–23.

Engel, G. L. (1977). The need for a new medical model: A challenge for biomedicine, *Science, 196*, 129–136

32. Durkheim, E. (1938; first pub. 1895). *The Rules of Sociological Method*, trans. Solovay, S. A., and Mueller, J. H., Chicago.

Nisbet, R., and Merton, R. (1971). Preface, in *Contemporary Social Problems*, 3rd ed., ed. Nisbet, R., and Merton, R., New York.

33. Lévi-Strauss, C. (1963). The sorceror and his magic, in his *Structural Anthropology*, New York, pp. 167–185.

Turner, V. (1967), *The Forest of Symbols*, Ithaca, N.Y.

Lieban, R. W. (1973). Medical anthropology, in *Handbook of Social and Cultural Anthropology*, ed. Honigman, J. J., Chicago, pp. 1031–72.

Landy, D., ed. (1977). *Culture, Disease and Healing: Studies in Medical Anthropology*, New York.

Fabrega, H. (1979). Elementary systems of medicine, *Culture, Medicine and Psychiatry*, 3, 27–49.34.

34. Glick, L. B. (1967). Medicine as an ethnographic category: The Gimi of the Guinea Highlands, *Ethnology, 6*, 31–56.

Jansen, G. (1973). *The Doctor–Patient Relationship in an African Tribal Society*, Atlantic Highlands, New Jersey.

Zola, I. (1975). In the name of health: On some sociopolitical consequences of medical influence, *Soc. Sci. Med.*, 9, 83–7.

35. Ashworth, H. W. (1958). Absence from work on a medical certificate, *Lancet, 1*, 732–3.

36. Field, M. (1958). *Doctor and Patient in Soviet Russia*, Cambridge, Mass.

37. Fox, T. F. (1951). Professional freedom, *Lancet, 2*, 115–119, 171–175.

Daniels, A. K. (1969). The captive professional: Bureaucratic limitations in the practice of military psychiatry, *J. Health and Social Behavior*, 10, 255–265.

38. Parsons, T. (1952). *The Social System*, London.

Freidson, E. (1970). *Professional Dominance: The Social Structure of Medical Care*, Hawthorne, N.Y.

Cole, S. and LeJeune, R. (1972). Illness and the legitimation of failure, *American Sociological Review*, 37, 347–56.

Shuvall, J., Antonovsky, A., and Davies, A. M. (1973). Illness: A mechanism for coping with failure, *Social Science and Medicine*, 1, 259–65.

Twaddle, A. (1973). Illness and deviance, *Social Science and Medicine*, 7, 751–762.

Waitzkin, H. (1979). Medicine, super-structure and micropolitics, *Social Science and Medicine*, 13A, 601–609.

39. Renaud, M. (1975). On the structural constraints to state intervention in health, *Int. J. Hlth. Serv.*, 5, 559–571.

Young, A. (1978). Mode of production of medical knowledge, *Medical Anthropology*, 2, 97–124.

Taussig, M. T. (1980). Reification and the consciousness of the patient, *Social Science and Medicine*, 14B, 3–13.

40. Ginsberg, M. (1932). *Studies in Sociology*, London.

Marshall, T. H. (1950). *Citizenship and Social Class and Other Essays*, London.

Drucker P. F. (1951). *The New Society*, London.

Lockwood, D. (1958). *The Blackcoated Worker*, London.

Curtis, R. F., and Jackson, E. F. (1977). *Inequality in American Communities*, New York.

Coleman, R. D., and Rainwater, L. (1978). *Social Standing in America: New Dimensions of Class*, New York.

Lewis, M. (1978). *The Culture of Inequality*, Amherst, Mass.

41. Pridan, D., and Navid, H. (1964). Health education in a clinic, *J. Coll. Gen. Practit.*, 7, 222–231.

42. Benstead, N., and Theobald, G. W. (1952). Iron and physiological anaemia of pregnancy, *Brit. Med. J.*, 1, 407–10.

Mohler, D. N., Wallin, D. G., and Dreyfus, E. G. (1955). Studies in home treatment of strepococcal disease: Failure of patients to take penicillin by mouth as prescribed, *New Eng. J. Med.*, 252, 1116–18.

Davis, M. S., and Eiochorn, R. L. (1963). Compliance with medical regimens: A panel study, *J. Hlth. Hum. Behav.*, 4, 240–9.

Gordis, L., Markowitz, M., and Lilienfeld, A. M. (1969). Studies in the epidemiology and preventability of rheumatic fever: IV. A quantitative determination of compliance in children on oral penicillin prophylaxis. *Pediatrics*, 43, 173–82.

Lipowski, Z. J. (1969). Psychosocial aspects of disease, *Ann. Int. Med.*, 71, 1197–1206.

Zola, I. K. (1972). The concept of trouble and sources of medical assistance, *Social Science and Medicine*, 6, 673–679.

Hayes, B. R., Taylor, D. W., and Sackett, D. C. (1979). *Compliance in Health Care*, Baltimore.

Mathews, J. J. (1983). The communication process in clinical settings, *Social Science and Medicine*, 17, 1371–78.

43. Rosenbluth, D., and Bowlby, J. (1955). The social and psychological backgrounds of tuberculous children, *Brit. Med. J.*, 1, 946–9.

Jenkins, C. D. (1966). Group difference in perception: A study of community beliefs and feelings about tuberculosis, *Amer. J. Sociol.*, 71, 417–29.

Sontag, S. (1978) *Illness as Metaphor*, New York.

44. Korsch, B. M., and Negrete, V. F. (1972). Doctor-patient communication, *Scientific American*, 227, 66–75.

Lorber, J. (1975). Good patients and problem patients: Conformity and deviance in a general hospital, *J. Health and Social Behavior*, 16, 213–25.

Shapiro, M. C., Najman, J. M., Chang, A., Keeping, J. D., Morrison, J., and Western, J. S. (1983). Information control and the exercise of power in the obstetrical encounter, *Social Science and Medicine*, 17, 139–46.

45. Waitzkin, H., and Stoeckle, J. (1972). The communication of information about illness, in *Advances in Psychosomatic Medicine*, ed. Lipowski, Z. J., Basel, vol. 8. pp. 180–215.

Stimson, G. V., and Webb, B. (1975). *Going to See the Doctor: The Consultation Process in General Practice*, Boston.

Wadsworth, M. and Robinson, D. eds. (1976). *Studies in Everyday Medical Life*, Totowa, N.J.

Kleinman, A., Eisenberg, L., and Good, B. (1978). Clinical lessons from anthropological and cross-cultural research, *Ann. Int. Med.*, 88, 251–258.

46. Fanon, F. (1965). Medicine and colonialism, in his *Studies in a Dying Colonialism*, New York.

47. Weaver, J., and Garret, S. (1978). Sexism and racism in the American health care industry: A comparative analysis, *Int. J. Hlth. Serv.*, 8, 677–703.

48. Scheff, T. J. (1966). *Being Mentally Ill: A Sociological Theory*, Hawthorne, N.Y.

Cockerham, W. C. (1979). Labeling theory and mental disorder: A synthesis of psychiatric and social perspectives, *Studies in Symbolic Interaction*, 2, 257–80.

Waxler, N. (1980). The social labeling perspective on illness and medical practice, in ed. Eisenberg, L., and Kleinman, A., *The Relevance of Social Science for Medicine*, Boston, pp. 283–306.

Gove, W. R. (1982). The current status of the labelling theory of mental illness, in ed. Gove, W. R., *Deviance and Mental Illness*, Beverly Hills, pp. 273–300.

Link, B. (1982) Mental patient status, work, and income: An examination of the effects of a psychiatric label, *Amer. Sociol. Rev.*, 47, 202–15.

Weinstein, R. M. (1983). Labeling theory and the attitudes of mental patients: A review, *J. Hlth. and Soc. Behav.*, 24, 70–84.

49. Edgerton, R. B. (1967). *The Cloak of Competence: Stigma in the Lives of the Mentally Retarded*, Berkeley.

Mercer, J. (1973) *Labeling the Mentally Retarded: Clinical and Social System Perspectives on Mental Retardation*, Berkeley.

50. Fabrega, H. (1972). The study of disease in relation to culture, *Behavioral Science*, 17, 183–293.

Mechanic, D. (1972). Social psychological factors affecting the presentation of bodily complaints, *New Eng. J. Medicine*, 286, 1132–36.

Douglas, M. (1975). *Natural Symbols*, London.

51. Suchman, E. A. (1964). Sociomedical variation among ethnic groups, *Amer. J. Sociol.*, 70, 319–31.

52. Geertsen, R., Klauber, M. R., Rindflesh, M., Kane, R. L., and Gray, R. (1975). A re-examination of Suchman's view on social factors in health care utilization, *J. Health and Social Behavior*, 16, 226–237.

53. Zola, I. K. (1972). Studying the decision to see a doctor, in *Advances in Psychosomatic Medicine*, vol. 8, ed. Lipowski, Z., Basel, pp. 216–36.

Hulka, B. S., Kuper L. L., and Cassel, J. C. (1972). Determinants of physician utilization, *Medical Care, 10,* 300–309.

54. Joint Committee of the Royal College of Obstetricians and Gynaecologists and the Population Investigation Committee (1948). *Maternity in Great Britain,* London.
    Spence, J., Walton, W. S., Miller, F. J. W., and Court, S. D. M. (1954). *A Thousand Families in Newcastle upon Tyne,* London.
    Marr, J. W., Hope, E. B., Stevenson, J. D., and Thomson, A. M. (1955). Consumption of milk and vitamin concentrates by pregnant women in Aberdeen, *Proc. Nutr. Soc., 14,* vii.
    Yankauer, A., Boek, W. E., Lawson, E. D., and Ianni, F. A. J. (1958). Social stratification and health practices in child-bearing and child-rearing, *Amer. J. Publ. Hlth., 48,* 732–41.
    Davis, K., Gold, M., and Makuc, D. (1981). Access to health care for the poor: Does the gap remain? *Ann. Rev. Publ. Hlth., 2,* 159–82.
    Mechanic, D. (1983). The experience and expression of distress: The study of illness behavior and medical utilization, in ed. Mechanic, D., *Handbook of Health, Health Care, and the Health Professions,* New York, pp. 591–607.

55. Kutner, B., Makover, H. B., and Oppenheim, A. (1958). Delay in the diagnosis and treatment of cancer: A critical analysis of the literature, *J. Chron. Dis., 7,* 95–120.
    Kutner, B., and Gordon, G. (1961). Seeking care for cancer, *J. Hlth. Hum. Behav., 2,* 171–8.

56. Taussig, M. (1978). Nutrition, development and foreign aid: A case study of U.S. directed health care in a Colombian plantation zone, *Int. J. Hlth. Serv., 8,* 101–121.

57. Cumming, E., and Cumming, J. (1957). *Closed Ranks: An Experiment in Mental Health Education,* Cambridge, Mass.

58. Hollingshead, A. B. and Redlich, F. C. (1958). *Social Class and Mental Illness,* New York.
    Eisenberg, J. M. (1979). Sociologic influences on decision-making by clinicians, *Ann. Int. Med., 90,* 957–964.

59. Rosenstock, I. M. (1960). What research in motivation suggests for public health, *Amer. J. Publ. Hlth., 50,* 295–302.
    Hochbaum, G. (1960). *Behavior in Response to Health Threats,* Department of Health, Education and Welfare, Washington, D.C.

60. Mechanic, D. (1962). The concept of illness behavior, *J. Chron. Dis., 15,* 189–94.
    Phillips, D. (1965). Self reliance and inclination to adopt the sick role, *Social Forces, 43,* 555–563.
    Kasl, S. V., and Cobb, S. (1966). Health behavior, illness behavior, and sick role behavior, *Arch. Env. Hlth., 12,* 245–266.
    Becker, M. H., and Maiman, L. A. (1983). Models of health-related behavior, in ed. Mechanic, D., *Handbook of Health, Health Care, and Health Professions,* New York, pp. 539–68.

61. Gabrielson, I. W., Levin, L. S., and Ellison, M. D. (1967). Factors affecting school health follow–up, *Amer. J. Public Hlth., 57,* 48–59.

62. Elling, R., Whitemore, R., and Green, M. (1960). Patient participation in a pediatric program, *J. Hlth. Hum. Behav., 1,* 183–191.

63. Feldman, J. (1966). *The Dissemination of Health Information: A Case Study in Adult Learning,* Chicago.

64. Marriot, M. (1955). Western medicine in a village of Northern India, in *Health, Culture and Community,* ed. Paul, B. D., New York, pp. 239–68.

Press, I. (1969). Urban illness: physicians, cures and dual use in Bogotá. *J. Hlth. Soc. Behav.*, 10, 209–218.

Leslie, C., ed. (1976). *Asian Medical Systems: A Comparative Study*, Berkeley.

Helman, C. G. (1978). Feed a cold, starve a fever—folk models of infection in an English suburban community and their relation to medical treatment. *Culture, Medicine and Psychiatry*, 2, 107–138.

Trostle, J. A., Hauser, W. A., and Susser, I. S. (1983). The logic of non-compliance: Management of epilepsy from the patient's point of view. *Culture, Medicine, and Psychiatry*, 1, 1–22.

Durkin-Longley, M. (1984). Multiple therapeutic use in urban Nepal, *Social Science and Medicine*, 19, 867–72.

65. Gurin, G., Veroff, J., and Feld, S. (1960). *Americans View Their Mental Health*, Joint Commission on Mental Illness and Health Monograph, Ser. 4, New York.

66. Strauss, A. L. (1969). Medical organization, medical care, and lower income groups, *Social Science and Medicine*, 3, 143–177.

Anderson, R., and Benham, L. (1970). Factors affecting the relationship between family income and medical care consumption, in *Empirical Studies in Health Economics*, ed. Karman, H. E., Baltimore, pp. 73–95.

Goering, J. M., and Coe, R. M. (1970). Cultural versus situational explanations of the medical behavior of the poor, *Soc. Sci. Quart.*, 51, 309–19.

McKinlay, J. B. (1972). Some approaches and problems in the study of the use of services—An overview, *J. Health and Social Behavior*, 13, 115–151.

Rice, T. W., Eichorn, R. L., and Fox, P. D. (1972). Socio-economic status and use of physician services: A reconsideration, *Medical Care*, 10, 261–271.

Riessman, C. K. (1974). The use of health services by the poor, *Social Policy*, 5, 41–49.

Dutton, D. B. (1978). Explaining the use of health services by the poor: Costs, attitudes, or delivery systems? *Amer. Sociol. Rev.*, 43, 348–368.

67. Pratt, L., Seligman, A., and Reader, G. G. (1958). Physicians' views on the level of medical information among patients, in *Patients, Physicians and Illness*, ed. Jaco, E. G., Glencoe, Ill., pp. 222–8.

Cartwright, A. (1964). *Human Relations and Hospital Care*, London.

Mumford, E. (1970). *Interns: From Students to Physicians*, Cambridge, Mass.

Bogdan, R., Brown, M. A., and Foster, S. B. (1982). Be honest but not cruel: Staff/ parent communication on a neonatal unit, *Human Organization*, 41, 6–16.

68. Mendelson, J. M., and Chafetz, M. E. (1959). Alcoholism as an emergency ward problem, *Quart. J. Stud. Alcohol*, 20, 270–5.

Chafetz, M. E., Blane, H. T., Abram, H. S., Golner, J., Lacy, E., McCourt, W. F., Clark, E., and Meyers, W. (1962). Establishing treatment relations with alcoholics, *J. Nerv. Ment. Dis.*, 134, 395–409.

69. Gajdusek, D. C., and Zigas, V. (1957). Degenerative disease of the central nervous system in New Guinea, *New Engl. J. Med.*, 257, 974–978.

70. Gajdusek, D. C. (1973). Kuru in the New Guinea Highlands, in *Tropical Neurology*, ed., Spillane, J. D., New York, pp. 376–383.

71. McArthur, N. (1964). The age incidence of kuru, *Annals of Human Genetics*, 27, 341–52.

72. Gajdusek, D. C., and Gibbs, Jr., C. J. (1975). Slow virus infections of the nervous system and the laboratories of slow, latent and temperate virus infections, in *The Nervous System, Vol. 2: The Clinical Neurosciences*, Tower, D. B. ed. New York, p. 113–135.

73. **Alpers, M.** (1970). Kuru in New Guinea: Its changing pattern and etiologic elucidation, *Amer. J. Trop. Med. Hyg., 19,* 133–137.

74. **Lindenbaum, S.** (1979). *Kuru Sorcery: Disease and Danger in the New Guinea Highlands,* Palo Alto, Calif.

75. **Baxter-Grillo, D. L.,** and **Lesi, F. E. A.** (1964). Factors influencing the occurrence of neonatal tetanus in Ibadan, *W. Afr. Med. J., 12,* 23–8.

76. **Holmes, E. G., Stanier, M. W.,** and **Thompson, M. D.** (1955). The serum protein pattern of Africans in Uganda: Relation to diet and malaria, *Trans. Roy. Soc. Trop. Med. Hyg., 49,* 376–84.

77. **Kuper, L., Watts, H.** and **Davies, R.** (1958). *Durban: A Study in Racial Ecology,* London.
    Kuper, H. (1960). *Indian People in Natal,* London.

78. **Kark, S. L.,** and **Chesler, J.** (1956). Survival in infancy, *S. Afr. J. Lab. Clin. Med., 2,* 134–159.

79. **Morris, J. N., Heady, J. A.,** and **Daly, C.** (1955). Social and biological factors in infant mortality, *Lancet 1,* 343–9, 395–7, 445–8, 449–502, 554–9.
    Shapiro, S., and **Moriyama, I. M.** (1963). International trends in infant mortality and their implications for the United States, *Amer. J. Publ. Hlth., 53,* 747–60.
    Chase, H. C. (1969). Infant mortality and weight at birth: 1960 United States birth cohort, *Amer. J. Publ. Hlth., 59,* 1618–28.
    Shapiro, S., and **Abramowicz, M.** (1969). Pregnancy outcome correlates identified through medical record–based information, *Amer. J. Publ. Hlth., 59,* 1629–50
    Susser, M., Marolla, F. and **Fleiss, J.** (1972). Birthweight, fetal age and perinatal mortality, *Amer. J. Epi., 96,* 197–204.

80. **Stein, Z. A.,** and **Susser, M. W.** (1958). A study of obstetric results in an underdeveloped community. Part I (a) The objects, materials and methods of the study; (b) some comparative rates, *J. Obstet. Gynaecol. Br. Emp., 75,* 763–768.
    Susser, M. W., and **Stein, Z. A.** (1958). A study of obstetric results in an underdeveloped community. Part II: The incidence and importance of certain factors with bearing on obstetric death rates, *J. Obstet. Gynaecol. Br. Emp., 65,* 769–773.
    Stein, Z. A., and **Susser, M. W.** (1959). A study of obstetric results in an underdeveloped community. Part III: The role of the hospital in the prevention of obstetric death, *J. Obstet. Gynaecol. Br. Emp., 66,* 62–67.
    Susser, M. W., and **Stein, Z. A.** (1959). A study of obstetric results in an underdeveloped community. Part IV: The causes and prevention of maternal and obstetric deaths, *J. Obstet. Gynaecol. Br. Emp., 66,* 68–74.

81. **Bradshaw, E.** and **Harington, J. S.** (1981). The cancer problem among Blacks: South Africa, in *Cancer Among Black Populations,* ed., Mettlin, C., Curtis, N. and Murphy, G. New York.

82. **Burrell, R. J. W.** (1957). Oesophaegeal cancer in the Bantu, *S. Afr. Med. J., 31,* 401–9.

83. **Brockington, C. F.** (1956). *A Short History of Public Health,* London.
    Rosen, G. (1958). *History of Public Health,* New York.

84. **Graham, S.** (1973). Studies of behavior changes to enhance public health, *Amer. J. Publ. Hlth., 63,* 327–34.
    Berkanovic, E. (1976). Behavioral science and prevention, *Preventive Medicine, 5,* 92–105.

85. **Kinsey, A. C., Pomeroy, W. B.,** and **Martin, C. E.** (1948). *Sexual Behavior in the Human Male,* Philadelphia.

Kinsey, A. C., Pomeroy, W. B., Martin, C. E., and Gebhard, P. H. (1953). *Sexual Behavior in the Human Female*, Philadelphia.

Ford, C. S., and Beach, F. A. (1953). *Patterns of Sexual Behaviour*, London.

86. Office of Population Censuses and Surveys (1978). Demographic Review: A Report on Population in Great Britain, Series DR no. 1, H.M.S.O., London.

Eversley, D., and Kollmann, W., ed. (1982). *Population Change and Social Planning*, London.

87. Gagnon, F. (1950). Contribution to the study of the aetiology and prevention of cancer of the cervix and of the uterus, *Amer. J. Obstet., Gynec., 60,* 516–22.

Kessler, I. I. (1976). Human cervical cancer as a venereal disease, *Cancer Research, 36,* 783–91.

88. Wynder, E. L., Cornfield, J., Schroff, P. D., and Doraiswami, K. R. (1954). A study of the environmental factors in carcinoma of the cervix, *Amer. J. Obstet. Gynec., 68,* 1016–46.

89. Rojel, J. (1953). The interrelation between uterine cancer and syphilis, *Acta Path. Microbiol. Scand.,* Suppl., *97,* 3–82.

90. Rotkin, I. D. (1967). Epidemiology of cancer of the cervix. II. Marital and coital factors in cervical cancer, *Amer. J. Publ. Hlth., 57,* 803–14.

Rotkin, I. D. (1967). Epidemiology of cancer of the cervix. III. Sexual characteristics of a cervical cancer population, *Amer. J. Publ. Hlth., 57,* 515–29.

Harris, R. W. C., Brinton, L. A., Cowdell, R. H., Skegg, D. C. G., Smith, P. G., Vessey, M. P., and Doll, R. (1980). Characteristics of women with dysplasia or carcinoma *in situ* of the cervix uteri, *Brit. J. Cancer, 42,* 359–69.

91. Westoff, C. F., and Ryder, N. B. (1969). Recent trends in attitudes towards fertility control and in the practice of contraception in the United States, in *Fertility and Family: A World View,* ed. Behrman, S. J., Corsa, L., and Freedman, R., Ann Arbor, Mich., pp. 388–412.

National Center for Health Statistics (1980). *Contraceptive Efficacy among Married Women Aged 15–44 Years, United States,* U.S. Department of Health and Human Services, Series 23, No. 5, Hyattsville, Maryland.

National Center for Health Statistics (1982). *Trends in Contraceptive Practice: United States, 1965–76,* U.S. Department of Health and Human Services, Series 23, No. 10, Hyattsville, Maryland.

92. U.S. Department of Health and Human Services (1982). *The Health Consequences of Smoking: Cancer. A Report of the Surgeon General,* U.S. Government Printing Office, Washington, D.C.

U.S. Department of Health and Human Services (1983). *The Health Consequences of Smoking: Cardiovascular Disease. A Report of the Surgeon General,* U.S. Government Printing Office, Washington, D.C.

93. Wynder, E. L. (1959). Laboratory contributions to the tobacco-cancer problem, *Brit. Med. J., 1,* 318–22.

94. Heath, C. W. (1958). Differences between smokers and non-smokers, *Arch. Intern. Med., 101,* 377–88.

Lilienfeld, A. M. (1959). A study of emotional and other selected characteristics of cigarette smokers and non-smokers as related to epidemiological studies of lung cancer and other diseases, *J. Nat. Cancer Inst., 82,* 259.

Freiberg, L., Kaij, L., Dencker, S. J., and Jonsson, E. (1959). Smoking habits of monozygotic and dizygotic twins, *Brit. Med. J., 1,* 1090–2.

Eysenck, H. J., Tarrant, M., Woolf, M., and England, L. (1960). Smoking and personality, *Brit. Med. J.*, *1*, 1456–60.

Reeder, L. (1977). Socio-cultural factors in the etiology of smoking behavior: An assessment, *Research on Smoking Behavior*, Monograph No. 17, National Institute of Drug Abuse, Washington, D.C., pp. 186–200.

95. MacArthur, C., Waldron, E., and Dickinson, J. (1958). The psychology of smoking, *J. Abnorm. Soc. Psychol.*, *56*, 267–75.

96. Morris, J. N. (1972). *Statistics of Smoking in the United Kingdom*, London.

Sterling, T. D., and Weinkam, J. J. (1976). Smoking characteristics by type of employment, *J. Occup. Med.*, *18*, 743–54.

Covey, L. S., and Wynder, E. L. (1981). Smoking habits and occupational status, *J. Occup. Med.*, *23*, 537–42.

Cummins, R. O., Shaper, A. G., Walker, M., and Wale, C. J. (1981). Smoking and drinking by middle-aged British men: Effects of social class and town of residence, *Brit. Med. J.*, *283*, 1497–1502.

97. Salber, E. J., and MacMahon, B. (1961). Cigarette smoking among high school students related to social class and parental smoking habits, *Amer. J. Publ. Hlth.*, *51*, 1780–9.

Horn, D. (1968). Current smoking among teenagers, *Publ. Hlth. Rep.* Wash., *83*, 458–60.

Holland, W. W., and Elliott, A. (1968). Cigarette smoking, respiratory symptoms and anti-smoking propaganda, *Lancet*, *1*, 41–3.

Banks, M. H., Bewley, B. R., Bland, J. M., Dean, J. R., and Pollard, V. (1978). Long-term study of smoking by secondary school children, *Arch. Dis. Child.*, *53*, 12–19.

Bachman, J. G., Johnston, L. D., and O'Mally, P. M. (1981). Smoking, drinking, and drug use among American high school students: Correlates and trends, *Amer. J. Publ. Hlth.*, *71*, 59–69.

Eckert, P. (1983). Beyond the statistics of adolescent smoking, *Amer. J. Publ. Hlth.*, *73*, 439–41.

98. Cartwright, A., and Martin, F. M. (1958). Some popular beliefs concerning the causes of cancer, *Brit. Med. J.*, *2*, 592–4.

Cartwright, A., Martin, F. M., and Thompson, J. G. (1960). Efficacy of an anti-smoking campaign, *Lancet*, *1*, 327–9.

99. Doll, R., and Hill, A. B. (1964). Mortality in relation to smoking: Ten years observation of British doctors, *Brit. Med. J.*, *1*, 1399–1410, 1460–7.

Hammond, E. C., and Garfinkel, L. (1968). Changes in cigarette smoking, 1959–65, *Amer. J. Publ. Hlth.*, *58*, 30–45.

100. Jacobs, M. A., Anderson, L. S., Champagne, E., Karush, N. M., Richman, S. J., and Knapp, P. H. (1966). Orality, impulsivity and cigarette smoking in man: Further findings in support of a theory, *J. Nerv. Ment. Dis.*, *143*, 207–19.

Stewart, L., and Livson, N. (1966). Smoking and rebelliousness: A longitudinal study from childhood to maturity, *J. Cons. Psychol.*, *30*, 225–9.

Burns, B. H. (1969). Chronic chest disease, personality, and success in stopping cigarette smoking, *Brit. J. Prev. Soc. Med.*, *23*, 23–7.

101. Freud, S. (1949; first pub. 1905). *Three Essays on the Theory of Sexuality*, trans. Strachey, J., London.

102. Levy, D. M. (1928). Fingersucking and accessory movements in early infancy, *Amer. J. Psychiat.*, *7*, 818–918.

103. Whiting, J. W. M., and Child, I. L. (1953). *Child Training and Personality: A Cross-Cultural Study*, New Haven.

Sears, R. S., MacCoby, E. E., and Levin, H. (1957). *Patterns of Child Rearing*, New York.

104. Orlansky, H. (1949). Infant care and personality, *Psychol. Bull.*, 46, 1–8.
Lindesmith, A. R., and Strauss, A. L. (1950). Critique of culture-personality writings, *Amer. Sociol. Rev.*, 15, 587–600.
Thurston, J. R. and Mussen, P. H. (1951). Infant feeding, gratification, and adult personality, *J. Personality*, 19, 449–58.
Sewell, W. H. (1952). Infant training and personality of child, *Amer. J. Sociol.*, 58, 150–9.
Caldwell, B. M. (1964). The effects of infant care, in *Review of Child Development Research*, ed. Hoffman, M. L., and Hoffman, L. W., New York.

105. Baumslag, N., Grace-Mason, L., Roesel, C., and Sabin, Z. (1979). *Breast is Best: A Bibliography on Breastfeeding and Infant Health*, U.S. Dept. of Health, Education and Welfare, Washington, D.C.
Taylor, B., and Wadsworth, J. (1984). Breastfeeding and child development at five years. *Developmental Medicine and Child Neurology*, 26, 73–80.
Forman, M. R., Graubard, B. I., Hoffman, H. J., Beren, R., Harley, E. E., and Bennett, P. (1984). The Pima infant feeding study: Breast feeding and gastroenteritis in the first year of life, *Amer. J. Epi.*, 119, 335–349.

106. Cassel, J. (1955). A comprehensive health program among South African Zulus, in *Health, Culture and Community*, ed. Paul, B. D., New York, pp. 15–42.

107. McLaren, D. S. (1966). A fresh look at protein-calorie malnutrition, *Lancet*, 2, 485–88.
Jelliffe, D. B. (1968). *Infant Nutrition in the Subtropics and Tropics*, 2nd ed., Wld. Hlth. Org., Monogr. Ser., No. 29.
Stein, Z. A., and Kassab, H. (1970). Nutrition, in *Mental Retardation*, ed. Wortis, J., New York.
Birch, H. G., and Gussow, J. D. (1970). *Disadvantaged Children: Health, Nutrition, and School Failure*, New York.

108. Davis, A., and Havighurst, R. J. (1946). Social class and color differences in child rearing, *Amer. Sociol. Rev.*, 2, 698–710.
Douglas, J. W. B. (1950). Breast-feeding, *J. Obstet. Gynaec. Brit. Emp.*, 57, 335–61.
Westropp, C. (1953). Breast-feeding in the Oxford Child Health Survey, (1) A study of maternal factors, *Brit. Med. J.*, 1, 138–40.
Spence, J., Walton, W. S., Miller, F. J. W., and Court, S. D. M. (1954). *A Thousand Families in Newcastle upon Tyne*, London.
Havighurst, R. J., and Davis, A. (1955). A comparison of the Chicago and Harvard studies of social class differences in child rearing, *Amer. Sociol. Rev.*, 20, 438–42.
Dykes, R. M. (1957). Vitamin supplementation and type of feeding in infancy, *Lancet*, 2, 230–2.
Yankauer, A., Boek, W. E., Lawson, E. D., and Ianni, F. A. J. (1958). Social stratification and health practices in child-bearing and child-rearing, *Amer. J. Publ. Hlth.* 48, 732–41.
Meyer, H. F. (1958). Breast feeding in the United States: Extent and possible trend, *Pediatrics*, 27, 116–21.
McGeorge, M. (1960). Current trends in breast feeding, *N.Z. Med. J.*, 59, 31–41.
Robertson, W. O. (1961). Breast feeding practices: Some implications of regional variations, *Amer. J. Publ. Hlth.*, 51, 1035–42.

109. Hytten, F. E., Yorston, J. C., and Thomson, A. M. (1958). Difficulties associated with breast-feeding, *Brit. Med. J.*, 1, 310–15.

110. **Kark, S. L.** (1957). The initiation of breast feeding in the puerperium, *Med. Proc., 3*, 404–9.

111. **Jelliffe, D. B.** (1952). The protein content of the breast-milk of African women, *Brit. Med. J., 2*, 1131–2.

   Welbourn, E. M. (1955). The danger period during weaning: A study of Baganda children who were attending child welfare clinics near Kampala, Uganda, *J. Trop. Paediat., 1*, 34–46, 98–111, 161–73.

112. **Hytten, F. E.** (1951). Observations on the vitality of the newborn, *Arch. Dis. Childh., 26*, 477–86.

113. **Firth, R.** (1959). Concepts of health and disease, in *Medicine and Anthropology*, ed. Galdston, I., New York.

   Troyat, H. (1967). *Tolstoy*, New York.

114. **Jelliffe, D. B.** and **Jelliffe, E. F. P.** (1981). Recent trends in infant feeding, *Ann, Rev. Publ. Hlth., 2*, 145–58.

   Martinez, G. A., and **Dodd, D. A.** (1983). 1981 Milk feeding patterns in the United States during the first 12 months of life, *Pediatrics, 71*, 166–70.

115. **Mead, M.** (1931). *Growing Up in New Guinea*, London.

   Dubois, C. A., and **Kardiner, A.** (1944). *The People of Alor*, Minneapolis.

   Kardiner, A. (1945). *Psychological Frontiers of Society*, New York.

   Benedict, R. F. (1947). *The Chrysanthemum and the Sword: Patterns of Japanese Culture*, London.

   Erikson, E. H. (1949). Childhood and tradition in two American tribes, in *Personality in Nature, Society and Culture*, ed. Kluckhohn, C., and Murray, H. A., London.

   Gladwin, T., and **Sarason, S. B.** (1953). *Truk: Man in Paradise*, New York, Viking Fund Publications in Anthropology, No. 20.

   Carstairs, G. M. (1957). *The Twice-Born*, London.

116. **Seligman, B. Z.** (1934). The part of the unconscious in social heritage, in *Essays Presented to C. G. Seligman*, ed. Evans-Pritchard, E. E., Firth, R., Malinowski, B., and Schapera, I., London.

   Goldenweiser, A. (1946). *Anthropology*, New York.

   Boyer, L. B., Klopfer, B., Brawer, F. B., and **Kawai, H.** (1964). Comparisons of the shamans and pseudoshamans of the Apaches of the Mescalero Indian reservation: A Rorschach study, *J. Projective Techniques and Personality Assessment, 28*, 173–180.

   Silverman, J. (1967). Shamans and acute schizophrenia, *American Anthropologist, 69*, 21–31.

   Handelman, D. (1968). The development of a Washo Shaman, *Ethnology, 6*, 444–464.

117. **Barnouw, V.** (1973), *Culture and Personality*, rev. ed., Homewood, Ill.

118. **Caudill, W. A.** (1973). The influence of social structure and culture on human behavior in modern Japan, *J. Nerv. Ment. Dis., 157*, 240–257.

119. **Whiting, B. B.,** and **Whiting, J. W. M.** (1975). *Children of Six Cultures: A Psycho-Cultural Analysis*, Cambridge, Mass.

120. **Geber, M.,** and **Dean, R. F. A.** (1957). The state of development of newborn African children, *Lancet, 1*, 1216–1219.

   Williams, C. D. (1957). The state of development of newborn African children, *Lancet, 2*, 93–94.

   Ainsworth, M. (1967). *Infancy in Uganda*, Baltimore.

121. **Segal, M. H., Campbell, D. T.,** and **Herskovits, M. J.** (1966). *The Influence of Culture on Visual Perception*, Indianapolis, Ind.

D'Andrade, R. G. (1973). Cultural constructions of reality, in *Cultural Illness and Health*, ed. Nader, L., and Maretzki, T. W., Washington, D.C., pp. 115–127.

Serpell, R. (1982). Measures of perception, skills, and intelligence: The growth of a new perspective on children in a Third World country, in *Review of Child Development Research*, ed. Hartup. W., Chicago, pp. 392–440.

122. Cooley, C. H. (1902). *Human Nature and the Social Order*, New York.

123. Mead, G. H. (1934). *Mind, Self and Society*, Chicago.

124. Goffman, E. (1959). *The Presentation of Self in Everyday Life*, New York.
Goffman, E. (1961). *Asylums*, New York.
Garfinkel, H. (1967). *Studies in Ethnomethodology*, Englewood Cliffs, N.J.
Burke, K. (1971). *Language as Gesture*, Berkeley.
Rock, P. (1974). *The Making of Symbolic Interactionism*, London.

125. Geertz, C. (1976). "From the native's point of view": On the nature of anthropological understanding, in *Meaning in Anthropology*, ed., Basso, K. H. and Selby, S. A., Albuquerque, pp. 221–237.

126. Parsons, T. (1964). *Social Structure and Personality*, New York, pp. 78–111.

127. Wolff, H. G. (1953). *Stress and Disease*, Springfield, Ill.

128. Wolf, S., and Wolff, H. G. (1947). *Human Gastric Function*, London.

129. Susser, M. W. (1967). Causes of peptic ulcer, a selective epidemiological review, *J. Chron. Dis., 20*, 435–56.

130. Beaumont, W. (1833). *Experiments and Observations on the Gastric Juice and the Physiology of Digestion*, Plattsburg, N.Y.
Pavlov, I. P. (1928). *Lectures on Conditioned Reflexes*, New York.

131. Mirsky, A., Kaplan, S., and Broh-Kahn, R. H. (1950). Pepsinogen excretion (Uropepsin) as an index of the influence of various life situations on gastric secretion, in *Life Stress and Bodily Disease*, Proceedings of the Association for Research in Nervous and Mental Diseases, Baltimore.

132. Von Bergmann, G. (1913). Ulcus duodeni and vegetatives Nervensystem, *Berl. Klin. Wschr., 51*, 2374.
Draper, C., and Touraine, G. A. (1932). The man-environment unit and peptic ulcers, *Arch. Intern. Med., 49*, 615–62.

133. Alexander, F. (1934). The influence of psychologic factors upon gastrointestinal disturbances: A symposium, *Psychoanal. Quart., 3*, 501–39.

134. Kellock, T. D. (1951). Childhood factors in duodenal ulcers, *Brit. Med. J., 2*, 1117–20.

135. Cohen, S. I., Silverman, A. J., Waddell, W., and Zuidema, G. D. (1961). Urinary catecholamine levels, gastric secretion and specific psychological factors in ulcer and non-ulcer patients, *J. Psychosom. Res., 5*, 90–115.

136. Goldberg, E. M. (1958). *Family Influences and Psychosomatic Illness*, London.

137. Spiegel, E. (1918). Beitrage zur Klinischen Konstitutions-pathologic. II. Organdisposition bei ulcus pepticum, *Dtsch. Arch. Klin. Med., 126*, 45–60.
Doll, R., and Buch, J. (1950). Hereditary factors in peptic ulcer, *Ann. Eugen.* (Lond.), *15*, 135–46.

138. Selye, H. (1950). *The Physiology and Pathology of Exposure to Stress*, Montreal.

139. Engel, G. L. (1962). *Psychological Development in Health and Disease*, Philadelphia.
Weiner, H. M. (1977). *Psychobiology and Human Disease*, New York.

140. *Some examples are provided by:*
Funkenstein, D. H. (1953). The relationship of experimentally produced asthmatic attacks to certain acute life stresses, *J. Allergy, 24*, 11–17.

Prugh, D. G., Staub, E. M., Sands, H. H., Kirschbaum, R. M., and Lenihan, E. A. (1953). A study of the emotional reactions of children and families to hospitalization and illness, *Amer. J. Orthopsychiat.*, 23, 70–106.

Coleman, R., Greenblatt, M., and Solomon, H. C. (1956). Physiological evidence of rapport during psychotherapeutic interviews, *Dis. Nerv. Syst.*, 17, 71–7.

Rees, L. (1956). Psychosomatic aspects of asthma in elderly patients, *J. Psychosom. Res.*, 1, 217–18.

Sainsbury, P. (1960). Psychosomatic disorders and neurosis in out-patients attending a general hospital, *J. Psychosom. Res.*, 4, 261–73.

Coppen, A., and Kessel, N. (1963). Menstruation and personality, *Brit. J. Psychiat.*, 109, 711–21.

Friedman, S. B., Choodoff, P., Mason, J. W., and Hamburg, D. A. (1963). Behavioral observations on parents anticipating the death of a child, *Pediatrics*, 32, 610–25.

141. Susser, M. W. (1968). *Community Psychiatry: Epidemiological and Social Themes*, New York.

142. Dohrenwend, B. S., and Dohrenwend, B. P., eds. (1981). *Stressful Life Events and Their Contexts*, New York.

143. Kasl, S. V., and Cobb, S. (1970). Blood pressure changes in men undergoing job loss: A preliminary report, *Psychosomatic Medicine*, 32, 19–38.

144. Kasl, S. V., Cobb, S., and Brooks, G. W. (1968). Changes in serum uric acid and cholesterol levels in men undergoing job loss, *J. Amer. Med. Ass.*, 206, 1500–7.

145. Naroll, R. (1962). *Data Quality Control*, New York.

Schwab, J. J., and Schwab, M. E. (1978). *Sociocultural Roots of Mental Illness: An Epidemiological Survey*, New York.

Leff, J. (1981). *Psychiatry Around the Globe: A Transcultural View*, New York.

146. Sainsbury, P. (1955). *Suicide in London: An Ecological Study*, Maudsley Monographs No. 1, London.

MacMahon, B., Johnson, S., and Pugh, T. F. (1963). Relation of suicide rates to social conditions, *Publ. Hlth. Rep.* (Wash.), 78, 287–93.

Massey, J. T. (1967). Suicide in the United States, 1950–1964, *Vital and Health Statistics*, Series 20, No. 5, United States Public Health Service, Washington, D.C.

Adelstein, A., and Mardon, C. (1975). Suicides, 1961–74, *Population Trends*, 2, 13–18.

Warshauer, M. E., and Monk, M. (1978). Problems in suicide statistics for whites and blacks. *Amer. J. Publ. Hlth.*, 68, 383–88.

147. Morselli, E. A. (1882) *Suicide: An Essay in Comparative Moral Statistics*, New York.

Halbwachs, M. (1930). *Les Causes du Suicide*, Paris.

Henry, A. F., and Short, J. F. (1954). *Suicide and Homicide*, Glencoe, Ill.

Maris, R. (1975). Sociology, in *A Handbook for the Study of Suicide*, ed. S. Perlin, New York, pp. 93–112.

Hopper, K., and Guttmacher, S. (1979). Rethinking suicide: Notes toward a critical epidemiology, *Intl. J. Hlth. Serv.*, 9, 417–38.

148. Durkheim, E. (1951; first pub. 1897). *Suicide: A Study in Sociology*, trans. Spalding, J. A., and Simpson, G., Glencoe, Ill.

149. Srole, L. (1951). Social dysfunction, personality, and social distance attitudes, unpublished paper read before American Sociological Society, cited in Merton, R. K. (1957) *Social Theory and Social Structure*, rev. ed., Glencoe, Ill., p. 164.

150. Seeman, M. (1958). On the meaning of alienation, *Amer. Sociol. Rev.*, 23, 783–91.

Merton, R. K. (1957). *Social Theory and Social Structure*, rev. ed., Glencoe, Ill.

151. **Selvin, H. C.** (1958). Durkheim's suicide and problems of empirical research, *Amer. J. Sociol.*, *63*, 607–19.

152. **Dublin, L.** (1963). *Suicide: A Sociological and Statistical Study*, New York.
     Maris, R. (1969). *Social Forces in Urban Suicide*, Homewood, Ill.

153. **Brook, E. M.**, ed. (1974). Suicide and Attempted Suicide, Public Health Papers, No. 58, Geneva.

154. **Weissman, M.** (1974). The epidemiology of suicide attempts, 1960 to 1971, *Arch. Gen. Psychiatry*, *30*, 737–746.

155. **Thomas, D. S.** (1927). *Social Aspects of the Business Cycle*, New York.
     Sainsbury, P. (1972). The social relations of suicide, *Soc. Sci. Med.*, *6*, 189–198.
     Dooley, D. and **Catalano, R.** (1980). Economic change as a cause of behavioral disorder, *Psychol. Bull.*, *87*, 450–68.

156. **Pokorny, A. D.** (1964). Suicide rates in various psychiatric disorders, *J. Nerv. Ment. Dis.*, *139*, 499–506.
     Temoche, A., Pugh, T. F., and **MacMahon, B.** (1964). Suicide rates among current and former mental institution patients, *J. Nerv. Ment. Dis.*, *138*, 124–130.

157. **Parrish, H. M.** (1957). Epidemiology of suicide among college students, *Yale J. Biol. Med.*, *29*, 585–95.
     Bruhn, J. G. (1962). Broken homes among attempted suicides and psychiatric outpatients: A comparative study, *J. Ment. Sci, 108*, 772–9.
     Tuckman, J., and **Youngman, W. F.** (1964). Attempted suicide and family disorganization, *J. Genet. Psychol.*, *101*, 187–93.
     MacMahon, B., and **Pugh, T. F.** (1965). Suicide in the widowed, *Amer. J. Epidem.*, *81*, 23–31.

158. **Monk, M. E.,** and **Warshauer, M.** (1974). Completed and attempted suicide in three ethnic groups, *Amer. J. Epidem.*, *100*, 333–345.

159. **Ogden, M., Spector, B.,** and **Hill, C.** (1970). Suicides and homicides among Indians, *Public Health Reports*, *85*, 75–80.
     Seiden, R. (1972). Why are the suicides of young blacks increasing? *HSMHA Health Reports*, *87*, 3–8.

160. **Watson, W.** (1958). *Tribal Cohesion in a Money Economy: A Study of the Mambwe people of Northern Rhodesia*, Manchester.

For psychological interpretations of suicide see:

161. **Menninger, K. A.** (1936). *Man Against Himself*, New York.
     Stengel, E. (1964). Suicide and attempted suicide, London.
     Perlin, S., and **Schmidt, C. W.** (1975). Psychiatry, in *A Handbook for the Study of Suicide*, ed. Perlin, S., New York, pp. 147–164.

162. **Bohannan, P.,** ed. (1960). *African Homicide and Suicide*, Princeton, N.J.

163. **Douglas, J.** (1967). *The Social Meanings of Suicide*, Princeton, N.J.

164. **Loudon, J. B.** (1959). Psychogenic disorder and social conflict among the Zulu, in *Culture and Mental Health*, ed. Opler, M. K., New York.
     Lambo, T. A. (1960). Further neuropsychiatric observations in Nigeria, *Brit. Med. J.*, *2*, 696–70.

165. **Dohrenwend, B. P., Dohrenwend, B. S., Gould, M. S., Link, B., Neugebauer, R.,** and **Wunsch-Hitzig, R.** (1980). *Mental Illness in the United States: Epidemiological Estimates*, New York.

166. **Reid, D. D.** (1960). Epidemiological methods in the study of mental disorders, *Wld. Hlth. Org. Publ. Hlth. Pap.*, No. 2.

Cassel, J. (1964). Social science theory as a source of hypotheses in epidemiological research, *Amer. J. Publ. Hlth.*, 54, 1482–88.

167. Stainbrook, E. (1952). Some characteristics of the psychopathology of schizophrenic behaviour in Bahian society, *Amer. J. Psychiat.*, 109, 30–5.

Edgerton, R. B. (1966). Conceptions of psychosis in four East African societies, *American Anthropologist*, 68, 408–25.

Waxler, N. E. (1979). Is outcome for schizophrenia better in nonindustrial societies?, *J. Nerv. Ment. Dis.*, 167, 144–58.

Warner, R. (1983). Recovery from schizophrenia in the Third World, *Psychiatry*, 46, 197–212.

168. Lucas, C. J. (1959). Social and familial correlates of schizophrenic delusions, *Proc. Roy. Soc. Med.*, 25, 1066–7.

169. Opler, M. K., and Singer, J. L. (1956). Ethnic differences in behaviour and psychopathology, *Int. J. Soc. Psychiat.*, 2, 11–22.

170. Roberts, B. H., and Myers, J. K. (1954). Religion, natural origin, immigration, and mental illness, *Amer. J. Psychiat.*, 110, 759–64.

171. Laubscher, B. (1937). *Sex, Custom and Psychopathology*, London.

Tooth, G. (1950). *Studies in Mental Illness in the Gold Coast*, Colonial Research Publications No. 6, London, H.M.S.O.

Yap, P. M. (1951). Mental diseases peculiar to certain cultures: A survey of comparative psychiatry, *J. Ment. Sci.*, 97, 313–27.

Lambo, T. A. (1955). The role of cultural factors in paranoid psychosis among the Yoruba tribe, *J. Ment. Sci.*, 101, 239–66.

Kennedy, J. G. (1973). Cultural psychiatry, in *Handbook of Social and Cultural Anthropology*, ed. Honigmann, J. J., Chicago, pp. 119–98.

172. Zubin, J. (1969). Cross-national study of diagnosis of mental disorders: Methodology and planning, *Amer. J. Psychiat.*, (Suppl.), 125, 12–20.

Cooper, J. E., Kendall, R. E., Gurland, B., Sartorius, N., and Tiborfarkas, T. (1969). Cross-national study of diagnosis of mental disorders: Some results from the first comparative investigation, *Amer. J. Psychiat.*, Suppl., 125, 21–9.

Gurland, B., Fleiss, J., Cooper, J. E., Kendall, R. E., and Simon, R. (1969). Cross-national study of diagnosis of mental disorders: Some comparisons of diagnostic critiques from the first investigation, *Amer. J. Psychiat.*, Suppl., 125, 30–9.

Kendall, R. E. (1969). Cross-national study of diagnosis of mental disorders: Discussion: The problems raised by cross–cultural studies, *Amer. J. Psychiat.*, Suppl., 125, 111–13.

Pope, H. G. Jr., and Lipinski, J. F. Jr. (1978). Diagnosis in schizophrenia and manic-depressive illness, *Arch. Gen. Psychiat.*, 35, 811–28.

World Health Organization (1979). *Schizophrenia: An International Follow-up Study*, New York.

Carpenter, W. T., Heinrichs, D. W., and Hanlon, T. E. (1981). Methodologic standards for treatment outcome research in schizophrenia, *Amer. J. Psychiat.*, 138, 465–71.

173. Leighton, D. C., Harding, J. S., Macklin, D. B., Macmillan, A. M., and Leighton, A. H. (1963). *The Stirling County Study of Psychiatric Disorder and Socio-Cultural Environment. Vol. III. The Character of Danger: Psychiatric Symptoms in Selected Communities*, New York.

174. Eaton, J. W., and Weill, R. J. (1955). *Culture and Mental Disorders*, Glencoe, Ill.

Egeland, J. A., and Hostetter, A. M. (1983). Amish Study, I: Affective disorders among the Amish, 1976–1980, *Amer. J. Psychiat.*, 140, 56–61.

5

Theories and indices
of social class

Systematic inquiry into the health consequences of social inequality dates from the pioneering work in the nineteenth century of Louis-René Villermé in France and of William Farr and his successors in the British General Register Office. Occupation provided a key index of social position. It soon became clear that many factors, including the hazards of work, poor housing, nutrition, and hygiene were necessary to account for observed differences in mortality. In 1911, the Chief Medical Statistical Officer in the General Register Office, T. H. C. Stevenson, used the concept of social class to arrange the British census data into five social classes. The basis of the division in the first instance appeared to be socioeconomic ranking of occupations.° This system of classification proved to be a powerful epidemiological tool, as well as an immense gain to comparative sociology. Since then, vital statistics and population statistics in Britain have continued to be presented in social class categories.

This scale, the General Register Office's Classification, was used to demonstrate that many diseases have a different prevalence among groups of people at different social levels. These social class gradients have helped to provide a deeper understanding of clinical phenomena and to affect decisions on questions of social policy. The poor had a higher incidence of some diseases, the rich of others, although the poor have always borne the brunt. Health practices, too, like the use of health services, welfare and

---

° Occupation had been recorded in the British census and death registration data from the mid-nineteenth century. Occupations were arranged in what was essentially a *nominal scale*, a mutually exclusive classification assigned to numbered categories, of which the International Classification of Diseases is also an example. Stevenson's contribution was to develop an *ordinal scale*, in which the numbers are ordered by the degree or order of magnitude of the property scaled. Stevenson specified the quality scaled as social class, a concept about which it was easier to obtain consensus in 1911 than it is now. His supposedly "socioeconomic" ranking gradually evolved, in the hands of the General Register Office, into a ranking of "prestige." In 1961, the scale was further defined to take into account different levels of responsibility accorded occupations.

maternity clinics, and methods of infant feeding, were found to be correlated with social class. Despite the advances in social welfare and preventive medicine and the enormous decline in mortality since social gradients in disease were first defined, disparities between the classes persist.

The term "social class" in common usage is given a number of meanings in different contexts, like the word "society" itself; even in sociological theory there are almost as many definitions as there are sociologists (1). These ambiguities have their roots both in the complexity of the phenomena which the term attempts to describe and in the theoretical dispositions of the observers of such phenomena. The analysis of social class is at once a difficult and contested endeavor; how it is conceived and applied depends upon one's understanding of the nature and exercise of power and privilege in society.

In all societies people are differentiated by biological and social criteria, ranging from the fundamental classifications by age and gender in hunting and gathering societies to the complex divisions by social class in contemporary capitalist societies. Such divisions are not merely functional. Categories of social distinction are assigned different degrees of importance and prestige. Gradations of esteem, in turn, reflect broader social values and circumstances. The near-universal esteem accorded the role of healer, for example, cannot be understood without recognizing how deeply threatening episodes of illness can be. In "simple" societies, even the primary divisions of gender and age derive their meaning from the culturally prized performances with which they are associated. Thus in some of the subsistence economies of precolonial Africa, where men and women were not necessarily unequal partners in productive activities, the social status of women more nearly approximated that of men. With the advent of wage-labor and the relegation of women's work to the domestic hearth their social status was devalued (2). (For discussion of roles and status, see Chapter 7.)

Although the varieties of social inequality are many (3), pronounced inequality in the possession of material goods appears to be a relatively late historical development. Disparities in social position were recognized in tribal societies and village communities, but the privileges of rank were not synonymous with wealth. In numerous instances, a village headman has been found to be materially poorer than his neighbors. Often the primary perquisite of rank was redistributive—to portion out the pooled surplus so that inequalities of wealth were kept minimal and did not in any event jeopardize survival. Regulation of the social order was achieved through the medium of the kinship system, and kinship ties served to offset potential conflict with cross-cutting obligations of mutual support (4).

A formal machinery of sanctions, separate from and overriding the control exerted by kinship systems, first appears in stratified societies, paramount among which are the state societies of today. In stratified societies, private property—in the sense of ownership and control of scarce means of production—restricts common access to resources. The exploitation of human labor becomes possible, for those denied free use of the raw materials needed for survival must purchase them with their labor, with a portion of their produce, or with military or other service. Distinctions of wealth, rank, and power are intensified. For our purposes, the notable feature of such developments is the division of society into social classes (5).

When Marx and Engels wrote in 1848 that all human history to that point was the history of class conflict, they were recognizing a feature of much recorded history. Social orders which permit the privation of many for the benefit of few must give rise to persisting conflicts of interest. Thus, a formal apparatus of social control, exercised by those who benefit from the division of society, becomes necessary. Control is never a matter merely of the availability of sufficient force. Ruling orders must be recognized as legitimate—that is, endowed with *authority*—if they are to endure. This need not be the mandate of heaven invoked by traditional Chinese rulers, nor the divine right claimed by European kings, but it must be rooted in a source higher than that of personal ambition or greed. Max Weber provided one scheme for analyzing methods of exacting obedience. He classified societies by three modes of authority: traditional, legal, or charismatic. While this remains an important insight into the workings of dominance and subordination in social relationships, it does not suffice to explain the exercise of *power* in modern societies (6).

Power has been defined as the ability of one person or group to shape the behavior of another in a situation where the interests of the two are in real or potential conflict. In stratified societies, there is always a presumption of conflict in that certain groups are denied access to essential resources. Power may be exercised by individuals, collectivities, or institutions; it may be embodied in established procedures; it may be exerted through inaction as well as action; and it may involve decisions not taken or considered as much as it does those actually made. Indeed, the subtlest exercise of power may well be in those circumstances in which the compliance of the subject is apparently voluntary (7).

For social scientists studying medicine, such considerations become important when analyzing the health-related behavior of subordinate classes, their access to clinical services, and social policies which have implications for health—such as, for example, the setting of health and safety standards at the workplace. In the United States, studies of pollution control, public transportation, national health insurance, and the growing corporate invasion of the health-service sector illustrate the utility of the concept of power (8).

Theories of social class

In its modern sense as a term of social division, "class" is a word that came into currency during the period of social dislocation brought about by the industrial revolution. It signaled in part a growing awareness that social position was created, not inherited, an awareness which was at least dimly available by 1705 when Defoe observed: "'tis . . . plain that the dearness of wages forms our people into more classes than other nations can show." In the centuries that followed, the lines of division the term was intended to designate were shifting and ambiguous. "Class" was used to denote sometimes an economic grouping (landowners, laborers), sometimes a social rank (the middle class) or, after Marx, a politically self-aware and active formation (in some uses, the working class). Preferred usage often corresponded with the political disposition of the user, a practice which continues to the present day. In the extreme, the term may be avoided altogether, as in much American sociological inquiry into the particularities of "socioeconomic status," rather than "class" (9).

Sociologists generally distinguish between two dimensions of stratification: a structural dimension that encompasses the demographic and economic differences of the various groupings (job and educational opportunities, health profiles, marriage and divorce rates, family size, etc.); and a cultural dimension that includes behavior, attitude, and habitat (dietary habits, leisure activities, political beliefs, relationships between the sexes and generations, place of residence, etc.). The first are usually referred to as aspects of life-chances; the second as mode of life (10). These are not merely scholarly distinctions, nor are they new ones. While drafting the *Federalist Papers* in 1787, James Madison remarked that managerial and manufacturing interests "grow up of necessity in civilized nations, and divide them into different classes, actuated by different sentiments and views."

In any classification scheme, the type of work an individual performs is of central importance. Modern industrial processes and their associated forms of organization have created an intricate structure of specialized occupations bearing certain relationships toward one another. This structure of relationships persists through time, although it is constantly modified as new productive processes or techniques of control are introduced (11). At one end of the occupational scale are those who own and direct productive activities; at the other end are laborers who have little direct control over the process of production. Between these extremes lies a highly differentiated middle layer of persons of many occupations.

Some occupations demand greater skill, longer training, and higher education than others and are better rewarded. These factors are significant in determining the social prestige given to an occupation, and are connected with income, education, residence, and mode of life. That is, people can be seen to belong to different economic groups, and these groups can be ranked into a system of stratification, each group having a different degree of power or prestige.

Such was the starting point for the analysis of social class formulated by Karl Marx as part of a general account of the origins, dynamics, and prospects of industrial capitalism.° Marx saw in class antagonism the animating force of historical development. His analysis of the forces at work in nineteenth-century England convinced him that the three great classes of wage-laborers, capitalists, and landowners were rapidly being reduced to two—bourgeoisie and proletariat—whose interests were fundamentally opposed. These two contending classes were defined by their relationship to the process of production. The bourgeoisie owned and controlled the means of production (the land, factories, mines, etc.), while the proletariat held title to little else than their labor. Selling that labor was the latter's sole means of livelihood. The "innermost secret" (as Marx called it) at the core of the modern economic apparatus was that the

---

°Marx left behind no full-scale study of social class. The manuscript of *Das Kapital* breaks off just as Marx is reaching his stride in his discussion of "the three great classes [of] wage-labourers, capitalists and landlords." From remarks scattered throughout his writings, however, it is possible to reconstruct a general theory of class and class struggle (12).

terms of exchange were unequal. Workers produced more value than they received as wages in return. Given this condition, conflict was endemic to modern society. Class struggle might be muted or strident, it might assume new forms as circumstances changed, but it could not disappear so long as the essential inequality in the production process persisted.

Subsequent writers have refined and extended Marx's analysis to incorporate features of contemporary society. Changes in the division of labor, technology of production, and standards of living; the expansion of capitalism to a global system of production; and the ascendancy of the state or public sector in the market have all required revisions in Marx's original scheme. For our purposes, the critical features of Marx's notion of class which have survived all such revisions are as follows: Class is a relational entity; capitalists cannot be defined without reference to wage-earners, and the same holds for the so-called middle strata. Economic class relations are inherently unstable, built as they are on a fundamental fact of inequality and the exploitation of labor. They are determined primarily by structural characteristics of the process of production, and therefore are discontinuous categories rather than gradations of prestige or status. Finally, since the class structure, engendered by economic relationships, is influenced by the prevailing state of class conflict, other factors become relevant to the definition of class. These include cultural traditions, informal associations, and forms of solidarity not directly related to the workplace. Thus in Marxian analysis, class is a theoretic term that refers to a complex force in social change. The manifestation of class is a historical phenomenon, however. As such it can be understood only by attending to the particularities of a given social context (13).

There is much more to Marx's theory of social class than this bald account, but it is in essence a theory based on the structure of relations of production. Other theorists have taken a more multifaceted view of social stratification and its causes. Max Weber, whose late-nineteenth-century ideas have stimulated a great deal of theorizing in modern sociology, took the view that three distinct systems of stratification existed in industrial societies: one system founded on *economic interest,* a second on *prestige* or honor, and a third on *power* (14). Weber did not disagree with Marx on the economic stratification of society in terms of property and income; indeed it has been said that he conducted a lifelong dialogue "with the ghost of Marx." But he observed, from his studies of Germany in particular, that certain groups of people derived social prestige or honor from the preindustrial past. Thus the prestige of the nobility and the learned professions was independent of their economic resources in an industrial society. Such *status groups,* as they are usually called, have proliferated in industrial societies. They take the form of a series of professional and other groups. By virtue of their skilled occupations, their elaborate education and culture, and their whole style of life, they are bound together by common interests. In turn, these status groups link together the two extreme economic classes of owners and unskilled workers along a continuum of prestige.

Moreover, Weber treated political power as a separate issue independent of the existence of economic classes, thus tempering the idea of discrete classes locked in opposition. He introduced intangible elements of judgment into the analysis of social class, and rather than a dichotomy postulated a series of status groups, not necessarily divided by a fundamental conflict over the question of the ownership of property. Weber did not deny that these three systems of stratification—by prestige, economic class, and power—could and did overlap, as it were, so that there could be a coincidence of status grouping, economic dominance, and access to political power. But he insisted that stratification in contemporary industrial society could be analyzed in at least three distinctive and separate ways.

Weber's influence on theories of social stratification has been pervasive. Many contemporary sociologists, particularly in the United States, have come to emphasize status groups in their analysis of the workings of the social system, and to consider these groups as more important than socioeconomic classes. One reason for this is the many conflicts between groups in society besides those that arise from social class interests (15). Talcott Parsons suggested that stratification be considered as the "ranking of units in a social system, in accordance with the standards of the common value system," a Weberian approach that allows for a number of differing stratifications (16). The present society of the United States, marked by comparative affluence and opportunities for social mobility, has given substance to this approach as an operational tool for analyzing the contemporary industrial system. The increase in the number of professional and technical occupations, and the decline in the proportion of manual workers as against other occupations, have changed and complicated the occupational structure of society. The proportions in particular occupations, and in turn in particular classes, shift as the economy changes. In the nineteenth century, manual workers were by far the largest single occupational category. By 1960 in the United States, white-collar workers comprised 43 per cent of the labor force, and manual workers 39 per cent (17). By 1981, 52.7 per cent were white collar, and 31.1 per cent were blue collar (18). The prestige of old and new occupations also changes as their relative importance to the economy changes. Finally, power relations change as workers, and in turn employers, organize for both economic and political purposes. The legalization of workers' organizations such as trade unions, and the influence on the political system of mass parties, have helped to redress the huge disparity in political power that marked the nineteenth-century class system.

Nevertheless, while the model of discrete social classes with distinct ideologies governed by their relations to the process of production may require modification, it remains true that people of similar occupation and income tend to share a common experience and mode of life. Income and occupation set bounds to the kinds of "lifestyles" that people can adopt. Although in the United States no less than 21,741 occupations were listed in the *Dictionary of Occupational Titles* (19), this vast number can be condensed into a smaller number of major occupational groups of similar skills and work. Earnings within each group tend to be similar so that broad economic categories emerge. Each of these categories could be considered as a discrete social class if it could be shown that the members of such groupings share a set of interests that are defined by their economic position and differ from the interests of other groupings; that they draw upon a common stock of traditions, values, and beliefs expressed in their formal and informal affiliations; and that certain circumstances may induce consciousness of their class position and impel them to act in the interests of that class.

The fact that a number of persons of similar occupations and income are grouped together in broad categories of this kind, however, does not necessarily mean that they will act in a class-conscious way. Other factors cut across such broad categories: how people choose to spend their money, what religious beliefs they hold, what degree of education they have acquired, what political party they vote for, or what occupational aspirations they hold for themselves or their children. All or any of these matters may unite them with persons in other economic groups and divide them from their economic peers.

Consciously and unconsciously, most individuals classify others by their speech, dress, and social behavior and rate themselves by certain criteria as equal, inferior, or superior to others. The way in which they interact differs according to this subjective rating of their own social position in relation to that of others (20). These variations in modes of social interaction express divergent values, but to the extent that reciprocal patterns of superordinate and subordinate behavior exist to which people respond appropriately, one may infer that certain values are common to them all. Accepted forms of behavior protect the exclusiveness of social classes, and distinguish particular modes of life. Each social class teaches its children how to behave; this acquired behavior tends to keep them in the same social class as their parents and also to exclude them from other classes. A person who moves from one social class to another must learn to modify his or her behavior.

The association of subjective class consciousness with a person's status and role has been demonstrated (21) and replicated (22,23), and can be considered as evidence for the validity of the existence of social class, though it is insufficient by itself to validate the concept. While all individuals have subjective feelings about their own social position in relation to others, such personal ratings, however definite they may appear to individuals, are unreliable criteria by which to define the objective existence and functions of social classes in society. People tend to generalize about their society as a whole on the basis of their own limited social experience of a small part of that whole, and hence what people understand by their social class position varies with their particular circumstances (24). Thus, when they think of others who are geographically or socially distant from them, and of whom they have little or no direct knowledge, they tend to lump them all together into a single category, although in fact these may be highly differentiated among themselves. This stereotyping of the socially distant occurs at all levels in industrial society, as well as in the attitudes of persons of one society toward those in another. For instance, white settlers in Africa almost invariably interacted with Africans only as master to servant, but this did not prevent whites from generalizing about all African tribal life, of which most of them had no direct experience or knowledge (25).

In the same way, a rag sorter in Britain may have seen a clear social class distinction between himself and a porter in the neighborhood where they both lived. But he may have found difficulty in recognizing any social distinction between a doctor and a pharmacist, and regarded both as equally "upper class." The Registrar General, on the other hand, while not recognizing social distinctions clear to the rag sorter, would have allocated both him and the porter to Social Class V as persons of "other lowly occupations," and graded doctors in Social Class I and pharmacists in Social Class II. In other words, both the rag sorter and the Registrar General conceive social class distinctions in terms of their own values, experiences, and necessities.

People in small communities tend to recognize only three social classes, and often assert that they themselves belong to the middle class, using certain other categories of persons whom they consider superior or inferior as "reference groups" to define their own position; although an estimate of their social class position in terms of the wider society might not bear out this classification (26). Most Americans today, however, recognize as many as five distinct classes (upper, lower-upper, middle, working, and poor), and can readily assign themselves and their neighbors to one of these. Feelings of class identification appear to run strong (23). Assignments of class membership are heavily dependent upon income (as evidenced by standard of living), less so upon occupational standing (valued primarily in terms of autonomy and job security), and much less so upon educational attainment (which is viewed chiefly as a means to an end) (22).

The varied social experiences of individuals in a complex society are responsible for the anomalies that occur when sociologists attempt to construct a single continuous scale of social class positions based on the subjective evaluations of individuals (27). Social class is thought of differently in Bath and in Bolton, in New York and in New Orleans, in a workingmen's club and in the Harvard Club; each neighbourhood, village, town, and metropolis has a unique experience. Although characteristics by which people in industrial society estimate the social class of others can be observed and recorded, these are multiple and subtle and cannot provide the measures for a usable definition of social classes. Nor do these characteristics explain the basis of class differences.

In the United States especially, where an early history of slavery and later waves of immigration from Europe, Asia, and Latin America have combined to produce a population of great cultural diversity, *ethnicity* is a potent source of social affiliation. Far from being mere vestigial loyalty to bygone "idols of the tribe," ethnic identity—whether ascribed or avowed—affects social behavior, politics, job opportunities, the composition of social networks, and views of the nature of the social system. Ethnicity denotes more than a secondary system of cross-cutting ties which modulate the effects of a primary division along class lines; ethnic identity has been championed, manipulated, and endured to produce the unique American version of a stratified society. Here again structural and cultural dimensions can be distinguished. At the cultural level, all ethnic groups may be described in terms of shared values, sentiments, symbolic heritage, and point of origin. It is at the structural level that critical differences emerge in the power positions of ethnic groups. The structural dimension of ethnicity follows from the two historic modes of entry to the United States. Africans arrived involuntarily into slavery. Since then, positions of deprivation and subordination for blacks have persisted throughout the country into modern times. For a century after the American Civil War blacks were generally excluded from all but menial and low-paying jobs, deprived of schooling, and barred from most trade unions; only political struggle gained them full civil rights and access to higher reaches of society. This struggle, which continues, is a class as well as an ethnic struggle (28).

By contrast, Europeans, Hispanics, and Asians of the nineteenth and twentieth centuries (like the early British, French, and Dutch settlers) arrived for the most part voluntarily. Each successive migratory group tended to move into a social position inferior to that of those already settled. But they retained their identities as groups that could be mobilized for mutual social support, for economic survival, and for political battles.

The differences in the social positions of ethnic groups point up the hazards of a simple model of multilayered or parallel systems of stratification. Ethnicity articulates with the class system in complex ways. It may reinforce, challenge, or deflect attention from economic differentiation (29).

Indices of social class

In epidemiological studies, the problems stemming from a lack of theoretical consensus on the meaning of social class are compounded by the variety of indices used to represent class standing. Ingenuity is needed to translate theoretical formulations into testable hypotheses and to devise a set of appropriate measures. Many researchers choose to employ stock indices of social class without any explicit rationale. Even when a particular formulation of class justifies an index, investigators may face a considerable problem—what may be termed "Durkheim's dilemma"—in having to rely on available data. As we discussed in Chapter 4, the empirical facts and figures Durkheim marshaled, were collected and classified by coroners in various regions, each with his own working definition of which deaths should be counted as suicides. There was no way of ensuring that such definitions were congruent with one another, let alone that they matched Durkheim's own definition (30).

Nonetheless, a number of Durkheim's original findings—the protective value of marriage, the family, and the "intense collective life" of religious communities, as well as the adversities of divorce, bereavement, and sudden economic disaster—have withstood both the test of time and refinements in research techniques. Where social phenomena bulk large enough so that trends are detected consistently or the same associations crop up repeatedly despite the variety of indices used, valid inferences may be drawn on the strength of corroborating evidence (31).

Such, in fact, appears to be the case with the effects of social class on many aspects of social life in modern industrial societies. Nowhere is this more evident than in the distribution of health and disease. Across broad groupings of occupations by social class, gradients have been stable and consistent over time in such matters as infant mortality rates, stillbirth rates, rheumatic heart disease, pneumonia and bronchitis, and death rates in general (32). Such gradients, persisting through dramatic declines in the rates of these conditions, have led to fresh understanding of many disorders and to their effective prevention.

For specific occupations grouped within any one social class, rates are more erratic because of the defects of crude classification and the effects of additional factors. A defect of classification is illustrated by the fact that a more regular distribution of the rates of health disorders appears when occupations that require rough manual labor are grouped together and separated from those that do not; such occupations may be spread widely through the broad social class grouping (33). The coexistence of regular social class gradients with intraclass anomalies also suggest that more than one system of stratification may affect health disorders. Since economic stratification, status stratification, and disparities in political power to a degree coexist independently, their relative importance in social and health matters can be expected to fluctuate with changes in technology, economic conditions, and government. Moreover, within each stratum wide variations in ways of life may exist.

Social class scales are convenient devices for analyzing and correlating social and medical phenomena. The difficulty lies in finding objective, measurable criteria by which the complex populations of industrial societies can be accurately and readily classified. Industrial society is a process of social interaction between individuals in time, during which values are constantly modified and relationships change. In the actual communities where people live, work, and meet one another, social standing or social prestige depends on a large number of social attributes. Some of these attributes have a value common to all members of society, but others have a particular value in particular residential areas or for particular social groups. Social class scales can be constructed to deal with these complexities, but the techniques of collecting the requisite data are laborious. They are uneconomic for use in large populations, and suitable only for small communities or limited groups.

For reasons of convenience, therefore, occupation has been commonly used as a basis for ranking large populations by social class. Occupation is an objective criterion easy to establish; it can be compared with other occupations within the same or a different community; and it provides a single criterion of socioeconomic class. For although one's social standing and patterns of health and disease may well vary according to the place where one lives and the social standing of the persons with whom one interacts, one's occupation often determines income, dwelling place, and social standing—in sum, one's socioeconomic position.

The several elements that enter into social stratification make clear that the use of occupation as the sole index for constructing a social class hierarchy must lead to oversimplification. Job assignments to one or other class are often made for males alone and are insensitive to variations in family status which are not fixed by occupation, while rapid changes in the technology of work make comparisons over time difficult. Moreover, assumptions about the nature of social class are easily smuggled in, and the underlying values by which the superiority or inferiority of occupations on the scale are determined may never be explicit. In some of the social class scales based on occupation now in use, occupations are rated by criteria that are held to be "obvious" or "self-evident."

The learned professions are usually given a high rating. Indeed, they are often put right at the top, and a cynic might observe that occupational prestige scales are in fact constructed by professional people. There are variations on the theme: some market researchers may choose to place business leaders first and professors second; professors of sociology may reverse this order; but on the inferiority of all other occupations they are agreed. Professions crucial in an individual's life at times of crisis—

physicians, lawyers, and the clergy, for example—are rated high. Occupations that have a predominantly mental-verbal function and demand a formal education are also rated high; hence schoolteachers are rated above bank clerks, and clerical workers above manual workers. Self-employment and clean occupations are considered superior and personal service demeaning. High financial rewards confer prestige and the importance of a position in business or other economic enterprise is related to size.

A broad consensus in rating occupational prestige seems to reflect a general value system underlying industrial societies everywhere. A study in the United States in 1946 asked a sample of the public to rank 90 occupations on a five-point class scale. Such occupations as justice of the Supreme Court, physician, and professor were all given high rank, while low rank was given to such occupations a street sweeper and garbage collector (34). Subsequent studies confirm the findings; indeed, rankings of occupational titles have proven quite robust. Assignments of occupational prestige scores by surveyed populations changed little between 1925 and 1965 (35). In 1956, a comparative study of ranking of similar occupations in Britain, the United States, New Zealand, Germany, Japan, and the Soviet Union showed that there was a great deal of agreement in all of these countries and the results have been repeated subsequently (36). Further studies in developing countries have shown that the ranking of occupations there appears to agree with the scale of values current in industrialized societies (37).

Agreement on the prestige of various occupations in industrial societies provides a basis for comparison between them. To compare their occupational structures, both the description of occupations and their rating should everywhere be made in the same manner, and the International Labor Organization has tried to provide a standard international classification of occupations (38). All this bristles with difficulties for the reasons set out previously, and also because scientific and technological discoveries constantly modify productive processes. The number, kind, and status of occupations change accordingly (see Table 5.1). Such changes in production in turn engender changes in social relationships.

When comparing population data, birthrates, or death rates, one must know that equivalents are being compared in order to obtain a valid result. Epidemiologists have striven since the mid–nineteenth century to standardize records of health disorders and vital events. Rules for standardizing records of vital events such as birth, for example, or premature birth, illegitimate birth, and stillbirth, have been developed and accepted by the World Health Organization. Yet problems of validity and reliability remain and the work continues. Social class scales based on occupation are far from having even this degree of precision.

Concordance on the prestige rating of occupations is the basis for many social class scales. Even within one society comparisons should be made with caution. It is an arduous task simply to keep abreast of the vast and growing number of occupations, and placing them within the complex structure of social and economic life leads to contradictions in classification. A single occupational category can comprise an extremely varied assortment of jobs. Both the president of a university and the youngest teacher in a nursery school could be classified as teachers, although today it is usual to differentiate teachers by the kind of academic establishment that employs them.

Table 5.1 Shifts in U.S. occupational structure

	Per cent				
	1900	1950[a]	1960	1970[b]	1981[b]
Professional, technical, and kindred workers	4.2	8.6	11.4	14.2	16.4
Managers, officials, and proprietors (except farm)	5.9	8.8	8.5	10.5	11.5
Clerical and kindred workers	3.0	12.3	14.9	17.4	18.5
Sales workers	4.5	7.0	7.4	6.2	6.4
Craftsmen, foremen, and kindred workers	10.6	14.2	14.3	12.6	12.6
Operatives and kindred workers	12.8	20.3	19.9	16.4	10.5
Laborers (except farm and mine)	12.4	6.5	5.5	4.7	4.6
Service workers (except private household)	3.6	7.8	8.9	10.4	13.4
Private household workers	5.4	2.6	2.8[c]	1.4	1.0[d]
Farmers and farm managers	19.8	7.5	3.9	4.0	2.7
Farm laborers and foremen	17.8	4.4	2.4	1.2	1.3[d]
Total	100.0	100.0	100.0	100.0	100.0
Number of economically active (in thousands)[e]	29,030	59,230	67,990	78,678	100,397

[a]These data include adjustments that take account of the differences between the 1950 and 1960 classification systems.

[b]U.S. Dept. of Commerce and Bureau of the Census (1983). *Statistical Abstract*, Washington, D.C.

[c]U.S. Dept. of Commerce and Bureau of the Census (1970). *Historical Statistics of the United States Colonial Times to 1970*, Washington, D.C.

[d]Bureau of Labor Statistics, New York Office (personal communication).

[e]The definition of economically active was not the same at each of these dates. For 1900, it refers to all those 10 years old or more who reported a gainful occupation whether or not they were working or seeking work at the time they were interviewed. For 1950 and 1960, it refers to all those 14 years old or more who had previously worked and who were either working for pay or looking for work during a specified week.

Sources: (1900, 1950, 1960) Gendell, M., and Zetterberg, H. L., eds. (1964). A *Sociological Almanac for the United States*, New York, p. 66 (Data taken from U.S. Bureau of the Census).

The manager of a supermarket could be classified with the owner of a corner store; in England, a duke who owns half a county and a commoner who cultivates half a hundred acres could both be classified as farmers; and the Director of the Bank of England and the director of a small local business can both be classified as company directors. Modern industrial society is too complex to enable simple class categorizations to correlate precisely with medical and other phenomena on a national scale.

One social class scale which is widely known and used in medicine is that of the Registrar General in Great Britain, which presently releases studies through the Office of Population Censuses and Surveys. Census material is used to group together occupations considered to be of the same kind, and all are arranged in five social classes (39). The general arrangement and numbers of the 1971 census are shown in Table 5.2.

Class I embraces a diverse collection of occupations and people. In a rough-and-ready way, this class may be said to include all those persons whom many people would regard as the "upper class" or the "upper middle class." This class therefore includes certain powerful social groups, such as the "captains of industry" and the socially eminent aristocracy. While a separate tabulation of these groups might be

Table 5.2   Distribution of population by occupation grouped in social classes, 1931,1951, and 1971 census, England and Wales: Per 1000 economically active and retired males

Social class		Age-group	1931	1951	1971
Nonmanual					
I	Professional occupations (e.g., doctors, lawyers, company executives)	16–44 45–64	18 32	31 33	50[a] 41
II	Managerial and lower professional occupations (e.g., sales managers, teachers)	16–44 45–64	100 183	119 175	143 195
IIIN	Nonmanual skilled occupations (e.g., clerks, shop assistants)	16–44 45–64	511 435	563 462	109 104
Manual					
IIIM	Manual skilled occupations (e.g., bricklayers, underground coal miners)	16–44 45–64	511 435	563 462	355 345
IV	Partly skilled occupations (e.g., bus conductors, postmen)	16–44 45–64	184 166	150 163	138 182
V	Unskilled occupations (e.g., porters, ticket collectors, general laborers)	16–44 45–64	163 171	98 153	61 81

[a]The lower age-group for 1971 was 15–44.

Source: Leete, R. and Fox, J. (1977). Registrar General's social classes: Origins and uses, *Population Trends*, 8 Table 3.

relatively unimportant for epidemiology, their economic, social, and political significance is out of all proportion to their numbers (40). Their special characteristics tend to disappear because of their inclusion with larger numbers of "middle-class" people.

Class II includes most of the people commonly described as "middle class," but again the span of occupations is even wider, and any one occupational category embraces people of different economic and social circumstances. Changes within an occupation may also affect its ranking. For instance, in the 1960 revision of the scale, airline pilots were reclassified from Class III to Class II in recognition of the professional training they undergo.

The nucleus of Class III was, until recently, the skilled manual occupations. These include a large proportion of foremen and supervisory workers, as well as clerical workers, clerks, and typists. So constructed, this class represented a weakness of the classification as a whole, for it was enormous in size compared with the others, and heterogeneous because of the arbitrary juxtaposition of so many varied occupations. For these reasons and others as well (differences in family structure, for example), Social Class III was split in the 1970 Classification of Occupations into manual and nonmanual components. This division has the additional advantage of allowing the five classes to be readily grouped along the manual/nonmanual axis.

Broadly speaking, Social Classes III, IV, and V contain that section of the population which most people would describe as "working class"—a category that includes many whose work is not primarily manual, especially with the growth in the postwar period of the service sector (41). The divisions between the three classes are anything but distinct, for technical changes in industry have altered the traditional division of labor, and often have rendered arbitrary the allocation of occupations to the skilled, unskilled, or semiskilled category.

Thus inconsistencies and difficulties abound. For instance, in the past, the directors of small local businesses could be assigned to Social Class I as company directors or to Social Class II as owners of small businesses. Their inclusion as company directors in Class I led to a serious anomaly in the mortality statistics for the period 1949–1953 (42), and produced an absurdly high death rate for company directors and their wives. The 1951 census provided the "denominator" for calculating these mortality rates, and many managers and small businessmen were then probably assigned to Class II. But the deaths among them, which comprise the "numerator" for the calculation, were assigned to Class I. The inconsistency between the two sets of data so inflated the deaths of Social Class I as to reverse the expected gradient between Classes I and II for mortality from all causes of men aged 20–64. This error illustrates how important it is to record, code, and classify occupations exactly when calculating rates, and further to proceed in the same way for both numerator and denominator—in other words, for cases and population at risk.

Anomalies are apparent particularly in the social classification of women who work. Relationships between classifications based on women's own occupations and those based on their husbands' occupations are subject to changes in the demand for their participation in the labor market. Women in industrial society have a lower economic standing than men, have less opportunity to achieve skilled occupations, and may seek work for motives and goals distinct from those of men (43). Until recently, married women were simply placed in the same social class as their husbands, for they were considered as "dependents" grouped with the head of the household. This is no longer a tenable assumption. One study of a national sample in the United States found that nearly 40 per cent of the working women surveyed ranked higher than their husbands in occupational prestige; primarily, white-collar jobs occupied by many such women ranked above the skilled manual jobs occupied by their husbands (44). (The U.S. Census Bureau currently shows some sensitivity to this fact by assigning family socioeconomic status on the basis of the occupation of the chief wage-earner.) Single women who work are classified by their occupations, although these may in fact conceal their actual social class positions. A woman with a father in Social Class I may take a job as a typist, an occupation allocated to Social Class III, but whether or not this alters her position in society will depend on factors other than her job. In Britain, class assignments based upon women's own occupations compared with assignments based on those of their husbands indicated that most but not all women fell within the same class as their husbands; mortality patterns, too, were similar (45).

Such difficulties are further complicated by the fact that many people change their occupations during their working life; the number of these changes is considerable and growing. During a 10-year period of the British National Survey of Children, which followed a sample including all those born during one week of 1946, about 18 per cent of the fathers moved up in the social class scale, while 8 per cent moved down. The number of fathers in the categories of large employers and foremen increased by more than 100 per cent (46). This social class movement had important medical implications, for the families of those who moved up had different medical histories from those who moved down. The occupational mobility of a parent may affect not only his or her own social class position and health, but also that of spouse and children. All such changes in occupation can lead to discrepancies in classification and therefore to errors in the calculation of death rates. For instance, in the late 1950s, recorded death rates among face workers in British coal mines were very high (47). When these rates were investigated in detail, they were found to be inflated by errors in the classification of certain kinds of colliers at death, although the corrected rate still remained high. Work at the coal face is a peak occupation in a collier's working life-cycle, and many relatives may be unaware of a collier's actual job in the pit at the time of death. In the re-analysis, face workers were allocated to Social Class III, while other colliery workers were allocated to Social Classes IV and V. A comparison of death certificates with employment records showed that many colliers who were not face workers had in fact been so recorded. This was partly due to men being described on death certificates as "coal miners," a general category which the Registrar General always recorded as face workers, and partly because the relatives of dead colliers upgraded them to the occupational category of face workers. The reasons for this upgrading involve the changing cycle of a single collier's work. Many men who work underground but not on the coal face have been face workers at some time, and many others have been trained for this work and hope to become face workers.

This instance emphasizes the importance of accurate recording of social data in medical records. Vague terms like "civil servant" or "scientist" are not sufficient. Classification of retired persons, widows, or orphans not yet at work needs special care. Much of the information collected by health workers in the British National Survey of Children had to be amended after repeat visits, and in 12 per cent of cases the occupational group to which families were assigned had to be altered (46). Measurement error of this sort plagues much social mobility research (48).

The Bureau of the Census in the United States does not publish occupational material in the form of a social class scale. The bureau does, however, group occupations in a prestige hierarchy, from professional occupations at the top to unskilled workers at the bottom (49). As can be seen by comparing Tables 5.1 and 5.2, the order resembles closely the British hierarchy of occupations, except for the separate classification of farmers and farm workers. In fact, it would be a simple matter to make a slight rearrangement in this hierarchy and set out the material in the form of five social classes in the British manner as follows:

SOCIAL CLASS I

Professional, technical, and kindred
   workers.

SOCIAL CLASS II

Managers, officials, and proprietors
Farmers and farm managers

SOCIAL CLASS III

Clerical and kindred workers
Sales workers
Craftsmen, foremen, and kindred workers

SOCIAL CLASS IV

Operative and kindred workers (semiskilled)

SOCIAL CLASS V

Laborers
Service workers
Private household workers

The main difference is that the British scale puts the proprietors and managers and the higher professions at the top, while the American scale puts all professional and technical workers at the top; this may possibly reflect a real difference in values between the two countries. The first scale devised to measure the relative social rank of occupations in the United States was drawn up by William C. Hunt of the Bureau of the Census in 1897. Hunt arranged all gainful workers into four social classes: proprietors, clerks, skilled workers, and laborers.

This may be regarded as the first of the long series of socioeconomic class scales devised by social researchers in the United States. Most of them can be criticized for the same weaknesses of conceptual validity and operational reliability that have already been set out for the British social class scale. Some occupations cover too wide a range of actual jobs to be placed together comfortably on the same point in the scale—for instance, salesmen, farmers, pharmacists, or librarians. Shopkeepers could be ranked either by the size of the businesses or by the type of goods they deal in; there is room for a great many anomalies.

To construct a valid unitary scale of the prestige of occupations in a modern industrial society presents undeniable difficulties (50). The equivalences or differences in prestige of occupations depend on subjective estimations on the part of respondents, and they are sometimes unable to distinguish between occupations. Nonetheless, despite wide variations in study methods and wholesale changes in the economy and labor force, consensus on the prestige ratings of occupations has proved remarkably constant over time. For purposes of indexing the relative social standing and way of life of families, it is probably the most useful measure (51).

Investigators have assembled scales of occupational prestige that reflect general social standing within a community. The *Duncan Socioeconomic Index* (or SEI) (52) used data from a 1947 opinion survey of occupational prestige in the U.S. to assign prestige scores to 45 job categories. These scores were weighted for the respective contributions of education and income (calculated to account for 83 per cent of the observed variance in ranking). The weightings were then applied to the remaining occupational categories to yield a standardized score for each of the more than 20,000 jobs grouped under 296 occupational titles in the U.S. Census Bureau's alphabetical *Index of Occupation and Industries* (1960). Prestige scores of occupations obtained in a 1963 survey correlated highly with those of the 1947 survey. Although certain anomalies are apparent (clergy and teachers, for example, may rank higher on sub-jective scales than they do on the basis of earned income and education), the relative simplicity of the scale and its use of easily obtainable, reliable information has led to wide use.

In the United States, official agencies in the health field have made only limited use of occupation as an index for assessing social class. The Health Department of New York City, for example, has long recorded occupation in registering births and deaths, and a readily available code exists by which to classify the multitude of par-ticular occupations into socioeconomic status, but occupation is not coded and used for analysis. Income appears on the surface to provide a reasonable index for a socio-economic class scale, but it is even more unreliable than occupation, and when iso-lated from other factors can be inadequate or misleading. Apart from this, the exact income of many people is difficult to establish. Many in industrial societies are secre-tive about their incomes and also about the way they spend their money. For the very rich, income is a most inexact measure of true wealth. Many others, like farmers, may not know their exact income; still others, such as authors or speculators, have fluc-tuating incomes. While the way income is spent indicates social standing more accu-rately than the amount spent, this too presents difficulties in collecting the requisite data.

Owing to its simplicity in use, educational level has found favor as an index of social class (53). Since the advent of higher education on a mass scale, educational level might be thought a more useful single index of social class than occupation. The pop-ulation can be readily stratified by level of education, from elementary school through high school, college, and university, and a correspondence made with social class. Moreover, in mature adults education is a less changeable attribute than occupation. Still, difficulties are met. Income and occupational returns from education are not consistent; they vary by social class of origin and are subject to changes in the com-position of the labor force (54). In the years 1962–1973, the percentage of white-collar and professional jobs in the United States grew quite slowly, while the number of qualified applicants increased sharply. The result was a decline in the value of edu-cation as measured by occupational attainment, especially among younger age groups (55). Moreover, as noted earlier, Americans' subjective ranking of their own and their neighbors' social class today relies only distantly upon years of schooling (22).

This points up a more general problem with all status indicators. Positional goods like education derive their value from their relative scarcity. Insofar as they become widely available, the differential advantage and prestige which they confer decline accordingly (56). The principal weakness in social class scales based on one index, such as occupation or education, is their simplification of reality. The Registrar General's scale, a model of such constructs, envisages industrial society as a hierarchy of social classes based on the relative prestige of occupations, and on the relations of individuals to production. At the time of its first appearance, at the beginning of this century, it doubtless reflected a social reality in which the divisions between the classes were much more evident than today. It closely resembles the type of stratification proposed by Marx. The model is of a social pyramid with lines of horizontal cleavage dividing the population into discrete social classes with differing degrees of power and prestige.

It is assumed that people throughout society, wherever they live, uniformly agree on the prestige of each occupation on the scale, recognize the divisions, and approve the rank assigned.

All unilinear scales necessarily represent industrial society as a static structure with uniform values, and therefore give both a misleading clarity to the definition of social class and an unsophisticated view of the relations between people in different social positions. To construct more accurate scales of social class, some sociologists have combined a number of criteria into a constellation: for example, occupation, income, education, and place of residence. Such ratings have long been used in community studies, as well as in medical investigations. In a New Haven study of mental illness, occupation and education were used as criteria to create what is now known as the *Hollingshead two-factor index of social position* (57). Occupation and education were scaled and weighted separately, then combined into a single score. The occupational scale used the 10 major occupational categories set out in the Bureau of Census hierarchy of occupations, and the educational scale was a seven-point measure based on the number of years completed in school and college. This method has the virtue of simplicity, and of combining two indices which bear some relation to each other. It has been widely adopted for subsequent sociomedical studies.

In another study, an elaborate six-rung scale of class structure used both respondents' subjective evaluations of their own and others' social position and the independent assessment by community experts of status symbols, prestige activities, and membership in certain associations (58). A built-in bias was thus unavoidable: the social system was in effect presented from the point of view of those at the top. In a different community where this method was applied, people at the bottom of the scale viewed the class structure simply as one in which some people at the top had money and power and those at the bottom did not. An effort was made to construct a more objective index, which aggregated measures of occupation, income, housing, and place of residence, each factor being weighted and ranked on a seven-point scale. The resultant orders of prestige conflate disparate elements in one score, making it impossible to separate out the economic, prestige, and power dimensions of stratifiction. Nor is it possible to analyze the interrelationships between these three aspects of social class.

The problem of consistency besets all attempts to define social class by using a number of dimensions of stratification. A high position on one index may be reinforced by a high position on the others; conversely, individuals may rank high on one index and low on others. These consistencies and inconsistencies may have significant social and psychological consequences. Thus, an early study examined the consistency between the rankings of four indices of social class position: occupation, income, education, and ethnic origin. The degree of consistency between the rankings on all four, called *status crystallization*, was found to be related to social behavior. In this instance, the behavior studied was political preference, and high crystallization and low crystallization were related to different voting behavior (59). More generally, studies of the interrelationships of the components typically used to construct composite measures of social class have shown them to be but weakly intercorrelated. The various items included in the composite measure may be related to the study variable of interest in quite different ways. The use of such aggregate measures not only perpetuates conceptual confusion but may conceal rather than reveal actual effects (51).

Table 5.3 Social area analysis in nineteenth century London applied to causation of cholera

Number of districts[a]	Elevation in feet above Trinity high-water mark	Annual mortality to 10,000 persons living		Observed average Number of persons to		Average annual value of		Poor rate in the £ of houserent 1842–1843
		Cholera 1849	All causes (1838–1844)	An acre	A house	Houses (£)	House and shop room to each person (£)	
16	Under 20 feet	102	251	74	6.8	31	4.645	.072
7	20–40	65	237	105	7.6	56	7.358	.071
8	40–60	34	235	184	8.5	64	7.342	.056
3	60–80	27	236	152	8.8	52	6.374	.049
2	80–100	22	211	44	7.7	38	5.183	.036
1	100	17	227	102	9.8	71	7.586	.043
1	350	8	202	5	7.2	40	5.804	—
Mean of 38 Districts		66	240	107	7.6	46	5.985	.064
All London		62	252	29	7	40	5.419	.063

[a]London Districts, arranged according to the elevation of their soil.

Source: Farr, W. (1852). *Report on the Mortality of Cholera in England, 1848–1849*, London.

Multivariate anlaysis of social position points the way to exploiting the inconsistencies of the several dimensions of stratification. Subsequent studies have used this method to seek out possible health effects of "status inconsistency" (see Chapter 7), and have classified individuals as high or low on each of such criteria as occupation and education. These dimensions have then been combined to construct subgroups, or types, on the model of the cells of a fourfold table. The combination of attributes or qualities in different degrees in different individuals, it is proposed, creates types distinct from each other; the distinction between the types resides in a combination of attributes that produces something new, something that cannot be derived merely from the sum of the attributes.

Another way of using multiple indices is the method of social area analysis developed for a study in the San Francisco Bay Area (60). Epidemiologists of the nineteenth century sometimes used a form of social area analysis to demonstrate the social distribution of diseases. Table 5.3 gives figures from which William Farr concluded that cholera was amost perfeclty correlated with "elevation of habitation," and not with a variety of indices of the social conditions of residential areas.° A similar "ecological" approach—combining such area indices as occupation, education, rent, and quality of housing—was used in a mortality study of two New England towns (61). An ensemble of ten "predictor" variables that describe the demographic, ethnic, and social environment of New York City neighborhoods has been shown to be highly correlated with a variety of health outcome variables (62). Studies of this sort may be more properly considered analyses of one of the effects of social stratification—poverty—rather than of social stratification itself.

To correlate social strata as precisely as possible with other phenomena such as health disorders may require several indices of social class to be grouped with occupation; even then, the investigator must pay attention to the constellation of occupations and the determinants of social prestige in particular communities. Yet epidemiologists and other sociomedical scientists may take comfort that, in the past, simple and crude methods have yielded rich results. Insistence on perfectly valid and reliable measures can only paralyze research. The prudent application of social class analysis continues to be valuable in the study of health, as the following chapter will show.

References

1. **Pfautz, H. W.** (1953). The current literature on social stratification: Critique and bibliography, *Amer. J. Sociol.*, 58, 391–418.
   Tumin, M. M. (1953). Some principles of stratification: A critical analysis, *Amer. Sociol. Rev.*, 18, 387–93.
   MacRae, D. G. (1953–54). Social stratification: A trend report and bibliography, *Current Sociol.*, 2,
   Ellis, R. A. (1958). The continuum theory of social stratification: A critical note, *Sociology and Social Research*, 42, 269–73.

° While Farr's observation was correct, his inference was faulty. John Snow, in his classic studies, soon after demonstrated the intermediate role of contaminated water in the transmission of cholera: waters at higher altitudes (above the city of London) would be expected to have been less contaminated.

Bottomore, T. B. (1966). *Classes in Modern Society*, New York.

Anderson, C. (1974). *The Political Economy of Social Class*, Englewood Cliffs, N.J.

Giddens, A. (1975). *The Class Structure of the Advanced Societies*, New York.

Rothman, R. A. (1978). *Inequality and Stratification in the United States*, Englewood Cliffs, N.J.

2. Rosaldo, M. Z., and Lamphere, L., eds. (1974). *Women, Culture and Society*, Stanford.

Etienne, M., and Leacock, E., eds. (1980). *Women and Colonization: Anthropological Perspectives*, New York.

3. Beteille, A., ed. (1969). *Social Inequality*, Baltimore.

4. Gluckman, M. (1955). *Custom and Conflict in Africa*, Oxford.

Sahlins, M. D. (1968). *Tribesmen*, Englewood Cliffs, N.J.

Sahlins, M. D. (1972). *Stone Age Economics*, Chicago.

5. Fried, M. (1967). *The Evolution of Political Society*, New York.

Carneiro, R. (1970). A theory of the origin of the state, *Science, 169,* 733–738.

Harris, M. (1975). *Culture, People, Nature*, 2nd., New York.

6. Gerth, H. H., and Mills, C. W. (1946). *From Max Weber: Essays in Sociology*, New York.

Bendix, R., and Lipset, S. M., eds. (1953). *Class, Status, and Power*, Glencoe, Ill.

Barber, B. (1957). *Social Stratification: A Comparative Analysis of Structure and Process*, New York.

Dahl, R. (1957). The concept of power, *Behavior Sciences, 2,* 201-15.

Dahrendorf, R. (1959). *Class and Class Conflict in Industrial Society*, Stanford.

Thomas, R. M. (1962). Reinspecting a structural position on occupation prestige, *Amer. J. Sociol., 67,* 565.

Ossowski, S. (1963). *Class Structure in the Social Consciousness*, New York.

Fried, M. H. (1968). State: The institution, in *International Encyclopedia of Social Science*, ed. Sills, D. L., vol. 15, pp. 143–150.

Coser, L. A., and Rosenberg, B., eds. (1969). *Sociological Theory: A Book of Readings*, London.

7. Schattschneider, E. E. (1960). *The Semi-Sovereign People: A Realist's View of Democracy in America*, New York.

Bachrach, P., and Barantz, M. (1962). Two faces of power, *Amer. Polit. Sci. Rev., 56,* 947–952.

Gramsci, A. (1970). *Prison Notebooks*, London.

Lukes, S. (1974). *Power: A Radical View*, London.

8. Krause, E. A. (1970). *The Lost Reform: The Campaign for Compulsory Health Insurance in the United States, from 1932–1943*, Cambridge, Mass.

Crenson, M. A. (1971). *The Un-Politics of Air Pollution: A Study of Non-Decision Making in the Cities*, Baltimore.

Navarro, V. (1977). *Health and Medical Care in the U.S.A.*, Farmingdale, N.Y.

Whitt, J. A. (1979). Toward a class–dialectical model of power: An empirical assessment of three competing models of political power, *Amer. Sociol. Rev., 44,* 81–99.

Starr, P. (1982). *The Social Transformation of American Medicine*, New York.

9. Williams, R. (1976). *Keywords*, New York.

10. Tumin, M. (1967). *Social Stratification, The Form and Functions of Inequality*, Englewood Cliffs, N.J.

Lipset, S. M., Hodge, R. W., Siegal, P. M., Stinchcombe, A. L., Rodman, H., and Barber, B. L. (1968). Social stratification, in *International Encyclopedia of Social Science*, ed. Sills, D. L., vol. 15, pp. 288–337. New York.

Rubin, L. (1977). *Worlds of Pain: Life in the Working Class Family*, New York.

11. **Marglin, S.** (1974). What do bosses do? The origins and functions of hierarchy in capitalist production, *Rev. Radical Political Economics*, 6, 60–112.
    Braverman, H. (1974). *Labor and Monopoly Capital*, New York.
    Noble, D. (1975). *America by Design*, New York.
    Gordon, D. M. (1976). Capitalist efficiency and socialist efficiency, *Monthly Review*, 28, 19–39.
12. **Marx, K.,** and **Engels, F.** (1947; first pub. 1846). *The German Ideology*, New York.
    Marx, K. (1962; first pub. 1867). Preface to the first German edition of *Capital*, in *Marx and Engels, Selected Works*, Moscow, vol. 1, pp. 448–52.
    Marx, K. (1975; first pub. 1869). *The Eighteenth Brumaire of Louis Bonaparte*, New York.
    Marx, K. (1981; first pub. 1893). *Capital: A Critique of Political Economy*, vol. 3, New York, translated by B. Fowkes.
13. **Thompson, E. P.** (1963). *The Making of the English Working Class*, New York.
    Ollman, B. (1968). Marx's use of class, *Amer. J. Sociol.*, 73, 573–80.
    Wallerstein, I. (1973). Class and class conflict in contemporary Africa, *Canadian J. African Studies*, 7, 375–80.
    Miliband, R. (1977). *Marxism and Politics*, New York.
    Thompson, E. P. (1978). Eighteenth century English society: Class struggle without class, *Social History*, 3, 133–65.
    Robinson, R. V., and **Kelley, J.** (1979). Class as conceived by Marx and Dahrendorf: Effects on income inequality and politics in the United States and Great Britain, *Amer. Sociol. Rev.*, 44, 38–58.
14. **Weber, M.** (1947). *The Theory of Social and Economic Organization*, trans. Henderson, A. R., and Parsons, T., rev. ed., London.
    Bendix, R. (1960). *Max Weber: An Intellectual Portrait*, New York.
    Miller, S. M. (1963). *Max Weber: Selections from His Work*, New York.
15. **Homans, G. C.** (1951). *The Human Group*, London.
    Loomis, C. P. (1960). *Social Systems: Essays on Their Persistence and Change*, Princeton, N.J.
    Lenski, G. E. (1966). *Power and Privilege*, New York.
    Runciman, W. G. (1966). *Relative Deprivation and Social Justice*, London.
16. **Parsons, T.** (1951). *The Social System*, New York.
17. **Vollmer, H. M.,** and **Mills, D. L.** (1966). *Professionalization*, Englewood Cliffs, N.J.
18. **Featherman, D. L.,** and **Hauser, R. M.** (1973). On the measurement of occupation in social surveys, *Sociol. Methods and Research*, 2, 239–51.
    U.S. Dept. of Commerce and Bureau of the Census (1983). *Statistical Abstract of the United States, 1982-3*, 103rd ed. Washington, D.C.
19. **Government Printing Office** (1965). *Dictionary of Occupational Titles*, Washington, D.C.
20. **Ginsberg, M.** (1947). *Reason and Unreason in Society*, London.
    Hatt, P. K., and **Reiss, A. J.,** eds. (1951). *Reader in Urban Sociology*, Glencoe, Ill.
    Bottomore, T. B. (1964). *Elites and Society*, London.
21. **Centers, R.** (1949). *The Psychology of Social Classes*, Princeton, N.J.
22. **Coleman, R. D.,** and **Rainwater, L.** (1978). *Social Standing in America: New Dimensions of Class*, New York.
23. **Jackman, M.R.,** and **Jackman, R. W.** (1982). *Class Awareness in the United States*, Berkeley.
24. **Thomas, W. I.,** and **Znaniecki, F.** (1927), *The Polish Peasant in Europe and America*, New York.

Martin, F. M. (1954). Some subjective aspects of social stratification, in *Social Mobility in Britain*, ed. Glass, D. V., London, pp. 51–75.

Miller, S. M., and Riessman, F. (1968). *Social Class in America*, New York.

25. Epstein, A. L. (1958). *Politics in an Urban African Community*, Manchester.

Leys, C., and Pratt, C. (1960). *New Deal in Central Africa*, London.

26. Merton, R. K., and Lazarsfeld, P. F. (1950). *Continuities in Social Research*, Glencoe, Ill.

Merton, R. K. (1957). *Social Theory and Social Structure*, rev. ed., Glencoe, Ill.

27. Hall, J., and Jones, D. C. (1950). Social grading of occupations, *Brit. J. Sociol., 1*, 31–55.

Kahl, J. A. (1957). *The American Class Structure*, New York.

Gordon, M. (1957). *Social Class in American Sociology*, New York.

28. Barth, F., ed. (1969). *Ethnic Groups and Boundaries*, Boston.

Vincent, J. (1974). The structuring of ethnicity, *Human Organization, 33*, 375–79.

Cohen, A., ed. (1976). *Urban Ethnicity*, New York.

Mullings, L. (1978). Ethnicity and stratification in the urban United States, *Ann. N.Y. Acad. Sci., 318*, 10–22.

29. Green, M. (1972). Behavioralism and class analysis, *Labor History, 13*, 89–106.

Massey, G. (1975). Studying social class: The case of embourgeoisement and the culture of poverty, *Social Problems, 22*, 595–608.

30. Durkheim, E. (1951; first pub. 1897). *Suicide: A Study in Sociology*, New York.

Douglas, J. (1967). *The Social Meanings of Suicide*, Princeton, N.J.

31. Susser, M. (1973). *Causal Thinking in the Health Sciences: Concepts and Strategies in Epidemiology*, Oxford.

Elinson, J., and Patrick, D. (1979). Methods of sociomedical research, in *Handbook of Medical Sociology*, 3rd. ed., Freeman, H. E., Levine, S., and Reeder, L. G., Englewood Cliffs, N.J., pp. 437–59.

Hopper, K., and Guttmacher, S. (1979). Rethinking suicide: Notes toward a critical epidemiology, *Int. J. Hlth. Serv., 9*, 417–38.

32. Fox, J. (1977). Occupational mortality 1970–1972, *Population Trends, 9*, 1–8.

33. Heady, J. A. (1959). Occupation and mortality: Filial mortality, *Brit. J. Industr. Med., 16*, 70–3.

34. National Opinion Research Center (1947). Jobs and occupations: A popular evaluation, *Public Opinion News, 9*, 3–13.

Reiss, A. J. (1961). *Occupations and Social Status*, New York.

Hodge, R. W., Siegel, P. M., and Rossi, P. H. (1964). Occupational prestige in the United States, 1923–63, *Amer. J. Sociol., 70*, 286–302.

35. Duncan, O. D. (1968). Social stratification and mobility: Problems in the measurement of trend, in *Indications of Social Change*, ed. Sheldon, E. B., and Moore, W., New York, pp. 675–719.

Featherman, D. L., and Hauser, R. M. (1973). On the measurement of occupation in social surveys, *Sociological Methods and Research, 2*, 239–51.

36. Inkeles, A., and Rossi, P. H. (1956). National comparisons of occupational prestige, *Amer. J. Sociol., 61*, 329–39.

Pineo, P. C., and Porter, J. (1970). Occupational prestige in Canada, in *The Logic of Social Hierarchies*, ed. Lauman, E. O., Siegel, P. M., and Hodge, R. W., Chicago, pp. 174–88.

37. Mitchell, J. C., and Epstein, A. L. (1959). Occupational prestige and social status among urban Africans in Northern Rhodesia, *Africa, 29*, 22–40.

Hodge, R. W., Treiman, D. J., and Rossi, P. H. (1961). A comparative study of occupational prestige, in *Class, Status, and Power,* ed. Bendix, R., and Lipset, S. M., New York, pp. 309–321.

38. United Nations (1956). *Index to the International Industrial Classification of all Economic Activities,* New York.
    International Labour Organization (1983). *Yearbook of Labor Statistics, 1982,* 42nd edition, New York.

39. Department of Employment (1982). *Classification of Occupations and Directory of Occupational Titles,* 3rd. supplement, Sheffield.

40. Mills, C. W. (1956). *The Power Elite,* New York.
    Lupton, T., and Wilson, C. S. (1959). The social background and connections of "top decision makers," *Manchester School of Economic and Social Studies, 27,* 30–51.
    von Barch, H. (1963). *The Unfinished Society,* trans. Ilford, M., New York.
    Useem, M. (1984). *The Inner Circle: Large Corporations and the Rise of Business Political Activity in the U.S. and U.K.,* New York.

41. Glass, D. V. (1954). *Social Mobility in Britain,* London.
    Lockwood, D. (1958). *The Blackcoated Worker,* London.
    Frankenberg, R. (1966). *Communities in Britain; Social Life in Town and Country,* London.
    Levison, A. (1974). *The Working Class Majority,* Baltimore.

42. Logan, W. P. D. (1959). Occupational mortality, *Proc. Roy. Soc. Med., 52,* 463–8.

43. Myrdal, A., and Klein, V. (1956). *Women's Two Roles,* London.
    Cantor, M., and Laurie, B., eds. (1977). *Class, Sex and the Woman Worker,* Westport.
    Kuhn, A., and Wolpe, A-M., eds. (1978). *Feminism and Materialism,* London.

44. Haug, M. (1972). Social class measurement: A methodological critique, in *Issues in Social Inequality,* ed. Thielbar, G. W., and Feldman, S. D., Boston, pp. 429–51.

45. Leete, R., and Fox, J. (1977). Registrar General's social class: Origins and uses, *Population Trends, 8,* 1–7.

46. Douglas, J. W. B. (1958). *Communication to the Society for Social Medicine,* Dublin.

47. Heasman, M. A., Liddell, F. D. K., and Reid, D. D. (1958). The accuracy of occupational vital statistics, *Brit. J. Industr. Med., 15,* 141–6.

48. Gintis, H. (1980). The American occupational structure eleven years later, *Contemporary Sociol., 9,* 12–16.

49. U.S. Employment Service (1977). *Dictionary of Occupational Titles,* 4th edition, Washington, D.C.
    Miller, A. R., Treiman, D. J., Cain, P. S. and Roos, P. A. eds., (1980). *Work, Jobs, and Occupations: A Critical Review of the Dictionary of Occupational Titles,* Washington, D.C.
    U.S. Department of Commerce and Bureau of Census (1981) *1980 Census of Population. Alphabetical Index of Industries and Occupations,* 2nd Edition, Washington, D.C.

50. Watson, W. (1964). Social mobility and social class in industrial communities, in *Closed Systems and Open Minds,* ed. Gluckman, M., London.

51. Otto, L. B. (1975). Class and status in family research, *Journal of Marriage and the Family, 37,* 315–32.

52. Duncan, O. D. (1961). A socioeconomic index for all occupations, in *Occupations and Social Status,* ed. Riess, A. J., New York, pp. 109–38.
    Blau, P. M., and Duncan, O. D. (1967). *The American Occupational Structure,* New York.

Van Dusen, R.A., and Zill, N., eds. (1975). *Basic Background Items for U.S. Household Surveys*, Social Research Council, Washington, D.C.

53. Kitagawa, E. M., and Hauser, P. M. (1968). Education differentials in mortality by cause of death, United States, 1960, *Demography, 5*, 318–53.
   Haller, A. O. (1970). Changes in the structure of status systems, *Rural Sociology, 35*, 469–87.

54. Freeman, R. (1976). *The Over-Educated American*, New York.
   Wright, E. O., and Perrone, L. (1977). Marxist class categories and income inequality, *Amer. Sociol. Rev., 42*, 32–55.

55. Featherman, D. L., and Hauser, R. M. (1978). *Opportunity and Change*, New York.

56. Hirsch, F. (1980). *Social Limits to Growth*, Cambridge, Mass.

57. Hollingshead, A. B., and Redlich, F. C. (1958). *Social Class and Mental Illness*, New York.

58. Warner, W. Ll., and Lunt, P. S. (1941). *The Social Life of a Modern Community*, New Haven.
   Warner, W. Ll., Meeker, M., and Eells, K. (1949). *Social Class in America*, Chicago.
   Pfantz, H. W., and Duncan, O. D. (1950). A critical evaluation of Warner's work in social stratification, *Amer. Sociol. Rev., 15*, 205–15.

59. Lenski, G. E. (1954). Status crystallization: A non–vertical dimension of social status, *Amer. Sociol. Rev., 19*, 405–13.
   Blalock, H. M. (1967). Status and consistency: Integration and structural effects, *Amer. Sociol. Rev., 32*, 790–801.

60. Shevky, E., and Williams, M. (1949). *The Social Areas of Los Angeles: Analysis and Typology*, Berkeley.
   Shevky, E., and Bell, W. (1955). *Social Area Analysis* Stanford.
   Sussman, M. B., ed. (1959). *Community Structure and Analysis*, New York.

61. Stockwell, E. G. (1963). A critical examination of the relationship between socio–economic status and mortality, *Amer. J. Publ. Hlth., 53*, 956–64.

62. Struening, E. L., and Lehman, S. (1969). A social area study of the Bronx: Environmental determinants of behavioral deviance and physical pathology, in *Social Psychiatry*, ed. Redlich, F. C., *Res. Publ. Ass. Nerv. Ment. Dis.*, no. 47, Baltimore.

6

Social class and
disorders of health

For social scientists, uneven distributions of disease, illness, and sickness in society are manifestations of social structure and culture that reveal variations in custom, disparities in resources, or differences among subgroups in the conditions of daily life. For epidemiologists, the discovery of such variations is a starting point; they must elucidate their medical significance, and through preventive medicine attempt to eliminate them (1). In this chapter, we take the social class variable as the starting point for epidemiological analysis.

By the Middle Ages it was already clear that wealth could mitigate, and poverty exacerbate, the distribution of disease through human society. As we have said, chroniclers of the plague in medieval Europe noted that it was among the poor that the Black Death exacted its highest toll. In part this was due to the ability of the rich in the cities to flee the epidemic, but the inadequate nutrition and weakened resistance of the poor probably also played its part.

The case of the Great Plague of London in 1665 is particularly instructive because of the quality of the records available which describe it. Plague had been endemic in England since the late 14th century. Four epidemics had occurred in the century preceding the outbreak of the Great Plague. A series of bad harvests, resultant famines, and numerous wars had driven rural people to urban areas in search of relief. With the people came rats, also in search of food. The heavy migration added to the overcrowding in the outskirts of the City of London. The intimacy of rats, fleas, domestic animals, and people in the households of the poor was the breeding ground for the plague. Fleas were the vectors that transmitted the plague bacillus, *Pasteurella pestis*, from infected rats to the human host.

When plague broke out, three quarters of the residents of the properous inner city fled. The weekly Bills of Mortality—which John Graunt used to perform the first epidemiological analysis of the mortality of a population over time (2)—were kept to give early warning of just such an epidemic to those classes who had the means to flee. As a result, that sector where half the city's population normally resided suffered only one-seventh of the total mortality. Here as elsewhere, plague was primarily an affliction of the indigent. As Defoe recorded in his *Journal of the Plague Year:* "The misery of that time lay upon the poor, who, being infected, had neither food nor physic, neither physician nor apothecary to assist them." Disease not only reflected class differences but could, at times, fan class frictions as well. Peasant uprisings, "crimes of sacrilege" and vandalism, and the sacking of the abandoned homes of the rich often followed in the wake of the plague. Flight, the only defense against infection, was not available to the poor (3).

Medical attention to the impact of class differences on health is of comparatively recent origin (4). The first and most striking relationship to be recognized was between disorders of health and low social class. One of the earliest users of a social class scale in medicine was Louis René Villermé. In the 1820s Villermé constructed a crude profile of poverty and wealth by looking at the connection between mortality and untaxed rents in Paris. Annual rents of more than 150 francs were taxed; rents under 150 francs, which were seen as indicators of poverty, were untaxed. Table 6.1 illustrates the percentage of untaxed renters in each Parisian arrondissement. Villermé noted that the districts with the higher percentages of untaxed rents had higher mortality rates. In 1840, with a more sophisticated approach, Villermé analyzed mortality by occupation and social class over a decade in the French textile city of Mulhouse.

In Britain, that manifesto of the public health movement, the *Report on the Sanitary Conditions of the Labouring Population of Great Britain*, compiled by Edwin Chadwick and published in 1842, contained many tables illustrating the connection between mortality and social class. These data were converted into tools of social crit-

Table 6.1 Average annual mortality for rich and poor in Paris as indicated by the taxation level of each *arrondissement*, 1817–1821

Arrondissement	Untaxed rents (%)	Deaths per 1000 inhabitants
2	7	16.1
3	11	16.7
1	11	17.2
4	15	17.2
11	19	19.6
6	21	18.5
5	22	18.9
7	22	19.2
10	23	20.0
9	31	22.7
8	32	23.3
12	38	23.3

Sources: Villermé, L. R. (1826). Rapport . . . sur une série de tableaux relatifs au mouvement de la population dans les douze arrondissements municipaux de la ville de Paris pendant les cinq années 1817, 1818, 1819, 1820, et 1821, *Archives générales de médecine, 10,* p. 227. Taken from Coleman, W. (1982). *Death Is a Social Disease,* Madison, p. 161.

icism by Friedrich Engels, who in *The Condition of the Working Class in England in 1844* argued the proposition that disease was a reflection of the relations of economic production. The report provided data equally cogent for the followers of Thomas Malthus, who in his *Essay on Population* of 1798 had contended that poor nutrition, unwholesome housing, hard labor, and lack of child care among the lowest orders of society were checks on population growth (5). Later it slowly emerged that the rich, too, had their particular disorders.

William Farr made the first analysis of national mortality rates by occupation; he used the deaths in 1851 as the numerator and the census data of that year as the denominator (6). The social class scale of 1911 made an advance in this type of analysis by ordering occupations into classes, and the 1931 census made yet another advance with an analysis by social class of mortality rates for married women. This helped to distinguish the occupational risks to which married men were exposed from the environmental risks which they shared with their wives (7). All these analyses revealed disparities in morbidity and mortality between the social classes (see Figures 6.1 and 6.2).

To conceive of these patterns of health and disease as static within each class is to misrepresent reality. Dispute about their interpretation is often the result (8). Changes take place in social and cultural relations, and these changes can be detected in health patterns. Within the general movement of society, each social class changes its way of life and its composition, the borders between classes alter, and members are exchanged between them.

Many dramatic changes in the social distribution of disease have occurred in the more than two decades since this book was first published. Death rates in older children have shown some trend toward equality between the social classes. As early as the late 1950s, deaths among children from rheumatic heart disease had fallen in all classes, but more in poorer than in prosperous communities (9). For deaths from all causes among children aged 1 to 2 years, the excess of Social Class V over Social Class I, which was more than 400 per cent in 1930–1932, was only 63 per cent in 1950–1951. The gap between the classes has diminished for infant mortality as well, although it remains wider for the age group of 9 to 12 months than for any other (10). The distribution of coronary heart disease—the main cause of mortality among men from middle age on—shifted from the upper toward the lower classes. A gradient from upper to lower classes where none previously existed emerged for lung cancer.

The patterns of health between classes will differ according to the index used. It must be borne in mind that disease refers to disordered physiological and psychological function; illness, to subjective awareness of disordered function; and sickness, to disrupted social roles (see Chapter 1). The sick role may be assumed or assigned either as a result of recognized inability to perform social roles—for instance, as measured in the "disability" surveys of the U.S. Public Health Service—or with entry to formal patienthood. Just as the separate criteria by which social class can be measured may not vary concomitantly with each other, so between the classes these three dimensions of health need not vary in lock step with each other. The root phenomena tapped by each dimension are determined by different factors distributed unequally between

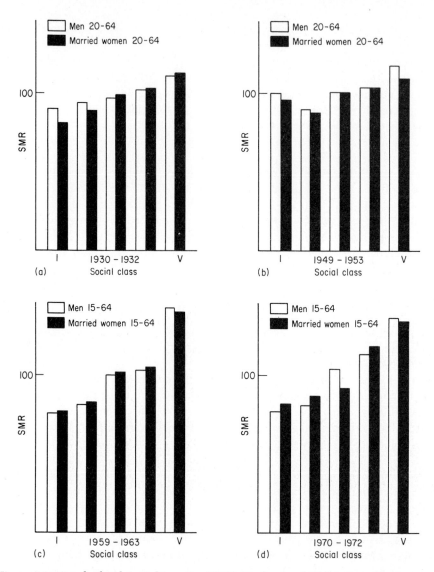

Figure 6.1 Standardized mortality ratios (SMR), England and Wales, for selected age and sex groups and time periods, by social class. *Source:* Adapted from Office of Population Censuses and Survey (1978). *Occupational Mortality, 1970–1972*, The Registrar General's Decennial Supplement for England and Wales, Series DS no. 1, H.M.S.O., London, p. 174; Antonovsky, A. (1967). Social class, life expectancy and overall mortality, *Milbank Mem. Fd. Quart.*, *45*, p. 63; and Townsend, P. (1974). Inequality and the Health Service, *Lancet, 1*, 1179–90.

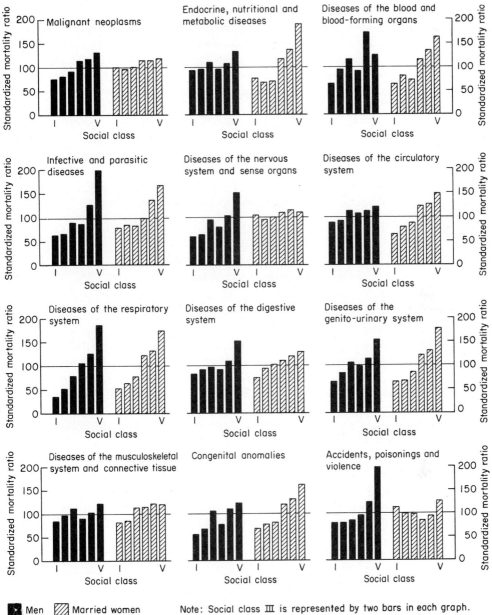

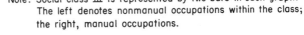

Figure 6.2 Occupational class and mortality from several causes in men and married women (15–64 years), by husband's occupation. *Source:* Adapted from Office of Population Censuses and Surveys (1978). *Occupational Mortality, 1970–1972*, The Registrar General's Decennial Supplement for England and Wales, Series DS no. 1, H.M.S.O., London, p. 41.

the classes. Disease is influenced by the physical and biological as well as the social environment. Illness, to the extent that it depends on psychological perception and not on the physical environment, will be influenced more than disease by personality and socialization. Sickness, to the extent that its expression depends on the capacity of economic, social, and technical resources to absorb it, will be influenced by culture and social structure to a greater extent than either illness or disease.

We turn first to consider in more detail a number of diseases—coronary heart disease, poliomyelitis, leukemia, and peptic ulcer—that made their first appearances in documented distributions as diseases of the higher classes. We then review in a more general way mortality patterns characteristic of the lower classes. More briefly, the place of work and of race and ethnicity in the social distributions of health are considered. Finally, we examine the relations of mental disorder to the social structure, and then offer an interpretation of persisting social inequalities in health.

Shifts in the social distribution of disease
Coronary heart disease

Coronary heart disease is an epidemic of our time that serves well to illustrate the use of the social class variable. In the United States, the diagnosis accounts for about one-third of all deaths among middle-aged men. In Britain, it causes a similar proportion of deaths: somewhat higher in Scotland and somewhat lower in England. The disease attained prominence as a scourge of middle-aged men of the upper classes. Even before it was firmly established as a disease entity in the medical literature with Herrick's description of 1912, William Osler had observed that angina pectoris (pain due to deficient blood supply to the heart muscle that often precedes or accompanies coronary heart disease) was an "affection of the better classes." Until quite recently, coronary heart disease remained a disorder of the privileged.

Coronary heart disease is a form of acute or chronic damage to the heart muscle that follows on deficient blood flow, or ischemia. This ischemia is caused by narrowing of the coronary arteries that supply the heart muscle, or myocardium. Narrowing occurs in arteries whose inner walls show the patchy degenerative changes of atheroma. Before damage to the heart muscle supervenes in the form of acute myocardial infarction—when a segment of the heart muscle dies because of the failure of the nutrient supply—an additional element is generally necessary, namely, clotting of blood in the lumen of the artery (11,12).

A striking social class gradient for coronary heart disease, declining from upper to lower social classes, was found in the analysis of mortality by occupations in Britain for the period 1930–1932. For the most part, data from American studies in the late 1930s and the 1940s confirmed the British finding (13). Recognition of this marked class disparity, coupled with the rising death toll from the disease, spurred the intensive search for environmental causes that continues to the present.

An early study found close correlations between the increase in motor vehicle licenses, radio and television ownership, and the rising death rate from coronary heart disease (14). This is not quite the lesson in statistical absurdity it may first appear to be: cars and modern media are indicators, admittedly crude ones, of a stage of economic development and a way of life associated with it. And coronary heart disease is notoriously a "disease of civilization" (15). Among men especially, the increase during the half century following clinical recognition of the disease in 1912 was sharp indeed. In the 1960s, prospective studies in the United States showed that the incidence of new events of angina, infarction and death in men in their forties and fifties had risen to about 1 per cent per year; in more than a fifth, death was the first manifestation.

There can be no serious doubt that the increase was real, and not the result merely of more accurate diagnoses, or of the shift in certification of deaths from nonspecific diagnosis such as myocardial degeneration to coronary heart disease, or of a present overdiagnosis of this disease (16). Mortality among men in both the United States and Britain continued to rise after the Second World War, a period when sensitivity to the diagnosis among physicians has been high. Before angiography became general in the 1970s, the instruments of diagnosis did not improve in any essential manner. Besides, diagnositc precision and fashions in nomenclature are unlikely to affect the sexes in a manner so grossly different as does coronary heart disease. The incidence in middle-aged women is about half that in men, and less before the menopause. In both sexes incidence rises regularly with age (17). Time trends emphasize the sex differences.

An analysis of mortality from *nonvalvular heart disease* (mainly coronary heart disease and hypertensive heart disease) reduces the likelihood that misclassification, or variation in classification through time, could account for the rising epidemic curve. In postwar Britain, the trend in mortality for this combination of disease categories among married women, in marked contrast to the trend among men, was actually in decline (see Figure 6.3). In the United States, mortality from heart disease among successive cohorts of women shows a similar steady decline in the period 1945 to 1975, again in contrast to the trend among men, which continued to rise into the mid 1960s (18). The trend for hypertensive heart disease may possibly contribute to these findings. Mortality from hypertension accounted for a substantial proportion of heart disease among women and may well have been declining throughout the period studied in Britain, as it was shown to do in Memphis, Tennessee (19).

That societies render their members more or less vulnerable to certain forms of disease is clear in the case of coronary heart disease. The disease has been linked with an affluent way of life; incidence is high in rich countries, and low in poor ones. This disparity is not simply the result of people living longer, nor of more effective diagnosis. Large differences are found across developed countries with roughly equivalent life spans and degrees of technological development (20). In Israel, marked differences in mortality from coronary disease occurred among successive waves of Yemenite Jewish migrants. Among the early immigrants, who in the period under study had been exposed to a Western way of life for 20 years or more, the mortality rate for degenerative heart disease in middle-aged men was more than six times that of recent immigrants (21). The difference, 3.3/1000 versus .49/1000, is almost identical to the changes in coronary mortality in England and Wales over the period 1931 to 1957, when the death toll rose from .49/1000 to 3.59/1000 (21). Similar changes in disease

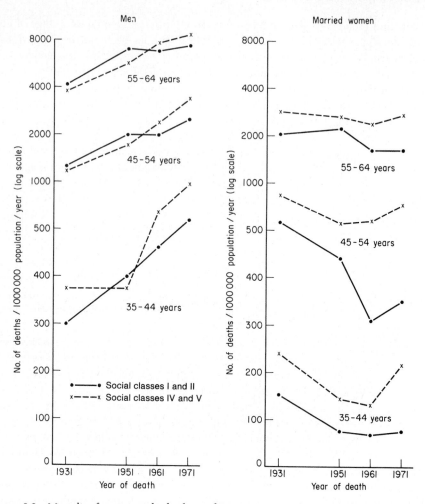

Figure 6.3 Mortality from nonvalvular heart disease in men and married women according to social class and age around four census dates, 1931–1971. *Source:* Marmot, M.G., Adelstein, A.M., Robinson, N. and Rose, G.A. (1978). Changing social class distribution of heart disease, *Brit. Med. J.*, 2, 1109–1112.

rates with environmental change occurred among Chinese- and Japanese-Americans; both groups have coronary heart disease rates that shift from those prevailing in their countries of origin toward those characteristic of their country of residence (22).

Such marked variation in coronary heart disease among different countries, at different times in the same country, and among people of the same ethnic stock with different experiences, underscores the importance of ways of life in shaping the distribution of disease. Even if the mode of operation remains obscure, the key must reside in the environment, including the social structure and cultural practices. The relation between social context and disease, we stress again, is a dynamic one. Societies change, their environments are modified, biological pathogens evolve, and physical agents appear or disappear; at the same time, the vulnerability of their people alters with the state of immunity and nutrition. Within industrial societies, although social classes may retain their relative positions, their size and composition fluctuate as both forms of production and the organization of the labor force change. All these changes enter into the quality and quantity of consumption, the styles of living, and the activities available to the members of the various classes. They may be expected also to enter into the distribution of mortality and morbidity from coronary heart disease.

An emerging shift in the social class distribution of coronary heart disease, noted in the second edition of this book, is now plainly apparent. In both Britain and the United States in 1950, mortality was already concentrated in the lowest social class among men under 45 years of age, although not among older men. Local mortality studies obtained similar results (23). In Britain, and probably in the United States as well, the social class shift is now present in all age groups (24). One new finding, remarkable for remaining so long unobserved, is that in the recorded statistics for women the mortality gradient for nonvalvular heart disease has always favored the higher social classes.

In the United States during the postwar period up to the early 1960s, most morbidity studies found a greater incidence of coronary disease in the higher social classes (13). At the same time, in different parts of the country, conflicting trends or an absence of a class gradient began to be observed. In a longitudinal study of Evans County in Georgia, high *prevalence* was observed in the higher social classes at the outset. As the population was followed through time, however, this observation was confounded by high *incidence* in the lower social classes equal to that in the higher classes (25). The change could not be explained by differences in case-fatality rates among the classes, nor by biased diagnostic criteria, by missed cases, or by competing causes of death. Further evidence that suggests a social class shift in coronary mortality and morbidity in the United States in the 1960s comes from studies of mortality in rich and poor states, from the results of the National Health Interview Survey, and from studies of selected metropolitan areas (26).

The concentration of coronary heart disease in the lower social classes has taken place in the face of the recent decline in death rates from coronary heart disease in the United States—amounting to about 30 per cent in the past decade (27). The meager data available suggest, therefore, that the higher social classes have been the main beneficiaries of the decline in coronary heart disease mortality in the United States. In Britain, the rise in coronary death rates has begun to slow but they have not yet begun to decline. The observed social class shifts in the disease, however, suggest that a decline beginning in the higher classes will follow in Britain. In the 1970s, a decline was already apparent in the coronary death rates of British physicians (28).

Logically, social class itself can be taken to explain a profile or pattern of disease—disease as a *group* characteristic—without falling into the ecological fallacy (see below). The manifestation of disease in the members of a class, however, requires the operation of intermediate agents that impinge on individuals. The search for factors that could explain the social class gradient first focused on diet and body weight and later on exercise, smoking, and emotional strain. These are all concomitants of ways of life that vary with social class.

In diet studies the consumption of fats has been extensively studied (20,29,30). Diets high in saturated fatty acids raise the levels of blood lipids, cholesterol in particular. Lipids, in turn, may be connected with coronary heart disease either through the deposit of atheroma plaques on the vessel walls—which impede blood flow—or through increased coagulability of the blood, resulting in clots that block the vessels either acutely or through slower processes that likewise narrow the vessel walls.

Dietary habits, either customary or enforced by poverty, together with blood cholesterol levels, have been correlated with the incidence of coronary heart disease across social groups. In South Africa, fat consumption, blood cholesterol levels, and the incidence of coronary heart disease have all shown a gradient declining across white, coloured, and black racial groups. In East Africa, similar gradients have been found between Asians and Africans. In Europe, Trappist and Benedictine monks vary in their prescribed dietary habits; the Benedictines regularly eat meat while the Trappists never do. As expected, the Benedictines have been found to have the higher blood choleserol levels and a higher incidence of coronary heart disease (31). In patients who suffer from either of two diseases, diabetes and familial hypercholesterolemia, cholesterol levels are abnormally high, and the incidence of coronary heart disease among those affected is also abnormally high.

Prospective surveys of persons free of coronary heart disease on recruitment have established that elevated cholesterol levels put individuals at higher risk of developing the disease (17,32,33). That the variability of cholesterol levels is, in the main, environmentally determined is indicated by twin studies, which point to the predominant influence of mothers rather than fathers on the intrafamilial associations found among twins and their offspring, an influence not readily explained by Mendelian inheritance. Familial patterns too vary with social situation (34): correlations of cholesterol levels are distinctly stronger for members of lower-class families than of higher-class families (35).

Refined measures of cholesterol and lipid fractions in the blood have begun to add precision to predictions of risk. An excess of *low-density lipoprotein* and the depletion of *high-density lipoprotein* are independently associated with higher risk (36). The associations of cholesterol and lipid levels with coronary heart disease apply across societies. High levels have been shown to predict a greater likelihood of developing coronary heart disease in far-flung populations: in rural Georgia and South Carolina, as well as in New York, Chicago, and San Francisco; in Hawaii, Puerto Rico, and Japan; in Yugoslavia and Israel as well as in France and Britain (36,37).

Still, perplexing questions remain. Certainly factors other than cholesterol levels enhance vulnerability to coronary heart disease. The risk attached to given levels of cholesterol, for instance, is consistently higher in city than in rural dwellers. In migrants to cities, too, the risk is lower than in the urban-born, but higher than in those who stay in the country. In international comparisons, coronary mortality can be made to correlate as highly with protein intake as with fat consumption. Changes over time too seem not always to conform with the cholesterol hypothesis. Mortality from nonvalvular heart disease in Britain correlates best not with fats, but with sucrose and whole-grain meal bread (38).

Cholesterol levels reflect other dietary factors than fat alone, however, and these anomalous findings do not necessarily contradict the association of cholesterol with coronary heart disease. A diet low in fat is usually low in protein, high in fiber and starch, and of variable mineral and vitamin content. Each of these components has been shown in animal studies to affect cholesterol levels; in humans, not only unsaturated fatty acids, but also low protein and low calorie intake have been reported to reduce cholesterol levels (14,39). The extent to which plasma cholesterol levels reflect lifelong dietary habits is thus an unresolved problem. The effect of current diet on cholesterol levels is not clear: the daily intake of free-living populations is difficult to measure and cholesterol levels themselves vary from day to day. Thus, an English study failed to uncover any relationship between blood cholesterol levels and dietary intake calculated from reported food consumption over a short defined period (40). The Framingham study in the United States did no better (33).

It could be that populations surveyed in developed countries are saturated with dietary cholesterol and that, consequently, much of the variation above the threshold for saturation is due to factors other than fat in the diet. A recent follow-up of a population of male workers in Chicago suggests that the problem may rather reside in the difficulties of measuring dietary intake. In this Western Electric study, dietary intake was recorded by study subjects over a 28-day period on entry. Intake of saturated fats correlated with raised cholesterol level, and unsaturated fats with lower levels (30).

Cholesterol may thus represent a link in the causal chain leading to coronary disease. Alternatively, cholesterol is closely linked to some factor which is the common cause of coronary disease and of raised blood cholesterol levels. In the Chicago Western Electric study, dietary intake of saturated fats was linked to *serum* cholesterol levels, as noted, and *serum* cholesterol level to coronary disease. The association of *dietary* cholesterol and saturated fats with coronary disease, a weak one, was strengthened with *serum* cholesterol controlled; this suggests that serum cholesterol may not be in the direct causal sequence leading from dietary cholesterol to coronary disease (41). The evidence of the role of dietary fats in coronary disease is neither unequivocal nor complete, and other cooperating causes play at least as great a part. Nonetheless, it is reasonable to suppose that dietary differences among social classes partly explain the social class differentials in coronary heart disease. The presumption is strengthened by changes over time in dietary habits and cholesterol levels on the one hand, and coronary disease on the other. The upper classes have changed their habits and cholesterol levels most, and have benefited most from the decline in mortality (42). The fact that efforts to lower cholesterol levels by "prudent" diets and other means have had a degree of success strengthens the notion of a direct causal effect (29,43). Most recently, large scale randomized trials of the cholesterol lowering drug cholestyramine have succeeded in lowering coronary mortality by about one-fifth (44).

Men who suffer from coronary heart disease are heavier than those who do not, and *relative weight* (i.e., weight controlled for height) is a function of diet intake and energy expenditure. In multivariate analysis with cholesterol and other factors con-

trolled, the association of weight and coronary heart disease disappears (45). This finding is compatible with a causal chain in which weight is antecedent to cholesterol and
the other factors controlled in the analysis, which would then appear as intervening
variables through which weight acts (41). In the Framingham study, weight changes
correlated highly with changes in cholesterol levels. Obesity, one might note, varies
with social class in the same manner as does coronary heart disease. Obesity once
symbolized wealth and affluence—as in the unflattering cartoons of capitalists early
in this century—and in parts of the underdeveloped world it still does. Now, like
coronary heart disease in recent times, obesity in the developed world has become a
manifestation of the poorer classes (46).

   Physical exercise, too, has been linked with blood cholesterol levels, a finding which
lends indirect support to the association between exercise and coronary disease. When
exercise is sufficient to prevent weight gain, high-fat diets have been found not to
increase cholesterol levels as they do with less exercise (47). The extraordinary physical fitness of Masai warriors, reported to take a diet of meat and milk with relatively
high fat content but at the same time to cover many miles a day following their cattle,
probably accounts not only for their low average cholesterol level of only 120 mg.,
but also for the low frequency of coronary heart disease among them (48). Exercise
may influence coronary heart disease through another pathway, for it also increases
the fibrinolytic activity of blood and thereby impedes clotting (49).

   Physical activity may also have been a significant factor in the earlier social class
gradient. The prevalence of coronary heart disease varies with occupations demanding different degrees of activity. In a national survey of consecutive autopsies of men
aged 45 to 70 in the mid-1950s, occupations were graded as "light," "active," or
"heavy." At autopsy, both infarcts and fibrosis of heart muscle caused by diminution
of the coronary blood flow were most common in "light" workers, less common in
"active" workers and least in "heavy" workers. Within these grades of occupations
the prevalence of coronary heart disease did not vary with social class (50). However,
occupations involving heavy work predominated in the lower social classes, and light
occupations in the upper classes, consistent with the social class distribution of the
disease at the time of the study. A number of other studies, although not all, have
been able to relate the physical activity of occupations to coronary heart disease. Vigorous leisure-time activity appears to protect against the disease and exhibits a social
class pattern compatible with the current gradient for the disease, declining from
upper to lower classes (51).

   Hypertension, another attribute that puts individuals at high risk of coronary heart
disease, shows a similar relationship to occupation and physical activity (52). Indeed,
in the United States, hypertension has had consistently higher prevalence rates among
persons of low income, whether male or female, white or black. Around this relationship contradictions multiply; among them is the distribution of coronary heart disease
and hypertension among racial groups and between the sexes. Whites engage in sedentary occupations much more than blacks, and coronary heart disease is more common among whites than blacks. It is also found more frequently among men than
women. Yet, although hypertension is well established as a precursor of coronary
heart disease, it is far more common among blacks than among whites, and, above

the mid-forties—at the peak ages for coronary heart disease—hypertension is more common among women than men. Moreover, while coronary heart disease has but recently begun to decline, hypertension has been on the decline for 30 years or more (19).

These contradictions call for a digression. They can be created by faults of inference as much as by weaknesses in data or methods. This particular problem involves a form of the "ecological fallacy" (41,53). Legitimate inferences can be drawn about causality from direct associations found between phenomena analyzed at the same level of organization of the social system; the level of organization is indicated by the unit of observation—for instance, nations, or areas, or population groups, or households, or individuals. It is hazardous to draw inferences when the associated phenomena are situated at different levels of organization and involve different units of observation. Such an example is the inverse association between coronary heart disease and hypertension at the ecological level of ethnic groups and occupation, and the direct association between them at the individual level of persons. Depending on the frequency and distribution between subgroups of the phenomena under study, it is quite possible for an association to be positive at one level of observation, and negative at another. For instance, although in individuals hypertension is positively associated with coronary heart disease, it may be so relatively infrequent a condition, and its partial contribution to coronary heart disease may be so small, that in ethnic groups other factors, more frequent, making larger causal contributions to coronary heart disease, and differently distributed between the ethnic groups, could so far outweigh hypertension as to give rise to the appearance of a negative association at the group level of observation.

A similar analytical problem underlies the findings relating to region-specific mortality from coronary heart disease across the United States. Coronary mortality (under the rubric arteriosclerotic heart disease) varies as widely as it does across Europe, being high on the east and west coasts, and low in the mountain states. These variations cannot be attributed merely to flaws in certification of death and diagnostic fashion (54). But overall mortality varies in parallel manner, so that deaths from arteriosclerotic heart disease form an almost constant proportion of all deaths in each state. Where crude mortality is high, coronary mortality is high also, and in New York State coronary mortality is higher than the total age-adjusted mortality of North Dakota. The same proportions hold throughout, even when the selected causes are narrowed down and smoking-related diseases are removed from the roster of all causes. These results of ecological studies do not invalidate other findings, obtained in studies of individuals, that specify the associations of particular attributes with coronary heart disease. Within the broad ecological pattern determined by the total social, biological, and physical environment there is ample room for the operation of specific factors that are closer, in the sequence of causal events, to the outcome in individuals.

To return to the question of exercise as a factor in coronary heart disease, its effect may be to protect relatively young men against acute occlusion of the coronary arteries by thrombosis. The factors related to coronary heart disease have a somewhat different form among the old and the young; the old have more atheroma but fewer of the acute infarctions and sudden deaths characteristic of rapid blocking of the coronary arteries by thrombi (55). Drivers of double-decker London buses were found to suffer more acute coronary deaths than the more active conductors, and sedentary office clerks and telephone operators suffered more than postmen (56); in the affected age-groups these acute fatalities have occurred especially in younger men. Rapid occlusion of atheromatous arteries by thrombosis may have been the underlying pathology of the upsurge of coronary heart disease in middle-aged men in the period through the 1960s, for over time the prevalence of atheroma alone did not seem to run parallel with coronary heart disease. Autopsy reports in a London hospital over the half century before that varied little in the frequency with which atheroma was recorded. Indeed, while atheroma and stenosis of the coronary arteries is an almost invariable condition for the occurrence of infarction, a high proportion of men in the most affected age groups have such arterial changes, only some of whom suffer infarcts. The factors that cause the atheroma and stenosis may not be the same as those that precipitate occlusion. It may be mainly the young in whom atheroma can be prevented by a reversal of those habits of exercise, diet, and smoking that have only recently appeared in our society, and that are associated with coronary heart disease.

One other factor associated with coronary disease, *smoking* (57), also varies with social class (58). The risk with smoking, although not as high for coronary disease as for lung cancer, is not negligible. Average male cigarette smokers, compared with nonsmokers, have a risk of about 1.7 to 1 for coronary heart disease, and 9 to 1 for lung cancer; middle-aged men who smoke more than 20 cigarettes per day have a risk compared with nonsmokers of between 2 and 4 to 1 for coronary disease, and of more than 20 to 1 for lung cancer (59). Coronary disease is much more common than lung cancer, however, and the death toll from coronary disease attributable to smoking (the *attributable risk*) is greater than that from lung cancer. The risk declines among those who stop smoking.

We noted in the first edition of this book that since the smoking habits of social classes change, the distribution of coronary heart disease could also be expected to change between the classes. Among women, despite the lower incidence of coronary heart disease, social class changes related to smoking are likely to be even more striking than among men, because of the conjoint effects of oral contraceptives. In one study, premenopausal women with acute myocardial infarction were 7 times more likely to have smoked heavily, 4 times more likely to have used oral contraceptives in the past month, and 39 times more likely to have done both than were those women with no infarction. Other studies are congruent (60). Both smoking and oral contraceptives use vary markedly among social classes through time.

Emotion and behavioral factors must also be considered as possible causes of the social class gradient in coronary disease. In an early uncontrolled series of a hundred young coronary patients, emotional strain was found to precede the attack in 91 cases (61). Many of these young men were described as ambitious, conscientious, and obsessional. They tended to work to exhaustion, and to be restless and nagged by guilt during their leisure time. Men of this type, particularly those beset by a sense of urgency and competitiveness, were found to have higher cholesterol levels than unambitious men in less exacting occupations (62). In this early study, such variables as social and occupational status went uncontrolled, and the characterization of the personality types was not done objectively nor strictly separated from the observations on the dependent variable (cholesterol) to exclude bias. Further studies, however, in a general way support its findings. When men are under pressure, cholesterol levels have been found to rise and whole-blood clotting times to accelerate. Two small groups of accountants, "tax" accountants and "corporation" accountants, were studied over a period of five months. For each group the period of most strenuous work was well defined and occurred at a different time of the year; at these times cholesterol levels were highest and clotting times shortest, without any accompanying changes in physical activity or diet (63). The same holds for medical students under the strain of examination.

Many relevant studies of stressors in coronary heart disease are of the retrospective case-control type. Histories of stressful states obtained after the fact of the acute coronary event are subject to unmeasured bias on recall as compared with controls; measures of mental state taken after the event are likewise always assailable because their existence prior to the event can be no more than a supposition. Thus the causal sequence remains an open question. Prospective studies have identified a number of stress factors as the precursors, not so much of acute myocardial infarction, as of angina pectoris. Thus, anxiety, depression, neuroticism, and interpersonal problems have been related in most studies to angina (64,65,66), and only in some studies to myocardial infarcts (66,67). A study in Sweden has added "workload" (a composite measure of job-related stresses) to the list of contributing factors to myocardial infarcts. In another analysis, those at highest risk were persons in jobs that combined limited freedom and control over decisions with tasks that placed high demands on the workers (68).

Types of personality and of behavior pattern, too, have been further investigated since the early studies mentioned above (69). In a two-way classification of behavioral patterns into Types A and B, only Type A was found to be "coronary prone." In a predictive study, the coronary prone complex carried a higher risk of coronary heart disease than did either a raised cholesterol or a raised blood-pressure level. An eight-and-a-half-year follow-up of the original Western Collaborative Group Study—which controlled for the influence of the major risk factors of age, cholesterol, blood pressure and smoking—showed that subjects classified as Type A were at twice the risk of developing coronary heart disease as their Type B counterparts. Other studies have confirmed that Type A behavior is largely independent of other risk factors (64,70,71). Besides these longitudinal studies of personality type and incidence, a number of cross-sectional studies support these associations between Type A personality and coronary heart disease.

Two pathophysiological mechanisms have been suggested as modes through which Type A behavior engenders coronary risk: hyperresponsiveness—as measured by increased blood pressure and noradrenalin output—to challenging situations (72), and some unknown process leading to atherosclerosis and obstructed coronary arteries as shown on angiography (73).

Type A describes an extreme if not atypical profile of a hard-driving, competitive member of the "achieving society," wedded to his job and always rushing (74). That the Type A behavior pattern is environmentally induced seems not improbable: identical twins have been found to be no more concordant for the typical repertoire of behavior than are fraternal twins (75). The question naturally arises as to whether this personality configuration is a specific response to demands of societies that induce the disease, and perhaps more particularly to modern American society. The coronary-prone behavior pattern was after all first described among white, middleaged, upper-middle-class Californians, and the self-administered questionnaire most often used in surveys was standardized among them. The Type A woman, though less common than her male counterpart, may illustrate the adaptive value of this behavioral style in fulfilling the demands of occupational roles once the preserve of males alone (76).

Among men in European countries the behavior pattern seems to be less common than in the Untied States (77). Among black Americans, too, the typical behavior pattern seems seldom to be found (78). Not only does its frequency vary across cultures, but also the degree of risk associated with it. Among Japanese-Americans, the Type A behavior pattern was found to be relatively rare, and was not in itself associated with significantly raised risk of coronary disease. Only those men who exhibited the modified Type A behavior pattern and at the same time led a highly Westernized way of life were found to be at heightened risk of coronary heart disease (79).

In short, the Type A behavior pattern may be a mode of response to particular emotional and social demands. The assembled evidence suggests that both emotional strain and the manner of coping with it could be related to the social class distribution of coronary heart disease. Although the amount and the type of strain in each social class are not easily measured, for each class the external sources of stress and the resources for dealing with it are manifestly dissimilar (80,81). Common observation, and several anthropological studies, suggest that behavior patterns and coping styles are also distinctive by class. Studies in the United States have shown repeatedly that in both men and women Type A behavior is characteristic of higher social class position, as measured by either education or occupation (76,82). Although this form of behavior runs contrary to the contemporary social class distribution of coronary heart disease, it is not thereby annulled as a source of the disease within classes.

For this distribution of Type A behavior there are several possible reasons. In a competitive market economy, Type A behavior can be expected to be an advantage. Aggression, competitiveness, and intense commitment to job demands boost production and are likely to facilitate upward mobility. Social class differences in childrearing practices may also play a part. The values emphasized by parents reflect the realities of their occupational positions. In Italy and the United States, for example, middleclass fathers emphasized self-control above obedience, working-class fathers the reverse. The difference between them, it was found on further analysis, could be accounted for by the degree of independence in the father's occupation (83). In the United States, middle-class parents are themselves more likely than working-class parents to embody Type A characteristics, tend to have higher, more open-ended ambitions for their children, and may actively encourage certain Type A behavior by their high performance standards (84).

In contrast with personality factors, the latter-day concentration of most other recognized risk factors for coronary heart disease among lower-class people suggests that, as individuals, working-class people lack resources to protect themselves against those forces of commerce, industry, mass communication, and culture that promote unhealthy practices which the upper classes are learning to avoid. Self-esteem and the sense of control and autonomy in shaping the course of one's life, like education and knowledge about health (85), diminish with the social class gradient (81). At the same time, many attitudes and values prevalent among the working classes are likely to reinforce their vulnerability to coronary heart disease and to most other diseases as well. By paths still ill-understood, the psychosocial complex characteristic of each class engenders risks peculiar to it.

The reasons for the social class distribution of coronary heart disease, and for changes in that distribution, plainly could be manifold. Epidemiologists concern themselves first with immediate causes, and must labor at length, painstakingly and with rigor, to establish the uncontaminated contribution of single factors, to measure interaction among them, and to recognize confounding. Yet the broader context within which these factors operate equally needs to be understood.

The ways in which both good and harm are distributed are not simply in the hands of affected individuals. In industrial capitalist societies, with the coming of mass communications media and near-universal literacy, a generic culture is ever more widely shared: the same processed foods and tobaccos are available to the large body of the people, and generated power and motor transport are at the ready command of the humble as well as the rich. Jobs of low prestige that once were physically strenuous are no longer so, and a multitude of new occupations are sedentary. On the other hand, jobs of high prestige that once were emotionally strenuous may have become less so, as more men and now women have moved into large and ever-growing organizational structures in the wake of the vanguard who defined and formalized the roles within them. In accord with such changes, in the 1960s studies of morbidity among employees of large corporations showed lower rates of coronary heart disease among high-level executives than among those of lower level (86). Similarly, the Type A pattern appears to be more prevalent among business managers and lower order professionals than among executives and higher order professionals (87).

Poliomyelitis

Until the early 1960s when poliomyelitis came under effective control in the United States and Britain, death and paralysis from this disease followed a declining class gradient (88). Epidemiology sheds some light on the process of infection and immunity which accounted for this pattern. Although small clusters of cases of poliomyelitis were reported early in the nineteenth century, the poliomyelitis epidemic was a relatively recent phenomenon of industrial societies. The first substantial epidemic was reported in Sweden in 1887; another probable early outbreak in Britain in 1891 was a group of cases of "cerebrospinal fever" in children, all of whom suffered paralysis while only two died (89). Epidemics appeared first in countries with high standards of living, and for 30 years were noted chiefly in northwestern Europe, especially Scandinavia, the northeastern United States and Canada, Australia, and New Zealand. After the First World War the disease gathered momentum, to reach a peak in the decade after the Second World War. This was contrary to the general declining trend for epidemic infectious disease. Together with the social class gradient, the trend emphasized the connection of paralytic poliomyelitis with good living conditions.

Where the virus exists in poor sanitary conditions, infection is probably almost universal, but unrecognized. People living in these conditions acquire an active immunity through symptomless infection in their early years, perhaps even in the early months of life while still protected by a passive immunity transferred from their mothers. People living in good sanitary conditions are protected from infection, hence do not have the opportunity to acquire active immunity in their early years (90). Prospective studies of black South Africans living in a slum in the 1950s showed that almost all infants were infected by the poliomyelitis virus in the fist year of life (91). The clustering of the infections over a short period of time revealed the presence of a silent epidemic in the township, yet there were no cases of paralytic poliomyelitis. Black people in general suffered much less paralytic poliomyelitis than neighboring whites living in good conditions. In Britain in the 1950s, children of the lower classes, who lived in overcrowded homes that lacked such necessities as hot water and indoor toilets, developed antibodies to the virus more often than children who had adequate living space and amenities. In the United States a similar social distribution of the serological pattern of poliomyelitis antibodies was also demonstrated (92). According to these various studies, the risk of paralysis and death varied inversely with poor sanitation. This contrasts with infant mortality rates, long regarded as a sensitive index of poor living conditions and bad sanitation.

Over time paralytic poliomyelitis shifted its target from younger to older age groups. In "virgin" unexposed populations, susceptibility to paralysis and death, like mortality from all causes, has been thought to decline from infancy to puberty, and then to rise with age. This hypothesis of individual susceptibility increasing with age does not hold up well under close scrutiny (93); the changing age-distribution accords better with a social explanation. Not long ago, the disease was known as "infantile paralysis." These epidemics among infants probably resulted from the introduction of virulent strains into populations where only infants had not yet acquired natural immunity. Later the disease began to attack older children and then young adults, especially during the epidemic period after the Second World War. The shift in infection from one age-group to another was also, no doubt, connected with improving sanitation. The improvement probably reduced exposure to infection among infants, who had been the first to suffer in the early epidemics, and thereby did not generate the immunity gained from symptomless infections. Older children, and later young adults, having passed through their earlier years without acquiring immunity from symptomless infection, thus became vulnerable to infection (94).

As predicted in the first edition of this book from the existing class patterns of health behavior, vaccination against poliomyelitis altered the social distribution of the disease. Following the introduction of this highly effective procedure in the mid-1950s, a reversal of the class gradient occurred owing to the preponderance of upper-class children among those who initially accepted vaccination (95). Intensive educational campaigns resulted in widespread acceptance of vaccination, however, and in the United States the annual incidence of paralytic disease has fallen from a peak of 10,000 cases to a level of a mere 10 or so cases today. Pockets of underimmunized persons still exist, susceptible to infection by imported viruses. Immunization levels actually declined between 1965 and 1981, particularly among minority groups (93,96).

Leukemia

Until recently, deaths from the leukemias also followed a gradient declining from the upper to the lower social classes, except among infants. Epidemiological investigation demonstrated the leukemogenic effects of irradiation, for example, the consistent dose-response relationship between the incidence of leukemia in adults and therapeutic irradiation for ankylosing spondylitis (97). The irradiation with radioactive phosphorus of patients with polycythemia vera (an excess of red blood cells) also contributed to the leukemia that was until recently thought to be an intrinsic part of the disease (98). During prenatal life even diagnostic x-rays brought a raised incidence of leukemia in children (99), although this may no longer be true because the amount of irradiation has been carefully controlled. Irradiation has been incriminated as a cause of leukemia by a number of other observations. Earlier generations of American radiologists had a high overall death rate, and the particular risk of leukemia ranked high among them (100). The incidence of leukemia was much increased in survivors of the nuclear bombing of Hiroshima and Nagasaki (101); again, the incidence of leukemia was consistent with the dose of radiation (a dose inferred from the survivors' distance from the explosion).

The proportionate increase in deaths from leukemia during the first half of this century was exceeded only by the increase in deaths from cancer of the bronchus and from coronary heart disease. Although more accurate diagnosis of leukemia could have given the appearance of an increase where one did not exist, the rising rates could plausibly have been related to increased exposure of the population to irradiation (102). A further likelihood is that the upper social classes, who made more use of medical services than the lower (103), were thereby at greater hazard of exposure to irradiation, and that this exposure contributed to the class gradient in leukemia deaths. More precise diagnosis in the upper social classes would be likely to compound the effect of service usage, by adding the appearance of a gradient to an actual gradient.

For some subsequent changes in leukemia mortality—for instance, an increase in acute lymphoid leukemia in children following a period of decline, and an increase in adult myeloid leukemia—no ready explanations have been offered (104). A tendency of social class differences in leukemia deaths in Britain (1970–1972) to level out, however, may reflect the effects of increased use of health services by working-class patients, thereby increasing both exposure to irradiation and the likelihood of the disease being diagnosed.

Peptic ulcer

Secular changes over time have profound effects on ways of life in a society that are subsequently reflected in disease patterns. These effects are rarely uniform and are registered at different rates in the various social classes. Peptic ulcers, both gastric and duodenal, illustrate the dynamics of these changes, throughout the whole society and between the social classes. Duodenal ulcer in particular earned a name as a "disease of civilization." This followed the recognition that perforations of ulcers near the duodenum had rapidly increased among young and middle-aged men during this century (105,106), that the disease in its common form is associated with urban rather than rural life, and that the disease was connected with "stress" (107). An analysis of the distribution of the disease through time by age and sex, and particularly by social class, shows that the correlation between the disease and "civilization," in the sense of the development of industrial societies, is not straightforward.

Gastric ulcers, as recognized by acute perforations, began to be noted with increasing frequency from the beginning of the nineteenth century. Half of all perforations seen in English hospitals then occurred in young women aged about 20, but by the end of the century, observations in medical records on gastric and duodenal ulcers in adult men began to replace those on gastric ulcers in women, and to increase with great rapidity (107). These are the common ulcers of today. However, the volume of peptic ulcers in Britain, first gastric and then duodenal, reached a plateau in the 1950s and then began to recede, contrary to the rising trend expected on the assumption that the disease could be ascribed to continuing processes in industrial society. The explanation which most closely corresponds with these facts is that it is a "generation effect"; that is, successive cohorts or generations have carried their own specific risk of acquiring ulcers throughout most of life (108). This risk now appears to be waning. We have discussed the method of cohort analysis which leads to this conclusion in Chapter 2.

Social-class mortality also shows a changing pattern with the upward age shifts throughout that are expected from a cohort effect with a declining disease. Such a shift is seen in successive time periods in each class as the decline affected that class. In the analysis of occupational mortality around the 1951 census, the British Registrar General noted the reversal of the gradient of duodenal ulcer by social class. In the 1921 and 1931 analyses of occupational mortality, the condition had been most frequent in the higher social classes. In the 1951 and 1971 analyses,[*] it was most frequent in the lower social classes, and particularly Social Class V. Elaboration of these analyses showed that this puzzling reversal of the social class gradient was consistent with the generation effect described above.

Figure 6.4 shows gastric ulcer and duodenal ulcer mortality in males by social class in the periods around the 1921, 1931, 1951, and 1971 censuses. The gastric ulcer mortality pattern displays age shifts compatible with each successive generation in each social class carrying forward its own level of risk from one period to the next. Thus, with each successive census, a more or less regular pattern of mortality recurred in the age groups older by the interval which had elapsed between the censuses. The reversal of the class gradient was seen in the period around the 1921 census at about 55 years, in the 1931 census around 65 years, and in the 1951 census among the oldest

---

[*] In 1941 there was no census because of the Second World War. No analysis of social class mortality was published for the 1961 census.

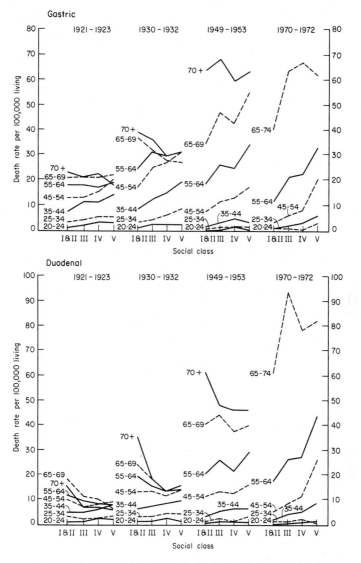

Figure 6.4 Death rates from gastric ulcer and duodenal ulcer in males by age and social class around four census periods, England and Wales. *Source:* Susser, M.W. (1982). Period effects, generation effects and age effects in peptic ulcer mortality, *J. Chron. Dis.*, 35, 29–40.

segment of the population. By the time of the 1971 census the gradient was reversed for all ages. The duodenal ulcer mortality pattern is similar to that of gastric ulcer from census to census, but follows some 10 years later. The reversals in the period around the 1921 census occur at 45 years, around the 1931 census at about 55 years, and around the 1951 census in the oldest segment of the population. By the time of the 1971 census, again the gradient was reversed for all age groups. These data suggest that for males, a recession of the wave of peptic ulcer began in the new generations of the higher social classes. The recession occurred first with gastric ulcer mortality in the cohorts born after 1885, and then moved to the lower social classes. With duodenal ulcer mortality, the same movement appears to have begun some 10 years later, in the 1895 cohort.

Such developments in the configuration of disease must always be considered in relation to a dynamic society in which not only modes of life are changing, but also medical care, and in particular the degree of diagnostic precision and the effectiveness and availability of treatment. Both types of changes are distributed unevenly throughout the social classes. The manner in which services and diagnostic facilities are distributed will necessarily affect the apparent incidence of diseases. The more facilities that are available, the more disease will be discovered, but the very presence of these facilities also reflects changes in the mode of life of the people concerned. Changes in diseases, whether real or apparent, also reflect social changes, and the pattern of ulcer mortality must be considered in relation to these.

Thus, one alternative explanation for the secular trend that comes at once to mind is that changes in diagnostic fashion influenced mortality rates. This explanation can be ruled out on two grounds. First, there was no doubt that as medicine advanced it had brought greater accuracy in diagnosis and in technical skills, and that these more accurate means of diagnosis were more widely applied than at earlier times. Such changes would almost certainly have contributed to an increase rather than to a decline in frequency. Second, it was apparent from the data that the prevailing beliefs of physicians, as expressed in the medical literature, followed the changing distributions of mortality and did not precede them. In 1901, Lord Moynihan's famous description of acute perforations was aimed at alerting the medical profession to a syndrome that was newly afflicting young men. After the Second World War, a 1947 survey of occupations showed that duodenal ulcer was a disease of middle age (109). Yet, in the realm of clinical medicine the condition was still considered a disease of younger men. Equally striking, in an incidence study of an English city of the late 1950s, was the interpretation by the author of the approximation of urban to rural rates which he observed. He inferred a rise in rural rates, in line with the prevailing belief that the disease was on the rise, when in fact the changes were owed to a decline in urban rates (110).

A second alternative explanation for the secular and social-class trends is that previous mortality and selective survival had affected the distribution of current mortality, so that current mortality did not reflect the distribution of previous morbidity. That is, those at high risk at younger ages died off and had selectively disappeared from the population remaining at risk at older ages. However, the cohort analysis shows that sex and social class cohorts which had high rates at younger ages also had high rates at older ages.

A third alternative explanation is that the trends were owed to a newly effective treatment, and that unequal distribution of effective treatment by age and social class affected survival by social class. In other words, the old, the poor, and the ill-educated might have higher mortality rates only because the young, the well-off, and the well-educated had access to effective treatment, especially surgical treatment, that had become available. The data run directly contrary to this expectation, unless the treatments available at the time had markedly adverse effects. Thus, at older ages, the highest mortality occurred in the highest social classes, and at that time the higher classes undoubtedly made greater use of available treatment than did the lower classes.

Each of the three alternative explanations suggested is less plausible than that of a generation effect—with the incidence of the condition itself on the decline—which is the result of environmental change. Similar change has been subsequently reported in local British data and also in morbidity in the United States. Disease is the result of interaction between host and environment, and explanations of the cohort phenomenon must include host responses as well as environmental exposures. The rise in ulcer mortality may have been related to an early phase of the population's involvement with industrialization; the subsequent decline may mark the end of a transitional period, and the better adaptation of large sections of the people to the demands of an open society. One attempt to test this hypothesis among a recently urbanized African population seems to support it; another attempt to test it in European mortality data is less compatible with it (111).

Although the specific factors underlying the dramatic changes in the disease over time remain obscure, some evidence relates duodenal ulcer to external strains that provoke anxiety. Strain frequently precedes the onset or recrudescence of symptoms, or of complications such as perforation and hemorrhage (112). During times of heightened anxiety, as in the bombing of Britain during the Second World War, peaks were found in the incidence of acute perforations and deaths from peptic ulcer (113). (Although in Northern Ireland during a period of marked civil strife, no increase in the incidence of peptic or duodenal ulcer was reported, the threat is of much lower order in scale and acuteness (114).) Conversely, troughs in incidence have been found during or after periods of rest from work, for instance, in the late summer, on Sundays and Mondays, and during the night.

Anxiety may bear some relationship to social class prevalence, more particularly of duodenal ulcer, through specific occupational strains. Certain occupations have long been held to carry a special risk for peptic ulcer, although such beliefs are often ill-founded—for instance, the alleged high risk incurred by bootmakers from external pressure on the stomach, by cooks from tasting hot spices, and by long-distance transport workers from irregular meals. Sea-pilots in Swedish ports comprise an occupational group that carries executive responsibility, however, and a well-founded liability to peptic ulcer. The same is true of air-traffic controllers, who have higher rates of peptic ulcer (and hypertension and diabetes) than do pilots; their rates are higher where the density of the air traffic they control is higher (115).

Occupational strain may be related also to the differences in prevalence that have been found among rural people; agricultural laborers had a low prevalence of duodenal ulcer, but not landowners and other rural dwellers. In industry, with fair consistency in a number of studies, managers and foremen share a moderate excess of duodenal ulcer morbidity; this is the more likely to be related to the common strains of their occupations, for their economic and social relations differ. Among foremen explicit anxieties about work have been found to be more common than among others, and to be more common also among patients with duodenal ulcer than among patients with gastric ulcer or controls. Nevertheless, the foremen's occupation might not have caused the anxiety associated with their duodenal ulcers because anxious, conscientious men might be at high risk both of becoming foremen and of falling sick with duodenal ulcers. Miners are also beset with special anxieties, however, and have been found to have a high rate of ulcers; these very different men take up their work for social rather than psychological reasons. Doctors have had a high prevalence, but at least in part this was caused by early and accurate diagnosis (108,109).

Diet has also been considered as a possible factor in the varying prevalence of peptic ulcer, and could relate to disparities between the classes, but as yet there is little direct evidence to incriminate particular diets, or such elements of diets as processed foods and hot spices. Smoking, too, is associated in moderate degree with the morbidity from ulcers and maintains their chronicity by delaying healing (116). The shifting pattern of smoking in each class over time bears a distinct similarity to the shifting pattern of peptic ulcer in each class, and smoking may well account for a part of the dynamics of the disease.

Persisting inequalities in the burden of disease

In the first half of this century in Britain, a miscellany of disorders such as alcoholism and cirrhosis of the liver, cancer of the colon, cancer of the breast, cancer of the prostate and, as just noted, duodenal ulcer, were more common in the upper social classes. As we showed above for coronary heart disease, poliomyelitis, the leukemias and peptic ulcer, however, several of these clusterings have either disappeared or reversed themselves in recent times (24,117). The unusually high rate for cirrhosis of the liver at the upper end of the class continuum is owed largely to the inclusion of certain occupations (notably publicans and innkeepers) in Social Class II. Today, upper-class males have higher mortality for malignant neoplasms of lymphatic and hematopoietic tissues (other than leukemia), melanoma of the skin, and cancers of a few specific sites (testis, eye, and brain); upper-class women have higher mortality for cancer of the breast, ovary, and body of the uterus, and for deaths attributed to mental disorders (probably organic brain syndromes) (24).

Historically, however, the toll of disease among the poor first drew attention to the striking disparities in prevalence between the social classes. In the wake of the Industrial Revolution, the poor contended daily with squalid living conditions, poor hygiene, inadequate nutrition, and hazardous work. Infant mortality rates were especially high in the lower classes, among whom a large number of infants died of gastroenteritis and the epidemic diseases of childhood. In the mid-nineteenth century one in two of all infants born in working-class districts in England could expect to die before reaching age five; the comparable figure for the children of the privileged classes was one in five. Thus for laborers in many districts, average life expectancy (at the time predominantly a function of infant mortality) was 20 years or less; that for the "gentry and professional classes" was 40 years or more. Tuberculosis, typhus, typhoid fever, scarlet fever, and diphtheria were rampant in the poorer sections of the Victorian city. Chroniclers of the period are unanimous in their horror at the lives

of the "lower order of society," their alleys and courts "rife with all kinds of enorm-
ity" (118).

Under the guidance of William Farr, the General Register Office began the regular
compilation of mortality statistics in 1839. Early figures provided abundant evidence
for the health effects of the hardships of poverty. Later, accumulated data enabled
the progress of the Sanitary Movement to be tracked in marked improvements in
adult mortality from mid-century onwards. Infant mortality remained high, averaging 150 per 1000 live births until late in the century. Indeed, the first official classification of social classes—the Registrar General's fivefold division of 1911—was constructed primarily as an aid in the analysis of infant mortality differences (119).

Beyond infancy, for as long as documentation has been available, mortality and
prevalence among the poor of all ages has been greater for epidemic and infectious
diseases, bronchitis, pneumonia and tuberculosis, rheumatic heart disease, and for
many others (4,120,121). Naturally these disorders were equated with poverty, and
the high rates were ascribed to poor living conditions, inadequate diet, bad sanitation,
and ignorance. Many people confidently expected therefore that if poverty were to
be abolished, and medical services made available to all, rates for various disorders
would eventually reach a single standard throughout society, irrespective of social
class. At a time when the dynamic relation of social change and the flux of disease
was not yet fully comprehended, they assumed that the upper classes had the lowest
incidence of such disorders that could be expected to result from good living conditions and the benefits of medical science and services. Hence, in Britain after the
Second World War, equalization of standards was expected to follow on the social
policies that introduced the welfare state.

This equalization did not occur. The grosser forms of poverty disappeared, free
social and medical services became available to all, and mortality rates at all ages
declined sharply—but large disparities in disease between the social classes remain.
The persistence of these large inequalities is the more remarkable given the universal
availability of health services in Britain since 1948 (122). In fact, evidence from the
United States as well as Britain indicates that by certain measures such disparities
have grown in the postwar years. Figure 6.1 illustrates the historical trend in the class
gradient of male and female mortality for the years spanning 1930 and 1972 in
England and Wales.

The British data provide a unique source for social class analysis of mortality. Analysis of historical trends is complicated, however, by changes in the class assignment
of certain occupations over time (especially since 1970 when job status was first used
in addition to occupational position in assigning class), and sometimes by inconsistencies between census and death certificates in the social class assignment of particular
occupational groups. Such classificatory problems, along with structural changes in
the occupational distribution of the labor force, make for difficulties in statements
about the absolute mortality differences over time of the members of a class. Adjustments to allow for the changes have usually had the effect of lowering the mortality
of the lowest class, and suggested that in the 1960s the gap between the social classes
was reduced. Even so, the gradient in mortality rates from Social Class I to Social
Class V remains marked (24,123).

Similar trends are apparent in the United States. Although the quality and representativeness of the data are not so high, and the definitions and indices of class vary considerably from study to study, social class differences are nevertheless consistently found (13,26,124). Studies between 1900 and 1940 showed a convergence in the mortality of socioeconomic groups. From 1940 to 1960 the trend is unclear. Some studies show a narrowing, others a widening, of the class gap in mortality over this period. Thus, the slope but not the existence of the gradient is in question. In the 1960s, however, socioeconomic differences in mortality appeared to widen. This growing inequality was evident in studies comparing metropolitan areas in different regions, social and geographic areas within a given region, and states grouped by income. The relative disparity grew despite a decline in mortality across all income groups, because the decline in low-income areas was significantly less than that in upper-income areas. In the state of Maryland, for example, heart disease mortality in the higher-income counties fell by 16.6 per cent, whereas in lower-income counties the decline was only 2.9 per cent.

In the United States and in Britain, strong gradients increasing from the higher to the lower classes have been found for infectious and parasitic diseases; malignant neoplasms, in particular cancers of the lung (for men), stomach, bladder, esophagus; diseases of the respiratory system, especially tuberculosis, for which the class gap has widened; diseases of the genitourinary system; and for fatal accidents, poisonings, and violence. The class gradients are moderately strong for diseases of the circulatory system as a whole (but striking for hypertensive disease and stroke), diseases of the digestive system, and for endocrine, nutritional, and metabolic diseases (where the gradient is quite marked for women) (24,125,126,127). Reports on the class distribution of cancer of the prostate are inconsistent: early evidence for a clustering among the professional classes may have been the sign of access to medical care with better diagnosis; later reports tend to show either no gradient or one increasing in the direction of the lower classes (128). Alcoholism no longer shows a clear pattern of class preference, although it is a chief cause of the high mortality due to cirrhosis found in Social Class II in Britain. Heavy drinkers in any social class tend to be at higher risk of death from all causes. In the United States, the rising mortality risk is more marked in the lower socioeconomic groups than in upper and middle groups (129).

Infant mortality rates have declined in a parallel manner across social classes, so that proportionately the gaps between them have altered little. In Britain the ratio today between Classes I and V remains roughly what it was before the institution of the National Health Service, though the rates are at a much lower absolute level. Indeed, for perinatal mortality the gap grew slightly wider: between 1951 and 1971 there was a 45 per cent decline for classes I and II and a 34 per cent decline for class V (see Figure 6.5 and Table 6.2). In the United States, similar disparities in infant mortality between social classes are apparent. In the second quarter of this century, postneonatal deaths declined and so did their contribution to the total infant death rate (130). The association between lower social class and high infant mortality did not change, however (131).

Attention shifted to perinatal mortality (stillbirths and deaths in the first week of life combined) as the relative contribution of this early period to total infant mortality

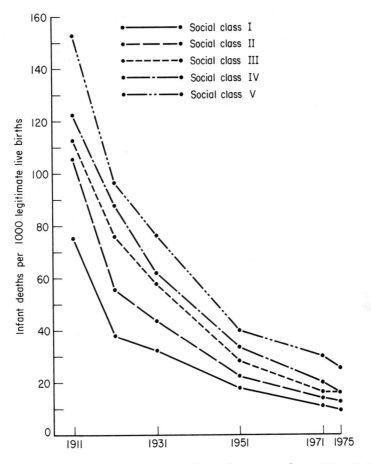

Figure 6.5 Social class trends in infant mortality at four census dates, 1911–71, England and Wales. *Source:* Leete, R., and Fox, J. (1977). Registrar General's social classes: Origins and uses, *Population Trends, 8,* 1–7.

increased. These early deaths are more often attributable to factors such as congenital defects or retarded fetal growth that have their origin prenatally and are irremediable postnatally. They too are subject to external forces, however, social as well as technical. Here, British data for the years 1950–1973 showed, against expectations, that the disadvantage of the lower social class in perinatal infant loss had actually increased (119).

Low birthweight, we observed in Chapter 3, is by far the most powerful determinant of perinatal survival and, to a lesser extent, of survival throughout infancy; adjusting for birthweight accounts for more than 90 per cent of the variation in perinatal mortality rates in the population (132,133). Indeed, if low birthweight is taken into account, the advantage in neonatal mortality rates of Sweden and several other

Table 6.2 Stillbirths and infant deaths by sex, age, and social class, England and Wales, 1970–1972

	Social class						All infants
	I	II	IIIN	IIIM	IV	V	
Stillbirths[a]							
Males	8.63	10.16	11.44	12.26	12.73	17.16	12.36
Females	8.92	10.01	11.54	12.81	13.41	17.82	12.67
Perinatal deaths[a] (stillbirths and less than 1 week)							
Males	17.44	19.79	22.02	23.16	25.27	33.93	23.80
Females	15.17	17.36	19.05	20.98	22.42	30.24	21.14
Early neonatal deaths[b] (less than 1 week)							
Males	8.89	9.73	10.70	11.04	12.70	17.06	11.59
Females	6.31	7.43	7.60	8.27	9.14	12.64	8.58
Late neonatal deaths[b] (1–3 weeks)							
Males	1.23	1.39	1.64	1.81	2.02	3.06	1.84
Females	0.99	1.29	1.27	1.53	1.84	2.41	1.57
Post neonatal deaths[b] (1–11 months)							
Males	3.47	4.09	4.57	6.20	7.31	14.61	6.48
Females	2.32	3.22	3.11	4.99	5.97	11.62	5.11
Total infant mortality (0–11 months)							
Males	13.60	15.21	16.91	19.06	22.03	34.73	19.91
Females	9.61	11.94	11.99	14.79	16.95	26.67	15.27

[a]Per 1000 live and stillbirths.

[b]Per 1000 livebirths.

Source: Office of Population Censuses and Surveys (1978). *Occupational Mortality, 1970–1972, England and Wales,* The Registrar General's decennial supplement, Series DS no. 1 H.M.S.O., London, p. 157.

countries over the United States largely disappears (134). The proportion of low birthweight babies born in the United States in the years 1950–1975 remained essentially unchanged. The improvement in infant mortality rates must therefore be attributed to other historical changes, not the least of which is greater technical efficacy in the care of the newborn (135, 136).

In a study of New York City births of the late 1970s which demonstrated the effectiveness of intensive care for the newborn in lowering mortality, access to the most effective forms of care varied little by social class or ethnic group (136). Thus, at this time the persisting effects of social class on perinatal mortality are mediated primarily through its association with low birthweight. The frequency of low birthweight in different social classes and ethnic groups runs parallel with the mortality gradient, and can account for virtually all the disparities between them in perinatal mortality (132). Other factors such as smoking and the presence of chronic and infective conditions in the mother play a role, possibly in combination with maternal nutrition, in large part through their effects in both slowing fetal growth and inducing premature delivery and thereby lowering birthweight (137). Social class is a complex measure that taps many dimensions of habits and ways of life, including access to health care, that are correlatives of relative deprivation (138).

Social class patterns of *morbidity* in general mimic those of mortality. In the United States for the years 1964 and 1973, the toll of sickness, whether measured by days of restricted activity, confinement to bed, or work loss, was consistently higher for the poor (defined by annual income under $3000) than for the nonpoor; with one exception (work loss), the differences grew in the period under study (139). The gradient of morbidity is consistent across income groups (see Table 6.3). Class gradients that disfavor the worse off classes are found for the prevalence of chronic conditions as a whole (see Figure 6.6), and for such specific disorders as hypertension, heart conditions, cerebrovascular disease, peptic ulcer, arthritis, and allergies (140).

The impact of unequal social class conditions is clearly discerned in the health and activity of old people. The survivors from the lower social classes are fewer, their disabilities are considerably greater in number and severity, and fewer lower-class men remain at work beyond the retirement age. That smaller numbers of lower-class men continue to work after the age of 65 seems to be largely the result of poor health and the strenuous nature of the work open to them. The aged of the lower classes have tended to live in poor houses with few amenities, their food is insufficient and ill prepared, and they often have inadequate domestic help and nursing care (141). High rates of disability add to these discomforts. Because current disability is a cause of low income but does not influence past education, mortality among old people shows a stronger gradient when income is used as the index of social class than when education is used (121).

Hazards of work

In general, physical hazards in the workplace arise in those occupations assigned to the lower reaches of the social class scale. In so far as work contributes to morbidity and mortality, therefore, the lower social classes carry the burden. The toll of work-

Table 6.3   Sickness by age and sex in occupational classes, Great Britain, 1974–1976

	Acute sickness: days of restricted activity (person/year)				Chronic sickness: long-standing limiting illness (rates per 1000)			
	Age-group				Age-group			
	0–14		15– 44	45– 64	0–14[a]		15– 44	45– 64
	M	F	M	M	M	F	M	M
Professional	12	8	9	13	92	76	60	168
Employers	14	8	11	13	106	73	75	161
Other nonmanual	13	11	11	21	95	78	84	261
Skilled	12	11	15	23	102	81	88	248
Semiskilled	12	11	14	21	108	70	91	275
Unskilled	10	11	19	29	123	107	109	380

[a]Limiting and nonlimiting, long-standing illness, disability, and infirmity.

Source: Morris, J. N. (1979). Social inequalities undiminished, *Lancet, 1,* 87–90.

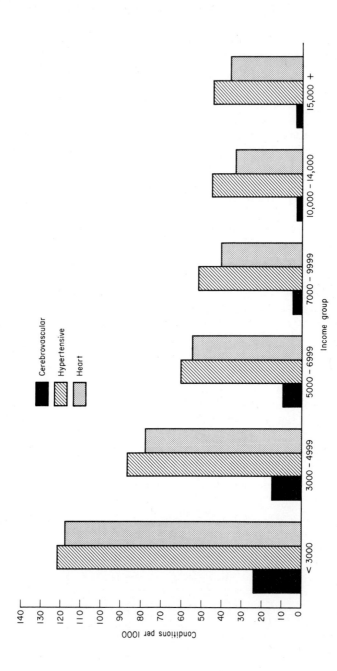

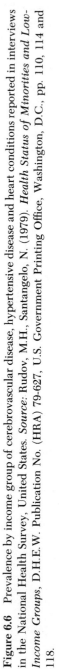

Figure 6.6 Prevalence by income group of cerebrovascular disease, hypertensive disease and heart conditions reported in interviews in the National Health Survey, United States. *Source:* Rudov, M.H., Santangelo, N. (1979). *Health Status of Minorities and Low-Income Groups,* D.H.E.W. Publication No. (HRA) 79-627, U.S. Government Printing Office, Washington, D.C., pp. 110, 114 and 118.

related injury and disease is a matter of growing concern in advanced industrialized societies such as Britain and the United States (142,143). Estimates of the hazards of work have been deflated by many factors: inadequate detection and underreporting of workplace accidents; lack of provision for independent monitoring of industrial and occupational disease; the skittishness of industry about acknowledging the toxicity of the huge number of chemicals constantly being added to its products; the difficulty of obtaining good measures of the exposure of workers to toxic substances from industrial sources; and the difficulties of establishing the often convoluted and insidious chains of cause and effect in occupational diseases of long latency, especially when relatively small numbers are exposed. In the late 1960s, however, the success of American coal miners in having black lung (pneumoconiosis) declared a compensable occupational disease stimulated much lobbying, advocacy, research, and legislation about occupational health and safety in the United States.

Estimates of the extent of work-related illness and death remain unreliable. There is confusion over the jurisdiction of regulatory bodies; the classification of occupational disease by compensation boards is narrow; and workers often underreport injury or illness for fear of loss of job or wages (144). In 1978, nearly 1 in 10 U.S. workers in the private sector reported an occupational injury or illness; work-related fatalities stand at 8 per 100,000 workers. Almost two million workers are presently estimated to be severely or partially disabled because of work-related diseases or accidents (145). Groups at particular risk include industrial workers, agricultural laborers, nonunion workers, and employees of small firms (30 per cent of the U.S. labor force work in shops with fewer than 25 employees; 75 per cent are nonunionized). Among migrant workers, most of whom belong to minority ethnic groups and many of whom reside illegally in the United States, the combination of poor working conditions with poor living conditions results in infant mortality rates at least 60 per cent above the national average and a life expectancy of only 49 years (142,146).

The source of hazards at work are multiple. Machines, materials, and processes give rise to such physical hazards as excessive noise, heat, tool vibration, dust, and toxic chemicals (142,143,147). The social organization of work may give rise to psychological strain in a variety of circumstances, such as speedup of the assembly line, simple and repetitive work with underutilization of skills, lack of control over the labor process, shift work, and job insecurity (148). When such factors increase fatigue and reduce attentiveness, they also increase the likelihood of accidents. Measures of alienation and dissatisfaction have shown that the objective organization of work is an important determinant of general well-being (149).

Hazards related to work need not be confined to the workplace, controversial as attempts to count them may be (150). Families of asbestos workers have developed mesothelioma, most likely the result of contamination by asbestos fibers adhering to work clothes brought home. Communities surrounding concentrated industries may experience high rates of specific cancers: bladder and liver cancers around petrochemical industries, respiratory cancers around foundries. Children living near copper smelters show raised body levels of arsenic; those living near lead smelters show raised levels of lead, with effects on the neural system that are certainly not healthy, although inconsistent and difficult to measure. Nor are such dangers confined within the national boundaries of industrial companies. In response to the militancy of unions around issues of safety and health and the accompanying government regulations, some firms have exported hazardous industries to Third World countries where opposition and regulation are less troublesome (151).

Race, ethnicity, and health

Although class remains the key to the social structure of advanced industrialized societies, in some societies race and ethnicity designate social groups that in varying degrees cut across the lines of class structure and pose problems for the collection and interpretation of health data. The meaning given here to race derives from established use rather than demonstrated validity. Race is an operational term, ostensibly based on skin color, that in fact specifies group membership, a social designation of uncertain reliability. Biologically, race can be no more than an indicator of the distribution of gene frequencies across populations, as we discussed in Chapter 4. Indeed, the distributions of genes across population groups are so deeply conflated with geographic, social class, and cultural distinctions that many physical anthropologists would prefer to dispense with the term.

In this section, when we refer to *race*, we follow the practice of the U.S. Census Bureau and the National Center for Health Statistics. In the published reports of these agencies,° the term race refers to a group affiliation assigned to a person or household. The racial classifications in use are white, black, Hispanic, native American and, for some purposes, Chinese-American and Japanese-American. The affiliation may be elicited in a survey directly from the respondent, or it may be inferred from the perception of an interviewer, a health professional, or an official of an agency making a record. Hence, the designation of Hispanic race may rest merely upon notice of a common Spanish surname. Problems arise in assigning an appropriate category to black Hispanic-Americans, or to "Ladino" immigrants from Mexico and Central America of mixed Spanish and Indian descent.

In its rudimentary meaning, *ethnicity* refers to a shared heritage. This heritage includes a common geographical origin and history, a distinctive language (in the past if not actively maintained), and a characteristic culture. Like social class and race, ethnicity is a word widely used and variously construed. Ambiguity resides in the fact that ethnicity is an analytic term describing a sector of the cultural landscape and, at the same time, a tool of political organization that is consciously manipulated and invoked under some circumstances but not under others. Ethnicity designates group membership, but membership may be assigned by others or declared by the individual, fixed or fleeting, manifest or latent. Ethnic affiliation, whether ascribed or avowed, is only one among many statuses available to an individual and must be analyzed within the specific circumstances under which it is activated. (See also discussions of group indices in Chapter 3 and associations in Chapter 7.)

° In the 1980 census, 15 different groups were listed on the questionnaire used; assignments were based on the self-identification of respondents. Published health data, however, generally use only the categories noted in this text.

The distinction between insiders and outsiders established by ethnicity typically takes form under conditions of confrontation, crisis, or ritual. Hence the way in which the boundaries of ethnic groups are drawn is as important as the culture they contain. Ethnicity itself cannot be taken as a comparable unit of analysis across social groups without paying attention to the specific contexts in which it occurs. A dominant culture may tolerate or assimilate a subordinate one, or may subject it to discrimination, segregation or persecution. Thus, in Britain, the situations of the Scots and the Welsh cannot be lumped together with that of the Irish without doing violence to the different circumstances under which each of their ancient identities persists. Nor, in the United States, can the social position of descendants of European immigrants and descendants of African slaves° be compared without taking into account the dual influence of racism and the class structure in restricting the opportunities of the latter (152).

In societies influenced by legacies of slavery or colonialism or both, racial and ethnic divisions tend to coincide with those of the class structure. But racial and ethnic divisions can cut across class divisions. Thus, distinctions of race or ethnicity are complex, and the health status of a minority group does not necessarily correspond to that characteristic of its class position. Where racial disadvantage is present, however, it can be largely explained by the close association of minority status—in the United States, being black especially—with lower-class membership. For such groups, the two types of status are conflated and, technically, confounded. Race may operate over and above class, however, usually exaggerating and occasionally suppressing the differences between groups. Black Americans and native Americans have predominantly lower-class status and markedly poor mortality profiles. By contrast, Japanese-Americans have an average income well above that of the general population and a favorable mortality profile. Chinese-Americans cover the range of social classes, but they have notably high birthweight and—if the vital statistics are correct and not distorted by omissions of illegal immigrants—infant mortality rates which are the most favorable in the country, distinctly better than would be expected from their overall social position (153).

Black Americans constitute 11 per cent of the U.S. population and make up the largest proportion of the nonwhite population. Black Americans have a lower life expectancy than whites, suffer significantly more disability from sickness, and are twice as likely to report their health as unsatisfactory. Excepting suicide, blacks have higher rates for each of the 10 leading causes of death, and twice the rate of death from cirrhosis of the liver. Maternal mortality of nonwhites is three times that of whites. Infant mortality is a third again that of whites, and postneonatal mortality is nearly twice as high. Infant mortality for nonwhites—as noted, predominantly blacks—has declined in parallel with that for whites, and thus the inequality persists (see Figure 6.7). In the postwar period (1950–1980), the gap between racial groups

---

° The term "Afro-American" adopted by some black Americans offers a good illustration of the equivocality of ethnicity. When designated simply by its color, the group is a minority. The African affiliation gives the same group ethnic identity, complete with cultural heritage, linguistic distinctions, and an expanded history.

in the rate of low birthweight increased steadily until the late 1960's when rates began to decline slowly in a more or less parallel manner; nonwhite rates remain twice as high as those for whites (154).

Prevalence rates among black Americans are higher than among whites for arthritis, diabetes and its long-term consequences, and the anemias. Hypertension and stroke reach very high rates among blacks and especially black women, a fact that cannot be attributed to genetic differences alone (155). Even with race held constant, lower social class communities with high rates of crime and marital breakup have higher rates of high blood pressure than better-off communities. Dark skin is associated with higher levels of blood pressure, but whether a hereditary or a social status is reflected in this association is not known (156).

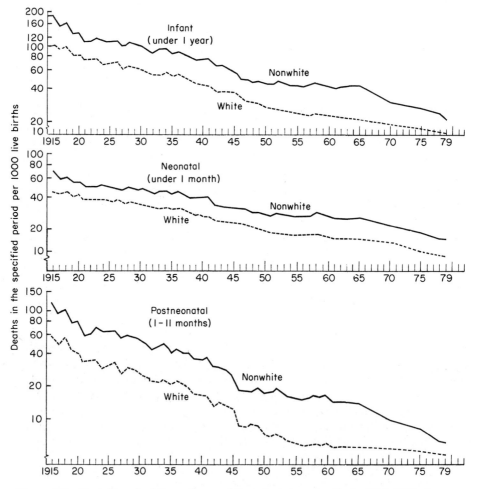

Figure 6.7 Mortality of white and non-white infants by age: U. S., 1915–1979. *Source:* United States Dept. of Health and Human Services (1982). *Health, United States, 1982,* Hyattsville, Maryland.

With respect to health, few data are available with which to establish the significance of ethnicity. Indeed, with a modest number of exceptions, ethnicity has been
applied more effectively either as an index of the health effects of environmental
change with migration, or as a marker for risk from particular genetic disorders, than
it has been in the description and adumbration of the nature of cultural differences
in health. Thus, the migration to the United States of ethnic groups—Norwegians,
Poles, Japanese, Chinese, Irish—has shed light on the influence of environmental factors in psychotic disorders, stomach cancer, breast cancer, coronary heart disease, and
neural tube defects (see Chapter 8, pp. 324 ff.). The tendency of ethnic groups to
endogamy has helped to identify a number of genetic syndromes attributed to single
major genes, for instance, Tay-Sachs among Jews from Central Europe and the Baltic,
and glucose-6-phosphate dehydrogenase deficiency and thallassemia among eastern
Mediterranean peoples (157,158). Other disorders or characteristics have shown con-
centrations among ethnic groups without that fact having as yet illuminated understanding of the condition to any notable degree. For example, alcoholism is relatively
common among the Irish and uncommon among Jews, but studies unrelated to ethnicity have identified both the environmental and genetic factors involved (159).
Birthweight, we have noted, exhibits a marked social gradient that has large implications for infant mortality, but the relatively high birthweight of both native Americans and Chinese-Americans remains an obscure phenomenon still to be elucidated
and interpreted (160).

In giving so brief a sketch of the ways in which race and ethnicity impinge on
health, we do not mean to downplay their significance for the social identity, the
political weight, and the life chances of the groups involved. We do mean to indicate
that their significance for health status is not universal, but particular and dictated by
parochial circumstance. As categorizations, race and ethnicity directly influence the
epidemiology of certain disorders. Their main influence, however, is an indirect one;
the influence is exercised through the consequences of race and ethnicity for social
position and opportunity, including access to health care and experience within health
facilities (161).

In the origins of some disorders cultural practices are also implicated (see Chapter
4), but in general it is the social position with which both race and ethnicity are conflated that has the predominant influence on the health experiences of a given ethnic
group. An example of recent concern in the United States is the high frequency of
teenage pregnancy among blacks. The adverse outcomes notoriously associated with
teenage reproduction can be shown to take origin, in the case of birthweight and
perinatal mortality, mainly in the social circumstances which precede such births.
Likewise, in the case of the mental performance, the deficits in the children of teenage mothers reside not in the mothers' age but in the social circumstances which
follow teenage maternity (162).

Mental disorders

The search for social and cultural factors in the genesis and course of mental disorders
was kindled early on by the recognition of their uneven distribution in society. Aside

from age and sex, social class is the social variable with the most marked and consistent relation to mental disorders. In 1855, Edward Jarvis reported that "the pauper class furnishes, in ratio of its numbers, sixty-four times as many cases of insanity as the independent class." Twentieth century studies continue to find striking disparities between the social classes. Understanding of the class relationship is complicated, however, by unresolved problems of selecting reliable and valid methods for identifying and classifying disorders and for measuring their frequency (163,164,165,166).

Variability in the extent and nature of the social class gradient occurs with the particular mode of case finding. When one takes a global view of all types of disorders, including undifferentiated psychological distress or "demoralization," studies of "true prevalence" show a gradient of rates increasing markedly toward the bottom of the social scale. These studies—conducted largely since the Second World War—do not rely on statistics that bring persons into the ken of services. Incidence studies, which must do so, also show the highest rates of psychiatric disorders in the lowest social class (166,167).

When attention shifts to specific disorders, however a limited group appears to account for the social class gradient: schizophrenia, personality disorders, and neurotic depression are most frequent in the lowest social class; manic-depressive psychoses, senility, and organic brain syndrome are more evenly distributed. When psychiatric cases are further differentiated on the basis of inception and duration of disorders, chronic disability measured by extended failure in social role performance shows a particularly high concentration at the lower end of the class structure (168).

Much debate has followed, not about the findings, which have proved consistent, but about their interpretation. The debate revolves around two questions. First, are the main determinants of the class relationship psychosocial or genetic? And second, within the social realm of explanation, what particular aspects of culture and society are pathogenic? Since this chapter focuses on social class, we shall do no more than note the gradual accumulation of evidence suggesting a complex interplay between genetic and social factors in the class relationship of mental disorders. Multiple causes are at work, but the relative contributions of specific factors remain to be demonstrated.

What then is it about the nature of societal arrangements and the corresponding cultural attitudes, behavior and symbolic meanings that produces high levels of generalized distress and high rates of particular mental disorders at the bottom of the class structure? Diverse aspects of society and culture differentiate the lives and experiences of groups at a social advantage from those at a disadvantage in a manner that could affect the occurrence of mental disorders among them. Hypotheses about causes range from the material conditions and consequences of poverty, such as dilapidated and overcrowded housing and poor physical health (169), to such social concomitants of low economic status as job loss, unrewarding conditions of work, disrupted relations with primary groups (owing to separation and divorce), and harsh socialization experiences in childhood (170).

During the 1970s, many investigators focused on stressful life experiences as a source of mental disorders and of their social class distribution in particular. A progression of experimental and clinical studies had earlier demonstrated a connection between noxious physical and emotional stimuli and consequent physiological or psychological dysfunction (171). Despite a host of methodological difficulties, these studies of stressful life events showed that lower-class persons were indeed heavily bombarded by environmental stressors. Yet more than the frequency of stressful life events was involved. For the same frequency of events, more mental distress was generated among lower-class than higher-class persons (80,172).

The unequal response to stressors among social classes appears to have its origin in resources that enhance or inhibit vulnerability. Resources may be external or environmental on the one hand, and internal or intrapsychic on the other. External resources encompass such things as finances and the support to be found in the person's network of social relationships. Internal or intrapsychic resources, by contrast, reside in the personality structure; these resources sustain an individual's adaptability in interpreting experience and in responding effectively (80,173,174). In the terms of the classic epidemiologic triad of agent, host, and environment, noxious life experiences would constitute the agents, and internal resources the host, while external resources would constitute the environment. Thus, psychological damage inflicted by psychosocial agents will vary in magnitude with intrapsychic susceptibility or resistance to particular stressors, and with the environmental social supports which buffer or cushion the consequences of exposure to stressors (173,175). Two discrete psychiatric conditions, depression and schizophrenia, will serve to illustrate the relationship between social class and mental disorders.

Depression. Symptoms of depression in the population at large, and episodes of clinical depression (those in need of clinical care), are more common among women and the lower classes (176), although psychotic depression is more evenly distributed across the class structure (166,167,168). A diverse set of risk factors in the community at large has been identified for episodes of clinical depression as well as for depressive symptoms. These include stressful life events—for instance, the loss of an accustomed role or relationship—and childhood emotional deprivation, often involving disruption of early attachments (177). They also include situations such as marriage in which housewives perform unskilled and unrewarding tasks or, if working, experience "role-overload" from dual family and occupational demands. Maternal roles, too, are often performed in isolation from other adults (178).

Research on women in Camberwell, London, points to a complex relationship of depression with sociocultural factors and social class (80). Women with a diagnosis of primary depression in hospital or psychiatric clinics were compared with women chosen at random from the same community. The incidence and prevalence of clinical depression was higher among working-class than middle-class women. Working-class women, especially those with children at home, also experienced a greater onslaught of severe environmental stressors, particularly those involving losses. But environmental stressors did not completely explain these social class differences in the incidence of depression. Thus, given equivalent experience of stressful life events, the frequency of clinical depression in women with children at home was four times as high in working-class as in middle-class women. Along with the burden of child care—working-class women were more likely to have three or more children under 14 at home—

two other factors increased the vulnerability of working-class women: they tended to lack close intimate relationships with a spouse or lover, and they were more likely to have suffered the loss of a mother through death before the age of 11. Only in relation to one risk factor for depression—lack of employment outside the home—were working-class women more favorably placed than middle-class women.

These results suggest a model of depression which combines stressful experiences, the absence of environmental supports, and internal psychological vulnerability (80). Stressful experience may induce in certain women the sense that they are helpless; perceiving themselves as unable to control their world, they cannot cope with loss and the blows of stressful events. This state of helplessness in the face of stress is supposedly the consequence on the one hand of low self-esteem and, on the other hand, of a lack of external resources. Important resources for coping are support from a close, significant relationship with another, and some means of relief from the continuous demands made by the care of young children at home. Low self-esteem often arises in childhood in response to emotional trauma, such as the loss of a parent. The difficulty of establishing true causal sequences among this array of factors should not be underestimated.

Schizophrenia. The epidemiologic evidence that schizophrenia is concentrated in the lowest social class is stronger and more consistent than the evidence with regard to social class and depression (164,179). Both inceptions (i.e., first episodes) and all reported episodes (including recurrences) occur more frequently at the bottom of the class structure. However, the most sizable social class gradient occurs with the total number of episodes, a measure that resembles prevalence (166). Prevalence measures exaggerate the gradient still further, that is to say, the element of duration of the disorder adds to disadvantage at the bottom of the social structure (180). These findings suggest a social class component in the genesis of schizophrenia, but an even more powerful class component in its subsequent course, especially the persistence of chronic disability.

Schizophrenia has been found to occur more often than expected among first-degree relatives of those affected: that is, in parents, offspring, and sibs. The cause of the distribution may be either genetic or environmental; more likely it is both. The genetic transmission of schizophrenia has been well documented over the past decade by studies of adoptive children and their biological and social parents and relatives. For example, the rate of schizophrenia and schizophrenia-related disorders in the relatives of adopted children with schizophrenia is greater than in the relatives of adopted control children without schizophrenia (181). However, genetic factors do not account for all the variability in schizophrenia, and the search for relevant sociocultural factors continues (182) (see Chapter 9, pp. 377–380.)

Early investigators found environments characterized by poverty and social isolation to be breeding grounds for schizophrenia. A pioneering study in the late 1930s in Chicago took first admissions to mental hospitals and related them by diagnosis to the social ecology of the areas from which the patients came (179). Depressive psychosis was evenly distributed across the city, but schizophrenia was concentrated in deteriorated areas. This result was consistent in other American cities, and in Bristol, England, as well (183,184,185).

The Chicago study gave rise to an initial hypothesis that schizophrenia was the consequence of situations of social isolation and alienation from society. Subsequent studies uncovered associations with schizophrenia that could be seen as potentiating factors in lower-class situations. Schizophrenic patients had occupations of low prestige that frustrated any aspirations to upward social mobility they might have shared with the dominant culture (183). In the areas in which they lived, isolated single-room lodging and tenements predominated (184,186). Finally, the schizophrenic patients in such areas lived separated from both the domestic support and the personal relations that families might have afforded them.

The additive and joint effects of all these factors together are likely to be reflected in the poor prognosis and prolonged course of schizophrenia (187). Thus, a cumulative process appears progressively to exaggerate the alienating attributes of schizophrenia. The situation of the patient who does not recover is seen to become more alienated as measures of successively greater severity of sickness are applied, beginning with the inception of psychiatric care, and moving to patients who have repeated episodes, then to those who are admitted to hospitals, and finally to those whose sickness becomes chronic and continues for a year or more. With each measure, schizophrenic persons are progressively more often in lower-class occupations, unemployed, or unmarried, and more often living away from families (180).

All these characteristic features of schizophrenia could come about through social selection, as well as through the force of adverse social situations. Individuals already predisposed to schizophrenia, or manifesting early symptoms, may "drift" into the occupations of the lower classes. The social correlates of schizophrenia could therefore arise from the intrinsic nature of the disorder and its effects on social performance. A British study, by an ingenious method which linked mental hospital records to registrations of birth, succeeded in establishing that drift did in fact occur. Occupations of schizophrenic patients drawn from a national sample were compared with the occupations of their fathers as recorded on their birth certificates. Most patients belonged to lower occupational categories than their fathers, and since the occupations of the fathers were normally distributed at the time of the patient's birth, downward drift between the generations must have taken place. Moreover, downward drift was evident in the patients' occupational histories; these were incongruous with their educations, which matched the status of their families (188). Subsequent studies have also produced support for the drift hypothesis (189).

The drift hypothesis does not, however, account for all the observed variation by class. One causal model for schizophrenia, like the model for depression described above, combines the triad of genetic susceptibility with stressful life experiences and maladaptive coping patterns, here arising from the lack of both external and internal resources (190). Each of the social components of this model is linked to lower-class position. Social stressors have been associated with both the onset and subsequent episodes of schizophrenia (191) and, as noted earlier, the frequency of stressors is greater at the bottom of the class structure. It is argued that people in the lower classes tend to lack both the external supports for coping with these stressors and a range of cognitive experience sufficient for the mastery of a daunting environment. Lower-class families may inculcate a belief in conforming with external authority and a fatalistic view of the world, and occupations that demand only simple repetitive work and limited responsibility may reinforce such a response.

Indeed, from comparisons of families of schizophrenics and psychoneurotics across social classes, some investigators have speculated that lower-class subculture could produce schizophrenia (192). Family-oriented research, in attempting to establish a convincing causal link between disturbed pattern of socialization, coping styles, and schizophrenic outcomes, faces profound difficulties of method and interpretation. Family dynamics, in which there is so much fluidity and reciprocity in the patterns of cognitive and affective communication and role relationships, are difficult to measure. It is not surprising that such studies have failed to establish that typical family patterns found with schizophrenia are antecedent in time to the onset of the disease (193).

In sum, many factors appear to be implicated in the onset and course of schizophrenia: together with genetic susceptibility, stressful life experiences, the lack of social resources, and maladaptive ways of coping learned through disturbed family socialization experiences may all contribute. Whatever the precise sociocultural factors involved, lower-class persons are placed at somewhat higher risk for the onset of schizophrenia. After onset, they are placed at distinctly higher risk for its persistence as a disabling condition.

Accounting for persisting class differences in health

When infections were the predominant agents of disease, debility, and death, the origins of the social gradient of mortality could be readily accounted for by the physical environment in which people dwelt. The poor suffered more and more often because poor nutrition rendered them susceptible to the agents of disease borne by food, water, and air, agents to which they were frequently exposed in their overcrowded dwellings and unsanitary environments. As the burden of infectious disease, morbidity, and mortality has eased in the course of this century and the chronic "degenerative" diseases have come to play the dominant role, the explanation of persisting class differences must shift as well. However, since the social classes in industrial societies do not have comparable modes of life or uniform culture, biological and social phenomena can be expected to continue to exhibit class differences.

While the grinding poverty of the past has been much alleviated, relative poverty continues in the United States and Britain (194). This relative deprivation is seen in the quality of the physical environment (crowded homes, lack of playground facilities, lead in the paint of old houses and in old water supply systems), in education, and in cultural amenities. Thus a multiplicity of social and cultural factors is available to contribute to the unfavorable health patterns of the lower social classes. Lower-class children suffer more deaths due to accidents, violence, and poisoning than do higher-class children. Lower-class women marry younger than upper-class women, conceive more often before marriage, bear more illegitimate children, and have tended to have larger families. As a result, there have been more young mothers with large families in the lower classes. Mothers of large families lose more infants from respiratory diseases and from accidents, and indeed from all major causes of death, including sudden infant death syndrome, now the leading cause in the postneonatal period (10,123,195). Although comparative youth favors the childbearing of lower-class women, frequent pregnancies and especially the low birthweight of their infants has contributed to their heavy losses. Smoking among women is now most common among the lower-classes and compounds the risks of their children from low birth-weight, from respiratory disease, and from sudden infant death syndrome.

Childhood accidents, now a leading cause of death in young children under five, are associated with such factors as overcrowding and fathers out of work as well as large family size. Poor health, financial problems, and marital tensions, all shown to be more common among working-class families in a South London community, were all also associated with higher rates of childhood accidents (196). Depression in the mother, also more common in working-class families, further heightened the risk.

Since social classes are defined largely by occupation, type of work by definition sharply discriminates among them. Although the dangerous trades tend to be located at the lower rungs of the occupational ladder, work hazards do not explain the larger part of the mortality differences among the social classes. In Britain, about 20 per cent of the variation in general death rates might be accounted for by occupation over and above social class. The conditions and the manner of daily life best explain the raised rates of sickness and death among the working class (197).

Besides being affected by work and environment, health is hostage to custom. The habitual practices that characterize the daily round of personal and social life are more than manifestations of individual preference. They are tied to the norms and sanctions not only of the larger culture, but of the subcultures of each class (see Chapter 4). Both health-promoting and health-jeopardizing behavior vary with social class. Upper-class women are more likely to breast-feed their children; cigarette smoking has declined first among the upper classes in both the United States and Britain; vigorous leisure exercise is more common among the better-off; and "prudent diets" are less likely to be the common fare of the poor (198,199). Surveys of health knowledge invariably find deficits among the poor and the ill educated (85); their espousal of health values is often lukewarm and their adherence to medical regimens unreliable. Finally, the poor have tended to make less use of preventive health services even in the face of more pressing needs, and even when financial barriers have been removed (200). These findings do not represent merely the quirks and quiddities of individuals; nor are they explained by the idea that a "culture of poverty" is self-perpetuating. Adequate explanation must take proper account of the social structure in which such a culture emerges, and of the patterned behavior of groups fostered by the larger social environment (201).

Social class inequalities have been found for so many causes of sickness and death and have proved so enduring that it is plausible to infer that a generalized susceptibility to disease is a condition of lower-class life (175,198,202). Just as poor nutrition increases the likelihood of infection and the severity of its effects, perhaps so the social environment of lower-class life may render people susceptible to a range of disorders. Economic hardship, frustrated aspirations, chronic insecurity about jobs, frequent disruption of social ties are all features of the lives of the working class and the poor. Unemployment has always been felt first and most among lower-class workers. Difficult as it is to prove its direct effects, current evidence points to an enhanced risk of disease (203). The cycle between disease and poverty persists in our own time (204). The mediating roles of psychosocial stressors, coping behavior, and supportive networks in this cycle, touched upon in Chapter 4, will be further examined in Chapter 8. One mediating factor, however, resides in the means society adopts to prevent disease.

The social effects of prevention

A paradox noted in the first edition of this book, with regard to the social distribution of disease, has become increasingly obvious in the succeeding decades. Prevention in many instances has widened the disparity in health between the social classes. The twentieth century has been an era in which many new preventive techniques have turned on personal behavior rather than on social engineering. In the nineteenth century, public regulation by law ensured the necessary precautions in segregating drinking water from sewage, in safeguarding the hygiene of foods and food handling, in the notification of infectious diseases and the control of rodents, in the limitation of child labor, and in the maintenance of housing standards. In the twentieth century, Western society has relied more on public exhortation toward private precaution. Health education aims to induce people to quit smoking, to drink alcohol moderately, to eat prudently, and to use seat belts. Public regulation, on the other hand, might for example remove subsidies for tobacco growing and abolish the advertisement of cigarettes, provide incentives for dietary changes, or require automatic restraints for car passengers. But regulation, where it has not been strenuously resisted, has on the whole taken second place to exhortation.

In such major chronic diseases as coronary heart disease, hypertension, diabetes, and lung cancer, we have noted that prudence in smoking, eating, and exercise can much reduce the risk, but as we have also noted, such prudence is chiefly espoused by the higher social classes. Screening for the early detection of disease can reduce the risks from cancer of the neck of the uterus and breast cancer, and prenatal screening can reduce the incidence at birth of Down's syndrome. Again the higher social classes have benefited first and most from these techniques. In the case of infectious diseases, the bellwether for these class trends was poliomyelitis. Paralytic poliomyelitis affected the higher social classes predominantly, but after vaccination became available in the mid-1950s, residual cases were concentrated among the poor and the ill educated in the lower classes. The same pattern has been repeated for measles.

In these matters, it can be argued that the effects to date testify not so much to the failure of health education to change behavior, as they do to the slowly growing success of a social movement (see Chapter 4) (205). Nothing less than a social movement is likely to have changed such ingrained behavior as smoking, diet, and exercise in the face of the many social and economic inducements to persist in such behavior. A social movement alone is usually not enough to effect change in an entire society. The ultimate diffusion through all social classes of the benefits of a social movement will require political action. The movement relating to such health behavior as smoking, diet and exercise—like the health values on which it rests—is class based. Its impetus comes from the better educated social classes, and the benefits of the movement are distributed in the same manner. The effect is thus to exaggerate the large existing disparities in health between the social classes. As a result, to the disproportionate burden of health disorders carried by the lower social classes, we must now add obesity, lung cancer, coronary heart disease, and the many other adverse consequences of smoking.

Unless political action so changes the economic and social forces that act to structure the behavior and exigencies of everyday life of the poorer classes, change among those classes towards behavior that promotes health is bound to be slow. Lack of education, lack of access to healthy foods and to places for exercise, and the pressures of advertising media, all combine with poverty—specifically, inadequate income to make use of what access may be provided—to sustain self-damaging behavior.

We have tried to show that health is one facet of the social system, and that few indices illustrate better than health the inequalities that reside in class societies. In early phases of industrialization the urban working class and the poor newly migrated from the country carried the main burden of disease and death. At later stages of capitalist development in Europe, resources, technology, productive systems, and wealth expanded, and made possible the control of many infectious and epidemic diseases. The food supply improved and probably enhanced host resistance. While the overall toll of disease and mortality among all social classes is, we have seen, now much less than in earlier phases, the affluence of modern society has not banished inequalities in health among social classes. The persistence of these inequalities makes apparent the social origins of the distribution of disease. Each of the social classes engendered by the production system of any given society encounters a different structure of opportunities and is subject to different exigencies of daily life. These realities are reflected in the culture of classes, embodied in parental values and behavior and, in turn, transmitted to children as part of their world view. Choices about consumption and what is consumed, patterns of family life, modes of recreation, images of self, and the shape of things hoped for—the entire body of practices and expectations that make up social life—are affected in subtle and intricate ways.

This pervasive culture of everyday life, although experienced as natural and inevitable, stems from the socioeconomic order (206). Thus, to the extent that inequalities in health reflect material deprivation, they can be considered as vestiges of the early stages of industralization. To the extent that inequalities in health result from stressful conditions at work, the disruption of family and community life and consequent loss of social support, maladaptive patterns of coping, and hazardous forms of consumption, they can be seen to reflect the molding of social and cultural life by contemporary economic relations. In the absence of data, it may be speculated that the health configurations across the strata of societies found in different economic systems will equally reflect their underlying economic forms. "Structural" explanations cannot be ignored by those concerned with the distributions and the changes in patterns of morbidity and mortality.

References

1. **Frost, W. H.** (1927). Epidemiology in Nelson Loose-Leaf Systems, Public Health-Preventive Medicine, 2, 163–190, reprinted in *Papers of Wade Hampton Frost*, ed K. F. Maxcy, 1941, New York.
   Morris, J. N. (1957). *Uses of Epidemiology*, 1st ed., Edinburgh.
2. **Graunt, J.** (1939; first pub. 1662). *Natural and Political Observations Mentioned in a Following Index, and Made Upon the Bills of Mortality*, London, reprinted, Baltimore.
   Glass, D. V. (1963). John Graunt and his natural and political observations, *Proc. Roy. Soc., Biology, 159*, 2–37.
3. **Defoe, D.** (1966; first publ., 1722) *A Journal of the Plague Year*, London.
   Roberts, R. S. (1966). The place of plague in English history, *Proc. Roy. Soc. Med., 59*, 101–105.
   Ziegler, P. (1969). *The Black Death*, New York.
   Braudel, F. (1973). *Capitalism and Material Life*, New York.
4. **Villermé, L. R.** (1826). Rapport fait par M. Villermé, et lu à l'Académie de médecine, au nom de la Commission de statistique, sur une série de tableaux relatifs au mouvement de la population dans les douze arrondissements municipaux de la ville de Paris pendant les cinq années 1817, 1818, 1819, 1820, et 1821, *Archives générales de médecine, 10*, 216–45.
   Villermé, L. R. (1840). *Tableau de l'état physique et moral des ouvriers employés dans les manufactures de coton, de laine et de soie*, 2 vol, Paris.
   Registratr General of England and Wales. (1855) *Fourteenth Annual Report, 1851*, London, H.M.S.O.
   Humphrey, N. A. (1887). Class mortality statistics, *J. Roy. Statis. Soc., 50* (Part II), 255–85.
   Daric, J. (1949). Mortalité, profession et situation sociale, *Population* (Paris), *4*, 671, trans. in U.S. Public Health Service (1951). *Vital Statistics*, Special Reports, Series 33, no. 10.
   Logan, W. P. D. (1954). Social class variations in mortality, *Brit. J. Prev. Soc. Med., 8*, 128–37.
   Coleman, W. (1982). *Death Is a Social Disease*, Madison, Wis.
5. **Engels, F.** (1958; first pub. 1845). *The Condition of the Working Class in England in 1844*, English trans. by Henderson, W. O., and Chaloner, W. H., Stanford.
   Flinn, M. W., ed. (1965). *The Report on the Sanitary Condition of the Labouring Population of Great Britain, 1842, by Edwin Chadwick*, Edinburgh.
   Malthus, T. (1983; 1798 originally published. *Essay on Population*, London.
6. **Farr, W.** (1975). *Vital Statistics: A Memorial Volume of Selections from the Reports and Writings of William Farr*, edited for the Sanitary Institute of Great Britain by Noel Humphreys, with an Introduction by Mervyn Susser and Abraham Adelstein, New York Academy of Medicine Library. History of Medicine Series, No. 46, Metuchen, NJ.

7. **Stocks, P.** (1938). The effects of occupation and its accompanying environment on mortality, *J. Roy. Stat. Soc., 101,* 669–708.

8. **Kadushin, C.** (1964). Social class and the experience of ill health, *Soc. Inq., 34:* 67–80.
   Antonovsky, A. (1967). Social class and illness: A reconsideration, *Soc. Inq., 37:* 311–322.
   Antonovsky, A. (1967). Social class, life expectancy and overall mortality, *Milbank Mem. Fd. Quart., 45,* 31–73.

9. **Morris, J. N.** (1959). Health and social class, *Lancet, 1,* 303–5.

10. **Fox, J.** (1977). Occupational mortality 1970–1972, *Population Trends, 9,* 1–8.

11. **Duguid, J. B.,** and **Rannie, I.** (1964). Mechanical factors in atherosclerosis, *Texas Rep. Biol. Med., 22,* 70–77.

12. **Crawford, T., Dextre, D.,** and **Teare, R. D.** (1961). Coronary artery pathology in sudden death from myocardial ischaemia, *Lancet, 1,* 181–85.

13. **Antonovsky, A.** (1967). Social class and the major cardiovascular diseases, *J. Chron. Dis., 21,* 65–106.
   Lehman, W. E. (1967). Social class and coronary heart disease; A sociological assessment of the medical literature, *J. Chron. Dis., 20,* 381–91.
   Marks, R. (1967). A review of empirical findings, in social class and cardiovascular disease, *Milbank Chem. Fd. Quart., 45,* 2, Part 2, 51–108.

14. **Yerushalmy, J.,** and **Hilleboe, H. E.** (1957). Fat in the diet and mortality from heart disease, *N.Y. St. J. Med., 57,* 2343–53.

15. **Sigerist, H. E.** (1943). *Civilization and Disease,* Chicago.
   Ryle, J. A. (1948). *The Natural History of Disease,* 2nd ed., London.
   Dubos, R. (1965). *Man Adapting,* New Haven.

16. **Morris, J. N.** (1951). Recent history of coronary disease, *Lancet, 1,* 69–73.
   Morris, J. N. (1975). *Uses of Epidemiology,* 3rd ed., Edinburgh.

17. **Kannel, W. B., Dawber, T. R.,** and **McNamara, P. M.** (1966). Detection of the coronary-prone adult: The Framingham Study, *J. Iowa St. Med. Soc., 56,* 26–34.
   Doyle, J. T. (1966). Etiology of coronary disease: Risk factors influencing coronary disease, *Mod. Conc. Cardiov. Dis., 35,* 81–86.
   Stamler, J., Berkson, D. M., Lindberg, H. A., Hall, Y., Miller, W., Mojonnier, L., Levinson, M., Cohen, D. B., and **Young, Q. D.** (1966). Coronary risk factors, *Medical Clinics of North America, 50,* 229–54.
   Kuller, L. H. (1976). Epidemiology of cardiovascular diseases: Current perspectives, *Amer. J. Epidem., 104,* 425–56.

18. **Patrick, C. H., Palesch, Y. Y., Feinleib, M.,** and **Brody, J. A.** (1982). Sex differences in declining cohort death rates from heart disease, *Amer. J. Publ. Hlth., 72,* 161–66.

19. **Paffenbarger, R. S., Milling, R. N., Poe, N. D.,** and **Krueger, D. E.** (1966). Trends in death rate from hypertensive disease in Memphis, Tennessee, 1920–1960, *J. Chron. Dis., 19,* 847–56.

20. **Keys, A.,** ed. (1970). *Coronary Heart Disease in Seven Countries,* American Heart Assoc. Monograph No. 29, New York.

21. **Kagan, A.** (1960). Atherosclerosis of the coronary arteries—epidemiological considerations, *Proc. Roy. Soc. Med., 53,* 18–22.

22. **Worth, R. M., Kato, K., Rhoads, G. G., Kagan, A.,** and **Syme, S. L.** (1975). Epidemiological studies of coronary heart disease and stroke in Japanese men living in Japan, Hawaii, and California: Mortality, *Amer. J. Epid., 102,* 481–501.
   King, H. (1975). Selected epidemiological aspects of major disease and causes of death among Chinese in the United States and Asia, in *Medicine in Chinese Culture: Com-*

parative Studies of Health Care in China and Other Societies, ed. Kleinman, A., et al., Dept. of Health, Education, and Welfare Pub. No. (NIH) 75–653, Washington D.C. pp. 487–550.

23. **Lilienfeld, A. M.** (1956). Variation in mortality from heart disease, *Public Health Reports, 71*, 545–70.

  Kent, A. P., McCarroll, J. R., Schweitzer, M. D., and **Willard, H. N.,** (1958). A comparison of coronary artery disease (arteriosclerotic heart disease) deaths in health areas of Manhattan, New York City, *Am. J. Publ. Hlth., 48*, 200–207.

  Pell, S., and **D'Alonzo, C. A.** (1958). Myocardial infarction in a 1-year industrial study, *J. Amer. Med. Assoc., 166*, 332–37.

  Breslow, L., and **Buell, L.** (1960). Mortality from coronary heart disease and physical activity of work in California, *J. Chron. Dis., 2*, 421–44.

  Stamler, J., Lindberg, H. A., Berkson, D. M., Shaffer, A., Miller, W., and **Poindexter, A.** (1960). Prevalence and incidence of coronary heart disease in strata of the labor force of a Chicago industrial corporation, *J. Chron. Dis., 2*, 405–20.

24. **Office of Population Censuses and Surveys.** (1978). *Occupational Mortality, The Registrar General's Decennial Supplement for England and Wales 1970–1972*, Series DS No. 1., London.

25. **Cassel, J., Heyden, S., Bartel, A. G., Kaplan, B. H., Tyroler, H. A., Cornoni, J. C.,** and **Hames, C. G.** (1971). Incidence of coronary heart disease by ethnic group, social class and sex, *Arch. Int. Med., 128*, 901–906.

26. **Wilson, R. W.,** and **White, E. L.** (1977). Changes in morbidity, disability, and utilization differentials between the poor and the non-poor: Data from the Health Interview Survey: 1964 and 1973, *Medical Care, 15*, 636–46.

  Lerner, M., and **Stutz, R. N.** (1978). Mortality by socioeconomic status, 1959–61 and 1969–71, *Md. State. Med. J.*, 35–42.

  Yeracaris, C. A., and **Kim, J. H.** (1978). Socioeconomic differentials in selected causes of death, *Am. J. Publ. Hlth., 68*, 342–51.

  Kraus, J. F., Borhani, N. O., and **Franti, C. E.** (1980). Socioeconomic status, ethnicity, and risk of coronary heart disease, *Amer. J. Epidem., 111*, 407–14.

27. **Havlik, R.,** and **Feinleib, M.** eds., (1979). *Proceedings of the Conference on the Decline in Coronary Heart Disease Mortality*, U.S. Dept. of Health, Education and Welfare, Publ. No. 79–1610, Washington, D.C.

28. **Rose, G.** (1981). Strategy of prevention: Lessons from cardiovascular disease, *Brit. Med. J., 282*, 1847–51.

29. **Stamler, J.** (1969). Prevention of atherosclerotic coronary heart disease, in *Trends in Cardiology, 2*, 88–132, New York.

30. **Shekelle, R. B., Shryock, A. M., Paul, O. Lepper, M., Stamler, J., Liu, S.,** and **Raynor, W. J.** (1981). Diet, serum cholesterol, and death from coronary heart disease: The Western Electric Study, *New Eng. J. Med., 304*, 65–70.

31. **Bronte-Stewart, B., Keys, A.** and **Brock, J. F.** (1955). Serum cholesterol, diet and coronary heart disease, *Lancet, 2*, 1103–7.

  Shaper, A. G., and **Jones J. W.** (1959). Serum cholesterol, diet and coronary heart disease in Africans and Asians in Uganda, *Lancet, 2*, 534–37.

  Groen, J. J., Tijong, K. B., Koster, M., Willebrands, A. F., Verdeonck, G., and **Pierloot, M.** (1962). The influence of nutrition and ways of life on blood cholesterol and the prevalence of hypertension and coronary heart disease among Trappist and Benedictine monks, *Amer. J. Clin. Nutr., 20*, 456–70.

32. Kinch, S. A., Gittlesohn, A. M., and Doyle, J. T. (1964). Application of a life table analysis in a prospective study of degenerative cardiovascular disease, *J. Chron. Dis.*, *17*, 503–14.

Morris, J. N., Kagan, A., Pattison, D. C., Garner, M. J., and Raffle, P. A. B., (1966). Incidence and prediction of ischaemic heart disease in London busmen, *Lancet*, *2*, 553–59.

33. Kannel, W. B., and Gordon, T., eds., *The Framingham Study, An Epidemiological Investigation of Cardiovascular Disease, Sections 1–33 (1968–1978)*, U.S. Dept. of Health, Education and Welfare.

34. Feinleib, M., Garrison, R. J., Fabsitz, R., Christian, J. C., Hrubec, Z., Borhani, N. O., Kannel, W. B., Rosenman, R., Schwartz, J. T., and Wagner, J. O. (1977). The NHLBI twin study of cardiovascular disease risk factors: Methodology and summary of results, *Amer. J. Epidem.*, *106*, 284–95.

Christian, J. C., Feinleib, M., Hulley, S. B., Castelli, R. R., Fabsitz, R. R., Garrison, R. J., Borhani, N. O., Rosenman, R. H., and Wagner, J. (1976). Genetics of plasma cholesterol and triglycerides: A study of adult male twins, *Acta. Genet. Med. Gemellol.*, Roma, *25*, 145–59.

Christian, J. C., and Kang, K. W. (1977). Maternal influence on plasma cholesterol variation, *Am. J. Human. Genet.*, *29*, 462–67.

35. Tyroler, H. A., Heiss, G., Heyden, S., and Hames, C. G. (1980). Family follow-up study of serum cholesterol in Evans County, Georgia, *J. Chron. Dis.*, *33*, 323–30.

36. Hsia, S. L., Chao, Y., Hennekens, C. H., and Reader, W. B. (1975). Decreased serum-cholesterol binding reserve in premature myocardial infarction, *Lancet*, *2*, 1000–1004.

Tyroler, H. A., Hames, C. G., Krisham, I., Heyden, S., Cooper, G., and Cassel, J. C. (1975). Black-white differences in serum lipids and lipoproteins in Evans County, *Preventive Medicine*, *4*, 541–49.

Rhoads, G. G., Gulbrandsen, C. L., and Kagan, A. (1976). Serum lipoproteins and coronary heart disease in a population study of Hawaii, Japanese men, *New Eng. J. Med.*, *294*, 293–98.

Castelli, W. P., and Morgan, R. F. (1977). Lipid studies for assessing the risk of cardiovascular disease and hyperlipidemias, *Human Pathology*, *2*, 153–64.

37. Gordon, T., Garcia-Palmieri, M. R., and Kagan, A. (1974). Differences in coronary heart disease in Framingham, Honolulu and Puerto Rico, *J. Chron. Dis.*, *27*, 329–44.

Marmot, M. G., Syme, S. L., Kagan, A., Kato, H., Cohen, J. B., and Belsky, J. (1975). Epidemiological studies of coronary heart disease and stroke in Japanese men living in Japan, Hawaii and California: Prevalence of coronary and hypertensive heart disease and associated risk factors, *Amer. J. Epidem.*, *102*, 514–25.

Marmot, M. G., and Syme, S. L. (1976). Acculturation and coronary heart disease in Japanese-Americans, *Amer. J. Epidem.*, *104*, 225–47.

Kozarevic, D., Pirc, B., Racic, Z., Dawber, T. R., Gordon, T., and Zukel, W. J. (1976). The Yugoslavia cardiovascular disease study, *Amer. J. Epidem.*, *104*, 133–50.

Garcia-Palmieri, M. R., Costas, Jr., R., Cruz-Vidal, M., Cortes-Alicea, M., Patterne, D., Rojas-Franco, L., Sorlie, P. D., and Kannel, W. B. (1978). Urban-rural differences in coronary heart disease in a low incidence area, The Puerto Rico Heart Study, *Amer. J. Epidem.*, *107*, 206–15.

Reed, D., McGhee, D., Cohen, J., Yano, K., Syme, L., and Feinleib, M. (1982). Acculturation and coronary heart disease among Japanese men in Hawaii, *Amer. J. Epi.*, *115*, 894–905.

38. Marmot, M. G., Adelstein, A. M., Robinson, N., and Rose, G. A. (1978). Changing social class distribution of heart disease, *Brit. Med. J.*, 2, 1109–12.

39. Olson, R. E. (1957). Dietary fat in human nutrition, *Am. J. Publ. Hlth.*, 47, 1537–41.
    Yudkin, J. (1967). Diet and coronary thrombosis, *Lancet*, 2, 115–62.

40. Morris, J. N., Marr, J. W., Mills, G. L., and Pilkington, T. R. E. (1963). Diet and plasma cholesterol in 99 bank men, *Brit. Med. J.*, 1, 571–76.

41. Susser, M. W. (1973). *Causal Thinking in the Health Sciences: Concepts and Strategies in Epidemiology*, New York.

42. Stamler, J. (1981). Primary prevention of coronary heart disease: The last 20 years, *Amer. J. Cardiol.*, 47, 722–35.

43. Christakis, G., Rinzler, S. H., Archer, M., Winslow, G., Jampel, S., Stephenson, J., Friedman, G., Fein, H., Kraus, A., and James, G. (1966). The anti-coronary club: A dietary approach to the prevention of coronary heart disease—a seven-year report, *Am. J. Publ. Hlth.*, 56, 299–314.
    Leren, P. (1966). The effect of plasma cholesterol lowering diet in male survivors of myocardial infarction: A controlled clinical trial, *Acta. Med. Scand. Supp.*, 466, 5–92.
    American Heart Association (1968). *The National Heart Study: Final Report*, Monograph No. 18., New York.
    Turpienen, O., Miettinen, M., Karvonen, M. J., Roine, P., Pekkarinen, M., Lehtosuo, E. J., and Alvirta, P. (1968). Dietary prevention of coronary heart disease: Long term experiment, *Amer. J. Clin. Nutr.*, 21, 255–76.
    Dayton, S., Pearce, M. L., Hashimoto, S., Dixon, W. J., and Tomiyasu, U. (1969). A controlled clinical trial of a diet high in unsaturated fat in preventing complications of atherosclerosis, *Circulation*, 40, Suppl. II, 1–63.
    Bierenbaum, M. L., Fleischman, A. I., Green, D. P., Raichelson, R. I., Hayton, T., Watson, P. B., and Caldwell, A. B. (1970). The 5 year experience of modified fat diets on younger men with coronary heart disease, *Circulation*, 42, 943–52.
    Glueck, C. J., Mattson, F., and Bierman, E. L. (1978). Diet and coronary heart disease: Another view, *New Eng. J. Med.*, 298, 1471–74.

44. Brensik, J. F., Levy, R. G., Kelsey, S. F., Passamani, E. R., Richardson, J. M., Loh, I. K., Stone, N. J., Aldridge, R. F., Battaglini, J. W., Fisher, M. R., Friedman, L., Friedwald, W., Dietre, K. M., and Epstein, G. E. (1984). I. Effects of therapy with cholestyramine: Results of the NHCBI Type II coronary intervention study, *Circulation*, 69, 313–24; and II. The influence of changes in lipid values introduced by cholestyramine and diet on progression of coronary artery disease: Results of the NHLBI Type II coronary intervention study, *Circulation*, 69, 325–37.

45. Sanders, K. (1959). Coronary artery disease and obesity, *Lancet*, 2, 432–35.
    Damon, A., Dammophon, S. T., Harpending, H. C., and Kannel, W. B. (1969). Predicting coronary heart diseae from body measurements of Framingham males, *J. Chron. Dis.*, 21, 781–802.
    Keys, A., Aravanis, C., and Blackburn, H. (1972). Coronary heart disease: Overweight and obesity as risk factors, *Ann. Int. Med.*, 77, 15–27.
    Ashley, Jr., F. W., and Kannel, W. B. (1974). Relation of weight change to change in atherogenic traits: The Framingham Study, *J. Chron. Dis.*, 27, 103–14.
    Weinsier, R. L., Fuchs, R. J., Kay, T. D., Triebwasser, J. H., and Lancaster, M. C. (1976). Body fat: Its relationship to coronary heart disease, blood pressure, lipids and other risk factors measured in a large male population, *Amer. J. Med.*, 61, 815–24.

46. Goldblatt, P. B., Moore, M. E., and Stunkard, A. J. (1965). Social factors in obesity, *J. Am. Med. Assoc.*, 192, 1035–44.

Stunkard, A., D'Aquili, E., and Fox, S. (1972). Influence of social class on obesity and thinness in children, *J. Am. Med. Assoc., 221,* 579–84.

47. Mann, G. V., Teel, K., Hayes, O., McNally, A., and Bruno, D. (1955). Exercise in the disposition of dietary calories, *New Eng. J. Med., 253,* 349–55.

48. Mann, G. V., Shaffer, R. D., and Rich, A. (1965). Physical fitness and immunity to heart disease in Masai, *Lancet, 2,* 1308–10.

49. Biggs, R., Macfarlane, R. G., and Pilling, J. (1947). Observations on fibrinolysis—experimental activity produced by exercise or adrenaline, *Lancet, 1* 402–405.

50. Morris, J. N., and Crawford, M. D. (1958). Coronary heart disease and physical activity of work, *Brit. Med. J., 2,* 1485–96.

51. Morris, J. N., Adam, C., and Chave, S. P. W. (1973). Vigorous exercise in leisure time and the incidence of coronary heart disease, *Lancet, 1,* 333–37.
    Paffenbarger, R. S., Hale, W. E., Brand, R. J., and Hyde, R. T. (1977). Work-energy level, personal characteristics, and fatal heart attack: A birth-cohort effect, *Amer. J. Epidem., 105,* 200–213.
    Brand, R. J., Paffenbarger, R. S., Sholtz, R. I., and Kamport, J. B. (1979). Work activity and fatal heart attack studied by multiple logistic risk analysis, *Amer. J. Epidem., 110,* 52–62.
    Morris, J. N., Pollard, R., Everitt, M. G., Chave, S. P. W., and Semmence, A. M. (1980). Vigorous exercise in leisure-time: Protection against coronary heart disease, *Lancet, 2,* 1207–10.

52. Brown, R. G., Davidson, L. A., McKeown, T., and Whitfield, A. G. W. (1957). Coronary artery disease, influences affecting its incidence in males in the seventh decade, *Lancet, 2,* 1073–77.

53. Robinson, W. S. (1950). Ecological correlates and the behavior of individuals, *Amer. Soc. Rev., 15,* 351–7.

54. Syme, S. L. (1967). Implications and future prospects in social stress and cardiovascular disease, *Milbank Mem. Fd. Quart., 45,* No. 2, Part 2, 175–80.

55. Acheson, R. M., and Jessop, W. J. E. (1961). Tobacco smoking and serum lipids in old men, *Brit. Med. J., 2,* 1108–11.
    Acheson, R. M. (1962). The etiology of coronary heart disease: A review from the epidemiologic standpoint, *Yale J. Biol. Med., 35,* 143–70.

56. Morris, J. N. (1959). Occupation and coronary heart disease, *Arch. Intern. Med., 104,* 903–7.

57. Hammond, E. C., and Horn, D. (1954). The relationship between human smoking habits and death rates, *J. Amer. Med. Assoc., 155,* 1316–28.
    Zukel, W. J., Lewis, R. H., Enterline, P. E., Painter, R. C. M., Ralston, L. S., Fawcett, R. M., Meredith, A. P., and Peterson, B. (1959). A short-term community study of the epidemiology of coronary heart disease, *Amer. J. Publ. Hlth., 49,* 1630–39.

58. Cartwright, A., Martin, F. M., and Thompson, J. B. G. (1959). Distribution and development of smoking habits, *Lancet, 2,* 725–27.
    U.S. Dept. of Health and Human Services (1981). *The Health Consequences of Smoking for Women. A Report of the Surgeon General,* Washington, D.C.

59. Advisory Committee to the Surgeon General of the Public Health Service (1964). *Smoking and Health.* Public Health Service Pub. No. 1103. Washington, D.C.
    U.S. Department of Health and Human Services (1982) *The Health Consequences of Smoking: Cancer. A Report of the Surgeon General,* Washington, D.C.

60. Oliver, M. F. (1970). Oral contraceptives and myocardial infarction, *Brit. Med. J., 2,* 210–3.

Mann, J. I., Doll, R., Thorogood, M., Vessey, M. P., and Waters, W. E. (1976). Risk factors for myocardial infarction in young women, *Brit. J. Prev. Soc. Med.*, *30*, 94–100.

Shapiro, S., Slone, D., and Rosenberg, L. (1979). Oral contraceptive use in relation to myocardial infarction, *Lancet*, *1*, 734–37.

61. Russek, H. I., and Zohman, B. L. (1958). Relative significance of heredity, diet and occupational stress in coronary heart disease of young adults, *Amer. J. Med. Sci.*, *253*, 166–77.

62. Friedman, M., and Rosenman, R. H. (1959). Association of specific behavior patterns with blood cholesterol, *J. Amer. Med. Assoc.*, *169*, 1286–96.

63. Friedman, M., Rosenman, R. H., and Carroll, V. (1958). Changes in the serum cholesterol and blood clotting time in men subjected to cyclic variation of occupational stress, *Circulation*, *17*, 852–61.

64. Jenkins, C. E. (1976). Recent evidence supporting psychologic and social risk factors for coronary heart disease, *New Eng. J. Med.*, *295*, 987–94, 1033–38.

65. Ostfeld, A. M., Lebovits, D. Z., Shekelle, R. B., and Paul, O. (1964). A prospective study of the relationship between personality and coronary heart disease, *J. Chron. Dis.*, *17*, 265–76.

Medalie, J. H., Kahn, M. A., Neufeld, H. N., Riss, E., and Goldbourt, U. (1973). Myocardial infarction over a five year period. I. Prevalence, incidence and mortality experience. II. Association of single variables to age and birth place, *J. Chron. Dis.*, *26*, 64–84, 329–49.

Medalie, J. H., Snyder, M., Groen, J. J., Neufeld, H. N., Goldbourt, V., and Riss, E. (1973). Angina pectoris among 10,000 men. 5 year incidence and univariate analysis, *Am. J. Med.*, *55*, 583–94.

66. Fløderus, B. (1974). Psychosocial factors in relation to coronary heart disease and associated risk factors, *Nord. Hyg. Tidskr.*, Supp. 6.

67. Bruhn, J. G., Peredes, A., and Adsett, C. A. (1974). Psychological predictors of sudden death in myocardial infarction, *J. Psychosomatic Res.*, *18*, 187–91.

68. Theorell, T., and Fløderus-Myrhed, B. (1977). Workload and risk of myocardial infarction, A prospective psychosocial analysis, *Int. J. Epidem.*, *6*, 17–21.

Karasek, R., Baker, D., Marxer, F., Ahlbom, A., Theorell, T. (1981). Job decision latitude, job demands, and cardiovascular disease: A prospective study of Swedish men, *Amer. J. Publ. Hlth.*, *71*, 694–705.

69. Review Panel on Coronary Prone Behavior and Coronary Heart Disease (1981). Coronary-prone behavior and coronary heart disease: A critical review, *Circulation*, *63*, 1199–1215.

70. Rosenman, R. H., Brand, R. J., Shortle, R. I., and Friedman, M. (1976). Multivariate prediction of coronary heart disease during 8.5 year follow-up in the Western Collaborative Group Study, *Amer. J. Cardiol.*, *37*, 902–10.

Jenkins, C. D., Zyzanski, S. J., and Rosenman, R. H. (1976). Risk of new myocardial infarction in middle-aged men with manifest coronary heart disease, *Circulation*, *53*, 342–47.

71. Haynes, S. G., Levine, S., and Scotch, N. (1978). The relationship of psychosocial factors to coronary heart disease in the Framingham Study. I. Methods and risk factors, *Amer. J. Epidem.*, *107*, 362–83.

Haynes, S. G., Feinleib, M., and Levine, S. (1978). The relationship of psychosocial factors to coronary heart disease in the Framingham Study. II. Prevalence of coronary heart disease, *Amer. J. Epidem.*, *107*, 384–402.

Haynes, S. G., Eaker, E. D., and Feinleib, M. (1983). Spouse behavior and coronary heart disease in men: Prospective results from the Framingham Heart Study. I. Concordance of risk factors and the relationship of psychosocial status to coronary incidence. II. Modification of risk in Type A husbands according to the social and psychological status of their wives, *Amer. J. Epi., 118*, 1–22, 23–41.

72. Dembrowski, T. M., MacDougall, J. M., and Shields, J. L. (1977). Physiological reactions to social challenge in persons evidencing the Type A coronary-prone behavior pattern, *J. Human Stress, 3*, (3), 2–9.

73. Zyzanski, S. J., Jenkins, C. D., Ryan, T. J., Flessas, A., and Everist, M. (1976). Psychological correlates of coronary angiographic findings, *Arch. Int. Med., 136*, 1234–37.
Frank, K. A., Heller, S. S., Kornfeld, D. S., and Sporn, A. A. (1978). Type A behavior and coronary angiographic findings, *J. Amer. Med. Assoc., 240*, 761–63.

74. McLellan, D. (1961). *The Achieving Society*, New York.
Johnson, D. W., and Johnson, R. T. (1976). Goal structures and open education, *Journal of Research and Educational Development, 8*, 30–46.
Bowles, S., and Gintis, H. (1976). *Schooling in Capitalist America*, New York.

75. Glass, D. C., ed. (1977) *Behavior Patterns, Stress and Coronary Disease*, Hillsdale, N.J.

76. Waldron, I. (1978). The coronary-prone behavior pattern, blood pressure, employment and socio-economic status in women, *J. Psychosom. Res., 22*, 79–87.

77. Zyzanski, S. J. (1978). The coronary-prone behavior pattern and coronary heart disease: Epidemiological evidence, *Coronary-Prone Behavior*, ed. Dembrowski, T. M., Weiss, S. W., Shields, J. L., New York, pp. 25–40.

78. Waldron, I., Zyzanski, S., and Shekelle, R. B. (1977). The coronary-prone behavior pattern in employed men and women, *J. Human Stress, 3*, (4), 2–18.

79. Cohen, J. B. (1978). The influence of culture on coronary-prone behavior, in *Coronary-Prone Behavior*, ed. Dembrowski, T. M., Weiss, S. W., and Shields, J. L., New York, pp. 191–98.
Jenkins, C. D., Zyzanski, S. J., and Rosenman, R. H. (1978). Coronary-prone behavior: One pattern or several? *Psychosom. Med., 40*, 23–43.

80. Brown, G. W., and Harris, T. (1978). *Social Origins of Depression: A Study of Psychiatric Disorders in Women*, New York.

81. Pearlin, L. I., and Radabaugh, M. (1976). Economic strains and the coping functions of alcohol, *Amer. J. Sociol., 82*, 652–63.

82. Keith, R. A., Lown, B., and Stare, F. J. (1965). Coronary heart disease and behavior patterns, *Psychosom. Med., 27*, 424–34.
Mettlin, C. (1976). Occupational careers and the prevention of coronary-prone behavior, *Soc. Sci. Med., 10*, 367–72.
Shekelle, R. B., Schoenberger, J. A., and Stamler, J. (1976). Correlates of the JAS Type A behavior pattern score, *J. Chron. Dis., 29*, 381–94.

83. Kohn, M. (1969) *Class and Conformity*, Homewood, Ill.

84. Matthews, K. A., Glass, D. C., and Richins, M. (1977). Behavioral interactions of mothers and children with the coronary-prone behavior pattern, in *Behavior Patterns, Stress, and Coronary Disease*, ed. Glass, D. C., Hillsdale, N.J.

85. Feldman, J. (1968). *The Dissemination of Health Information, A Case Study in Adult Learning*, Chicago.

86. Pell, S., and D'Alonzo, A. (1963). Acute myocardial infarction in a large industrial population, *J. Amer. Med. Assoc., 185*, 31–38.
Lehman, E. W., Schulman, J., and Hinkle, L. E. (1967). Coronary deaths and organizational mobility, *Arch. Environm. Health., 15*, 455–61.

87. **Williams, C. A.** (1968). The relationship of occupational change to blood pressure, serum cholesterol, a specific overt behavior pattern and coronary heart disease, Ph.D. thesis, Department of Epidemiology, University of North Carolina. As cited by Waldron et al. (ref. 78).

88. **Registrar General.** (1966) *Decennial Supplement, England and Wales. Parts I and II: Occupational Mortality,* H.M.S.O., London.

89. **Gale, A. H.** (1959). *Epidemic Disease,* Harmondsworth.
   Paul, J. R. (1971). *A History of Poliomyelitis,* New Haven.

90. **Maxcy, K.F.** (1944). A review of the epidemiology of acute anterior poliomyelitis, *J.-Lancet, 64,* 216–23.
   Paul, J. R. (1949). Poliomyelitis attack rates in American troops, 1940–48, *Amer. J. Hyg., 50,* 57–62.
   Ames, W. R. (1951). Variations in the age selection of poliomyelitis associated with differences in economic status in Buffalo, N.Y., 1929, 1944, and 1949, *Amer. J. Publ. Hlth., 41,* 388–95.

91. **Gear, J., Measroch, R., Bradley, J.,** and **Faerber, G. I.** (1951). Poliomyelitis in South Africa, *S. Afr. Med. J., 25,* 297–301.
   Gear, J. (1952). Immunity to poliomyelitis, *Ann. Intern. Med., 37,* 1–22.

92. **Melnick, J. L.,** and **Ledinko, N.** (1951). Social serology: Antibody levels in a normal young population during an epidemic of poliomyelitis, *Amer. J. Hyg., 54,* 354–82.
   Backett, E. M. (1957). Social patterns of antibody to polio virus, *Lancet, 1,* 778–83.
   Winkelstein, W. (1959). Factors in participation in the 1954 poliomyelitis vaccine field trials, Erie County, New York, *Amer. J. Publ. Health, 49,* 1454–66.

93. **Nathanson, N.,** and **Martin, J. R.** (1979). The epidemiology of poliomyelitis: Enigmas surrounding its appearance, epidemicity, and disappearance, *Amer. J. Epidem., 110,* 672–92.

94. **Burnet, F. M.** (1953). *Viruses and Men,* London.

95. **Clausen, J., Seidenfeld, M.,** and **Deasy, L.** (1957). Parent attitudes toward participation of their children in polio vaccine trials, in *Patients, Physicians and Illness,* ed. Jaco, E. G., Glencoe, Ill., 119–28.

96. **Brandt, A.** (1978). Polio, politics and duplicity: Ethical aspects in the development of the Salk vaccine, *Int. J. Hlth. Serv., 8,* 257–70.
   U.S. Department of Health and Human Services (1983). *Health. United States, 1983,* Hyattville, Md.

97. **Court-Brown, W. M.,** and **Doll, R.** (1957). Leukemia and aplastic anaemia in patients irradiated for ankylosing spondylitis, *Spec. Rep. Ser. Med. Res. Counc. (Lond),* No. 295, London, H.M.S.O.

98. **Modan, B.,** and **Lilienfeld, A.** (1965). Polycythemia and leukemia—the role of radiation treatment, *Medicine, 44,* 305–44.

99. **Stewart, A., Webb, J.,** and **Hewitt, D. A.** (1958). A survey of childhood malignancies, *Brit. Med. J., 1,* 1445–1508.
   MacMahon, B. (1962). Prenatal-X-ray exposure and childhood cancer, *J. Nat. Cancer Inst., 28,* 1173–91.

100. **March, H. C.** (1950). Leukemia in radiologists in a twenty-year period, *Amer. J. Med. Sci., 220,* 282–6.
   Peller, S., and **Pick, P.** (1952). Leukemia and other malignancies in physicians, *Amer. J. Med. Sci., 224,* 154–9.
   Seltser, R., and **Sartwell, P.** (1965) The influence of occupational exposure to radiation on the mortality of American radiologists and other medical specialists, *Amer. J. Epidem., 81,* 2–22.

101. **Folley, J. H., Borges, W.,** and **Yamawaki, T.** (1952). Incidence of leukemia in survivors of the atomic bomb at Hiroshima and Nagasaka, Japan, *Amer. J. Med., 13*, 311–21.

102. **Hewitt, D.** (1955). Some features of leukemia mortality, *Brit. J. Prev. Soc. Med., 9*, 81–8.

   United Nations (1958). *Report of the United Nations Scientific Committee on the Effects of Atomic Radiation*, General Assembly Official Records, Thirteenth Session, Suppl. No. 17 (A/3838), New York.

   Medical Research Council. (1960). *The Hazards to Man of Nuclear and Allied Radiations*, Second Report, Cmnd. 1225, H.M.S.O., London.

103. **Barr, A.** (1958). Hospital admissions and social environment, *Med. Offr., 100*, 351–4.

   Bergner, L., and **Yerby, A. S.** (1968). Low income and barriers to use of health services, *New Eng. J. Med., 278*, 541–6.

104. **Adelstein, A.,** and **White, G.** (1976). Leukemia 1911–1973: Cohort analysis, *Population Trends, 3*, 9–13.

   Birch, J. M., Swindell, R., Marsden, H. B., and **Morris Jones, P. H.** (1981). Childhood leukemia in North West England 1954–1977: Epidemiology incidence and survival, *Brit. J. Cancer, 43*, 324–29.

   Stiller, C. A. and **Draper, G. J.** (1982). Trends in childhood leukemia in Britain 1968–1978, *Brit. J. Cancer, 45*, 543–51.

105. **Bager, B.** (1929). Beitrag zur kenntris uber Vorkommen, Klinik und Behandlung von perforierten Magen und Duodenalgeschwuren nebst einer Untersuchung uber die Spatresultate, nach Verschiedenen Operations-methoden, *Acta. Chir. Scand., 64*, Suppl. II.

106. **Jennings, D.** (1940). Perforated peptic ulcer, *Lancet, 1*, 395–98, 444–47.

107. **Hurst, A. F.,** and **Stewart, M. J.** (1929). *Gastric and Duodenal Ulcer*, London.

   Alexander, F. (1934). The influence of psychologic factors upon gastrointestinal disturbances: A symposium, *Psychoanal. Quart., 3*, 501–39.

   Davies, D. T., and **Wilson, A. T. M.** (1937). Observations on the life-history of chronic peptic ulcer, *Lancet, 2*, 1353–60.

   Stewart, D. N., and **Winser, D. M. de R.** (1942). Incidence of perforated peptic ulcer, *Lancet, 1*, 259–61.

108. **Susser, M. W.** (1961). Environmental factors and peptic ulcer, *Practitioner, 186*, 302–11.

   Susser, M. W., and **Stein, Z.** (1962). Civilization and peptic ulcer, *Lancet, 1*, 115–19.

   Susser, M. (1982). Period effects, generation effects, and age effects in peptic ulcer mortality, *J. Chron. Dis., 35*, 29–40.

109. **Doll, R., Jones, F. A.,** and **Buckatzsch, M. M.** (1951). Occupational factors in the aetiology of gastric and duodenal ulcers, *Spec. Rep. Series. Med. Res. Coun., 276*, 1–96.

110. **Pulvertaft, C. N.** (1959). Peptic ulcer in town and country, *Brit. J. Prev. Soc. Med., 13*, 131–38.

111. **Monson, R.,** and **MacMahon, B.** (1969). Peptic ulcer in Massachusetts physicians, *New Eng. J. Med., 281*, 11–15.

   Langman, M. (1974). The changing nature of the duodenal ulcer diathesis, in *Chronic Duodenal Ulcer*, ed. Wastell, C., London, pp 3–15.

   Mendeloff, A. I. (1974). What has been happening to peptic ulcer? *Gastroenterology, 67*, 1020–22.

   Sturdevant, R. A. L. (1976). Epidemiology of peptic ulcer: Report of a conference, *Amer. J. Epidem., 104*, 9–14.

   Segal, I., Dubb, A. A., Tim, L. O., Solomon, A., Sottomayor, M. C. C. G., and **Zwane, E. M.** (1978). Duodenal ulcer and working-class mobility in an African population in South Africa, *Br. Med. J., 1*, 469–72.

Sonnenberg, A., Fritsch, A. (1983). Changing mortality of peptic ulcer disease in Germany, *Gastroenterology, 84*, 1533–37.

112. Davies, D. T., and Wilson, A. T. (1939). Personal and clinical history of haematemesis and perforation, *Lancet, 2*, 723–27.
Mittlemann, B., and Wolff, H. G. (1942). Emotions and gastroduodenal function, *Psychosom. Med., 4*, 5–61.

113. Spicer, C. C., Stewart, D. N., and Winser, D. M. de R. (1944). Perforated peptic ulcer during the period of heavy air raids, *Lancet, 1*, 14.

114. Clyde, R. J., Collins, J. S. A., Compton, S. A., Cooper, N. K., and Friel, C. M. (1975). Peptic ulcer and civil disturbances, *Lancet, 2*, 1302.

115. Cobb, S., and Rose, R.M. (1973). Hypertension, peptic ulcer, and diabetes in air traffic controllers, *J. Amer. Med. Assoc., 224*, 489–92.

116. Doll, R., Jones, F. A., and Pygott, F. (1958). Effect of smoking on the production and maintenance of gastric and duodenal ulcers, *Lancet, 1*, 657–62.

117. Cohart, E. N., and Miller, C. (1955). Socioeconomic distribution of cancer of the gastrointestinal tract in New Haven, *Cancer, 8*, 379–88.
Office of Population Censuses and Surveys. (1958). *The Registrar General's Decennial Supplement for England and Wales, 1931–51*, London, H.M.S.O.
Wynder, E. L., and Shigematsu, T. (1967). Environmental factors of cancer of the colon and rectum, *Cancer, 20*, 1520–61.
Krain, L. S. (1972). Racial and socioeconomic factors in colon cancer mortality, *Oncology, 26*, 335–44.
Goldblatt, P.O., and Fox, A. J. (1978). Household mortality from the OPCS Longitudinal Study, *Population Trends, 14*, 21–27.
Fox, A. J., and Goldblatt, P. O. (1982). *Longitudinal Study: Socio-Demographic Mortality Differentials, 1971-1975*, Office of Population Censuses and Surveys, Series LS no. 1, H.M.S.O., London.

118. Griscom, J. H. (1970; first pub. 1845). *The Sanitary Conditions of the Labouring Population of New York, With Suggestions for Its Improvement*, New York.
Rosen, G. (1973). Disease, debility, and death, in *The Victorian City: Images and Realities*, ed. Dyos, H. J., and Wolff, M., 2 vols., London, pp. 625–68.
Brockington, C. F. (1979). The history of public health, in *The Theory and Practice of Public Health*, ed. Hobson, W., New York, pp. 1–8.

119. Lambert, P. (1976). Perinatal mortality: Social and enviromental factors, *Population Trends, 4*, 4–8.

120. Young, M. (1926). Variation in mortality from cancer of differing parts of the body in groups of men of different social status, *J. Hyg. (Lond.), 25*, 209–17.
Registrar General (1927). *Decennial Supplement, England and Wales, 1921, Part II: Occupational Mortality, Fertility and Infant Mortality*, H.M.S.O., London.
Sydenstricker, E. (1929). Economic status and the incidence of illness: Hagerstown Morbidity Studies, No. 10., *Public Hlth. Rep. (Wash.), 44*, 1821–33.
Titmuss, R. M. (1943). *Birth, Poverty and Wealth: A Study of Infant Mortality*, London.
Clemmesen, J. and Nielsen, A. (1951). Social distribution of cancer in Copenhagen, 1943–47, *Brit. J. Cancer, 5*, 159–71.
Graham, S., Levin, M., and Lilienfeld, A. M. (1960). The socioeconomic distribution of cancer of various sites in Buffalo, N.Y., *Cancer, 13*, 180–91.

121. Kitagawa, E. M., and Hauser, P. M. (1973). *Differential Mortality in the United States*, Cambridge.

122. **Cartwright, A.,** and **Anderson, R.** (1981). *General Practice Revisted: A Second Study of Patients and Their Doctors,* New York.
123. **Report of a Research Working Group** (1980). *Inequalities in Health: The Black Report,* H.M.S.O., London.
      Gray, A. M. (1982) Inequalities in Health. The Black Report: A summary and comment, *Inter. J. Hlth. Serv., 12,* 349–80.
124. **Lerner, M.,** and **Anderson, O. W.** (1963). *Health Progress in the United States, 1900–1960,* Chicago.
      Nagi, M. H., and **Stockwell, E. G.** (1973). Socioeconomic differentials in mortality by cause of death, *Hlth. Serv. Rep., 88,* 449–56.
      Jenkins, C. D., Tuthill, R. W., Tannenbaum, S. I., and **Kirby, C. R.** (1977). Zones of excess mortality in Massachusetts, *New Eng. J. Med., 296,* 1354–56.
      Kitagawa, E. M. (1977). On mortality, *Demography, 14,* 381–90.
125. **Brown, S. M., Selvin, S.,** and **Winkelstein, W.** (1975). The association of economic status with the occurrence of lung cancer, *Cancer, 36,* 1903–11.
126. **Leff, A., Lester, T. W.,** and **Adington, W. N.** (1979). Tuberculosis: A chemotherapeutic triumph but a persistent socioeconomic problem, *Arch. Int. Med., 139,* 1375–77.
      Editorial (1979). Tuberculosis and social class, *Tubercle, 60,* 191–4.
127. **Acheson, R. M.,** and **Sanderson, C.** (1978). Strokes: Social class and geography, *Population Trends, 12,* 13–17.
128. **Richardson, I. M.** (1965). Prostatic cancer and social class, *Brit. J. Preven. Soc. Med., 19,* 140–42.
      Editorial. (1975). The epidemiology of cancer of the prostate, *J. Chron. Dis., 29,* 343–8.
      Hakky, S. I., Chisholm, G. D., and **Skeet, R. G.** (1975). Social class and carcinoma of the prostate, *Brit. J. Urol., 51,* 392–396.
      Ernster, V. L., Selvin, S., and **Sacks, S. T.** (1978). Prostatic cancer: Mortality and incidence rates by race and social class, *Amer. J. Epidem., 107,* 311–20.
      Ross, R. K., McCurtis, J. W., and **Henderson, N. C.** (1979). Descriptive epidemiology of testicular and prostatic cancer in Los Angeles, *Brit. J. Cancer, 39,* 284–92.
129. **U.S. Dept. of Health, Education and Welfare** (1978). *Third Special Report to the U.S. Congress on Alcohol and Health.* Washington, D.C.
130. **U.S. Bureau of the Census** (1936). Live births and deaths of infants in the United States and each state: 1933–1934, *Vital Statistics—Special Reports,* Vol. 1, No. 12.
      National Office of Vital Statistics (1954). *Vital Statistics of the United States, 1951,* Vol. II—*Mortality,* Washington, D.C.
131. **Donabedian, A., Rosenfeld, L. S.,** and **Southern, E. M.** (1965). Infant mortality and socioeconomic status in a metropolitan community, *Pub. Hlth. Rep., 80,* 1083–94.
      MacMahon, B., Kovar, M. G., and **Feldman, J. J.** (1972). *Infant Mortality Rates: Socioeconomic Factors,* Vital and Health Statistics, Series 22, No. 14, U.S. Dept. of Health, Education and Welfare, Washington, D.C.
      Markides, K. S., and **Barnes, D.** (1975). A methodological note on the relationship between infant mortality and socioeconomic status with evidence from San Antonio, Texas, *Social Biology, 24,* 38–44.
      Brooks, C. H. (1975). The changing relationship between socioeconomic status and infant mortality: An analysis of state characteristics, *J. Hlth. Soc. Behav., 16,* 291–303.
      Brooks, C. H. (1975). Path analysis of socioeconomic correlates of county infant mortality rates, *Int. J. Hlth. Serv., 5,* 499–514.

Antonovsky, A., and Bernstein, J. (1977). Social class and infant mortality, *Soc. Sci. and Med.*, *11*, 453–70.

132. Bergner, L., and Susser, M. W. (1970). Low birthweight and perinatal nutrition: An interpretive review, *Pediatrics*, *46*, 946–66.
Susser, M. W., Marolla, A., and Fleiss, J. (1972). Birthweight, fetal age and perinatal mortality, *Amer. J. Epidem.*, *96*, 197–204.

133. Hemminki, E., and Starfield, B. (1978). Prevention of low birthweight and pre-term birth, *Health and Society*, *56*, 329–61.

134. Geijerstam, G. (1969). Low birthweight and perinatal mortality, *Pub. Hlth. Rep.*, *84*, 939–48.

135. Chase, H. C. (1977). Time trends in low birth weight in the United States, 1950–74, in *The Epidemiology of Prematurity*, ed. Reed, D. M., and Stanley, F. J., Baltimore and Munich, pp. 17–38.
Lee, K. S., Paneth, N., Gartner, L., Pearlman, M. (1980). The very low birthweight rate: principal predictor of neonatal mortality in populations, *J. Pediat.*, *97*, 759–64.
Lee, K. S., Paneth, N., Gartner, L. M., Pearlman, M., and Gruss, L. (1980). Neonatal mortality: An analysis of recent improvements in the United States, *Amer. J. Publ. Hlth.*, *70*, 15–21.
Lee, K. S., Gartner, L. M., Paneth, N., and Tyler, L. (1982). Recent trends in neonatal mortality: The Canadian experience, *Can. Med. Assoc. J.*, *126*, 373–76.

136. Paneth, N., Kiely, J., Wallenstein, S., Marcus, M., Pakter, J., and Susser, M. W. (1982). Newborn intensive care and neonatal mortality in low birthweight infants, *New Eng. J. Med.*, *307*, 149–55.

137. Rush, D., and Kass, E. M. (1972). Maternal smoking: A reassessment of the association with perinatal mortality, *Amer. J. Epidem.*, *96*, 183–96.
Meyer, M. B., Jonas, B. S., and Tonascia, J. A. (1976). Perinatal events associated with maternal smoking in pregnancy, *Amer. J. Epidem.*, *103*, 404–76.
Sever, J. L., Ellenberg, J. M., and Edmonds, D. (1977). Maternal urinary tract infections and prematurity, in *The Epidemiology of Prematurity*, ed. Read, D. W., and Stanley, F. J., Baltimore, pp. 193–96.
Niswander, K. K. (1977). Obstetric factors related to prematurity, in *The Epidemiology of Prematurity*, ed. Read, D. W., and Stanley, F. J., Baltimore, pp. 249–68.

138. Dott, A. B. N., and Fort, A. T. (1975). The effect of maternal demographic factors on infant mortality rates; the effect of availability and utilization of perinatal care and hospital services on infant mortality rates. Summary of the findings of the Louisiana mortality study, Parts I and II, *Amer. J. Obstet. Gynec.*, *123*, 847–60.
Miller, H. C., Hassanein, K., Chin, T. D. Y. and Hensleigh, P. (1976). Socioeconomic factors in relation of fetal growth in white infants, *J. Pediat.*, *89*, 638–43.

139. Wilson, R. W., and White, E. L. (1977). Changes in morbidity, disability, and utilization differentials between the poor and the nonpoor: Data from the Health Interview Survey: 1964 and 1973, *Medical Care*, *15*, 636–46.

140. Wan, T. (1972). Social differentials in selected work-limiting chronic conditions, *J. Chron. Dis.*, *25*, 365–74.
Conover, P. W. (1973). Social class and chronic illness, *Int. J. Hlth. Serv.*, *3*, 357–68.
Graham, S., and Reeder, L. G. (1979). Social epidemiology of chronic disease, *Handbook of Medical Sociology*, ed. Freeman, H. E., Levine, S., and Reeder, L. G., 3rd. ed., Englewood Cliffs, N.J., pp. 71–96.
Department of Health and Human Services. (1980). *Health of the Disadvantaged: Chart Book II*, Washington, D.C.

141. **Edwards, F., McKeown, T.,** and **Whitfield, A. G. W.** (1959). Contributions and demands of elderly men, *Brit. J. Prev. Soc. Med., 13,* 59–66.
     Brockington, F., and **Lempert, S. M.** (1966). *The Social Needs of the Over-Eighties,* Manchester.
     Siegel, J. S. (1980). Recent and prospective demographic trends for the elderly population and some implications for health care, in *Second Conference on the Epidemiology of Aging,* ed. Haynes, S. G., and Feinleib, M., U.S. Dept. of Health and Human Services, NIH Pub. No. 80-969, Washington, D.C., pp. 289–316.
142. **Ashford, N.** (1976). *Crisis in the Workplace: Occupational Disease and Injury: A Report to the Ford Foundation,* Cambridge, Mass.
143. **Page, J.,** and **O'Brien, M.** 1972. *Bitter Wages,* New York.
     Special Task Force (1973). *Work in America,* Report to the Secretary of Health, Education and Welfare, Cambridge, Mass.
     Brodeur, P. (1973). *Expendable Americans,* New York.
     Kinnersly, P. (1973). *The Hazards of Work: How to Fight Them,* London.
     Stellman, J., and **Daum, S.** (1973). *Work Is Dangerous to Your Health,* New York.
     Berman, D. (1978). *Death on the Job: Occupational Health and Safety Struggles in the United States,* New York.
144. **Gordon, J. B., Akman, A.,** and **Brooks, M. L.** (1971). *Industrial Safety Statistics: A Recommendation,* New York.
     Barth, P. S., and **Hunt, H. A.** (1980). *Workers' Compensation and Work-Related Illnesses and Diseases,* Boston.
145. **Bureau of Labor Statistics.** (1980). *Occupational Injuries and Illnesses in 1978: Summary,* U.S. Department of Labor, Washington, D.C.
146. **U.S. Senate Hearings.** (1972). Hearings on Health Services for Domestic Agricultural Migrant Workers: Joint Hearing before the Sub-Committee on Health and Sub-Committee on Migrant Labor (Labor and Public Welfare Committee), 92nd Congress, 2nd Session, August 1, 1972, (Senate) S.3762.
147. **NIOSH Report.** (1975). *Job Demands and Worker Health,* Publication #75-160, U.S. DHEW, Washington, D.C.
     Mancuso, T. (1976). Prevention and Control of Occupational Exposures: An Overview, in *Third Conference of the International Symposium on Detection and Prevention of Cancer,* ed. Nieburgs, H. E., Part I, Vol. 2, pp. 1847–65.
148. **Shepard, J. M.** (1977). Technology, work and job satisfaction, *Ann. Rev. Sociol., 3,* 1–21.
     Baker, D. (1980). The use and health consequence of shift work, *Int. J. Hlth. Serv., 10,* 405–20.
149. **Coburn, D.** (1978). Work and general psychological and physical wellbeing, *Int. J. Hlth. Serv., 8,* 415–35.
150. **Lieban, J.,** and **Pistawka, H.** (1967). Mesothelioma and asbestos exposure, *Arch. Environ. Hlth., 14,* 559–63.
     Wagoner, J. K. (1976). Occupational carcinogenosis: The two hundred years since Percival Pott, *Annals of New York Academy of Sciences, 271,* 1–4.
     Davis, D. L., and **Magee, B. H.** (1979). Cancer and industrial chemical production, *Science, 206,* 1356–58.
     Epstein, S. (1979). *The Politics of Cancer,* New York.
     Rutter, M. (1980). Raised lead levels and impaired cognitive/behavioral functioning: a review of the evidence, *Dev. Med. Child Neurol.* (Suppl.), *42,* 1–36.
     Doll, R., and **Peto, R.** (1981). The causes of cancer: quantitative estimates of avoidable risks of cancer in the United States today, *J. Nat. Can. Inst., 66,* 1191–308.

Goldsmith, R. (1981). Mortality in a steelmaking community, PhD. Dissertation, Columbia University, unpublished.

Davis, D. L., Bridbord, K., Schneiderman, M. (1982). Cancer prevention: Assessing causes, exposures, and recent trends in mortality for U.S. males, 1968-78, *Teratogen. Carcinogen. Mutagen.*, 2, 105–35.

151. Elling, R. (1977). Industrialization and occupational health in underdeveloped countries, *Int. J. Hlth. Serv.*, 7, 209–35.

Butler, J., Giovannitti, D., Hainer, M., and Shapiro, H. (1978). Dying for work: Occupational health and asbestos, *NACLA Report on the Americas*, 12, 2–39.

Castleman, B. (1979). The export of hazardous factories to developing nations, *Int. J. Hlth. Serv.*, 9, 569–606.

152. Wagley, C. and Harris, M. (1958). *Minorities in the New World*, New York.

Barth, F., ed. (1969). *Ethnic Groups and Boundaries*, Boston.

Hannerz, U. (1974). Ethnicity and opportunity in urban America, in *Urban Ethnicity*, ed. Cohen, A., New York, pp. 37–76.

Vincent, J. (1974). The structuring of ethnicity, *Human Organization*, 33, 375–79.

Mullings, L. (1978). Ethnicity and stratification in the urban United States, *Annals of the New York Academy of Sciences*, 318, 10–22.

Steinberg, S. (1981). *The Ethnic Myth: Race, Ethnicity and Class in America*, New York.

Banton, M. (1983). *Racial and Ethnic Competition*, Cambridge.

153. Yu, E. (1982). The low mortality rates of Chinese infants: Some plausible explanatory factors, *Social Science and Medicine*, 16, 253–65.

154. Chase, H. C. (1977). Infant mortality and its concomitants, 1960–1972, *Medical Care*, 15, 662–74.

Rudor, M. H., and Santangelo, N. (1979) *Health Status of Minorities and Low Income Groups*, U.S. Department of Health, Education and Welfare. Publication No. (HRA) 79–627.

Erickson, J. D., and Bjerkedal, T. (1982). Fetal and infant mortality in Norway and the United States, *J. Amer. Med. Assoc.*, 247, 987–91.

155. McDonough, J. R., Garrison, G. E., and Hames, C. G. (1964). Blood pressure and hypertensive disease among negroes and whites, *Ann. Int. Med.*, 61, 208–28.

Henry, J. P., and Cassel, J. C. (1969) Psychosocial factors in essential hypertension, *Amer. J. Epidem.*, 90, 171–200.

Syme, L., Oakes, T. W., Friedman, G. D., Feldman, R., Siegelaub, A. B., and Collen, M. (1974). Social class and social differences in blood pressure, *Amer. J. Publ. Hlth.*, 64, 619–20.

Gillum, R. F. (1979). Pathophysiology of hypertension in blacks and whites: A review of the basis of normal blood pressure differences, *Hypertension*, 1, 468–75.

156. Harburg, E., Erfurt, B., and Hauenstein, L., Chape, C., Schull, W. J., and Schork, M. A. (1973). Socioecologic stress, suppressed hostility, skin color and black-white male blood pressure: Detroit, *Psychosomat. Med.*, 35, 276–96.

Keil, J., Tyroler, H. A., Sandifer, S. H., and Boyle, E. (1977). Hypertension: Effects of social class and racial admixture: The results of a cohort study in the Black population of Charleston, S.C., *Amer. J. Pub. Hlth.*, 67, 634–9.

Tyroler, H. A. (1977). The Detroit Project studies of blood pressure: A prologue and review of related studies and epidemiological issues, *J. Chron. Dis.*, 30, 613–24.

Harburg, E., Gleibermann, L., Roeper, P., Schork, M.A., and Schull, W. J. (1978). Skin color, ethnicity and blood pressure. I. Detroit Blacks, *Amer. J. Publ. Hlth.*, 68, 1177–83.

Harburg, E., Gleibermann, L., Roeper, P., Schork, M.A., and Schull, W. J. (1978). Skin color, ethnicity and blood pressure. II. Detroit Whites, *Amer. J. Publ. Hlth.*, 68, 1184–88.

Tyroler, H. A., and James, S. A. (1978). Blood pressure and skin color, *Amer. J. Publ. Hlth.*, 68, 1170–2.

157. Goldschmidt, E. (1963) *The Genetics of Migrant and Isolate Populations*, Baltimore.
Motulsky, A., and Goodman, A., eds. (1978) *Genetic Diseases Among Ashkenazi Jews*, New York.

158. Fraser, F. C., and McKusick, V. A., eds. (1970). *Congenital Malformations. Proceedings of the Third International Conference, The Hague, 1969*, New York.

159. Goodwin, D. W., Schulsinger, F., Hermansen, L., Guze, S. B., and Winokur, G. (1973) Alcohol problems in adoptees raised apart from biological parents, *Arch. Gen. Psych.* 28, 238–43.

160. Reed, D. M., and Stanley, F. J., eds. (1977). *The Epidemiology of Prematurity*, Baltimore.

161. Ford, A. B. (1976). *Urban Health in America*, New York.

162. Belmont, L., Cohen, P., Dryfoos, J., Stein, Z., Zayac, S. (1981). Maternal age and children's intelligence, in *Teenage Parents and their Offspring*, ed., Scott, K. G., Field, T., Robertson, E., New York, pp. 177–94.
Sandler, H. M., Vietze, P. M., O'Connor, S. (1981). Obstetric and neonatal outcome following intervention with pregnant teenagers, in *Teenage Parents and their Offspring*, ed. Scott, K. G., Field, T., Robertson, E., New York, pp. 249–63.
Rothenberg, R. B., and Varga, P. E. (1981). The relationship between age of mother and child health and development, *Amer. J. Pub. Hlth.*, 71, 810–17.

163. Dohrenwend, B. P. (1966). Social status and psychological disorders: An issue of substance and an issue of method, *Amer. Sociol. Rev.*, 31, 4–34.

164. Dohrenwend, B. P., and Dohrenwend, B. S. (1969). *Social Status and Psychological Disorder*, New York.
Dohrenwend, B. P. (1975). Sociocultural and sociopsychological factors in the genesis of mental disorders, *J. Hlth. Soc. Behav.*, 16, 365–92.

165. Jarvis, E. (1971; first publ., 1855). *Insanity and Idiocy in Massachusetts: Report of the Commission on Lunacy*, Cambridge, Mass.

166. Adelstein, A. M., Downham, D. Y., Stein, Z. A., and Susser, M. W. (1968). The epidemiology of mental illness in an English city, *Soc. Psychiat.*, 3, 47–59.

167. Hollingshead, A., and Redlich, F. (1958). *Social Class and Mental Illness*, New Haven.
Jaco, E. (1960). *Social Epidemiology of Mental Disorders: A Psychiatric Survey of Texas*, New York.

168. Susser, M. W. (1968). *Community Psychiatry: Epidemiologic and Social Themes*, New York.

169. Booth, A., and Edwards, J. N. (1976). Crowding and family relations, *Amer. Sociol. Rev.*, 41, 308–21.
Gove, W. R., Hughes, M., and Galle, O. R. (1979). Overcrowding in the home: An empirical investigation of its possible psychological consequences, *Amer. Sociol. Rev.*, 44, 59–80.

170. Goode, W. (1956). *Women in Divorce*, New York.
Kornhauser, A. (1965). *Mental Health of the Industrial Worker*, New York.

Rutter, M. L., Quinton, D., and Yule, B. A. (1976). *Family Pathology and Disorder in the Children*, New York.

Cobb, S., and Kasl, S. V. (1977). *Termination: The Consequences of Job Loss*, Washington, D.C.

171. Lindemann, E. (1944). Symptomatology and management of acute grief, *Amer. J. Psychiat.*, *101*, 141–48.

Wolf, S., and Wolff, H. G. (1947). *Human Gastric Function*, London.

Selye, H. (1950). *The Physiology and Pathology of Exposure to Stress*, Montreal.

Meyer, A. (1951). The life chart and the obligation of specifying positive data in psychopathological diagnosis, in *The Collected Papers of Adolf Meyer, Vol. III, Medical Teaching*, ed. Winters, E. E., Baltimore.

Grinker, R. (1953). *Psychosomatic Research*, New York.

Hill, Jr., S. R. (1956). Studies on adreno-cortical and psychological response to stress in man, *Arch. Int. Med.*, *97*, 269–98.

Engel, G. L. (1962). *Psychological Development in Health and Disease*, Philadelphia.

172. Langner, T. S., and Michael, S. T. (1963). *Life Stress and Mental Health*, New York.

Brown, G. W., Ni Bhrolchain, M., and Harris, T. O. (1975). Social class and psychiatric disturbance among women in an urban population, *Sociology*, *9*, 225–54.

Kessler, R. C. (1979). Stress, social status and psychological distress, *J. Hlth. Soc. Behav.*, *20*, 100–8.

Kessler, R. C., and Cleary, P. D. (1980). Social class and psychological distress, *Amer. Sociol. Rev.*, *45*, 463–78.

173. Myers, J. K., Lindenthal, J. J., and Pepper, M. P. (1975). Life events, social integration and psychiatric symptomatology, *J. Hlth. Soc. Behav.*, *16*, 421–27.

174. Pearlin, L. I., and Schooler, C. (1978). The structure of coping, *J. Hlth. Soc. Behav.*, *19*, 2–21.

175. Cassel, J. (1976). The contribution of the social environment to host resistance, *Amer. J. Epidem.*, *104*, 107–23.

176. Srole, L., Langner, T. S., Michael, S. T., Opler, M. K., and Rennie, T. A. C. (1962). *Mental Health in the Metropolis*, Vol. I., New York.

Leighton, D. C., Harding, J. S., Macklin, D. B., MacMillan, A. M., and Leighton, A. H. (1963). *The Character of Danger*, New York.

Weissman, M. M., and Klerman, G. L. (1977). Sex differences and the epidemiology of depression, *Arch. Gen. Psych.*, *34*, 98–111.

Weissman, M. M., and Myers, J. K. (1978). Rates and risks of depressive symptoms in the United States urban community, *Acta. Psychia. Scand.*, *57*, 219–31.

177. Paykel, E. S. (1974). Life stress and psychiatric disorders, in *Stressful Life Events*, ed. Dohrenwend, B. S., and Dohrenwend, B. P., New York, pp. 135–49.

Jacobsen, S., Fasman, F., and DiMascio, A. (1975). Deprivation in the childhood of depressed women, *J. Nerv. Ment. Dis.*, *160*, 5–14.

Brown, G. W., Harris, T., and Copeland, J. R. (1977) Depression and loss, *Brit. J. Psychiat.*, *130*, 1–18.

Rutter, M. (1979). Maternal deprivation, 1972–1978: New findings, new concepts, new approaches, *Child Develop.*, 283–305.

Bowlby, J. (1980). *Attachment and Loss*, Vol. 3, New York.

178. Gove, W., and Tudor, J. (1973). Adult sex roles and mental illness, *Amer. J. Sociol.*, *77*, 812–35.

Gove, W., and Geerken, M. (1977). The effect of children and employment on the mental health of married men and women, *Social Forces, 56*, 66–76.

Richman, N. (1978). Depression in mothers of young children, *J. Roy. Soc. Med., 71*, 489–93.

Richman, J. (1978). *Psychological and psychophysiological distress in employed women and housewives: Class, age and ethnic differences*, Ph.D. thesis, Columbia Univ., New York.

179. Faris, R. E. L., and Dunham, H. W. (1939). *Mental Disorders in Urban Areas: An Ecological Study of Schizophrenia and Other Psychoses*, New York.

180. Susser, M. W., Stein, Z. A., Mountney, G. H., and Freeman, H. L. (1970). Chronic disability following mental illness in an English city. Part I. Total prevalence in and out of mental hospital, *Soc. Psychiat., 5*, 63–68.

Susser, M. W., Stein, Z. A., Mountney, G. H., and Freeman, H. L. (1970) Chronic disability following mental illness in an English city. Part II. The location of patients in hospital and community, *Soc. Psychiat., 5*, 69–76.

181. Heston, L. L. (1966). Psychiatric disorders in foster-home-reared children of schizophrenic mothers, *Brit. J. Psychiat., 112*, 819–25.

Kety, S. S., Rosenthal, D., Wender, P. H., Schulsinger, F., and Jacobsen, B. (1975). Mental illness in the biological and adoptive families of individuals who have become schizophrenic: A preliminary report based on psychiatric interviews, in *Genetic Research in Psychiatry*, ed., Fieve, R. R., and Rosenthal, D., Baltimore, pp. 147–66.

182. Kidd, K. K., and Cavalli-Sforza, L. L. (1973). An analysis of the genetics of schizophrenia, *Social Biology, 20*, 254–65.

183. Clark, R. E. (1949). Psychoses, income and occupational prestige: Schizophrenia in American cities, *Amer. J. Sociol., 54*, 433–40.

184. Hare, E. H. (1956). Mental illness and social conditions in Bristol, *J. Ment. Sci., 102*, 349–57.

185. Stein, L. (1957). Social class gradient in schizophrenia, *Brit. J. Prev. Soc. Med., 11*, 181–95.

186. Gerard, D. L. and Houston, L. G. (1953). Family setting and the social ecology of schizophrenia, *Psych. Quart., 27*, 90–101.

187. Brown, G. W., Bone, M., Dalison, B., and Wing, J. K. (1966). *Schizophrenia and Social Care*, London.

188. Goldberg, E. M., and Morrison, S. L. (1963). Schizophrenia and social class, *Brit. J. Psychiat., 109*, 785–802.

189. Dunham, H. W. (1965). *Community and Schizophrenia: An Epidemiologic Analysis*, Detroit.

Turner, R. J., and Wagenfeld, M. (1967). Occupational mobility and schizophrenia: An assessment of the social causation and social selection hypotheses, *Amer. Sociol. Rev., 32*, 104–13.

190. Kohn, M. L. (1972). Class, family, and schizophrenia: A reformulation, *Social Forces, 50*, 296–304.

Mechanic, D. (1972). Social class and schizophrenia: Some requirements for a plausible theory of social influence, *Social Forces, 50*, 305–9.

Kohn, M. L. (1972). Rejoinder to David Mechanic, *Social Forces, 50*, 310–13.

191. Birley, J. L. T., and Brown, G. W. (1970). Crisis and life change preceding the onset or relapse of acute schizophrenia: Clinical aspects, *Brit. J. Psychiat., 116*, 327–33.

192. **Myers, J. K.,** and **Roberts, B. H.** (1959). *Family and Class Dynamics in Mental Illness,* New York.

193. **Liem, J. H.** (1980). Family studies of schizophrenia: An update and commentary, *Schiz. Bull., 6,* 429–55.

194. **Townsend, P.** (1979). *Poverty in the United Kingdom,* Berkeley.
     Ryan, W. (1981). *Equality,* New York.

195. **Morris, J. N.,** and **Heady, J. A.** (1955). Social and biological factors in infant mortality. I. Objects and methods, *Lancet, 1,* 343–49.
     Heady, J. A., Daly, C., and **Morris, J. N.** (1955). Social and biological factors in infant mortality. II. Variation of mortality with mother's age and parity, *Lancet, 1,* 395–97.
     Daly, C., Heady, J. A., and **Morris, J. N.** (1955). Social and biological factor in infant mortality. III. The effect of mother's age and parity on social class differences in infant mortality, *Lancet, 1,* 445–48.
     Heady, J. A., Stevens, C. F., Daly, C., and **Morris, J. N.** (1955). Social and biological factors in infant mortality. IV. The independent effects of social class, region, the mother's age and her parity, *Lancet, 1,* 499–502.
     Morris, J. N., and **Heady, J. A.** (1955). Social and biological factors in infant mortality. V. Mortality in relation to the father's occupation 1911–50, *Lancet, 1,* 554–59.
     Morrison, S. L., Heady, J. A., and **Morris, J. N.** (1959). Social and biologic factors in infant mortality. VIII. Mortality in the post-neonatal period, *Arch. Dis. Childh., 34,* 101–14.
     Illsley, R. (1967). The sociological study of reproduction and its outcome, in *Childbearing—Its Social and Psychological Aspects,* ed., Richardson, S.A., and Guttmacher, A. F., Baltimore, pp. 75–141.
     Shannon, D. C., and **Kelly, D. H.** (1982). SIDS and near-SIDS, Parts I and II, *New Eng. J. Med., 306,* 959–65, 1022–28.

196. **Adelstein, A. M.,** and **G. C. White** (1976). Causes of children's death analysed by social class, in *Child Health: A Collection of Studies,* London, H.M.S.O., pp. 25–40.
     Brown, G. W., and **Davidson, S.** (1978). Social class, psychiatric disorder of mother, and accidents to children, *Lancet, 1,* 378–80.

197. **Fox, A. J.,** and **Adelstein, A. M.** (1978). Occupational mortality: Work or way of life? *J. Epidem. Comm. Hlth., 32,* 73–78.

198. **Morris, J. N.** (1979). Social inequalities undiminished, *Lancet, 1,* 87–90.

199. **Pratt, L.** (1971). The relationship of socioeconomic status to health, *Amer. J. Pub. Hlth., 61,* 281–291.
     Khosla, T., and **Lowe, C. R.** (1972). Obesity and smoking habits by social class, *Brit. J. Prev. Soc. Med., 26,* 249–56.
     Coburn, D., and **Pope, C. R.** (1974). Socioeconomic status and preventive health behavior, *J. Hlth. Soc. Behav., 15,* 67–78.
     Kirk, T. R. (1978). Breast-feeding and mother's occupation, *Lancet, 2,* 1201–02.
     Ashwell, M., North, W. R. S., and **Meade, T. W.** (1978). Social class, smoking, and obesity, *Brit. Med. J., 2,* 1466–67.
     Kraus, J. F., Borhani, N. O., and **Franti, C. E.** (1980). Socioeconomic status, ethnicity, and risk of coronary heart disease, *Amer. J. Epidem., 111,* 407–414.

200. **Riessman, C. K.** (1974). The use of the health services by the poor, *Social Policy, 5,* 41–49.
     Davis, K. (1976). Medicaid payments and utilization of medical services by the poor, *Inquiry, 13,* 122–35.

Dutton, D. B. (1978). Explaining the low use of health services by the poor: Costs, attitudes or delivery systems, *Amer. Social. Rev.*, 43, 348–68.

Rundall, T. G., and Wheeler, J. R. C. (1979). The effect of income on use of preventive care: An evaluation of alternative explanations, *J. Hlth. Soc. Behav.*, 20, 397–406.

201. Valentine, C. (1968). *Culture and Poverty: Critique and Counter Proposals*, Chicago.

Leacock, E. B., ed. (1971). *The Culture of Poverty: A Critique*, New York.

Brenner, M. H. (1976). Estimating the social costs of national economic policy: Implications for mental and physical health, and criminal aggression, Joint Economic Committee of Congress, Paper No. 5, G.P.O., Washington, D.C.

Elinson, J. (1977). Discussion of papers presented at the session, Have we narrowed the gaps in health status between the poor and nonpoor, *Medical Care*, 15, 675–77.

McKinlay, J. (1979). A case for refocusing upstream: The political economy of illness, in *Patients, Physicians and Illness*, 3rd ed., ed. Jaco, E. G., New York, pp. 9–25.

202. Syme, S. L., and Berkman, L. F. (1976). Social class, susceptibility and sickness, *Amer. J. Epidem.*, 104, 1–8.

Eyer, J., and Sterling, P. (1977). Stress-related mortality and social organization, *Rev. Rad. Polit. Econ.*, 9, 1–44.

Najman, J. M. (1980). Theories of disease causation and the concept of a general susceptibility: A review, *Soc. Sci. and Med.*, 14A, 231–37.

203. Kasl, S. V., Gore, S., and Cobb, S., (1975). The experience of losing a job: Reported changes in health, symptoms and illness behavior, *Psychosomatic Medicine*, 37, 106–22.

Draper, P., Dennis, J, Griffiths, J., Partridge, T., and Popay, J. (1979). Micro-processors, macro-economic policy, and public health, *Lancet*, 1, 373–75.

Dooley, D., and Catalano, R. (1980). Economic change as a cause of behavioral disorder, *Psychol. Bull.*, 87, 450–68.

204. Kosa, J., and Zola, I. K., eds. (1975). *Poverty and Health: A Sociological Analysis*, rev. ed., Cambridge, Mass.

Antonovsky, A. (1979). *Health, Stress and Coping*, San Francisco.

205. Susser, M. (1980). Prevention and cost containment, *Bull. New York Acad. Med.*, 56, 45–52.

206. Gramsci, A. (1970). *Prison Notebooks*, London.

Navarro, V. (1976). *Medicine under Capitalism*, New York.

Williams, R. (1977). *Marxism and Literature*, London.

Stark, E. (1977). The epidemic as a social event, *Int. J. Hlth. Serv.*, 7, 681–705.

7

Community: status, roles, networks, mobility

Much has been made in recent times of "community" medicine, "community" psychiatry, and "community" participation. These concepts imply the emergence of health and medical services beyond the walls of established institutions. Such services can cover the whole population of defined areas without exclusion, and they aim to exploit local resources outside the institutions to better people's health and strengthen the supportive care available to them. Effective community health care requires an appreciation of the social structure of the local communities to be served, of social standing and modes of interaction, and of the motives and values that underlie them. Moreover, understanding of community structure and relations contributes also to a better understanding of the distribution and the causes of the disorders of health that create the need for community health care. Whether or not by design, the work of health professionals relates to communities. Practitioners deal with patients drawn from one local area; most hospital physicians draw their patients from limited, if wider, districts; and health officers employed by local government deal with the people of defined administrative areas.

So far we have discussed the division of the whole population in terms of social classes founded on the categories of occupation and education. This chapter will continue the discussion of the structure of developed Western societies. But the variation in the types of residential aggregates that compose such societies, from single families living in isolated farmhouses to families massed in cities, makes any simple means of representing social divisions a crude approximation. Some hamlets and villages may have homogeneous populations marked by persistence of residence, distinctive customs, habits, and modes of speech, and common values (1). The activities of one individual are known to all, and local interests are judged by a more or less uniform scale of values. But others may be residential suburbs for a nearby town, with socially heterogeneous populations many of whom work elsewhere (2). Even when villagers work on the land it does not follow that they will have rural values and attitudes. Intensive farming may be carried out in close proximity to towns, and even within the boundaries of large towns, and in these circumstances farm workers take part in urban activities; their estimation of their interests may well differ from that of farm workers in the remote countryside.

Towns also vary in character, from older communities dependent on one economic activity, such as coal or cotton or marketing (3), to new towns planned to house a socially heterogeneous population. Several patterns have been discovered in cities across the United States. In Washington, D.C., for instance, lower-class people were concentrated in the center and the higher classes on the outskirts. This pattern is typical of a metropolis that is large and long settled. In cities like Tucson, Arizona, higher-class people were found in the center and lower-class on the outskirts. In cities like Los Angeles, both the highest- and the lowest-class people were overrepresented in central areas. These Tucson and Los Angeles patterns were associated with smaller and newer cities. Other cities showed no distinctive arrangement (4).

The evolution of modern urban spatial forms cannot be separated from that of economic and social function. Historically, cities were catchments for labor in the commercial, industrial and service sectors of the economy, producing specific kinds of wealth. Migrants who had been forced off the land or drawn to better prospects in cities swelled the labor pool. The harnessing of this labor force lay behind the early growth of industrial cities. Cultural considerations entered as well, sometimes in unobtrusive ways. Engels, for example, showed how the configuration of nineteenth century Manchester, the textile capital of England—with working-class dwellings and business districts concentrated in the inner city, affluent housing in the outlying areas, and access to the center provided by thoroughfares lined with shops—shielded genteel upper-class eyes from many aspects of working-class life. In the United States, distinctive urban forms appeared at different stages of industrial development: mercantile port cities in the colonial era; industrial factory towns in the nineteenth century; and corporate cities in the postwar period. Each urban form is characterized by typical patterns of land division (as between residence and workplace), transport, marketing, communication, and social class interaction (5).

Within the great conurbations in which the families of industrial societies live, activities are often segregated, and areas are specialized into industrial, commercial, and residential districts. Residential districts vary in social composition, from old established working-class neighborhoods near the centers of towns to new housing estates in the suburbs (6). Some housing estates are purely residential areas set at a distance from factories and workshops; others have factories sited within their boundaries or nearby. Others accommodate only the well-to-do, who work over a much wider area; and still others contain a heterogeneous population of many occupations.

Some observed patterns are the unplanned consequences of larger economic forces acting in a given geographic area. Thus, in the postwar period in the United States, waves of blacks leaving the south and of rural migrants leaving depressed farming regions led to pronounced changes in some northern cities. The poorest, lowest status groups tended to congregate in the inner city core, many of which slowly deteriorated or were already collapsing. The more privileged classes moved to "bedroom" community suburbs which were linked to the center city (where finance and commerce were still located) through rail and highway arteries (7). In Latin America, squatter settlements (or "land invasions" as they are known locally) have been conceived by some as the exploitation by the poor of unused ecological niches. Such "marginal" dwellings are also in fact an integral part of the local polity and economy (8).

Other changes are the deliberate result of planning. The systematic eradication of "skid row" areas and renovation of old single-room-occupancy dwellings, which took place in the United States in the 1960s and 1970s, represented the combined interests of city administrators and private developers. Upgrading property values raises both local tax revenues and rental income. The housing and population composition of metropolitan neighborhoods can be strongly influenced by restrictive zoning ordinances. New York City today still bears the imprint of a 1929 Regional Plan that set clear guidelines for urban land use. Priority was given to capacity to pay rent, a principle reflecting the dominance of real estate and finance capital on the planning board. As a result, choice areas of Manhattan are restricted exclusively to high-rise office buildings, expensive retail stores, and elegant residences. Older manufacture, like the garment industry, was confined to well-demarcated enclaves. Working-class residential districts have for the most part been pushed to the outer boroughs (9).

Administrative boundaries of local authorities create further complexities. They may include all residential areas; in others, the boundary between two local authorities may run down the middle of a street and divide an otherwise homogeneous residential area. In most metropolitan areas political boundaries are anachronistic: in England, the Manchester conurbation is divided into a patchwork of 52 separate units (10); New York City abuts on three states, and there are at least 1200 local authorities within 50 miles of Times Square.

Thus there is wide variation in the coincidence of homes, places of work, shopping and marketing centers, administrative and political units, and the general amenities of life. For many people in urban areas the "local community" simply comprises the group of homes and families in a restricted neighborhood, the place where they feel "at home" within urban society. These places are a focus of emotion or sentiment, and they have lost or failed to acquire other functions and purposes of communities (11).

On the other hand, some people live in areas with a sufficient concentration of workplaces, shops, schools, churches, and places of entertainment to enable them to live their lives wholly within them, there to find all their social relationships. In such places, the people usually tend to be culturally homogeneous, and to have a strong sense of common identity and community. These places are usually small towns or the older neighborhoods of large ones; but similar communities are also found in rural and fishing areas. The persistence of the sense of identity and loyalty depends on continuity of occupation and residence between successive generations, continuities still common in Britain although less so in the United States. Many miners' sons in the Lancashire town of Ashton, dockers' sons in London's Bethnal Green, and farmers' sons in Gosforth also became miners, dockers, and farmers. In these communities, when jobs and homes were hard to get, the older people were able to use their established social networks to obtain jobs and homes for young people. Thus they preserved continuity of occupation across generations.

The context of community itself undergoes constant evolution. An unusual opportunity to observe how much changes and how much remains the same is provided by three successive studies of a midwestern community, given the name of "Middletown" (12). The first and third study are separated by half a century. This interval of time saw accelerating change in the structure of the economy and labor markets, in communication and transportation, in the level of schooling of the populace at large, in the social relations of the family and composition of households, in religious affiliation and sexual attitudes and behavior. Yet Middletown, it seems, resisted, modified, and adapted to many such changes.

Class inequalities in Middletown have diminished in the last 40 years, reversing a trend begun in the late 1800s. Labor unions have firmly established themselves in the blue-collar community. Gross disparities in the living styles of different social classes have all but disappeared. Access to health care, ability to own a home, and leisure time are all more equitably distributed than before.

A major change took place in the economic base of the community. The large glassworks that had been a major employer in Middletown is now a diversified multinational corporation. The firm curtailed its local operations, and located its chief interests and corporate headquarters elsewhere. Employment patterns changed substantially. The proportion of skilled craftspeople in the labor force fell by more than 50 per cent, and blue-collar work too declined. At the same time, the proportion of working wives nearly doubled, almost solely owing to the addition of middle-class women who elected to work out of interest as well as for economic advantage. The counterpart to an eroding local industrial base was a growing federal government presence. In 1925, nearly all Middletown families earned their livelihood in the private sector. Even in the grip of the Great Depression, a minority of families (one in four) were on relief rolls. By 1977, the form, the distribution, and the amount of public support had changed markedly. Today, the day-to-day operations of local government are dependent upon state and federal funds. At least half of Middletown's families were receiving public support in some form, the bulk subsidized in the main indirectly by the federal government. Many of these indirect subsidies do not go to support the poor; benefits like government subsidized medical care, housing, and welfare are more than balanced by tax remissions on home mortgages, federal pensions, and the like.

Middletown beliefs and values had lost some of the insular quality that formerly typified midwestern towns. Regulations governing racial integration in schools, safety standards in factories, and the conduct of court proceedings testify to the federal presence in other than financial matters. Through newspapers, radio, and television, everyone in society is in touch with the course of events and opinions. Middletowners spent an average of 28 hours a week watching television, read more out-of-town newspapers, listened to more radio, and saw more movies than ever before. To take but one index of the effect of the multiplication of communications from the outside: while Middletowners were no less religious than before, they were much more tolerant of other people's beliefs.

Family life appeared to be the most enduring feature of Middletown's culture. The decisive shift from a traditional to a modern family (where children stay in school rather than go out to earn or learn a trade) occurred in the first three decades of the century. Since then Middletown families have exhibited unanticipated stability. Marriage·and divorce rates, family size and, among working-class families, proportion of working wives, did not change markedly in the ensuing years. Relations between the generations seemed no more strained than they had been 50 years before. If anything, observers found that the quality of home life, as measured by such indices as the amount of time parents spend with children, had improved.

How typical an American town Middletown might be remains open to question. Some of the continuities detected may have been artificially enhanced through the use of the same questionnaires used by earlier researchers. For other communities, the loss of local economic autonomy has been less benign (13). As blue-collar work and wage levels dropped in the late 1960s and throughout the 1970s more and more family members were forced into the labor market, family networks were disrupted and households migrated in order to survive. Dependence on social service agencies increased. In a Massachusetts community, two distinct patterns of service use were found. High unemployment rates were associated with increased use by the jobless of outpatient mental health services; high employment rates, on the other hand, were found to be associated with high rates of psychiatric hospitalization (14). The author proposed that the increased number of working household members weakened the family's own resources of support and diminished its capacity to care for disabled members. Interviews with hospital staff tended to corroborate this impression. Of course other factors, such as the greater availability of such services and a change in public attitudes about mental disorder, must be taken into account as well.

No study of a single community can encompass the whole range of the relationships of its members. The web of social interaction is extended beyond residential boundaries by "communities of affiliation." Thus most adults, wherever they live, are also members of associations that serve many vital interests; even in the most homogeneous neighborhoods such affiliations unite people with other members of society who reside elsewhere. Separation of home from place of work and multiplicity of roles fractionalizes community experience, and extends it into the larger society. Outside associations and activities enhance the influence on behavior of external events and cultural styles. Hence, a bus driver in a small village may go on strike in support of trade unionists at the other end of the country with whom he has no personal contact, despite the inconvenience that his action may cause to his relatives, friends, and neighbors, and in the face of their expressed disapproval.

Forms of behavior and their consequences for health care are a central concern of medicine and public health. These forms vary with occupation, skill, and education, yet much individual behavior anticipates or responds to the expectations of others. For these controls of behavior to operate effectively, they must take place within some kind of community life. In societies where communities are so variable, and the process of social mobility can change the social position of an individual many times during a lifetime, the controls over behavior are correspondingly complex and variable.

Status, role, and values

Interests and pursuits that cut across communities can be conceived in terms of status, role, and values. In each field of activity in which a person interacts with others, he or she acquires a *status*, and with this social position go certain expected forms of behavior, particular *roles* one is expected to play. Role is the dynamic aspect of status, and provides the link between individual behavior and social structure. A woman may be at one and the same time a wife, mother, daughter, sister, aunt, and grandmother, an official in a political party, the chairperson of a neighborhood organization, a lay preacher, and a physician, and each activity carries its own status. Performance of the multiple roles associated with each status will contribute to the estimate of social standing in the eyes of the person and of others. People anticipate predictable responses in specific situations according to the status of the parties involved; this *role expectation* is the habitual behavior that guides the forms of social intercourse.

Social statuses, singly or combined, will differ in significance for different social situations. They may be important in a man's social relations within his home town, but quite unimportant if he moves to a capital city; as a house physician or an intern for example, he may not count for much compared with his senior colleagues in the hospital, whereas in his home town his social standing may be high. The social standing of an individual is thus not a fixed quantity, but a variable that alters from one social situation to another.

Role expectation exists in all societies, together with the sanctions to ensure compliance with the expected behavior. Patterns of expected behavior are learned, and hence biological and social factors can be disentangled from one another; the behavior appropriate to a status may be acquired by anyone of the proper age and sex. Even the "natural" emotional responses considered appropriate to a relationship may be acquired. Adoptive parents, for instance, can feel as strongly about their children as biological parents feel about theirs. Biological ties are formally irrelevant to status in many economic and social activities—for instance, the relationship of employer and employee, teacher and student, shopkeeper and customer, doctor and patient. Even in statuses that would seem to be organically determined by age or sex, or by physical handicaps like deafness, blindness, and paralysis, many elements of status and role are in truth socially determined. Thus, for example, there is nothing inherent in biological sex that affects an individual's performance of domestic chores, clerical duties, or clinical responsibilities; yet the gender of the participants in a relationship is a pervasive social determinant of roles, whether in households between husbands and wives, in offices between secretaries and executives, or on hospital wards between nurses and doctors. With physical impairments, social definitions of role as handicapped may exaggerate dysfunction and limit the emergence of an individual's full potential (15).

A status, as distinct from the individual designated to hold it, is in essence a collection of rights and duties, defined by social usage and understood by others. Two types of status, *ascribed status* and *achieved status*, correspond with the nature of certain attributes of individuals (16). An ascribed status does not depend on innate ability or arise from the social rewards of individual performance; it is usually assigned at birth, and thereby the role can be predicted and the individual trained in the appropriate behavior. The simplest and most obvious of these attributes is age or generation; a more complex example is gender. In all societies, familial relationships are used as reference points for ascribed statuses, the most universal being the relationship of mother and child, which in turn determines a whole series of future statuses. In many peasant societies the majority of statuses are ascribed, and given to individuals on the basis of their gender, age, and familial relationships (17,18).

In contrast, an achieved status is not assigned at birth, but is acquired to the extent that social and cultural structure permit, through specific ability and individual effort in the course of life; in principle, the status must therefore be achieved through competition or other methods of selection. The separation of ascribed from achieved statuses is a major distinction between industrial societies and the simpler societies. In traditional societies, for example, the elementary family is usually a unit of a larger kinship structure, and kinship relations are basic to ascribed statuses and to most activities, domestic, economic, legal, religious, and political (19). In industrial society kinship is concerned primarily with domestic relations, and achieved statuses pervade most other fields of activity. Occupation is a basic achieved status, for it helps to determine in turn the acquisition of other statuses, and hence of social position or social class. Even in industrial society, however, achieved statuses do not replace ascribed statuses, but instead supplement them and help to define the social positions of individuals more clearly.

This is not to say that family statuses have no effect on other statuses. While formally irrelevant to achieved status, social advantage or disadvantage can be crucial. In those family businesses in which a son is trained as a "Crown Prince" to succeed his father, a family status determines an occupational status (20). These are special cases, where the adoption of an occupational status is related to the eventual inheritance of property; most people work for salaries or wages, and fathers, mothers, sons, and daughters often have different occupations. Where relatives do have the same occupation, their familial relationship is supposed to be subsidiary in the context of work.

The multiplicity of personal statuses and roles with different values and obligations is the basis of many conflicts in society. At the same time, conflict may be avoided when in a particular situation one or another role can be assigned salience. No individual can exercise all roles simultaneously, so at any moment one has both *active* and *latent* statuses (18,21). Accordingly, any particular status among the many that each individual holds can be ignored in circumstances where it has no direct bearing. In a game of tennis, it is of no account that a player is a son or mother or cousin; in principle, the familial status of each player has no bearing on the game.

On the other hand, the demands of social structure are not always consistent, and a person may be called on to choose between two courses of action, each of them appropriate in terms of a particular status, but irreconcilable in a social situation where both statuses are active. An academic physician often has the statuses of practitioner and research scientist: in caring for patients in an ethical manner, ideally he or she should act in their interests alone, yet as scientist he or she may wish to subject them to risky procedures to gain information that can be in the interests only of other future patients. In the modern-day practice of medicine this conflict is acute (22,23).

Role conflict has other, subtler sources as well. It may stem from the inconsistencies in the role itself, as, for example, when physicians are called upon to be both gentle healers and aggressive combatants against disease. It may arise from discrepancies between one's self-image and the demands of the role one assumes. Role conflict can be especially acute when the social setting in which a given role is active gives rise to expectations and obligations from disparate sources. Anyone will experience role conflict who occupies an intercalary status in which he or she must respond to the different interests and expectations of groups, each with a legitimate claim on one's performance. Typical instances of such situations are the industrial medical officer who stands between management and workers, the military medical officer who must care for soldiers and take orders from superior officers, or the college physician positioned between students and administration. These physicians treat patients in the confidence enjoined by the Hippocratic ethic, but with the information gained it may seem to their employers and sometimes themselves that they can help managers, staff officers, and administrators make "better" decisions about workers, soldiers, and students (24).

Social roles and the demands attendant upon them are not immutable, however. Analysis of the conduct of everyday social intercourse reveals a high degree of ambiguity in the actual performance of roles. Individuals temper their investment in a given role and devise *ad hoc* solutions to resolve untenable situations. Conversely, the social structure is usually flexible enough to accommodate these departures. For the sake of ordered function in formal organizations, bureaucrats maintain a ritual of rules that are often meaningless to themselves as well as their clients (25).

In a clinical setting, the concepts of status and role can help the physician to frame questions relevant to the life problems of patients. Some individuals may be quite unable to fulfill their expected roles; for instance, the person suffering from chronic, almost asymptomatic schizophrenia may not be able to fulfill the roles appropriate to the status of husband or wife. Family "intolerance" can then send him or her back to the hospital (26). Any chronically handicapped patient may be in the same situation. Difficulties can also arise in situations that are, at least in part, of the individual's own making. Males in unconventional occupations (such as nursing) may experience unusual strain. The stereotypical "skid row" man rejects all roles usually expected of adult males and inhabits a sort of social limbo as a result. A transvestite rejects the role appropriate to ascribed gender status, and assumes behavior appropriate to the opposite sex. A woman who has statuses both as a professional worker and a mother may be frustrated in her desire to combine the obligations of wife, mother, and a career, a situation not uncommon among women doctors (27). This last example serves also to illustrate the necessity to conceive of status and role in historical as well as current context. It is as much the traditional exclusion of women from positions of power in Western society as it is the conflict between their responsibilities as wives or mothers and those incurred as professionals that makes their position difficult. Consider as well how the situation would change were it not assumed that parenting was essentially "mothering" and woman's work.

Roles are never defined in isolation; they require the consistent confirmation of others. Thus, the degree to which handicapped persons are made exceptional, even alien, can be compounded rather than alleviated by "helping" agencies. The interest of such agencies is often to maintain the distinctive status and the dependency of their clients in order to promote public recognition of their function. The benefits such a public interest group may bring to the class for whose interests it stands may run counter to the individual interests of those being served (28).

Regulation of social relations

Many aspects of the roles associated with ascribed and achieved statuses are regulated by law as well as by custom, particularly in such fundamental institutions as the family. Familial roles are diffuse and charged with emotion: a mother does not render her child a single service; parents are expected to love and favor their children; and, in general, all family relationships are fraught with the complexities that attend long-standing relations of intimacy and obligation. Still, the status of husband implies a pattern of expected behavior in which, as a last resort, the appropriate roles can be legally enforced; a father, for example, can be compelled by the court to support his child. Other roles may be regulated by custom, as in the allocation of household tasks or in the intricacies of courting (29). The nature of the sanctions used to enforce appropriate behavior depends on the system of values associated with statuses and roles.

The relationship of employer and employee is by contrast contractual, and kin relationship is formally irrelevant. The qualifications required by many occupational statuses in industrial society are technical, and must be obtained through training and education. Relations governed by contract are typical of the large-scale organizations in industrial society that have come to dominate industrial, commercial, educational, and administrative activities. In these organizations managers, technicians, supervisors, accountants, administrators, and other specialists are ranked in a hierarchy of positions of greater or lesser authority and prestige.

Entry and promotion depend in principle on individual capacity and merit exercised in free competition. These statuses must therefore be achieved, and cannot be ascribed. The role appropriate to a formal status is impersonal and anonymous; each incumbent of the status and actor of the role is deemed to be replaceable, and to act solely in terms defined by the functional requirements of the situation. Thus, formal roles are described as discrete and "affectively neutral," unlike familial roles (30). Nevertheless, many individuals in formal roles gain emotional and social satisfactions through the approbation given for their service, and such individuals are not solely dependent on the diffuse satisfactions gained from personal relations within family or neighborhood. Indeed, emotional involvements and impulsive desires may hinder the striving for achievement often expected in performing formal roles. This dichotomy between the impersonal values and expectations of formal roles and the emotional values and expectations of personal relations has been indicted by some as a factor in the *malaise* of industrial society (31). The revolt against reduction to sheer function has deep historical roots; it is at the heart of what Marx and others termed the *alienation* of the modern worker (32).

Relations between friends, neighbors, and acquaintances are based on personal qualities and attractions, usually take place between persons of roughly equal social status, and are informal and emotional (33). Although less fundamental to the continuance of society than economic and family relationships, these informal relations concern others not engaged in them and, here too, the appropriate roles and obligations are subject to regulation, if only by informal sanctions of gossip and public opinion. In preliterate societies, the degree of regulation exercised by such sanctions can be strict (34). In the industrial world, these loosely regulated relations are more variable, transient, and replaceable than the contractual relations of industry or marriage.

The behavior appropriate to the multiple roles of each person is therefore defined by different standards and regulated by controls of varying severity. These standards and controls range from the military and police power of the state, through the formal rules that govern bureaucratic organizations and functional associations, to the rules agreed upon by members of recreational clubs, and the sanctions of gossip over personal relations. The variety of available sanctions, and the range and degree of control each exerts, are functions of the sway of tradition, and the stage of political and economic development a society has reached. The modes of social control serve to resolve the conflicts that spring from opposed aims and values, and that threaten disruption to personal, domestic, economic, and social life (35).

The conflict of values and interests appears in the functional associations that serve and protect specific economic and other interests (for instance, trade unions, professional organizations, employers' federations, and political parties). They now play a significant part in the social lives of people in all industrial societies. These associations imply a common aim, and common values among members, that may not be shared with others, even with members of their own families (11). Where interests and aims are irreconcilable, society at large intervenes through the agency of the state. When these conflicts are between associations they are often about ends and not means, and therefore inherent and continuous. When the conflicts arise within functional associations, such as a trade union or professional institute, they are often about means and not ends, policy and not purpose, and are therefore reconcilable. It falls to the state to coordinate and protect the activities of other associations, and to mediate disruptive conflict between them.

It is the obligation of the state as well to uphold "law and order"—a successful political slogan because it describes the primary system of social rights, obligations, and values that in theory stand for the common interest, and not for anyone's specific interests. To carry out its mediating function, the state must maintain a certain autonomy from the claims of even powerful interests in society. It alone is invested with the ultimate coercive powers of imprisonment and death. These coercive powers confer other powers that go far beyond regulations. In modern capitalist society, the state increasingly assumes an interventionist role in the economy, and seeks to control disruptive market forces. The ideal democratic state that uses its power in the common interest of all has never been realized, and the political process at any level, local or national, can be represented as the struggle of particular groups to legitimize their special interests as the common interest. Groups who hold power try to retain it for the "common good," and groups excluded from power resist it for the same reason. Social expectations and the sanctions that ensure compliance with them are based on systems of value that have an affective as well as an ideological content and a material base; they express feelings and they also rationalize behavior (36).

In previous chapters the range of values common to a whole society was distinguished from other values special to individuals and groups, for instance those reared in the same neighborhood or subculture, so that a social class could be defined in part by the special values that underlie common attitudes, behavior, and the choice of friends and neighbors (37). For example, in the 1960s, a "good" husband in a working-class community was still one who gave his wife a fixed sum of money each week, who drank moderately, didn't "run around" with other women, and who did not interfere in household matters; he was not expected to help his wife at home (29,38). On the other hand, a "good" husband among professional people was one who shared household tasks and the rearing of children, who discussed his spending with his wife, and treated her as an intellectual equal and companion.

Social class differences in marital styles seem to have widened in some areas but diminished in others (12,39). Local circumstance plays a role in certain instances. When the economic situation worsens, working-class families become more than ever hostage to the chances of employment. The relationship of a young man and woman may be severely strained, for example, if the only work available is military service that will take a spouse away from home for extended periods of time. Middle-class couples tend to conform less with traditional gender stereotyping than do working-class couples—the male presumed to be cool and rational unless provoked; the female, vulnerable and ruled by emotion. Children learn early to emulate their parents, with working-class boys tending to be more controlled and less emotional than their middle-class counterparts. On the other hand, compared with earlier generations, husbands of both classes spend more time with their children and are more likely to help out with household chores. In Middletown, communication between working-class wives and husbands—including such once-taboo subjects as finances and sex—had improved markedly when compared to marriages thirty and fifty years ago.

In a given social situation some values take priority over others. Within formal organizations the status of individuals derives from the functions assigned to them, and judgments of their merit from efficiency in carrying out functions (40,41). Although clients of the organization, say the patients in a hospital, may give more weight to other values, and complain about the impersonality or inhumanity of the service (42), within the organization, promotion is supposed to depend on efficient performance. But since status in one sphere influences both role performance and the regard of others, an individual might gain favor with a superior because of kinship, shared schooling, or common values. Nepotism, and its modern equivalent the "old-boy network," involve the manipulation of formal roles in terms of roles appropriate to other situations.

The intrusion of informal values into formal organizations is not always deprecated. Some economic organizations employ only men with certain social characteristics, for instance, Roman Catholics or Episcopalians (43), or persons of the same ethnic group, or the relatives of employees. Industrial enterprises try to mitigate the affective neutrality and impersonality of formal roles in the interests of efficiency and profitability (44). Managers strive for "good human relations" by treating workers as "human beings," providing them with sympathetic advice about personal problems, and seeing to the welfare of their families. Japanese corporations are especially solicitous in this regard, to the possible benefit of the health of their employees (45). Policies of this kind draw on common values shared by all in the organization to reconcile inferiors to their situation. These common values are exhibited on such ritual occasions as Christmas parties, dances, and workshop outings, when people appear as "themselves" and not in their formal roles. The medieval institutions of the pilgrimage and the "feast of fools" and the role reversals practiced at Zulu "tribal" festivals (also practiced in the Roman holiday of Saturnalia) served much the same purpose, albeit on a grander scale (34,46).

Social mobility

Within communities in which people live and work a person, without changing occupational status, can be socially mobile through status acquired in other fields—in religion, for instance, or in local politics or sport (47). Social mobility in terms of a local prestige sytem is based on the unique combination of history, customs, social standards, and evaluation of occupational prestige that distinguishes one community from another. Residential movements within the community may keep in step with such social mobility.

Social standing and social mobility are therefore relative. An individual can rise and fall in terms of the values common to the whole society when he or she enters an occupation about whose standing there is broad agreement. Or one can rise and fall in terms of the values of the local community, without achieving a high-status occupation, through multiple statuses and roles. Place of residence, possessions, and mode of life all contribute to one's social standing. These local prestige systems are based on the competition of individuals and groups for prestige in terms of *reference groups* who set the standard for competition (41,48). As discussed previously, people use the term "class" to refer to these social differences in terms of local ratings of social position and social standing. They use it to refer simultaneously to common ratings of high-status occupations that set the standards for the upper levels of prestige. In the vernacular of local prestige systems, social classes cannot be defined in terms of occupations with much validity. Here the class concept describes relative success and failure in a competitive local system. Extra-occupational factors weigh heavily among the many manual workers whose job functions and earnings do not draw sharp lines between them. A skilled worker who owns a home and automobile, is active in church affairs, and has a daugher in college regards himself, and is regarded by others, as "middle class," and conforms to that mode of life in all but education and occupation.

In society at large, the greater potential for mobility possessed by persons in professional occupations is the outcome of two connected processes: the growth of science and technology, and the specialization of techniques now used by large-scale organizations. Since civil engineers first applied the theoretical principles of mechanics to practical purposes in early-nineteenth-century Britain, and monopolized their function by forming a professional association that required qualifications of competence, the number and variety of professional skills have continued to grow. The number of managers, supervisors, and administrators also proliferated (49), and they too began to claim professional status.

These salaried professionals are employed by large-scale organizations of all kinds—economic, productive, administrative, and commercial—both private and public. Many of these organizations operate on a national or even an international scale, and now link communities and regions together. Large-scale organizations absorb small local concerns and turn them into branches or departments, so that there is a movement away from local ownership to centralized control and direction (50). The state, too, has extended its services since the Second World War to include even the smallest and most remote community. In England, almost every community, from village to conurbation, has sited within it a branch, workshop, department, or office of several large-scale organizations, and almost certainly some branch of central government. The town of Glossop in Derbyshire, for instance, had only one civil servant before the First World War; in 1951, for a population no larger than before, it had about twenty senior civil servants, and many junior ones, as well as the managers and specialists of large-scale private industries (51).

Medical institutions, too, have experienced expansion and specialization. This is well illustrated by a comparison of the record of a typical cardiac patient at the Presbyterian Hospital in New York in 1908 with that of a similar patient in 1938. The 1908 patient was attended by two physicians and one specialist in all, and had two and a half pages of case notes; the 1938 patient was attended by eight physicians and ten specialists, and had 29 pages of notes (52).° The consequences for relations between patients and doctors are profound.

The balance between the traditional professions of medicine, law, and religion and the new professions mentioned above has altered considerably: engineering, building, and scientific professions outnumber the traditional ones by more than two to one in Britain whereas, before the Second World War, they amounted to less than half. Whether the new professions are scientific or nonscientific, they all show certain common characteristics, and these characteristics foster both social and residential mobility. They are all organized in the same way into professional associations or institutions, they qualify by university training, they attempt to achieve a monopoly of their function, and they all have similar careers, although their rewards might not be the same (53). Professional individuals tend to work for salaries, and not for fees, with the legal—and, to some extent, medical—professions being notable exceptions. Typically,

---

°A cursory review in 1984 in the same hospital suggests that despite still greater specialization and technical complexity, an organizational limit might have been reached. A 1984 cardiac patient was attended by 6 to 12 physicians and 1 to 4 specialists, depending on the nature and duration of hospital course. The case notes ranged in length from 13 to 45 pages, although they included only physician and specialist notes. (The 1908 and 1938 record also included nurses' notes, laboratory reports, medication sheets, physicians' orders, and vital sign charts.)

professions exert substantial control over the terms and conditions of their work, although with the growing conglomeration into hospitals and organizations of modern clinical practice, the autonomy of the medical profession may be waning (54). The process of professionalization can be observed in operation in many special fields associated with the practice of medicine, for example, with technical personnel in clinical pathology and radiology in the hospital, with hospital administrators, and with social workers.

The formal hierarchy of statuses of large-scale organizations provides the new professionals with a ladder of promotion through which to advance their careers (55). The similarity of bureaucratic structure in these organizations allows a professional to start as a junior in one and climb through intermediate positions in several, to a senior position in yet another. But even if a professional remains in the same organization, it may operate on such a large scale that he or she is obliged to move upon leaving one branch for another. Thus, mobility in status and responsibility is often accompanied by residential movement. Between 1965 and 1970, almost one-third of the U.S. work force changed occupations; two-thirds of those who changed were under 35 years old (56). This mobility in career and residence is characteristic of persons with scientific, technical, and administrative professions, and for this reason they have been termed "spiralists" (57).

Spiralists are clearly distinguished by function, education, culture, earning power, and potential mobility from the wage-earning worker. Educated at universities, they share a generic culture based partly on common liberal values, but with a wide range of diversity, so that it can support a number of subcultures without losing a common identity. Their life careers follow a typical path. Whatever precisely their work and salaries may be, they climb the ladder of promotion through competition for more responsible posts with higher salaries and prestige. Skilled manual workers earn their maximum wage soon after completing training, and most often continue at the same standard throughout their working lives, except when the wages of the whole trade go up. Spiralists, on the other hand, usually have built-in increments in their salaries, even without promotion.

Many spiralists are also occupationally mobile, in the sense that the demarcation of skills between many professions is not yet so rigid as among other occupations. A spiralist who acquires certain key qualifications can move from one profession to an allied one. Moreover, every professional qualification, whatever its basic skill, carries with it the potentiality of achieving high managerial or executive position: a schoolmaster can become an administrator in the educational system; a general, a bank director; a chemist, the chairman of a railway system; and a university professor, an ambassador. The career of a general manager in large-scale industry may have begun in any one of the specialized departments, as an engineer, accountant, administrator, or chemist. The abilities considered necessary for the top executive positions in bureaucratic organizations are not ascertained by examination, as are professional skills; promotion depends on such imponderables as "administrative ability," "qualities of leadership," "drive," and "personality" (57).

Physicians in settled local practice, like other upper- and middle-class people bound to one location by their occupations, are "burgesses" more than spiralists. Other doctors may be spiralists, for instance, those in academic life and research, or in public health and medical administration, or in the armed forces. Doctors in training in the hospitals also have some of the characteristics of spiralists; the system of training appointments with limited tenure enforces mobility. The process comes to an end for them when they attain full professional status, go into practice, and localize their interests.

These distinctions between physicians who are burgesses rooted in local communities, and those who are spiralists and socially mobile, lead to distinctions also between their modes of practice. The differences between "personal" and "technical" medicine rest in part on professional specialization. General internists, pediatricians, and obstetricians, whose focus is defined by the attributes of persons, can be differentiated from dermatologists, cardiologists, and nephrologists, whose focus is defined by organs and not whole persons, and from radiologists and surgeons, whose focus is defined not by persons at all but by techniques (58). But other factors also affect the form of practice: social situations and reference groups are no less potent for physicians than for patients in determining their forms of interaction.

A study in the Health Insurance Plan of Greater New York showed that the closer to primary care in the community physicians were, the more sensitive to the personal aspects of care patients found them (59). In a national study of house-officers in training, the young physicians' views of their seniors were consistent with those elicited from patients (60). The decisions of the general practitioner, who stands close to the community, are subject to lay pressures from that community. Although trained to act by professional criteria, the doctor must consider the wishes and circumstances of the patient and of those close to the patient. If the doctor's practice is to flourish, what he or she does must be acceptable to the people served. Patients reach community practitioners through the recommendations of other patients; their reputations are built up through each consultation and each decision. The content of these exchanges is carried back and reported by the patient, to be sifted within his or her social network. This process of referral and recruitment has been described as a "lay referral system."

Through lay referral networks—essentially reference groups for the interpretation of symptoms—the social world mediates individual decisions to seek clinical attention. Symptoms alone, unless they are extreme, are often insufficient to compel the sufferer to seek professional assistance (61). Instead, the degree to which symptoms disrupt everyday life seems to be crucial. This, in turn, depends upon the ability of the social network to accommodate irregular behavior that stems from illness (62). Would-be patients themselves influence this accommodation. Especially when chronic ailments are involved, they may slowly learn to endure as "normal" ever greater levels of pain or dysfunction (63). In general, kin try first to provide succor from their own internal resources; they tend to discourage early recourse to outside care, while friends and acquaintances are more likely to encourage it. A close group of friends and kin may become active participants in the treatment process, accompanying the patient through the stages of seeking care, consulting with physicians and providing counsel in decisions about treatment (64).

A lay referral network may also mediate professional behavior, and serve to press the practitioner into conformity with the expectations of patients. Thus, even the free prescription of medicines in the National Health Service in Britain varied greatly according to area, and bore as much relation to local cultures as to any recognizable "medical" need (65). Patients confront the community practitioner with problems that cover the whole range of medical competence, including its social and psychological components, and exert further pressure to maintain the healer's traditional responsibility for the whole person (66).

By contrast, full-time hospital physicians have been little subject to lay pressure, especially where a chain of referrals within the professional system, as from peripheral to teaching hospitals, puts social distance between them. The frame of reference of hospital staff comprises their professional colleagues and the values they share with them. Typically the staff consider the patient in hospital, with necessary if concerned detachment, as a case and an object of scientific study. Decisions about the management of this case must display technical competence and be justifiable to colleagues on scientific grounds. The hospital encapsulates the patient, whose set of associations and ideas is thereby strictly limited, and the behavior expected from the patient is accepting, submissive, and dependent. Patient needs tend to be assessed within this restricted framework. Thus, decisions about patients are often made with perfunctory attention to the latent roles relinquished in the world outside, in family, work, and leisure; the resultant dependency is beyond appeal to those outside. Dissatisfied hospital patients cannot effect change through the mechanics of the market place as they can with the practitioner in office or surgery (67). Only dissatisfied community groups, by resorting to political pressure on the institution, can effect such change from without.

In sum, the pressures in the community situation of the practitioner direct attention to the personal needs and social situations of patients. At the same time, that situation may isolate the practitioner professionally, and preclude constant reference to the scientific judgment of colleagues. On the other hand, the pressures in the hospital situation of the specialist maintain technical competence, but divert attention from the personal needs of patients. These orientations among doctors have material consequences for their patients. For while the mistakes of general practice often seem to arise from technical failures, the mistakes of hospital practice often do so from failures of communication with patients and among staff (68). (This is not to say that difficulties in communication do not occur in general practice (23,69).)

Social networks

Complex social forces cause individuals and families to choose where they will live and with whom and how they will interact. The social structure permits idiosyncrasy in role specialization, and hence variations in behavior. But this behavior is not arbitrary; choice is limited by economic and social factors, as well as by personal characteristics. Occupation and marriage are determinants of residence, and the scale and quality of a family's social life increase with occupational skills, education, and income. These attributes are reflected in the nature and extent of the voluntary social interaction and the web of social relations from which each person builds a *social network* (33).

All of the persons within a social network will not necessarily know one another, and each will have his or her own network of social relations with others; they do not form an organized group. The social network forms the actual or primary social environment of an individual; it is the means whereby people fit themselves into society as a whole. Networks in which most of the persons with whom an individual interacts also know and interact with each other independently of that individual are termed *close-knit;* networks in which few of the persons know and interact with one another independently are termed *loose-knit* (29).

Other characteristics of social networks relevant to patterns of disease and help-seeking include *size*—the number of people with whom one is, or when the need arises could be, in contact; *diversity*—the range of age, experience, external contacts, education, and income represented by members of a network; *intensity*—the strength of ties between members; *content* of typical interactions, ranging from the quotidian to the intimate; *frequency* of contacts; and *symmetry* of relationships— the degree to which transactions or support are reciprocal (70). An additional attribute might be the ease with which certain networks are reconstituted once the individual moves elsewhere.

To illustrate the point, the social networks built up by the families of an unskilled laborer and a spiralist, both working in the same firm and living in the same town, will be quite different. The laborer, who resides in the neighborhood in which he was born and has married a woman also born and reared there, has a close-knit social network comprised of persons who live nearby. Many of these persons are either related to the husband or wife, or have been known to them since childhood. They are distinguished by their local speech, habits, customs, and values, and are members of the same associations, religious, political, and recreational. They meet one another in many shared activities that bind them together in a community of interests. Loyalty to family and to place coincide; social interaction with kin, centered on mothers, tends to predominate over social interaction with others, and strengthens "in-group" feelings of belonging. This close-knit and geographically contained social network provides emotional and material support, and establishes the norms of behavior. Often there is no escape from the actual or supposed surveillance of kin and neighbors, and this may lead to conformity, lack of individuation, and susceptibility to the social control of gossip.

Spiralist couples, who were born and reared elsewhere, have a loose-knit network. They have no or few kin nearby, and a slight acquaintance with neighbors and fellow residents. Their social activities are with persons from a wide area, and even range abroad. Functional associations are a more significant element in the social life of the spiralist than of the laborer, and where these associations are socially heterogeneous, the spiralists tend to take over leadership (71). They work with one set, play golf with another, entertain others, and live beside yet another. To operate their dispersed networks they make use of expensive material objects, large homes, automobiles, and telephones, as well as appropriate social skills.

As they share a generic culture and a common set of liberal values, they can readily interact in these terms with colleagues, friends, and other associates who are their economic and social equals. The nearest equivalent to a close-knit network the spiralist family possesses is possibly the professional association or institute to which the spiralist belongs, particularly where highly specialized skills are shared. For although colleagues are dispersed throughout the country, they tend to meet regularly to discuss professional matters, read about each other in journals, and soon learn about changes in status and residence among their associates. Spiralist families seek emotional satisfactions and social support in a less direct way, have more varied demands, and are less dependent on kin. Indeed, they may view kin with cool detachment.

Since their social networks are loose knit and dispersed, and their loyalties widespread, social control depends on many sanctions other than those exercised by local residents. Such dispersed networks facilitate residential mobility. The spiralist who moves from one post to another quickly builds up a new local network of friends and acquaintances; some of his or her new colleagues may already be known or known of, and active social relations may be resumed with old friends while new ones are being made.

Physical proximity need not determine social proximity. The family in an isolated farmhouse may have a great deal of social interaction with kin and friends (1), whereas "house-centered" families in densely populated cities may have a minimum of voluntary social interaction (2). People thus interpret the terms "neighbor" and "neighborhood" in varied ways. The working class tend to consider the ideal relationship between persons who live nearby to be one of mutual interdependence and material assistance (38,72), whereas spiralists stress the material and social self-sufficiency of each household, adopt formal attitudes toward people who live nearby, and depend on persons dispersed over a wide area for friendship and the sharing of mutual interests.

The structure of social networks exhibits the interplay between the diffuse personal forces that engage people in primary groups as family and neighbors, and the functional economic forces that engage them in outside secondary groups. Distinctive social networks form in the context of the material and cultural resources at hand; each form is a typical resolution of the forces that beset people of different social groups. While sociological studies of urban populations in Britain in such varied areas as Oxford, Aberdeen, Liverpool, Bethnal Green, Banbury, Scotland, and some London suburbs all showed that close-knit networks tend to be found among the working class, and that families with loose-knit dispersed networks tend to be found among the middle class, all working-class families do not have close-knit networks nor all middle-class families loose-knit networks. The structure of networks is influenced not only by the social attributes of occupation, residence, class, and personal choice, but also by the fixed attributes of age, gender, birth rank, and the size of families of origin. In addition, the composition of a family's social network varies over time, with age and mobility, and with the progress of its own developmental cycle and those of other families with whom it interacts (73). The particular constellation of these factors at a given moment in a family's life history limits the choice of persons with whom they will interact, and the nature and purpose of their interaction, and hence the character of the social network.

The social uncertainty and loneliness that result from being torn from a contained network, where every nuance of social behavior was understood, have seemed severe enough to bring on neurosis and emotional disarray, particularly among spouses who lack the interest outside the home that work offers (74). British studies that looked for "suburban neurosis" in people removed from settled urban places in London to housing estates strange to them, however, failed to demonstrate it (75). The result could possibly have been falsely negative. Countervailing forces cancel out, and the effect of better living conditions could have balanced the social disruption of the move.

So far, research has succeeded poorly in eliciting effects of losing or altering social networks. As new research gains sophistication in measuring this complex variable, we may better understand the ways networks contribute to health and state of mind. An American social experiment that allocated poorly housed families at random to new housing found meager effects on disorders of health, except that those rehoused enjoyed greater optimism and more tranquil family relations than before, and than the comparison group enjoyed (76). In a Boston study, adjustment among working-class people who had to move was better if they had shown signs of preparedness for upward social mobility before the move. Adjustment was poorer if they were uprooted from close-knit social networks (77). A recent study of forcibly relocated elderly persons in three Connecticut cities did not detect such effects, however (78). Still, even though relocation was not found to be a socially uprooting experience, there was some evidence of adverse health effects on those who moved as compared with controls who did not. These results present some problems of interpretation: all "cases" in the study had the advantage of moving to better quality, federally subsidized housing for the elderly, and there was significant variation within the sample as to the reason for the move. Curiously, the majority of the "cases" saw the move as voluntary even though, by objective measures, the move was precipitated by external circumstances ranging from redevelopment to eviction, financial hardship, social service intervention, and combinations of these.

Attempts to study large samples with total mortality or coronary heart disease as an endpoint have yielded inconsistent results. A long-term prospective study of nearly 7000 people in Alameda County, California, showed that persons with a lack of contacts had higher mortality than those with extensive contacts. Ties with friends and relatives yielded better protection than those with church and other social groups. Another long-term prospective study in Tecumseh, Michigan, also showed higher mortality for persons with low scores on several measures of social relations; once age and other risk factors were controlled, the increase in mortality was still apparent for men, but not in general for women. In Tecumseh, low risk attended social contact with organized groups and, to a lesser degree, with friends and relatives. A third long-term prospective study in Honolulu of coronary heart disease in nearly 5000 Japanese men found an association between the strength of social networks and the prevalence of disease. The association did not hold, however, for incident disease. One must therefore entertain the idea that the onset of disease may have reduced social interaction rather than the reverse. Similar confounding may beset the favored idea that social networks protect only in the presence of stressors. Many stressful life events in themselves result in the depletion of social networks, as, for instance, with bereavement, divorce, change of residence, and loss of employment; the depleted network is a consequence, not a cause. The most consistent finding among these three studies is that the highest risk occurred among the most isolated persons (79).

The supportive strength of families, one may say in general, depends on their external relations as well as their internal structure. Internal structure comprises the array of family statuses, the allocation of roles to each status, and the ordered relationships among them. Since structure is not constant, and varies with the development of the family cycle, its supportive capacity for dependent members fluctuates with the progress of the cycle (see Chapters 9 and 10). The supportive strength of the family's external relations is founded on its social network. This strength derives from formal obligations between kin, informal obligations between kin and between kin and others, and from material resources. A close-knit network may compensate for poor material resources (2,80,81).

These external relations are mediated by the family's social position and the culture attendant upon that position. Position governs access to social and material resources, culture the use to which these resources may be put. For instance, English working-class cultures have enjoined home care for their dependent relatives, rather than removal to institutions. Families that shared this culture were reluctant to give up the care of subnormal children and old people even in the most difficult circumstances (82,83). These attitudes were tenable so long as mutual aid could be exchanged through local close-knit networks. In the presence of disease and illness, the combined elements of culture, social position, family structure, and social networks in each type of community will have a profound influence on the manifestation of sickness and the assumption of the sick role.

The sick role

The concepts of mobility, status, role, and social network all assume medical significance in the assessment of the social support available to dependent persons—and dependency is the condition of many patients. In medical practice the ability of a family to provide social support and material aid to dependent members is of obvious importance. When patients who are disabled by sickness are reintroduced to normal social life, for example, their family relationships and attitudes help to determine the outcome, and sometimes the clinical as well as the social prognosis. Schizophrenia is one disorder in which family response and family adjustment have been studied.

The extent to which the family with a member diagnosed as schizophrenic will tolerate disordered behavior and consider it a symptom of real illness, as well as the standards of performance they expect, affect the person's chances of maintaining himself or herself in the community. An early British study of chronic schizophrenic men discharged from the hospital estimated their social adjustment by their ability to keep out of the hospital (26). Success was found to be related not so much to the severity of their symptoms as to the social environment to which they returned. Some patients returned to their wives and parents; some returned to a sibling's home or to lodgings; and some took up residence in "common lodging-houses." The most successful patients were those who lived with siblings or in lodgings, and the least successful were those who returned to their wives or parents. The clinical state of the patient appeared to determine the outcome only among those who took up residence in "common lodging-houses."

This study, however, had several limitations; for instance, the sample included only the unrepresentative group of schizophrenic persons who had entered and then been discharged from the hospital, the effect of previous family relations could not be controlled, and the criterion of adjustment was a crude one. But these findings, and parallel ones (84), illustrate the different demands made on patients by various types of households and social relations. (They also suggest that the classical withdrawal of the person with schizophrenia from social contact and his or her inability to sustain affectional relations were best suited to relative social isolation.) The men who returned to their wives had to assume the roles of husband, father, and breadwinner, a complex of roles that made strenuous demands on their intellectual, emotional, and physical capacities. Only one-half of the men in this group were successful. The men who returned to parental homes had less strenuous demands made on them, although all of them had to fill the roles of sons or brothers. Their familial circumstances were more varied, however, for some returned to homes where their capacity to work was important. About two-thirds in this group were successful. On the other hand, those men who went into lodgings had the least demands made on them, and all were successful in avoiding rehospitalization. They performed their minimal social roles adequately so long as they could work and and pay their rent and behave quietly, however lurid their delusions and hallucinations. The men who took up residence with siblings were in a similar situation.

Within each domestic situation the behavior expected from the patient helped to determine his response. Those who lived with their wives and stayed out of hospital tended to do well, apparently because they were able to live up to high expectations. Many of those who lived with their parents were successful in the sense that they did not return to hospital, but they were allowed to assume childlike dependent roles because of the devoted care of a mother or of some other member of the family. The degree of tolerance of their condition shown by members of their families appeared to be important in setting the standard of expected behavior that confronted patients, and this was related to three interwoven social factors: first, the economic necessities of domestic situations; second, the accepted social standards of what was regarded as tolerable behavior in the mentally disabled; and third, the personalities of other members of the family. The quality of the emotional relationship between persons diagnosed as schizophrenic and their family members appears to bear critically on prospects for recovery. Subsequent British studies (85) found that the index of expressed emotion (a composite measure of criticism, hostility, and emotional overinvolvement) on the part of the relative at the time of admission was the best predictor of the likelihood of the patient's relapse after discharge. Maintenance drug therapy and reduced face-to-face contact did, however, mitigate the effect.

Outside the immediate household, the ability of psychiatric patients to sustain life in the community is also influenced by social intercourse and the networks they join. Thus, even people severely disabled by chronic schizophrenia, in a rundown Manhattan single-room-occupancy hotel, adapt better when they are part of a network than when they are not. Other ex-patients, "normals," and relatives—not professional service workers—form the effective core of such networks (86).

In rehabilitation following any serious sickness, the patient's medical condition and apparent normality may not be the main preconditions for success: the kind of social roles the patient will be expected to play in the familial and social environment may be crucial. In the same way, age, gender, and marital status have meaning in medicine as indices of social roles. The social role of a sick person is important in physical disorders as well as mental. To be sick is more than a medical condition. The patient has a customary part to play in relation to the doctor, to the family, and to other members of society, all of whom in turn expect patients to behave in certain prescribed ways.

Four aspects of the *sick role* have been emphasized. First, the sick person is exempt from normal social responsibilities, depending of course on the severity of the illness; the malingerer is punished because this exemption is fraudulently claimed. For similar reasons, the hysteric with conversion symptoms has often been harshly and angrily treated by doctors. Second, the sick person cannot help himself and must be cared for. When a neurotic man is instructed to "pull himself together," he is being denied the sick role and is in effect being regarded as though he did not suffer from illness. Third, the sick role is regarded as a misfortune, so it is assumed that the sick person will desire to get well, and is under an actual obligation to do so. A hypochondriac provokes resentment because he or she refuses to get well, and therefore risks losing the exemption from normal social obligations. The fourth aspect is the obligation of the sick person to seek competent help, usually from a doctor, and to cooperate with the doctor in the process of getting well (30,87).

The typical sick role is temporary; society expects that most patients will get well, as indeed they do: better than 90 per cent of illness for which primary care is sought is self-limiting. This appears most clearly in traditional societies, where all sickness is temporary, in the sense that there are no permanent bedridden sick. Among the Mambwe of central Africa, for instance, "natural" sickness is considered to make someone ill for only two or three days. If the person continues to feel sick after this time, it is suspected that someone is using sorcery against the sufferer, and the curer is called in. If the curer confirms that sorcery is the agency at work, the patient pays to turn the sorcery away and to provide a cure.

In the outcome the patient either recovers within a short period, or else dies, for the environmental conditions are too harsh to favor protracted crises (88). Under conditions of scarcity, there is seldom place for the bedfast patient, for neither the economy, the technology, nor the culture of tribal communities has developed in a way to support nonproductive individuals for any length of time. The majority of the Mambwe, like millions of other tribal Africans, suffer constantly from chronic diseases like malaria, treponemal infections, tuberculosis, and malnutrition. But such chronic disorders are so commonplace that they do not qualify a sufferer to be treated as "sick"; one must carry out one's social obligations and duties. In Uganda in the period after the Second World War, the European doctors rarely encountered the symptoms and the diagnosis of peptic ulcer among Africans, but at necropsy the scars of peptic ulcers were no less common than in Britain (89).

Chronic sick roles can be institutionalized only under specific conditions: they appear where there is an economy to support unproductive patients, a technology to cure or aid them, and a system of values that insists that they should be cared for. All these preconditions are not necessarily present in all industrial societies. Nazi Germany, for instance, adopted as a national policy the extermination of the bedridden and mentally disabled. Nor can the classical formulation of the sick role be extended from the situation of acute to that of chronic illness without modification (90).

Two kinds of chronic sick role can be recognized, the bedridden and the ambulant; each has its own problems. In industrial societies, the bedridden and dependent invalid has long had a recognized role. The ambulant invalid, on the other hand, had no such special role in the past: to be on one's feet and at work was usually considered healthy. Lepers° provide a long-standing exception, but although in the West they have been recognized as sick persons ever since Biblical times, most societies could not provide them with a positive social role and tended to exclude them altogether from normal life (91).

The distinction between the ambulant and the bedridden is no longer clear-cut. In Britain this came prominently to public notice during the Boer War in South Africa at the turn of the century, when the army was forced to reject a large number of young recruits on medical grounds. It became evident that many apparently healthy people were in fact in need of medical care and attention. Standards of health have been raised since then, and the expectation of life increased. A large and increasing number of people now survive to suffer from such chronic disorders as hypertension, coronary disease, heart failure, diabetes, and rheumatoid arthritis. They are kept on their feet and at work by continuous medical treatment. Such persons do not fit the stereotyped sick role, and their families often experience difficulty in according them the necessary relief from normal obligations warranted by their condition, for they appear to be neither ill nor well, and their condition is not temporary but permanent.

The chronic sick role offers a prolonged escape from everyday responsibilities, and for this reason some patients may prefer this role, despite the disadvantages of disablement and unemployment that follow. In such a case, the patient's personal preference is influenced by his or her family situation, and in any given illness the threshold of disordered function that produces disablement and unemployment varies accordingly. Personality factors, such as a reluctance to see oneself as seriously ill before surgery, may also influence the course of recovery and resumption of normal social obligations. Variations in the threshold are bound up with the social norms and values that define malingering, hypochondria, and neurosis, for these norms and values determine whether certain forms of behavior are tolerated or rejected. Many self-

---

°Those designated as lepers in earlier times are thought to have suffered from a variety of disfiguring diseases, and not necessarily from leprosy caused by Hansen's bacillus.

confessed witches in Britain in the past, as in contemporary Ghana, would be diagnosed in contemporary Britain as suffering from depression (92).

Family norms and values, and their material resources, govern the initial interpretation of the nature of the individual's problem, the recognition of it as an illness, and
the decision to seek and comply with treatment (62,93). The chance of a diabetic
child surviving, for instance, may depend on these factors; certain families may fail
to appreciate the full importance of the physician's instructions, or to equate them
with their own view of the illness, or else their material and social resources may be
inadequate to sustain the exacting regime of diet and medication. Rarer conditions
that require complicated diets, for instance, coeliac disease, phenylketonuria, and
galactosemia, make similar exacting demands on patients' families.

Treatment of adult ambulant patients with chronic disease makes increasing
demands on patients and their families. The hypertensive patient may have to maintain a carefully regulated dose of a ganglion-blocking agent or similar drug, the coronary patient of agents that suppress irregular cardiac rhythms, and if either is in
heart failure, he or she must keep to a regimen of digitalis, diuretics, and a salt-free
diet as well. In the same way, the patient with severe rheumatoid arthritis must keep
to steroids and balance the intake of potassium and sodium ions. All these conditions
require that the family adjust its customary routines to the patient's needs and to his
or her role as a partial invalid, at the risk of social and psychological problems. The
varying demands made by patients on their families must be considered in treatment,
no less than the varying demands made by families on patients (83).

The economic and social resources of the family are limited, and at almost all social
levels these restrict the possibilities of successful home care. Both husband and wife
have extensive commitments, as parents and wage-earners; each is dependent on the
other for economic, emotional, and social support. In most families these two are the
sole effective adults available to nurse a sick person, and the material and psychological economy of the family is at once unbalanced if one partner or a child falls ill.

Hence, a serious or long-term illness throws a strain on family relations, quite apart
from its twin threats of poverty and bereavement (94). Children make continuous
demands on their parents because of their dependence and need for constant care. A
parent who falls ill displaces the children through his or her own dependence, which
reduces the time, care, and attention that the well parent can devote to the children.
This may well intensify the conflict inherent in a parent's dual obligations to spouse
and to children, and at the same time disturb the children whose demands are not
met in the expected way. If the parent is not capable of accepting the additional
burden, he or she may respond to the situation either by resenting the sick spouse's
dependence, or by encouraging it excessively. The sick parent is also subject to
another form of strain, for he or she must accept a regression to a childlike role of
dependence and passivity, the penalty that accompanies the privileges of the sick role.
So long as a spouse accepts the sick role, and the exemptions from formal duties and
obligations that this entails, including tolerance of one's whims, he or she must also
accept deposition from normal authority and status.

The strain that a permanent sick role imposes on a family, with the continuing dependence of the member, is exemplified by parents who find they have a severely retarded child. Clinical observation points to a characteristic response pattern. At first, when the abnormality is discovered, there is a period of shock. Typically, the parents have a dominant feeling of guilt. This guilt has sources in the cultural stigma and hereditary taint that attaches to mental disorder, and in the personal problems of accepting a child who cannot fulfill the hopes and aspirations that parents project onto their children. Shock is followed by a period of turmoil, with a search for reassurance from whomever might give it, whether medical or lay. Finally an adjustment is made, which may be more or less stable, because the mentally retarded child always remains a potential focus of disturbance.

A poor adjustment may grow in time into a situation of intolerable and continuous strain, for when the child reaches an age when he or she should be a free-running schoolchild such a child still needs the care suitable for an infant, and may be competing for it with younger siblings. As the family comes slowly to face the prospect that the child's dependence is permanent, the feelings of guilt are intensified by feelings of resentment. It is common for one or both parents then to develop compensatory emotional reactions such as protectiveness and restrictiveness, or to blame each other for the situation. Such families can enter a state of chronic emotional crisis from which all members suffer (83).

For example, mothers of retarded children over the years may exhibit neuroses, with phobias, hypochondria, or somatic symptoms. Fathers sometimes display disorders in conduct or become unstable in employment. The retarded child may regress to infantile levels of behavior, with symptoms such as incontinence, tantrums, head-banging, or destructiveness (95). Often these family situations can be relieved by removing the child from the home into an institution. This removal need not be permanent or continuous, and a temporary removal often alleviates the symptoms in mother, father, and child. Thus, a mentally retarded child sometimes shows regressive behavior in the home but not in a training center that he or she attends every day, and in these cases the chronic family crisis may only become acute during the vacations when the training center is closed and the child is constantly at home. The particular needs of a severely subnormal individual therefore impose a sick role which in turn necessitates typical forms of behavior in the relations between the afflicted individual and other family members.

If, as also happens, a disturbed child is made the focal point of existing tensions in the family, his or her designated "sickness" may help stabilize an otherwise volatile situation. Sometimes the child takes on the role of scapegoat for unacknowledged conflicts between the parents. Similar observations have been made as well about alcoholics in families (96). Indeed, in a number of institutional settings (the mental hospital, prison, totalitarian state, and armed services) assignment to the sick role can function as a means of quelling dissidence or deviance that is otherwise disruptive. Alternately, access to the sick role can offer a way out of objectionable duties. In the United States during the Vietnam War, for example, a large number of young men who were politically opposed to the war obtained medical disqualifications for military service (97).

Social support

The social support provided by the families of all types of sick patients tends to be in inverse proportion to the care demanded of such social agencies as hospitals and public health authorities. Hospitals are now the dominant agency for medical care. Even midwifery, traditionally conducted in the home and concerned with an essentially normal process, has become centered on the hospital and not on the home. Hospitals were founded in the first place to provide a substitute home in which destitute and dependent persons could find shelter, food, and clothing; nursing and medical care for the indigent sick came later (98). Special hospitals also assumed a custodial function for those persons who were either mentally ill or socially deviant and could not be disciplined by the normal processes of the law. Hospitals of various kinds still have all these functions, but the principal purpose now is to provide specialized skills in the treatment of disease, and to relieve families of the strain of caring for the chronic sick. These services are used by families in all social classes, and not only by the indigent.

The turn to the hospital for treatment was influenced by the changes in family relations and expectations that have accompanied economic and social developments, as well as by the concentration of skill and technique. Rates of admission are still influenced by these factors, over and above the amount and type of sickness in the population. The separation of adults from their families of origin by mobility in occupation, social class, and residence increases the flow of patients into hospitals, for the isolated household whose members have dispersed social networks is less able to cope with the strain imposed by the sick role. Hence the public concern about the growing demand for hospital care, particularly for the chronic sick, the aged, and the mentally disordered.

If the strain on families and on hospitals of caring for the chronic sick is to be relieved, other agencies, no less effective than hospitals, must be provided. For example, to carry out a policy of keeping mental patients within their local communities, separate agencies at once become necessary to provide specialized medical care, day nursing, training centers, material support and equipment, family counseling from the first recognition of the diagnosis, and residential homes as a substitute for families—a fact never adequately recognized in the deinstitutionalization practices of U.S. mental hospitals. Consequently, the living situation of ex-patients tends to be characterized by the same isolation and segregation from the nonpatient community; their social relations remain dominated by the modes of custodial care, with the torpor and dependency that follow. Culturally, the move from mental hospital to "community" has meant for many the reproduction of the social space of the mental hospital ward (83,99).

In crises or disasters that produce total social dependence, as in incapacitating illness, people usually turn first for help to those who have a legal relationship with them. Legal kinship obligations are limited, with few exceptions, to the two generations of elementary families; a child relies on parents, one spouse on the other. The next call is likely to be made upon extra-familial kin and friends who constitute the family's social network. We have seen that the support provided by the social network depends on its composition and resources, and on the obligations and values that attach to social relations of different kinds. Relations within social networks imply reciprocal obligations and exchange of services. A system of reciprocal personal services where people's financial resources do not suffice for crises and contingencies is characteristic of close-knit contained networks (81).

Family and social support may be inadequate, leaving agencies as the only resort. In such failures, three principal conditions can be distinguished: first, when the patient makes demands on the family that exceed its resources; second, when there are no available kin; and, third, when there are no effective kin (100). For example, the excessive demands presented by the lack of development of a mentally retarded child may disrupt relations in families that have sufficient material and psychological resources to cope with the ordinary demands of normal children; these families may need additional social support. The material resources of a family are closely related to its social class position, and inadequate resources in money, housing, and paid help are acute in working-class families. Psychological resources may be inadequate in any social class, although family tolerance, with which these resources are connected, may be limited by attitudes toward mental illness customary in particular social groups.

Availability and effectiveness of kin are relative. Spiralist families can give effective help to relatives at a distance, for they usually command the needed money, accommodation, transport, and modes of communication. On the other hand, kin may be ineffective when they are physically nearby and available, because they are under some handicap or because they reject kinship obligations. The effectiveness of kin support is also limited by the phases of the family cycles of kindred at a given time (see Chapter 9). These phases determine the age and social status of the members of interacting families. A young parent can scarcely expect help from aged parents who are themselves dependent on outside support, or from a sister who is herself an unmarried youngest daughter caring for the parents. Siblings will be more effective at certain phases of their lives than at others; married sisters and brothers in the phase of family expansion are preoccupied with rearing and maintaining their own children. In contrast, parents whose children are dispersed can often help a married child and grandchildren.

Kin may not be available at all, either because they are dead or because they live at such a distance that they cannot help the patient. The need for agency support arises most often with patients at the extremes of life. Children without relatives invariably require a substitute home, usually provided by state or voluntary agencies. They may need support because of the desertion or separation of parents, or because of the early death of a mother or father. If substitute parenting can be provided, the remaining members of a disrupted nuclear family can maintain their relations with one another, and young children may then experience the continuing relations necessary to normal personality development (101). Step-parents or grandparents or other relatives can be adequate substitutes for a missing mother or father or for both.

The availability of kin, like their relative effectiveness, is also connected with the cycle of family development. Adults who are dependent because of mental or physical disability are likely to need agency support in middle age when their parents die, for siblings who might otherwise help are then preoccupied with their own families and careers. Old people, too, may outlive their close relatives; problems of support arise in particular for widows, and for individuals who have no children or who never married. We shall return to this later (see Chapters 10 and 12).

Birth rank, family size, and kinship customs set a fixed limit to the number of kin that an individual has, whether or not they live nearby or interact socially. When husband and wife are both "only children," the number of relatives must be few and the kin network small. Eldest children have younger parents at their birth than youngest children, and at a given age are more likely to have both parents surviving; they are also likely to have more unmarried siblings able to help them. In contrast, youngest children are less likely to have living mothers or living fathers, and are more likely to have widowed, aged, and dependent parents and to be their readiest support (81); older siblings with their own young children will be less able to care for dependents.

Social networks function as a social support, and a patient from a functioning network is likely to call on a limited number of agencies and only for short periods—for instance, the general practitioner, the district nurse, or unemployment insurance. The full services of social and welfare agencies are needed only when the social network breaks down, either through death, migration, or isolation.

In the absence of a functioning network, the family in trouble is likely to need considerable assistance from social agencies and for long periods. For example, one Lancashire family involved the simultaneous attentions of five agencies. The wife came from a broken home and had no available kin; her husband was estranged from his own family of origin because they disapproved of his wife. The wife subsequently deserted the family, leaving her husband to care for five children who ranged in age from two to ten. The two youngest children were admitted to a day nursery maintained by the Local Health Authority; a "home help" attended daily to provide domestic services; a public health nurse called daily to oversee the children; the School Attendance Officer kept a check on the family at the same time; and, finally, the Children's Department inspected the home at regular intervals. In spite of this attention, the children eventually had to be taken into residential care by the Children's Department of the local authority. When the family has a close-knit social network, a crisis of this kind can sometimes be met. For close-knit networks can provide replacements to substitute for members of the elementary family, and to some degree perform their roles; the network is a "self-balancing and self-correcting" institution (81). In general, social services are used less by families with close-knit networks than those with dispersed networks (29).

The focal point of social interaction in a close-knit network is usually a mother whose married children live nearby, and it is through her that family exchanges are regulated (81). Wives also turn to their sisters and to their mothers-in-law, but the main axis of relations is between daughter and mother. Daughters give more direct help than sons to their parents, as might be expected from traditional male and female roles. The dissolution of a close-knit contained network tends to follow upon the death of the mother who was the focal point, and wives then in turn become the focus of their own networks as their own children grow up and disperse. Reliable information about the role of men in family support is scanty. Family problems in our society have commonly been studied in terms of the problems of women and children, perhaps because the division of labor has taken most husbands and fewer wives away from their families during the interviewing day.

Working-class wives in contained networks pay a price in a narrowed range of social interaction, particularly in those areas where married women have few opportunities to work for wages and a tradition exists that married women do not work (102). Before marriage a young woman associates with friends and colleagues, both at work and in her leisure time. On marriage, when in the past many retired from work, a woman's social network contracted; her whole interest was concentrated on her home, on the care of her husband and children, and on attachments to mother and sisters. Her knowledge of the outside world and her responses to outside events became minimal. We observed working-class wives who were reluctant to travel beyond the bounds of their own neighborhood, apparently imprisoned by an emotional attachment to home and family. Although this resembles the symptoms of certain phobias, these women appeared to be prepared to travel anywhere on a visit to one relative as long as they were accompanied by another. Such travel did not pry them out of their close-knit networks. Similarly, working-class families tend to migrate to places where a pioneer has paved the way, as with the great European migration to the United States, and with Irish and West Indian immigrants to Britain, and within Britain in migration to new housing areas (103).

The wide dispersal of spiralist networks, by contrast, ensures connections that smooth the way into new places. Reciprocal help between generations is of a kind that can ignore distance. One study shows how this happens in middle-class American families, in which grandparents and parents often live in different towns (104). Help from the parents was seldom given directly, for the young couple were inhibited by their values and desire for independence from accepting this. Instead, the grandparents, in their phase of independence having already discharged their heavy commitments such as the education of their own children, sent presents of clothing, toys, and other things for grandchildren, provided common holidays by taking a holiday house, and made loans for house-buying. The grandparents added the indulgences of life— the "cakes and ale"—for the growing young family. Reciprocation is likely to occur when the grandparents themselves eventually become socially dependent.

In summary, social networks provide social support for people, place constraints on their behavior, and affect the nature of the environment to which they are exposed. The nature of the social network depends on its external relations in the community, the larger social context in which the network is established. At the same time, the functioning of a particular network will depend on its internal relations, the statuses and roles of the people who comprise it, their age, gender, kin relationships, associations, and occupations. All these elements together (the larger social context of the community, the networks of relations within it, and the statuses and roles within the networks) determine the experiences and the behavior of the individuals who occupy the statuses, perform the roles, relate in the networks, and are members of the community. These experiences of individuals are expressed in part in their diseases, their illnesses, and their sicknesses (a subject we take up in the next chapter). Thus, community experiences contribute to good or bad health, and they establish the norms and expectations for behavior about health.

References

1. **Arensberg, C. M.,** and **Kimball, S. T.** (1948). *Family and Community in Ireland,* Cambridge, Mass.
   Rees, A. D. (1950). *Life in a Welsh Countryside,* Cardiff.
   Williams, W. N. (1956). *The Sociology of an English Village: Gosforth,* London.
2. **Willmott, P.,** and **Young, M.** (1960). *Family and Class in a London Suburb,* London.
3. **Dennis, N., Henriques, F.,** and **Slaughter, C.** (1956). *Coal Is Our Life,* London.
   Stacey, M. (1960). *Tradition and Change: A Study of Banbury,* London.
4. **Schnore, L. F.** (1967). Measuring city-suburban status differences, *Urban Affairs Quart., 2,* 95–108.
5. **Engels, F.** (1956; first pub. 1845). *The Condition of the Working Class in England in 1844,* Stanford, CA.
   Mumford, L. (1961). *The City in History,* New York.
   Marcus, S. (1974). *Engels, Manchester and the Working Class,* New York.
   Sternlieb, G. and **Hughes, J. W.,** eds. (1976). *Post-Industrial America: Metropolitan Decline and Inter-Regional Shifts,* New Brunswick, N.J.
   Gordon, D. (1976). Capitalism and the roots of urban crisis, in *The Fiscal Crisis of American Cities,* ed. Alcaly, R. E., and Mermelstein, D., New York, pp. 82–120.
   Molotch, H. (1976). The city as a growth machine: Towards a political economy of place, *Amer. J. Sociol., 82,* 309–32.
6. **Lupton, T.,** and **Mitchell, C. D.** (1954). *Neighbourhood and Community,* London.
   Young, M., and **Willmott, P.** (1957). *Family and Kinship in East London,* London.
   Brennan, T. (1959). *Reshaping a City,* Glasgow.
7. **Tucker, C. J.** (1976). Changing patterns of migration between metropolitan and non-metropolitan areas in the United States: Recent evidence, *Demography, 13,* 435–43.
   Choldin, H. M., and **Hansen, C.** (1982). Status shifts within the city, *Amer. Sociol. Rev., 47,* 129–41.
8. **Perlman, J. E.** (1976). *The Myth of Marginality: Urban Poverty and Politics in Rio de Janeiro,* Berkeley.
   Collier, D. (1976). *Squatters and Oligarchs: Authoritarian Rule and Policy Change in Peru,* Baltimore.
   Eckstein, S. (1977). *The Poverty of Revolution: The State and the Urban Poor in Mexico,* Princeton.
9. **Fitch, R.** (1976). Planning New York, in *The Fiscal Crisis of American Cities,* ed. Alcaly, R. E., and Mermelstein, D., pp. 246–84.
   Legates, R. T., and **Hartman, C.** (1981). Displacement, *Clearinghouse Review, 15,* 207–49.
   Schlay, A. B., and **Rossi, P. H.** (1981). Keeping up the neighborhood: Estimating net effects of zoning, *Amer. Sociol. Rev., 46,* 703–16.
   Hartman, C., Keating, D., and **LeGates, R. T.** (1982). *Displacement: How to Fight It,* Berkeley.
   Werner, F. E., and **Bryson, D. B.** (1982). Guide to the preservation and maintenance of single-room occupancy (SRO) housing, *Clearinghouse Review, April,* 2–25, *May,* 999–1008.

10. **Glass, R.** (1948). *The Social Background of a Plan*, London.
    Freeman, T. W. (1959). *The Conurbations of Great Britain*, Manchester.
    Green, L. P. (1959). *Provincial Metropolis*, London.
11. **MacIver, R. A.** (1949). *The Elements of Social Science*, rev. ed., London.
12. **Lynd, R. S.,** and **Lynd, H. M.** (1929). *Middletown: A Study in American Culture*, New York.
    Lynd, R. S., and **Lynd, H. M.** (1937). *Middletown in Transition: A Study in Cultural Conflicts*, New York.
    Caplow, T., Bahr, H. M., Chadwick, B. A., Hill, R., and **Williamson, M. H.** (1982). *Middletown Families*, Minneapolis.
13. **Goldschmidt, W.** (1946). Small business and the community: A study in Central Valley of California on effects of scale of farm operation, in *Report of the Special Committee to Study Problems of American Small Business*, U.S. Senate, Washington, D.C.
    Lowenthal, M. (1975). The social economy in urban working class communities, in *The Social Economy of Cities*, ed. Gappert, G., and Rose, H., Beverly Hills, Calif. pp. 447–69.
14. **Sclar, E. D.** (1980). Community economic structure and individual well-being, *Int. J. Hlth. Serv.*, *10*, 563–80.
15. **Richardson, S. A.** (1963). Some social psychological consequences of handicapping, *Pediatrics*, *32*, 291–97.
16. **Linton, R.** (1936). *The Study of Man*, New York.
    Gerth, H., and **Mills, C. W.** (1953). *Social Structure and Character*, New York.
17. **Nadel, S. F.** (1951). *The Foundations of Social Anthropology*, London.
18. **Merton, R. K.** (1957). The role-set: Problems in sociological theory, *Brit. J. Sociol.*, *8*, 106–20.
19. **Radcliffe-Brown, A. R.,** and **Forde, C. Daryll** (1950). *African Systems of Kinship and Marriage*, London.
20. **Clements, R. V.** (1958). *Managers: A Study of Their Careers in Industry*, London.
21. **Rock, P.** (1974). The sociology of deviancy and conceptions of moral order, *Brit. J. Criminol.*, *14*, 139–49.
22. **Beecher, H. K.** (1966). Ethics and clinical research, *New Eng. J. Med.*, *274*, 1354–60.
    Rutstein, D. D. (1970). The ethical design of human experiments, in *Experimentation with Human Subjects*, ed. Freund, P., New York, pp. 383–401.
    Barber, B., Lally, J. J., Makarvahk, J. L., and **Sullivan, D.** (1973). *Research on Human Subjects: Problems of Social Control in Medical Experimentation*, New York.
    Gray, B. H. (1975). *Human Subjects in Medical Experimentation: A Sociological Study of the Conduct and Regulation of Clinical Research*, New York.
    Tancredi, L. R. (1975). The ethics quagmire and randomized clinical trials, *Inquiry*, *12*, 171–79.
    Fried, C. (1975). *Medical Experimentation, Personal Integrity and Medical Policy*, New York.
    Byar, D. P., Simon, R. M., Friedewald, W. T., Schlesselman, J. J., DeMets, D. L., Ellenberg, J. H., Gail, M. H., and **Ware, J. H.** (1976). Randomized clinical trials: Perspective on some recent ideas, *New Eng. J. Med.*, *295*, 74–80.
    Walters, L. (1977). Some ethical issues in research involving human subjects, *Perspectives in Biology and Medicine*, *20*, 196–99.
    Meisel, A., and **Roth, L.** (1981). What we do and do not know about informed consent, *J. Amer. Med. Assoc.*, *246*, 2473–77.

Schafer, A. (1982). The ethics of the randomized clinical trial, *New Eng. J. Med., 307,* 719–24.

23. Waitzkin, H., and Stoeckle, J. D. (1972). The communication of information about illness, *Adv. Psychosom. Med., 8,* 180–215.

Brody, D. S. (1980). The patient's role in clinical decision-making, *Ann. Int. Med., 93,* 718–22.

Cassileth, B. R., Zupkis, R. V., Sutton-Smith, K., and March, V. (1980). Information and participation preferences among cancer patients, *Ann. Int. Med., 92,* 832–36.

Beauchamp, T., and Childress, J. (1980). *Principles of Biomedical Ethics,* 2nd ed., New York.

Miller, B. L. (1981). Autonomy and the refusal of life-saving treatment, *Hastings Center Report, 11,* 22–28.

Veatch, R. M. (1981). *A Theory of Medical Ethics,* New York.

24. Daniels, A. K. (1969). The captive professional. Bureaucratic limitations in the practice of military psychiatry, *J. Hlth. Soc. Behav., 10,* 255–65.

25. Goffman, E. (1962). *Asylums: Essays on the Social Situation of Mental Patients and Other Inmates,* Chicago.

Blau, P. M., and Meyer, M. W. (1971). *Bureaucracy in Modern Society,* 2nd ed., New York.

26. Brown, G. W., Carstairs, G. M., and Topping, G. (1958). Post-hospital adjustment of chronic mental patients, *Lancet, 2,* 685–89.

Brown, G. W. (1959). Experiences of discharged chronic schizophrenic patients in various types of living group, *Milbank Mem. Fd. Quart., 37,* 105–31.

27. Siegel, A. E., and Haas, M. B. (1963). The working mother: A review of research, *Child Develop., 34,* 513–42.

Kosa, J., and Coker, R. E. (1965). The female physician in public health: Conflict and reconciliation of the sex and professional roles, *Sociol. Soc. Res., 49,* 294–305.

Bahr, H. M. (1973). *Skid Row: An Introduction to Disaffiliation,* New York.

28. Scott, R. A. (1969). *The Making of Blind Men,* New York.

Illich, I., Zola, I. K., McKnight, J., Caplan, J. London, and Shaikan, H. (1977). *Disabling Professions,* London.

Zola, I. K., ed. (1982). *Ordinary Lives: Voices of Disability and Disease,* Philadelphia.

29. Bott, E. (1971). *Family and Social Network,* 2nd. ed., New York.

30. Parsons, T. (1951). *The Social System,* Glencoe, Ill.

31. Popper, K. R. (1952). *The Open Society and Its Enemies,* London.

32. Garson, B. (1977). *All the Livelong Day: The Meaning and Demeaning of Routine Work,* New York.

33. Barnes, J. A. (1954). Class and committees in a Norwegian parish island, *Hum. Relat., 7,* 39–58.

34. Gluckman, M. (1956). *Custom and Conflict in Africa,* London.

Gregor, T. (1973). Privacy and extra-marital affairs in a tropical forest community, in *Peoples and Cultures of Native South America,* ed. Gross, D. R., Garden City, N.Y., pp. 243–60.

35. Coser, L. A. (1956). *The Function of Social Conflict,* London.

Cumming, E. (1968). *Systems of Social Regulation,* New York.

36. Firth, R. (1951). *Elements of Social Organization,* London.

Moore, B. (1967). *Social Origins of Dictatorship and Democracy,* New York.

Miliband, R. (1969). *The State in Capitalist Society,* New York.

Poulantzas, N. (1975). *Classes in Contemporary Capitalism*, London.
Williams, R. (1982). *Sociology of Culture*, New York.

37. Kohn, M. (1971). Bureaucratic man: A portrait and an interpretation, *Amer. Soc. Rev.*, *36*, 461–74.
Domhoff, G. W. (1971). *The Higher Circles*, New York.
Blum, A. A., Estey, M., Kuhn, J. W., Wildman, W. A., and Troy, L., eds. (1971). *White Collar Workers*, New York.
Fried, M. (1973). *The World of the Urban Working Class*, Cambridge, Mass.
LeMasters, E. E. (1974). *Blue Collar Aristocrats*, Madison.
Jackman, M. R., and Jackman, R. W. (1982). *Class Awareness in the United States*, Berkeley.

38. Rainwater, L., Coleman, R., and Handel, G. (1959). *Workingman's Wife*, New York.
Komarovsky, M. (1964). *Blue-Collar Marriage*. New York.
Howell, J. T. (1973). *Hard Living on Clay Street*, New York.

39. Sennett, R., and Cobb, J. (1973). *The Hidden Injuries of Class*, New York.
Rubin, L. (1976). *Worlds of Pain: Life in the Working-Class Family*, New York.
Susser, I. (1982). *Norman Street: Politics and Poverty in an Urban Neighborhood*, New York.

40. Roethlisberger, F. J., and Dickson, W. J. (1939). *Management and the Worker*, Cambridge, Mass.
Devons, E. (1950). *Planning in Practice*, Cambridge.

41. Merton, R. K. (1957). *Social Theory and Social Structure*, Glencoe, Ill., pp. 195–207.

42. Haug, M. R., and Sussman, M. B. (1969). Professional autonomy and the revolt of the client, *Social Problems*, *17*, 153–61.
Sussman, M. B. (1972). A policy perspective on the United States rehabilitation system, *J. Hlth. Soc. Behav.*, *13*, 152–61.
Haug, M. R., and Lavin, B. (1981). Practitioner or patient—who's in charge? *J. Hlth. Soc. Behav.*, *22*, 212–29.

43. Warner, W. L., and Srole, L. (1945). *The Social Systems of American Ethnic Groups*, New Haven.

44. Moore, W. E. (1951). *Industrial Relations and the Social Order*, New York.
Jacques, E. (1952). *The Changing Culture of a Factory*, London.

45. Matsumoto, Y. S. (1970). Social stress and coronary heart disease and stroke in Japan. A hypothesis, *Milbank Mem. Fd. Quart.*, *48*, 9–36.

46. Cox, H. G. (1969). *The Feast of Fools: A Technological Essay on Festivity and Fantasy*, Cambridge, Mass.
Turner, V., and Turner, E. (1978). *Image and Pilgrimage in Christian Culture*, New York.

47. Frankenberg, R. (1957). *Village on the Border*, London.

48. Srinivas, M. N. (1966). *Social Change in Modern India*, Berkeley.

49. Chester, T. E. (1961). *A Study of Post-War Growth in Management Organizations*, Paris.

50. Robinson, J. (1946). *The Economics of Imperfect Competition*, London.
Chamberlain, E. H. (1954). *Monopoly and Competition and Their Control*, London.
Barnet, R., and Müller, R. E. (1974). *Global Reach*, New York.

51. Birch, A. H. (1959). *Small-Town Politics*, London.

52. Dochez, A. R. (1939). President's address, *Transactions of the American Clinical and Climatological Association*, *54*, 19–23, cited by Rosen, G. (1963), in *The Hospital in Modern Society*, ed. Freidson, E., London, p. 27.

53. Carr-Saunders, A. M., and Wilson, P. A. (1933). *The Professions*, London.
    Lewis, R., and Maude, A. (1952). *Professional People*, London.
    Marsh, D. C. (1958). *The Changing Social Structure of England and Wales, 1871–1951*, London.
    Larson, M. S. (1977). *The Rise of Professionalism: A Sociological Analysis*, Berkeley.
54. Freidson, E. (1970). *Profession of Medicine*, New York.
    Freidson, E. (1970). *Professional Dominance*, New York.
    Starr, P. (1982). *The Social Transformation of American Medicine*, New York.
55. Copeman, G. H. (1955). *Leaders of British Industry*, London.
56. U.S. Department of Commerce, Bureau of the Census (1983). *Statistical Abstract of the United States, 1982–83*, Washington, D.C.
57. Watson, W. (1964). Social class and social mobility in industrial communities, in *Closed Systems and Open Minds*, ed. Gluckman, M., London.
58. Fox, T. F. (1960). The personal doctor and his relation to the hospital, *Lancet, 1,* 743–60.
    Smith, A. (1962). The future of general practice, *Lancet, 1,* 38–40.
    Susser, M. W. (1963). Further thoughts on the future of medical practice outside the hospital, *Lancet, 1,* 315–19.
    Balint, M. (1964). *The Doctor, His Patient and the Illness*, 2nd ed., New York.
    Powles, J. (1973). On the limitations of modern medicine, *Science, Medicine and Man, 1,* 1–30.
    Fuchs, V. (1975). *Who Shall Live?*, New York.
59. Freidson, E. (1960). Client control and medical practice, *Amer. J. Sociol., 65,* 734–82.
    Freidson, E. (1961). *Patients' Views of Medical Practice*, New York.
60. Kendall, P. L. (1961). Impact of training programs on the young physician's attitudes, *J. Amer. Med. Ass., 176,* 992–7.
61. Koos, E. L. (1946). *Families in Trouble*, New York.
    Mechanic, D. (1962). The concept of illness behavior, *J. Chr. Dis., 15,* 189–94.
    Zola, I. K. (1964). Illness behavior of the working class: Implications and recommendations, in *Blue Collar World*, ed. Shostak, A. B. and Gomberg, W., Englewood Cliffs, N.J., pp. 350–61.
    Fabrega, H. (1974). *Disease and Social Behavior*, Cambridge, Mass.
62. Litman, T. J. (1974). The family as a basic unit in health and medical care: A social behavioral overview, *Soc. Sci. Med., 8,* 495–519.
    Mauksch, H. O. (1974). A social science basis for conceptualizing mental health, *Soc. Sci. Med., 8,* 521–8.
    Douglas, M. (1975). *Natural Symbols*, London.
    Finlayson, A. (1976). Social networks as coping resources, *Soc. Sci. Med., 10,* 97–103.
    Hammer, M. (1983). "Core" and "extended" social networks in relation to health and illness, *Soc. Sci. Med., 17,* 405–11.
    Hammer, M., Gutwirth, L., and Phillips, S. L. (1983). Parenthood and social networks. A preliminary view, *Soc. Sci. Med., 16,* 2091–2100.
63. Wadsworth, M. (1974). Health and sickness: The choice of treatment, *J. Psychosom. Res., 18,* 271–276.
64. Kadushin, C. (1958–59). Individual decisions to undertake psychotherapy, *Administrative Science Quarterly, 3,* 379–411.
    Salloway, J. C., and Dillan, P. (1973). A comparison of family networks and friend networks in health care utilization, *J. Compar. Fam. Stud., 4,* 131–42.

Gottlieb, B. H. (1976). Lay influence on the utilization and provision of health services, *Canad. Psychol. Rev., 17*, 126–36.

Horwitz, A. (1978). Family, kin, and friend networks in psychiatric help-seeking, *Soc. Sci. Med., 12*, 297–304.

Janzen, J. (1978). *The Quest for Therapy in Lower Zaire*, Berkeley, Calif.

65. Martin, J. P. (1957). *Social Aspects of Prescribing*, London.

Logan, R. F. L. (1964). Studies in the spectrum of medical care, in *Problems and Progress in Medical Care*, ed. McLachlan, G., London.

66. Berger, J. (1967). *A Fortunate Man*, London.

67. Halberstam, M., and Lestier, S. (1978). *A Coronary Event*, New York.

Anonymous (1978). The death of a colleague, *Man and Medicine, 3*, 229–66.

Lear, M. W. (1980). *Heartsounds*, New York.

68. Stanton, A. H., and Schwartz, M. S. (1954). *The Mental Hospital*, New York.

Caudill, W. (1958). *The Psychiatric Hospital As a Small Society*, Cambridge, Mass.

Stein, Z. A., and Susser, M. W. (1964). Hypothesis: Failures in medical care as a function of the doctor's situation, *Med. Care, 2*, 162–6.

Sheehan, S. (1982). *Is There No Place on Earth for Me?*, New York.

69. Pratt, L., Seligmann, A., and Reader, G. (1957). Physicians' views on the level of medical information among patients, *Amer. J. Publ. Hlth., 47*, 1277–83.

Siegel, E., and Dillehay, R. C. (1966). Some approaches to family planning counseling in local health departments, *Amer. J. Publ. Hlth., 56*, 1840–46.

Cartwright, A. (1968). General practitioners and family planning, *Med. Offr., 120*, 43–6.

Francis, V., Korsch, B. M., and Morris, M. J. (1969). Gaps in doctor-patient communication, *New Eng. J. Med., 280*, 535–40.

70. Mitchell, J. C., ed. (1969). *Social Networks in Urban Situations*, Manchester.

Granovetter, M. S. (1973). The strength of weak ties, *Amer. J. Sociol., 78*, 1360–80.

Craven, P., and Wellman, B. (1974). The network city, in *The Community: Approaches and Applications*, ed. Effrat, M. P., New York.

71. Mogey, J. M. (1956). *Family and Neighbourhood*, London.

72. Thompson, B. (1954). Housing of growing families in Aberdeen, *Med. Offr., 91*, 235–9.

Gans, H. (1962). *The Urban Villagers*, New York.

Fried, M. (1973). *The World of the Urban Working Class*, Cambridge, Mass.

Stack, C. (1974). *All Our Kin*, New York.

73. Fortes, M. (1958). The developmental cycle in domestic groups, Introduction to *Cambridge Papers in Social Anthropology*, ed. Goody, J., Cambridge.

74. Martin, F. M., Brotherston, J. H. F., and Chave, S. P. (1957). Incidence of neurosis in a new housing estate, *Brit. J. Prev. Soc. Med., 11*, 196–202.

75. Taylor, Lord, and Chave, S. P. W. (1964). *Mental Health and Environment*, London.

Hare, E. H., and Shaw, G. K. (1965). *Mental Health on a New Housing Estate*, Maudsley Monograph No. 12, London.

76. Wilner, D. M., Walkley, R. P., Pinkerton, T. C., and Tayback, M. (1962). *The Housing Environment and Family Life: A Longitudinal Study of the Effects of Housing on Morbidity and Mental Health*, Baltimore.

77. Fried, M. (1965). Transitional functions of working class communities: Implications for forced relocation, in *Mobility and Mental Health*, ed. Kantor, M. B., Springfield, Ill., pp. 123–65.

78. Kasl, S. V., Ostfeld, A. M., Brody, G. M., Snell, L., and Price, C. A. (1980). Effects of involuntary relocation on the health and behavior of the elderly, *Second Conference*

on the Epidemiology of Aging, ed. Haynes, S. G., and Feinleib, M., U.S. Dept. Health and Human Services, Washington, D.C., pp. 211–32.

79. **Berkman, L. F.,** and **Syme, S. L.** (1979). Social networks, host resistance, and mortality: A nine year follow-up study of Alameda County residents, *Amer. J. Epidemiol., 109,* 186–204.

    Gore, S. (1981). Stress-buffering functions of social supports: An appraisal and clarification of research models, in *Stressful Life Events and their Contexts*, ed., Dohrenwend, B. S. and Dohrenwend, B. P., New York, pp. 202–22.

    House, J. S., Robbins, C., and **Metzner, H. L.** (1982). The association of social relationships and activities with mortality: Prospective evidence from the Tecumseh Community Health Study, *Amer. J. Epidemiol., 116,* 123–140.

    Reed, D., McGee, D., Yano, K., and **Feinlieb, M.** (1983). Social networks and coronary heart disease among Japanese men in Hawaii, *Amer. J. Epidemiol., 117,* 384–96.

    Berkman, L. F., and **Breslow, L.** (1983). *Health and Ways of Living: The Alameda County Study*, New York.

80. **Dahrendorf, R.** (1981). *Life Chances: Approaches to Social and Political Theory*, Chicago.

81. **Townsend, P.** (1957). *The Family Life of Old People*, London.

82. **Tizard, J.,** and **Grad, J.** (1961). *The Mentally Handicapped and Their Families*, Maudsley Monograph No. 7, London.

83. **Susser, M.** (1968). *Community Psychiatry: Epidemiologic and Social Themes*, New York.

84. **Freeman, H. E.,** and **Simmons, O. G.** (1958). Mental patients in the community: Family settings and performance levels, *Amer. Sociol. Rev., 23,* 147–54.

    Freeman, H. E., and **Simmons, O. G.** (1959). The social integration of former mental patients, *Int. J. Soc. Psychiat., 4,* 264–71.

    Waxler, N. E., and **Mishler, E. G.** (1963). Hospitalization of psychiatric patients: Physician centered and family-centered influence patterns, *J. Hlth. Hum. Behav., 4,* 250–7.

    Miller, D. (1967). Retrospective analysis of post hospital mental patients' world, *J. Hlth. Soc. Behav., 8,* 136–40.

    Greenley, J. R. (1972). The psychiatric patient's family and length of hospitalization, *J. Hlth. Soc. Behav., 13,* 25–37.

85. **Brown, G. W., Birley, J. L. T.,** and **Wing, J. K.** (1972). Influence of family life on the course of schizophrenic disorders: A replication, *Brit. J. Psychiat., 121,* 241–58.

    Vaughn, C. E., and **Leff, J. P.** (1976). The influence of family and social factors on the course of psychiatric illness, *Brit. J. Psychiat., 129,* 125–37.

    Leff, J. P. (1976). Schizophrenia and sensitivity to family environment, *Schiz. Bull., 2,* 566–74.

86. **Hammer, M.** (1963–64). Influence of small social networks as factors on mental hospital admission, *Human Organization, 22,* 243–51.

    Cohen, C. I., Sichel, W. R., and **Berger, D.** (1977). The use of a mid-Manhattan hotel as a support system, *Commun. Ment. Hlth. J., 13,* 76–83.

    Estroff, S. (1981). *Making It Crazy*, Berkeley.

    Hammer, M. (1983). Social networks and the long term patient, in *The Chronic Psychiatric Patient in the Community: Principles of Treatment*, ed. Barofsky, I. and Budson, R. D., New York, pp. 49–82.

87. **Sigerist, H. E.** (1929). Die Sonderstellung des Kranken, *Kyklos, 2,* 11–20, trans. in *The Sociology of Medicine*, ed. Roemer, M. I. (1960). New York.

    Twaddle, A. C., and **Hessler, R. M.** (1977). *A Sociology of Health*, St. Louis.

88. **Watson, W.** (1958). *Tribal Cohesion in a Money Economy: A Study of the Mambwe People of Northern Rhodesia*, Manchester.

89. **Raper, A. B.** (1958). The incidence of peptic ulceration in some African tribal groups, *Trans. Roy. Soc. Trop. Med. Hyg.*, 52, 535–46.

90. **Cogswell, B. E.,** and **Weir, D. D.** (1964). A role in process: The development of medical professionals' role in long-term care of chronically diseased patients, *J. Hlth. Soc. Behav.*, 5, 95–103.

    Freidson, E. (1965). Disability and social deviance, in *Sociology and Rehabilitation*, ed. Sussman, M. B., Washington, D. C., pp. 71–99.

    Zahn, M. A. (1973). Incapacity, impotence and invisible impairment: Their effects upon interpersonal relations, *J. Hlth. Soc. Behav.*, 14, 115–23.

    Parsons, T. (1975). The sick role and the role of the physician reconsidered, *Health and Society*, 53, 257–78.

    Strauss, A. (1975). *Chronic Illness and the Quality of Life*, St. Louis.

    Gallagher, E. B. (1976). Lines of reconstruction and extension in the Parsonian sociology of illness, *Soc. Sci. Med.*, 10, 207–18.

    Dimond, M. (1983). Social adaptation of the chronically ill, in *Handbook of Health, Health Care and the Health Professions*, ed. Mechanic, D., New York, pp. 636–54.

91. **Richards, P.** (1977). *The Medieval Leper and His Northern Heirs*, London.

92. **Field, M. J.** (1960). *Search for Security*, London.

    Brown, J. S. and **Rawlinson, M.** (1975). Relinquishing the sick role following open-heart surgery, *J. Hlth. Soc. Behav.*, 16, 12–27.

93. **McKinlay, J. B.** (1980). Social network influences on morbid episodes and the career of help seeking, in *The Relevance of Social Science for Medicine*, ed., Eisenberg, L., and Kleinman, A., London, pp. 77–107.

94. **Parsons, T.,** and **Fox, R.** (1952). Illness, therapy and the modern urban American family, *J. Soc. Issues*, 8 (4), 31–44.

95. **Adams, M.** (1956). Social work with mental defectives. I. *Case Conference*, 3, 4.

    Adams, M. (1957). Social work with mental defectives. II. *Case Conference*, 4, 1.

    Leeson, J. E. (1960). A study of six mentally handicapped children and their families, *Med. Offr.*, 104, 311–14.

96. **Watzlawick, P., Beavin, J. H.,** and **Jackson, D. D.** (1967). *Pragmatics of Human Communication*, New York.

    Roman, P. M., and **Trice, H. M.** (1968). The sick role, labelling theory and the deviant drinker, *Int. J. Soc. Psychiat.*, 14, 245–51.

    Bateson, G. (1971). The cybernetics of "self": A theory of alcoholism, *Psychiatry*, 34, 1–18.

97. **Karpinos, B. D.** (1967). Mental test failures, in *The Draft*, ed. Tax, S., Chicago.

    Waitzkin, H. (1971). Latent functions of the sick role in various institutional settings, *Soc. Sci. Medi.*, 5, 45–75.

98. **Clay, R. M.** (1909). *The Mediaeval Hospitals of England*, London.

    Rosen, G. (1963). The hospital: Historical sociology of a community institution, in *The Hospital in Modern Society*, ed. Freidson, E., London, pp. 1–36.

    Rosner, D. (1982). *A Once Charitable Enterprise: Hospitals and Health Care in Brooklyn and New York, 1855–1915*, New York.

99. **Edgerton, R. B.** (1967). *The Cloak of Competence*, Berkeley, Calif.

    Chu, F., and **Trotter, S.** (1974). *The Madness Establishment*, New York.

    Kirk, S. A., and **Therrien, M. E.** (1975). Community mental health myths and the fate of former hospitalized patients, *Psychiatry*, 38, 209–17.

Wolpert, J., and Wolpert, E. (1976). The relocation of released mental patients into residential communities, *Policy Sciences*, 7, 31–51.

Scull, A. T. (1977). *Decarceration: Community Treatment and the Deviant—A Radical View*, Englewood Cliffs, N.J.

Talbott, J. A. (1979). Care of the chronically mentally ill—Still a national disgrace, *Amer. J. Psychiat.*, 136, 688–89.

Wing, J. K., and Olsen, R., eds. (1979). *Community Care for the Mentally Disabled*, New York.

U.S. Department of Health and Human Services, Steering Committee on the Chronically Mentally Ill, (1980). *Towards a National Plan for the Chronically Mentally Ill*, Washington, D.C.

Mechanic, D. (1980). *Mental Health and Social Policy*, 2nd ed., Englewood Cliffs, N.J.

Estroff, S. (1981). Psychiatric deinstitutionalization: A sociocultural analysis, *J. Soc. Issues*, 37, 116–32.

Baxter, E., and Hopper, K. (1982). The new mendicancy, *Amer. J. Orthopsychiat.*, 52, 393–408.

100. Stein, Z., and Susser, M. W. (1960). Estimating hostel needs for backward citizens, *Lancet*, 2, 486–88.

Stein, Z., and Susser, M. W. (1960). The families of dull children: a classification for predicting careers, *Brit. J. Prev. Soc. Med.*, 14, 83–88.

101. Burlingham, D., and Freud, A. (1944). *Infants Without Families*, London.

Lewis, H. (1954). *Deprived Children*, London.

102. Zweig, F. (1952). *The British Worker*, Harmondsworth.

Oakley, A. (1974). *The Sociology of Housework*, New York.

103. Banton, M. (1959). *White and Coloured: The Behaviour of British People Towards Coloured Immigrants*, London.

104. Sussman, M. B. (1953). The help pattern in the middle class family, *Amer. Sociol. Rev.*, 18, 22–28.

Sussman, M. B. (1959). The isolated nuclear family: Fact or fiction, *Soc. Probl.*, 6, 333–40.

8

Social mobility, stress, and disorders of health

Adults in industrial society are all legally free to choose where they will live, and with whom they will interact and in what manner. Even their relations with adult kin are optional. This legal freedom is restricted by personal and social characteristics. Age, sex, occupation, race, education, and religion limit the choice of activities, and narrow the avenues to desired social positions. The kinds of skill an individual has limit the choice of jobs and of colleagues; social class, income, and ethnicity limit the choice of neighborhood and neighbors. In other words, although class societies foster variation and idiosyncrasy in individual behavior and achievement, these variations are systematic and not fortuitous. Even in the most democratic societies, vertical mobility from one social class to another has never been entirely free. There is always some channeling of movement and resistance to it, and insofar as equality of opportunity exists, it is a means of stratifying society on the criterion of particular valued abilities (1). Indeed, changes in the labor market, with a growing proportion of the workforce employed in skilled jobs and, consequently, an increasing proportion of occupations assigned to higher social classes, account for the great part of intergenerational mobility in a class society such as the United States (2).

Social mobility can be horizontal as well as vertical. It is horizontal when an individual exchanges affiliation with one church for another, or moves from one family to another through divorce and remarriage, or leaves a job in one factory to take up similar work in another. Nor is mobility confined to people. Social objects or values, those things that have been created or modified by human activity, can move from one country to another, and upwards or downwards from one social class to another (3).

Mobility and the health of individuals

In medicine, social mobility characterizes diseases, methods of treatment, and patients. Diseases show social movement; syphilis was introduced to South Africa by

314

Europeans, who then transmitted it to the subordinate Africans. Treatment, too, followed the same course (4). In Britain this kind of social movement has been traced for surgical operations; tonsillectomy and circumcision have moved from the higher to the lower social classes (5). In previous chapters we noted several examples of social mobility in health disorders: peptic ulcer probably followed a downward social course, and coronary heart disease appears to have done so as well. In the wake of the diffusion of cigarette smoking between the social classes, the sexes, and the age-groups of successive generations, a trail of morbidity and mortality from smoking-related diseases has been laid.

Infant feeding practices have shown similar downward social mobility, abetted by the market, with unhappy results in underdeveloped countries when taken up by poor mothers who must go out to work and lack the resources to prepare the formula properly. Contraceptive practices, too, have passed between the social classes, and in turn have helped alter the sexual relationships and the spacing and size of families, their economic capacity, and their health and socialization patterns. In Britain with the introduction of contraception on a wide scale, the so-called "male" method of the working-class (i.e., simple withdrawal before ejaculation) was superseded by the condom sheath, while among the middle and upper classes the diaphragm, a "female" method, superseded the condom, as it had earlier done in the United States (6). Subsequently, the advent of oral hormonal contraceptives and intrauterine devices has quite altered the picture of contraception and, we have good grounds to surmise, of sex behavior and the many facets of health related to it. The distribution of contraceptives across the world is now further affected not only by silent diffusion, but by active propagation of a variety of family planning methods in underdeveloped countries.

The social mobility of diseases invites both theory and action. As we saw with social class, an uneven and dynamic social distribution calls for explanation, and forms the base for many hypotheses about the causes of disease. At the same time, variation points to the possibilities of prevention, and demonstrates which social groups are most in need of treatment and care. The social mobility of persons has import not only for the uneven distribution and diffusion of disease but also as a potential source of stress and strain. Social mobility is not frictionless, and the burden may account for some of the variation in the distribution of disorders among social classes and migrant groups.

Social movement enforces a series of transitions into new environments, and the mobile individual must make personal adjustments as he or she passes through each. In social encounters strangers are confronted; at work new obligations and new responsibilities are contracted. Mobility by definition creates discontinuity in status and role and, in consequence, often in culture and values. The new behavior required in an unfamiliar position must be learned, and the novel customs and idiom of other reference groups must be understood. Extreme social mobility is exemplified by the immigrant, who must face not only unfamiliar situations, but also familiar situations demanding unfamiliar responses. In migrating families, effects of cultural conflict appear to be most acute for children of school age, although the evidence for this presents difficulties of interpretation (7).

A change in social situation entails some disruption of past relationships. At the same time, the statuses freshly acquired by the mobile person create incongruities in those new relationships that must replace or supplement the old. Aside from the new status that signals the mobility of the individual—say marriage or occupation—the array of statuses already possessed by the mobile individual might have little in common with the statuses of those with whom he or she must habitually relate. Some degree of *status inconsistency* is thus inevitable for the mobile individual. This disparity of station, standing, and background may exist not only between the individual and those he or she relates with in the new situation, but also among the individual's own statuses and attributes—for example, between high-ranking occupation and low income, or between high social standing and low income (8,9).

It was an early clinical impression that certain illnesses were likely to occur at a time when a patient must adapt to a life crisis (10). Evidence has been scanty, and the hypothesis hard to test. Nevertheless, some research has encouraged this view. Laboratory studies first demonstrated a clear link between noxious stimuli and physiological or psychological dysfunction. Epidemiological studies soon followed. The timing of perforations of duodenal ulcer, for instance, has been related to external sources of anxiety, and the timing of sickness has been related to adversity as it appears from the clustering of reported episodes of sickness and personal problems among employees (11). Episodes of schizophrenia and of depression have been shown to be preceded by some disturbing family event much more often than expected (12). The crisis may be a mass as well as an individual phenomenon: after pit disasters or mass dismissals, Scottish miners during the interwar period reacted with falling work output, absenteeism, strikes, and a burst of claims for disablement because of nystagmus (13).

This patchwork of knowledge has been built into a theory of *transitional crises,* changes in social situation that are believed to underlie or precipitate emotional and psychosomatic disorders. To discover and establish these hypothetical effects requires the spelling out of the precise elements of the transition that may cause them as well as of the effects themselves; in other words, specification of the independent as well as the dependent variables (14). The transition itself must be separated from the penumbra of experiences, values, and feelings bound up on the one hand with past statuses, and on the other with the newly acquired statuses. Associations between a history of particular transitions and existing health disorders have been found in a number of cross-sectional prevalence studies at a point in time, but it is another matter to extract from them the timing of the transitional and subsequent elements of such a change and the onset of a disease, especially an insidious chronic disease. The onset of sickness can be determined with somewhat greater confidence, but because sickness designates a social role, what is being measured as a dependent variable may be help-seeking behavior rather than the onset of disorder (15). Moreover, although transitions have in common sharp discontinuities in status and role, the social and emotional effects of these discontinuities can be difficult to separate from the effects of the continuing state that follows. Some transitions enlarge and others diminish a person's standing, competence, and control over life circumstances. Some convert him or her to membership in more or less valued minorities, others to membership in majorities. Some transitions are voluntary and desired, others involuntary and feared.

Transitions, being so diverse, can best be treated in classes, for instance, subdivided according to the two dimensions of the phase of the life arc and the direction of mobility. The particular phase of the life-arc dictates whether status and roles expand or contract; the direction is a function of the social standing of the new statuses relative to the old in a chosen frame of reference, and can be movement upward, downward, or horizontal. Thus, transitions can be *normal steps of recruitment* in the expanding phase of the life-arc, but their form and the probability of this occurrence are determined by the phase in which they occur. Such transitions as entering and leaving school, or taking up an occupation, or marrying and becoming a mother are steps of recruitment into enhanced statuses and an increment of roles. Bereavement and retirement are no less norms for all, but they are universally *steps of displacement* into diminished statuses and a decrement of roles. On the other hand, the premature separation of children, migration between and within countries, and switches of affiliation between equivalent groups are particular and not universal, that is, unpredictable *extranormal steps*, and these steps may either enhance or diminish statuses and roles (14,16).

With any of these transitions, the change in social standing that accompanies the change in statuses is combined and summarized in the dimension of social mobility as upward, horizontal, or downward. Unpredictable transitions tend to involve sharper discontinuities than do those normal transitions that are made by all who can make them. But the failure to negotiate a normal transition—whether to achieve schooling, or an occupation, or marriage, or reproduction—may in some settings carry the mark of continuing deviant status, and may even exact a heavy emotional penalty. Long-continued failure to negotiate a culturally normalized transition can produce one form of status inconsistency. For instance, youths who fail to obtain employment on leaving school combine adult status with a jobless status and economic dependency inappropriate for their age group in society. Premature transitions have similar results in discordant statuses—for instance, schoolgirls who become pregnant, or students who marry and raise families immediately on leaving school, and hence take on roles difficult to satisfy at the same time as the other role demands of that phase of life.

This framework alone cannot clearly separate the transition crisis from what went before and what follows. Nor does it attend to sometimes determinative changes in the larger social setting (for instance, a decline in employment prospects) within which normal transitions are expected. But it does help to focus the scattered evidence about the stresses of transitions, individual social mobility, and resulting inconsistency and incongruity.

Normal steps of recruitment

Upward steps of recruitment have been associated, in a few instances, with an excess of morbidity at the time of the step. Schoolchildren are referred to psychiatric services most frequently, according to a large American and a small British study, at an age that coincides with transfer from primary to high school, and some British authors have attributed the rare peptic ulcers found in children to strain arising from the competitive transition entailed by the effort to gain entry to academic secondary schools. Causal links are far from established, however.

At adolescence, the syndrome of the "identity crisis" has achieved wide currency (17). Much adolescent behavior can be explained in terms of having to relinquish dependent roles in family and school, and to search for an identity with suitable adult roles among those available. Industrial societies offer, at least in the standard perception, latitude of choice among a wide, ill-defined, and changing array of such roles. The adolescent is denied the security of the *rites de passage* that in traditional societies prescribe the terms of entry into adulthood and a well-defined life career.

These are normal experiences that affect everyone. There is as yet little evidence to show that health disorders have their onset more commonly at this time of life than before or after. Exceptions are age-peaks for leukemia and malignant bone tumors, appendicitis (or, more precisely, appendectomies) and menarcheal disorders in girls. Most notable are manifestations of "acting out": in adolescence and young adulthood, accidents, juvenile delinquency, and the use of narcotics, as well as suicides, tend to be common to many urban subcultures today (18).

The marital transition of itself produces no known health effects. Certainly the actual married state and the building of a family have many indirect, and probably some direct, consequences for the health of the conjugal partners. The single state is associated with high rates of sickness from many disorders, including alcoholism, schizophrenia, coronary heart disease, and perforated peptic ulcer (14,19). Rates of mortality are uniformly higher than for married people for a large number of listed causes of death (see Chapter 10). So far, however, there is probably more evidence to show that disease and its consequences (dependence, disability, and confinement in institutions) cause this failure in social transition than there is to show the reverse. Divorce, too, is associated with high rates of mental disorder, but again interpretation is complicated because the rates are probably inflated by a residue of mentally ill divorcees who fail to remarry. Maternity with its complications is one condition that does directly give rise to health disorders. In the period immediately postpartum, mild depression is common. While considerable physiological strain and adaptation accompany parturition and the end of pregnancy, psychological as well as physiological strains probably contribute both to this mild depression and to episodes of severe postpartum depression (20).

The normal upward transitions of occupation and employment have given rise to a number of studies, but to many more speculative hypotheses. Failure to find work on leaving school has been the common condition of black youths in the slums of American cities in the decades after the Second World War. This status inconsistency is put into social context by the concept of *anomie*, especially as it refers to disjunction between cultural norms that prescribe approved goals and a social structure that prevents the goals from being attained (see Chapter 4.) Competitiveness and striving for success are built into a mobile class society, but equal success is not allowed to everyone; there are always more losers than winners in a competititon. In a newly industrializing America, the ideology of mobility served to reconcile workers to the discipline of the factory, turning their potential resentment into a kind of self blame—a phenomenon still much in evidence among the disenfranchised today (21).

People of the lowest social classes are most exposed to these effects of *anomie*, since they have least chance to acquire social standing or wealth. Thus, they have been found more likely to report the feelings of alienation elicited by a questionnaire devised to measure the individual subjective state of *anomia* (22). The postulated outcomes or responses are group delinquency, gang violence, the use of narcotics, and other forms of deviant social behavior. Mental disorder has been studied directly: among blacks in Philadelphia, just such a discrepancy between occupational aspirations and low achieved status could explain the unexpectedly high rates of entry to psychiatric services among the Philadelphia-born compared with migrants from the South (23); but other explanations such as unequal service usage have not been ruled out.

Although the values of competitive achievement are widespread, they are not accepted by all individuals or all subcultures. The precise effects are mediated by the reference groups to which people affiliate directly or by aspiration, as well as by their individual personalities. The British working class, and parts of the American working class, have had a strong class loyalty that has inhibited aspirations to upward mobility (24). Robert Merton's model of the types of response that can be expected rests on two dimensions: the degree of acceptance, on one side of cultural goals, and on the other of the institutionalized means to attain them (25). Some accept both goals and means and conform; some accept goals but not means and innovate or rebel; others deny goals but comply with means, in a form of ritualism. Still others deny both goals and means; they may either retreat or revolt. Revolutionaries are those who seek to change the social and cultural structure and to substitute both new goals and new means of attaining them.

	Means	Goals
Conformism	+	+
Innovation/Rebellion	−	+
Ritualism	+	−
Retreat/Revolution	−	−

Anomia describes the subjective sense of alienation or status inconsistency of all those who do not conform, though many do conform. Durkheim suggested long ago that upward as well as downward social mobility results in high suicide rates by increasing the number of people in anomic situations. Hypotheses about the effects of vertical social mobility on health tend to consider two components of mobility: psychological and social. These are seldom separated, although only one or the other is usually emphasized. The psychological component refers to personality and mind set, the social to status inconsistency and its implicit psychological consequences.

The personality component most usually postulated is a competitive mental and behavioral set. This set is held to be elicited or intensified by the goals of individual achievement in mobile class societies, whereas it might remain latent in societies that put less store by achievement. Striving, energetic qualities have been found to mark even the play and leisure pursuits of those who move up the social scale, although this trait cluster has not been entirely consistent (26). The personality hypothesis has been advanced, implicitly or explicitly, as a factor in schizophrenia, mental disorder, and duodenal ulcer and, most prominently, in coronary heart disease. As a corollary, socially mobile persons have been considered more psychologicaly "deprived" than others (27). We noted in a previous chapter that ambitious, striving men beset by deadlines have seemed more prone both to attacks of coronary heart disease and to some of the precursors associated with the disease (see Chapter 4). In a Connecticut study, some investigators have looked to the so-called Protestant ethic of individual achievement to explain the finding of a much higher incidence of coronary heart disease among Protestants than Catholics. With upward mobility, however, risk was indeed raised solely among Protestants, but only modestly. Upward mobility, in keeping with the Protestant ethic, may be as rewarding as it is stressful. With downward mobility, risk was markedly raised among Protestants, and slightly among Catholics (28).

The social status component of stress in social mobility relates to status inconsistency. Social mobility produces status inconsistencies. One interpretation compatible with the results of this Connecticut study is that cultural background generates internal conflict about status inconsistency and thereby contributes to risk. Some other studies also suggest that such inconsistencies, placed in social and cultural context, may be relevant to coronary heart disease. A California study found raised risks for the disease with the intergenerational mobility for one particular group. These were college graduates who were the sons of foreign-born fathers; their risks were high compared with two groups presumed to be less mobile and to have fewer inconsistent statuses, namely the nongraduate sons of foreign-born fathers and the graduate sons of native-born fathers (29). Another study of a nationwide American corporation compared two types of *spiralists*. Executives without a college education, who had been recruited to the lower ranks of the company and worked their way up, had a higher incidence of coronary heart disease than those with a college education, who at the outset had been recruited to the managerial cadres. The executives recruited from the lower ranks also had a higher incidence than those who had remained in the ranks of craftsman (30). These relationships held for hypertension as well. The Connecticut data, too, on subsequent analysis revealed that the coronary heart disease rates of lower-class men were more affected by intergenerational mobility than those of their middle- or upper-class counterparts (31).

These various studies suggest that a form of status incongruity that carries high risk is the combination of low education with high occupation (32). Some class-related predispositions may play a part in this risk. Thus a study of upwardly mobile Bell telephone executives found that those who were not college educated differed from their college-educated co-workers in several attributes such as smoking, social background, and leisure activities (33).

The postulated effect of mobility may be owed to the demands of the new work situation, or to the disruption of social supports it brings about as much as to the mismatch of statuses (34). For example, job demands might simply outstrip personal skills or abilities or the new job itself might be inherently stressful. Elevated peptic ulcer rates are found among foremen (35). An increased frequency of peptic ulcer among assembly-line workers who become foremen—and who are thereby subjected to the cross-cutting loyalties to fellow workers and management inherent in such intercalary positions—is as likely to be a result of job demands as a result of promotion. Again, job stresses may be tempered, and dull repetitive work made tolerable, by positive social relations with co-workers (36). The actual work situation must be examined (37).

Status consistency as a variable has given mixed results (38). In the instance of mental states, the Philadelphia study mentioned above found no relationship between patients' entry to psychiatric care and dissonance between their coexisting statuses of occupation, education, and income. But a national questionnaire survey did discover an association between psychophysiological symptoms and dissonance between occupation and education. Thus, both women of high education married to men in occupations of low standing, and men of low education in occupations of high standing, had high symptom scores (9). In Israel too, dissonance between occupation and education among immigrants yielded high scores on a symptom inventory (39).

Status incongruence between an individual and those with whom the person relates impinges directly on such intimate relationships as marriage, where differences in background between spouses enforce accommodation in behavior and values. Marital strains of this kind have been explored for their contribution to rheumatoid arthritis, a chronic and insidious disorder more common among the lower social classes than the higher. Status incongruence between parents of rheumatoid patients and those of their variously chosen controls was measured by incongruity of the occupation and education of fathers compared with the education of mothers. In both sons and daughters the degree of incongruity was related to the amount of reported anger and irritation (which was taken in turn to be an index of contained hostility and resentment). Status incongruence between parents was also related to the frequency of rheumatoid arthritis in their daughters, although not in their sons: a repetition of this pattern of status incongruence between spouses was also discovered among the affected daughters (40). Thus, among women with rheumatoid arthritis, anger and hostility arising out of status incongruity could be an intervening psychological variable in a sociogenic causal chain. Among men who suffered from the disease, however, the predominant emotions or states were more often submissiveness and passivity. This gender difference in the emotional state of patients with rheumatoid arthritis could reflect modes of dealing with conflict that are typical for each gender. In turn, this emotional difference could lead to different manifestations of disease, illness and sickness in each gender. The direction of causal effects must remain at issue, however, since it is equally possible that the different emotional states are the typical responses of each gender to the disease.

An analysis of 269 couples in the Framingham study found that, regardless of their own social status, men married to women of higher standing than their own (defined by white-collar job or college education) were at significantly greater risk (RR = 2.6) of developing coronary heart disease than were men married to women of lower standing. In this study, it was not status incongruity in general but "exposure" to a higher status wife that was associated with elevated risk. The greater risk persisted after controlling for the usual coronary risk factors, and also when separate clinical end-points (angina, myocardial infarction) were used. A similar finding was reported in a San Diego study of 1698 couples, aged 45 to 79 years, which examined coronary deaths among husbands over a nine-year period. Educational attainment of each spouse was measured at the outset. Men less educated than their wives were at greater risk for coronary death than men who were as well or better educated than their wives The effect was especially pronounced in cases where educational discordance was greatest, that is, in high-school educated men married to college-educated women. Again, the risk was still elevated after controlling for the difference in age, social class, blood pressure, or other risk factors (41).

Normal steps of displacement

Normal transitions that diminish individual status include *retirement* and *bereavement*. (Some of the consequences of these displacements are discussed at greater length elsewhere; see Chapter 10.) Retirement has had psychological effects attributed to it on the basis of clinical case studies (42), but epidemiologic studies to demonstrate serious long-term consequences are lacking. Although morbidity at the time of retirement is high, the most that can be said is that retirement increases readiness to assume the sick role (43). Retirement selects the ill disproportionately. Illness is an important cause of retirement among men in the later decades of life, and many who feel fit and can find or keep jobs continue to work (see Chapter 12). This "healthy worker" effect can thus give rise to the spurious appearance of high morbidity rates among the retired.

Bereavement is one transitional crisis in which the transitional event itself, and its immediate consequences, can be taken to produce an effect. Indeed, clinical studies of disaster, bereavement, and grief first gave rise to the hypothesis of transitional crisis as a cause of emotional disorder (44). *Widowhood* offers a paradigmatic example of a stressful life event, and one that has the advantage of having been studied with a variety of research designs (45). At the turn of the century, Karl Pearson and his colleagues culled parish registers and tombstones to study the question of assortative mating, and found evidence of an association of age at death between spouses (46). In the early 1940s, an American study compared the death certificates of spouses in a single county and found associations between them, not only for age at death, but for specific causes of death as well (47). A later study of national statistics in the United States showed that the widowed, especially those widowed early, had excessive death rates from several causes; a number of causes such as pneumonia, tuberculosis, and vascular diseases of the heart and central nervous system were associated with the same cause of death in the spouse. These associations can be interpreted in at least three ways: first, that the selection of mates joins those with a mutual high risk already existing before marriage; second, that the shared environment of the marriage renders both spouses vulnerable to the same disorders; third, that after the dissolution of the marriage, the survivor was affected by the material, psychological, and social consequences of bereavement (48).

These early studies gave way to testing of specific hypotheses. Thus, the role of widowhood in suicide was demonstrated in a case-control study, using the death certificates of suicides and controls and examining the status of their spouses. Suicides were found to cluster in the first months following bereavement (49). At the same time, a British study linked widowhood to psychiatric hospital admissions by comparing the bereavement experience of Maudsley Hospital inpatients with that expected from age- and sex-specific national mortality rates (50). Since both widowhood and hospital admissions are associated with lack of social support, however, and since the comparison group was so imprecise, this study was vulnerable to confounding. The result was subsequently confirmed in a study that demonstrated the clustering of recent bereavement among new psychiatric admissions in a community register of all referred psychiatric patients, as compared with people with chronic psychiatric disability, and with a local census population (51).

Unpredictable extranormal steps

Among the irregular transitions that have been studied in health terms are premature separations of children from their families, changes of occupation and job, and migration.

To localize the effect of *premature separation* is complicated, because the separation is very often preceded by family disorder, and followed by abnormal socialization experiences in institutions and homes (see Chapter 11). The immediate emotional effects of the removal of a child from an intact home to the hospital are familiar to any sensitive parent or pediatrician. Effects over the longer term have proved difficult to demonstrate, even with the long separations that were once required for treatment in tuberculosis sanatoria (52).

In this regard enuresis, which is generally a facet of child development and socialization, is a symptom convenient to measure. Among children who were all separated from their homes and in institutional care, the frequency of the symptom at later ages was higher, the earlier the separation (53). Among another group of boys, all of whom were separated from their homes and living in a residential "approved" school because of delinquency, enuresis was more common among those who had lost their mothers because of her active departure from the home (54). Similarly, the active departure of mothers from the home, but not their death, has been related to attempted suicide (55). These findings, taken together, suggest that the separation itself may have effects on psychological and social development that emerge only under specific conditions. But in these studies the separate contributions of the periods of socialization before and after the separation have not been fully controlled.

Studies of coronary heart disease again provide data relating to the accidental extranormal transitions of changes in job status and occupation. In the California study referred to above, men who had held three or more different jobs in a lifetime, and in a North Dakota study men who had experienced four or more major changes of occupation, had a significantly increased risk of coronary heart disease (29,56). Another more complex result of the North Dakota study showed that men raised on farms, who had moved away into white-collar occupations, had a higher risk than both those who had moved away into blue-collar or manual occupations and those who had remained on farms. Evidently, migration was not alone responsible for the higher risk of the white-collar workers; the combination of upward mobility with migration was required. In these studies, diet, body weight, blood pressure, and parental longevity were controlled, and the comparison group was randomly selected and then matched for age, sex, and race. The numbers proved somewhat small for such refined analysis.

Migration between and within societies is a common, if sporadic, transition of modern society. When people uproot themselves and migrate to a new life in another society, the transition inevitably exposes them to status incongruity. The process of acquiring the culture of the new society, *acculturation*, is also a process of reducing marginal status. Full assimilation of an immigrant group may be spread over several generations. The ease or difficulty of acculturation experienced by immigrants depends to some extent on their social origin and on the degree to which their own culture resembles that of the host society. It also may depend on the extent to which ethnic enclaves can be created in the new culture, providing refuge and support among like-situated individuals facing the demands of unfamiliar surroundings (7,57). Hence immigrants vary in their manner of response and speed of adjustment (58).

Attempts have been made to describe and measure the effects of immigration on the personality of individuals, on their psychological adjustment, and on the incidence of mental and somatic disorders. Long ago, Hippocrates noted that whenever people were sent to another country "a terrible perturbation always followed." In 1685 Hofer coined the term *nostalgia* for a condition among immigrants characterized by persistent thoughts of home, melancholia, insomnia, lack of appetite, weakness, anxiety, palpitation, smothering sensations, and stupor.

Many pitfalls attend superficial comparisons of immigrant and native populations. Immigrant populations are often highly selected, and thereby share particular characteristics that influence the rates of illness among them. For instance, in past migrations overseas from Europe, young adult males from the poorer social classes in Europe tended to predominate. In the United States the immigration laws of 1921 and 1924 stemmed the flow of the poor and the peasantry of Europe, and subsequent immigration from abroad drew more on social classes of higher rank and greater education and wealth. The large contemporary mass of poor immigrants is Hispanic and crosses the borders from Mexico and Central America.

Immigrant groups in general are likely to have an age and sex and social class composition sufficiently different from parent or host populations to distort comparisons between them. In special circumstances, as with refugees, these distortions are exaggerated. When comparing populations, therefore, data need to be standardized, at a minimum, for age, sex, and the social attributes of education and occupation. When this was done for newly arriving immigrants in turn-of-the-century San Francisco, their supposed overrepresentation in the ranks of the insane disappeared (59). Account must be taken as well of the selective effect of immigration laws, the comparability of diagnoses, and availability of medical care. All these factors lead to unequal chances between social groups of health disorders becoming manifest.

Statistical corrections alone cannot eliminate certain biases. Counts of health disorders are influenced by cultural attitudes towards seeking and accepting medical treatment or admission to the hospital; the association of personal attributes with health disorders is influenced by the probability that persons with certain attributes, for example, a predisposition to schizophrenia, select themselves as immigrants. Selection must be sorted from reaction. In a pioneering study of mental illness and migration, self-selection was the explanation favored for the high rate of schizophrenia found among Norwegian male immigrants in Minnesota (60).

Even given a reactive phenomenon, and with racial and ethnic factors excluded by confining the study to a single ethnic group such as the Norwegians, the status incongruities and culture conflicts engendered by transition are not the only causes to be considered for the excess of mental disorders in immigrants. Reaction to accompaniments of the transition not intrinsically connected with it can also play a part. For example, difficult social conditions seemed to contribute to the high rates of psychoses of old age among the immigrant Norwegian women.

Some evidence has accrued to suggest that reaction to situational change can produce persisting psychopathology. Among migrants between the states of a single country, the United States, the risk of hospital admission for psychosis has usually been higher for recent arrivals (61). This finding associates mental disturbance with adaptation to migration, but does not rule out, as cause of the association, either lack of social support or a disposition of disturbed people to move.

Selection alone cannot account for two additional findings relating to hospitalized mental illness: among immigrants to the United States, the most affected age-groups have been too young themselves to have made the decision to migrate; and in the second generation offspring of migrants, rates have been lower than for first generation migrants. Clinical case studies suggest that immigration may provoke a psychosis labeled "alien's paranoid reaction." This is allegedly "cured" by repatriation, that is, by a return to the culture in which the migrants were reared, and to which they are adjusted (62).

The importance of the context in which migration takes place, and the social and psychological distance the migrant must traverse, are likely to mediate the effects of migration (63). Some of the studies that could discover no effects of horizontal mobility on mental illness or psychiatric symptoms examined groups that had made moves within one society or subculture, a transition not to be compared in magnitude with the move to a foreign land (23,64).

Interpretation of all the findings remains difficult because the main data sources are mental hospitals or prevalence surveys. The chance of admission to mental hospital is unequal among people with dissimilar social and personal characteristics: in the past, the chance of admission among mentally ill people was probably higher for immigrants than for natives. Prevalence surveys have two main problems in the study of transitions: the criteria used to identify illness, and the execution of the survey at one point in time. With regard to all the usual criteria used to identify illness in community surveys, validity remains doubtful if they are taken as equivalent to the conventional entities of mental disorder; with regard to the nature of prevalence as a cross-sectional measure at one point in time, surveys face notorious difficulty in pinpointing the time sequence, and therefore the causal relations, between past events and the onset of a chronic illness.

Besides mental disorders a number of diseases have been shown to vary with migration. At the population level, epidemic disease may be carried and transmitted by immigrants. The occurrence of three such epidemics (smallpox in the 1870s and 1880s, influenza in the 1890s) has been advanced as the underlying explanation for the correlation between fluctuations in mortality and the business cycle in 18 large American cities in the period 1871–1900. Sometimes immigrants are more affected than either the host or the parent population: among Polish male immigrants in the United States esophageal cancer was found to be more frequent than among native Americans or native Poles. Sometimes immigrants are affected in much the same way as their home population, and differ from the host population: among both Polish and Japanese immigrants in the United States death rates from cancer of the stomach were much the same as in their homeland but higher than in the United States, and Japanese women in the United States maintained the low frequency of breast cancer characteristic of Japan. More often, however, the rates for immigrants are intermediate between those of the parent and the host population: among Polish and Japanese immigrants to the United States the rates of cancer of the colon rose towards the level of those found among United States whites; among Japanese immigrants the death rate from arteriosclerotic heart disease has been found to rise in similar fashion, while that from cerebrovascular disease, high in Japan, declined (65,66).

For many of these disorders of health the source of the variation between migrants and their parent and host populations must be sought in elements of the environment unconnected with the social and psychological strains of migration. Such interpretations are reinforced when frequencies among the offspring of immigrants begin to approximate those of the host population. Thus, the discovery that migrants varied from the norms of host or homeland has been fruitful of hypotheses and studies relating to diet, climate, weather and air pollution, "substance abuse," and infection. Diet has been a focus of hypotheses about coronary heart disease (see Chapter 6) and colon cancer. Climate, weather and air pollution have been a focus of hypotheses about lung cancer: with the amount of smoking controlled, British emigrants to New Zealand and South Africa had higher mortality rates from lung cancer than the host populations and thus some factor over and above smoking seemed to be at work (67). Tobacco and alcohol use have been a focus of hypotheses about esophageal cancer.

Infection has been a focus of hypotheses about multiple sclerosis: in South Africa multiple sclerosis occurs occasionally among European immigrants but rarely among natives black or white. One postulate is that this disease is the deferred outcome of virus infection in childhood, and that like poliomyelitis, immunity acquired from infection early in life is general among the native and not the migrant population. Studies of migration and multiple sclerosis within the United States also demonstrate different frequencies in migrants, but the relationships are complex (68). Similar hypotheses about susceptibility explain the much higher risk of malignant melanoma of the skin in native or immigrant populations exposed to the sun in childhood than in immigrants exposed only as adults. Skin color, which reflects the skin's capacity for producing protective melanin and may be genetically determined, mediates this susceptibility.

Many processes accompany migration and proceed hand-in-hand with it. The discovery of variations cannot of itself single out the part played by acculturation, or the reordering of social roles, or new occupations, or changed economic standards, nor separate them from the part played by psychological and physiological adaptations to unfamiliar social situations and an altered physical environment. Studies of migration among populations resident in the same country somewhat reduce the contrasts of international comparisons by controlling some of these extraneous variables. Both parent and host populations are then accessible to study, enumerated by the same statistical systems, and available for tests of selective bias, and they can be of the same stock and social background. Such studies may control the factors of race and ethnicity by comparing immigrants of different generations from the same country, or migrants who move between rural and urban areas.

Thus, as mentioned above and discussed in Chapter 6, the comparison of first- and second-generation Japanese immigrants in California and in Hawaii has done much to clarify the contributions of cultural change to coronary heart disease, and the comparison of immigrants who migrated at different ages opened up new etiological possibilities for multiple sclerosis. In North Carolina, a study of the effects of acculturation in a factory town could at the same time compare first generation workers from a remote region with second generation workers of the same stock and social and geographic origin (69). The first generation workers—the recent migrants—reported higher rates of symptoms on a standardized inventory than the second generation, and a different pattern of sickness behavior was reflected in their work absences.

A study among the Zulu of Natal, South Africa, likewise related migration from country to city to hypertension, determined from blood pressure readings obtained in a sample survey (70). Hypertension was more frequent among urban than among rural dwellers. Among urban dwellers and notably women, however, hypertension was most frequent among those who had most recently left the country for the city. These complicated findings can be better attributed to the urban-rural transition and the acculturation process than to urban life per se. The hypothesis of failure to adapt to transitional strain was given further support by the higher prevalence of hypertension found among those town dwellers who manifested the closest affiliation with the styles of tribal life in such matters as family size, extended family ties, religious practice and witchcraft beliefs. These manifestations were in harmony with the traditional life in the country, and among country dwellers they were not associated with high frequencies of hypertension. Hence, retention of traditional ways may complicate rather than buffer the stressful effects of migration. Other factors, too, such as relative density of the ethnic populations, may play a role (7,57). Although the findings of a large array of studies can be taken to support the hypothesis of an urban factor in blood pressure levels (71,72), the intermediate processes that underlie changes in blood pressure have seldom been tested at the same time as the observations of acculturation. Hence such factors as obesity and diet remain equal contenders with psychosocial stress narrowly defined. Nor can personality differences in the perception of and response to stress be discounted (73).

In recent years, progress has been made in delineating the various elements of social mobility relevant to health. The results described above emphasize the complicated nature of the phenomenon. Social mobility is not a single homogeneous variable that will produce one class of effects. Before the effects produced by transition and mobility can be inferred, the conditions in which the variable acts must be specified, preceding and subsequent social experience must be controlled, and the form and direction of mobility must be differentiated. Uniformly favorable or unfavorable effects cannot be assumed. Transitions may generate strain, but many successful transitions bring countervailing rewards and compensations. This complexity does not preclude the possibility that social transitions have a common core that produces predictable psychosomatic effects in given conditions.

Stress and disease

The idea of "stress" as a cause of disease pervades the illustrative material in this and preceding chapters. At the ecological level, there can be no dispute that particular social structures generate particular patterns of health disorders. Put another way, the distribution of health in a society is one dimension of the social structure and an indicator of its nature and impact on people's lives.

When one turns to the individual level, however, and to the question of how the impact of the social structure is translated into pathology, much that is said rests on assertions of authority and faith. It is four or five decades since the "stress" hypothesis gathered momentum and began to displace the fashionable hypothesis of that time, which attributed a gallimaufry of obscure ills to foci of infection. Many excellent sets of teeth and many pairs of tonsils suspected of harboring hidden infection were sacrificed to that hypothesis. We can count ourselves fortunate that the stress hypothesis does not require surgical intervention. The assumption of this hypothesis is that stress in the individual mediates a major common pathway through which societal and psychological factors are expressed in the form of health disorders. An external stimulus implicit in the social situation—a *stressor*—impinges on the individual to cause *stress*—which is a heightened and persisting psychological and physiological reaction. Ultimately, if the stress is sufficiently prolonged and chronic, the maladaptation or *strain* results in one or several *stress disorders*.

These ideas are central to much current sociological research in health. In addition to the notion discussed above of specific life crises and transitions as precipitants of health disorders, a parallel notion of "stressful life events" as a cumulation of transitory disturbances gained currency. A spate of studies followed the development of interview instruments that provided stress scores based on the frequency of such events (74). These include such seemingly beneficial events as marriage, job promotion, and birth of a child, as well as those that are clearly traumatic like death of a spouse, or job termination, or involuntary displacement. The disturbances presumed to result have ranged from physical disabilities such as athletic injury to clinical episodes of shipboard illness, coronary heart disease, psychiatric disorder, the course of recovery from illness and, simply, generalized distress (75,76,77,78).

The cumulative corroboration of results is far from the norm in stress research. Even experiences which intuition suggests will require difficult adjustments—such as retirement—have not been shown to yield consistently negative effects (7). Conceptual difficulties abound. In the first place, events are never simple units; they derive their meaning and import from the present circumstances and past history of the affected individual (76,79). Nor is it clear which of many aspects of an event should be measured and tested for effect. Studies of residential moves have so far proved inconclusive, owing in part to their failure to separate the health benefits of improved housing from the adverse effects of disrupted social networks, unfamiliarity with new neighborhoods, and the like (80).

The epidemiological triad of agent-host-environment (see Chapter 6) can be useful in discussing conditions that mediate the impact of stressful experiences. With respect to the host, it is axiomatic in epidemiology that not all who are exposed to health hazards succumb to ill effects; the same is true of stress (79,81). In the Midtown Manhattan Study, for example, lower-class individuals did not only experience a greater frequency of stressful life events than their upper-class counterparts; they also manifested higher levels of distress in response to the same frequency of events (22). Similarly, some individuals appear to be able to insulate themselves emotionally against potentially traumatizing experience, such as captivity or forced exile, and fare better than their counterparts who lack that ability (82). The decisive factor then must be not the avoidance of stress, but the ability to cope with it. Individuals who learn to manage tension or master challenges are better able to meet the demands of unfamiliar situations (83). Their adaptability or resilience appears to be a function both of internal coping resources and of such "surface" characteristics as age, gender, and social class. In other words, individuals with different constitutions and experiences vary in susceptibility and immunity. No agent of disease is uniform in its effects upon a diverse population.

Host resistance is affected by the quality of the environment. The action of any agent or stimulus or stressor cannot meaningfully be considered free of context and situation. A social variable like population density will have different meanings for crowding and its effects when measured in terms of persons per room, or per household, or per area. Within families, the likelihood of common respiratory infections, for instance, is quite altered by the presence of children of schoolgoing age—as every new parent invariably learns. Likewise with persisting chronic sickness or with recurrent psychotic episodes, family environment must be expected to cushion or exacerbate the impact of stressful events (84).

Social support is a determinant of environmental quality that may mediate the impact of the stressor on the host. Social support may be defined as the extent to which social needs (love, esteem, belonging, identity, security, and material provisions) are met through interaction with others. Needs can be met through instrumental assistance (advice, information, financial aid) or through emotional sustenance (sympathy, acceptance, "moral support," affection), although the two domains of relief are not independent (85,86). The availability of such social and affective resources has been reported in several studies to buffer the effects of a wide range of stressful circumstances (87). Individuals with strong social support systems have seemed to withstand better "the slings and arrows of outrageous fortune" than those with weak or no support systems. They cope with adverse life changes (88) and negotiate their way through ongoing difficulties (89,90).

In other studies, however, a buffering effect of social support could not be demonstrated (91). The inconsistencies reside to some extent in weak methods of study (7,86,92). Definitions and measures of support are characteristically vague. This has led to confusion in operationalizing the concept; the supposed measures of support tend to be confounded with the measures of allegedly stressful life events. Many such events (gain or loss of a spouse, residential moves, change in job situation) directly or indirectly lead to changes in the individual's support network. The direction of effect then becomes impossible to disentangle in retrospect: one cannot tell whether support or its absence is antecedent to the disorders under study, whether it mediates the process, or whether it is a consequence of the disorder. When appropriate controls are introduced to correct this potential confounding the strength of the effect of social support is diminished (86).

The impact of social support is likely to be modified by the stability or instability of support over time. Thus in one longitudinal study of a representative sample of Manhattan children, scores for stressful life events correlated poorly with later behavioral disturbances; in contrast, characteristics of the life situation at home (poverty, quarreling, punitive parents, or disabled parents) correlated significantly (92). Equally important, the locus of support needs to be related to those effects that can most reasonably be anticipated. One study found that the support of co-workers appears to be more effective in cushioning the mental and physical impact of job-related stresses than support at home; neither kind of support was found to have much effect on the individual's experience of boredom or dissatisfaction with work (93).

Many of these problems with research into the effects of stressful life events relate to the instruments of measurement and to the design of the studies. The many efforts to measure the cumulative impact of stressful life events point to serious shortcomings of the most popular instrument (79,94), which is a simple cumulative score of a list of weighted events (95). We have noted the spate of studies about the impact of life events stimulated by the instrument. Typically, with new scientific techniques a hundred flowers bloom, but much weeding and culling must usually be done to refine them before notable growth can follow. Thus, researchers have come to recognize and correct for a number of obvious problems with the technique. To achieve this, specific stressors and specific outcomes must be studied. The use of a compendium of stressful events, it should be noted, is essentially a test of just one plausible hypothesis, namely, that stress is a response to the cumulation of events. There are as many other possible hypotheses as there are specifiable types of stressors and specific outcomes. If we aim to separate cause from consequence, a single scale that combines events not certainly antecedent to the manifestations under study is disqualified. For instance, many supposed stressors are transitional events. For any one event, say divorce or any other, the task of separating a stress reaction to an event from self and social selection for exposure to that event has proved difficult. The history of studies in the area makes this plain. Divorcées may not only become divorced and confound inference because they are physically or mentally ill; like the single, once divorced they may remain unmarried for that reason. Scales have contained numerous examples of similar confounding by contamination of the independent and the dependent variables, as when a supposed stressor, like disrupted sleep pattern or a state of low self-esteem, can well be a manifestation of a supposed outcome, like depression.

The instruments commonly used in stress research raise additional difficulties. Too often, the characteristics of stressors have remained poorly specified. Efforts to classify events by their desirability, novelty, predictability, intensity, and duration have somewhat sharpened the instruments (79,96). Besides such improvements in weighting scales, efforts have been made to differentiate singular events or classes of events, and also to measure unremarkable quotidian frustrations, or "daily hassles" (97). Understanding of inflammation was much advanced when causative agents were disaggregated: chemicals, heat, ultraviolet and ionizing radiation, bacteria, and multicellular parasites all cause inflammation. By analogy in the field of stress, specified events are likely to yield more convincing evidence than undifferentiated ones—loss, for example, has emerged as the peculiar antecedent of depression (98). Certain occurrences (say, death of a spouse) are much more easily marked in time and classifiable as events than are other, perhaps equally disruptive, developments (such as dissolution of a marriage) (7). Moreover, there is no need to presume that a situation must change in order to generate stress. Ill effects can be expected from noxious circumstances that persist or, indeed, that may be noxious simply because they persist (89,92).

Categorization of events is necessary in order to clarify the contributions of both host susceptibility and environment. As we have discussed, susceptiblity can be expected to vary with stages in the life-cycle that differentiate certain universal transitions, rites of passage, and normal role changes as incremental or decremental (see p. 317). Context and situation too are bound to be important. Experiments teach us that among animals the social context determines the impact of a biological stimulus or insult. For instance, nutritional deprivation has detectable effects on associative learning in rhesus monkeys or in rats when they are socially isolated and not when they interact socially (99). Finally, since psychosocial stressors of necessity are mediated by the psyche, we need to find the means to take into account the perception or denial of stress by the subject (76,100).

These are problems of the logical construction of indices, measures, and scales. Dangers also arise from the fundamental technical difficulty of establishing validity. The basic problem these instruments have shared with many other social instruments is their weakness as measures of reality. In simplest terms: if the instrument fails to measure the hypothetical causal variable, no association (causal or otherwise) can be demonstrated. One research team has developed a method that takes account not only of circumstances but also of a person's perceptions of those circumstances in assessing events, which are listed in a standardized dictionary (101,102); the gains in sensitivity must compensate for losses in neutrality, simplicity, and portability.

Reliability studies are also under way (103). Compared with reliability, however, the validity of measures of stressors has had little attention. An effort has been made in one study to test whether the events reported did in fact happen, and as many as 80 per cent could be confirmed. This indicates a degree of validity in measuring exposure to events, but whether they are in fact stressful events is another question. The discovery of an association tends to be taken as in itself validating for an instrument. Where events that carry much freight besides affective stress are under study, this is not a safe assumption. For example, a change in marital state often implies marked changes in income, in diet, in exposure to infectious disease, in life-style and habits as well as in emotional state.

With regard to measurement of the dependent variable, health disorders, the problems are more tractable. Mental disorder seemed at first to be the most obvious and likely, if not the sole, outcome of stressful experience. In psychiatric epidemiology, where the definition of a case has been a central problem for decades, a good distance has been traveled. The unidimensional scales used in many prevalence surveys created problems that resemble those of undifferentiated lists of stressful life events. The differentiation in the diagnosis of mental state attained through the research of more recent years (104) has made a distinct advance on unidimensional or conglomerate approaches (105,106). Other workers have begun to exploit and develop these diagnostic instruments for population survey work. So long as it had to be to acknowledged that a "case" of mental disorder was defined with difficulty, it also had to be acknowledged that one could not be precise about the effects of exposure to life stresses on mental states.

To turn now to the question of research design, major problems in the case-control design for the study of stress are to establish time-order, to recognize selective bias where there is a long time interval from exposure to manifestation, to select truly comparable controls, and to recognize the multiple outcomes of a single type of exposure. In case-control studies of the effects of life events, the outstanding unsolved problem is the bias likely to inhere in the *post hoc* reports of events by the cases: their recollection is colored by the outcomes that have befallen them and made them cases. A notorious unwitting example was the demonstration of an association of Down's syndrome births with "stressful" pregnancies. There can be no doubt that the chromosomal anomaly that produces Down's syndrome—trisomy 21—occurs before embryogenesis and the events of a recognized pregnancy. Another source of bias, contamination by the investigator's subjective judgment when either the potential stressors or the hypothesized effects are assessed or scored, is amenable to control by standardized techniques that keep the assessors of the effects blind to knowledge of stressors and vice versa. In reports of even the best studies it is not always clear that such precautions have been rigorously applied.

On the other hand, the case-control design is efficient and parsimonious; it allows the estimate of the odds ratio as an equivalent of relative risk even though it cannot yield a direct estimate of attributable risk. It also permits the simultaneous study of several independent variables, and often it offers the only possible way to study rare diseases (107).

The cohort design is superior in theory with regard to establishing both time-order and the starting population. There is no problem of restrospective bias in eliciting exposure, and observer bias in making observations of outcome is amenable to control. One can also recognize the multiple outcomes of a single type of exposure, such as a psychosocial stressor, and the design is likely to be superior for the study of rare causal variables, for example, wartime bombing or famines (108,109). In practice, the design may be less satisfactory than in theory. During years of laborious prospective observation, the nature of the problem may undergo change with the advent of new knowledge; expense may restrict observation to a single cohort or generation without the advantages of quick replication; rare outcomes may be impossible to study. Cohort studies tend to be most advantageous when cohorts can be reconstructed from existing historical data (109), or when they can exploit existing longitudinal data sets (110), or when they permit repeated follow-up and amendment of the questions studied.

The kinds of factors that are sought in stress research have some bearing on the prevention and control of the disorders that are found to result. Many observations relevant to controlling the effects of stress would require individual behavior change. Aside from the difficulty, and sometimes the questionable desirability, of inducing such change, much current life-stress research can add little to our ability to control health disorders. The demonstration that the cumulation of a wide array of undifferentiated stressful events can generate stressful states does not point to the means of prevention or treatment. On the other hand, the study of *specific major events* can point the way to prevention. If the immediate aftermath of widowhood puts a person at risk for suicide, for death from cirrhosis of the liver (presumably owed to alcoholism) and for other causes, as well as for entry to psychiatric care, a target group has been defined and various interventions can be tested (45). Some potential for intervention may also reside in demonstrating the effects of lack of social support, and possibly even those of malfunctioning social networks (111). The availability and effectiveness of the family networks of children can have crucial effects on their subsequent careers and behavior, and supportive networks may protect the health of adults as well. For specified vulnerable groups, it is not fanciful to think that health and social agencies could intervene effectively, as has been done with recently bereaved persons (112).

Mobility and the health of populations

Social ascent or descent takes place in time, and any consideration of the rate and direction of movement must therefore take historical change into account. The relative sizes of social classes change: in Britain between the censuses of 1921 and 1981 Social Classes I, II, and III grew larger, while Social Classes IV and V grew smaller. These changes accompanied advances in technology and production, and the concentration of public and private industries into large concerns with a bureaucratic form; large-scale organizations employ at least one-quarter of the working population (113,114). In 1981 more people were employed in commerce, finance administration, and in technical and clerical occupations, and fewer people in agriculture, mining, quarrying, and fishing. There was a redistribution from farm to city, and from manual to nonmanual and technical work.

Over a period of time, birthrates and death rates within the social classes affect their rate of recruitment. For example, in Britain between the two world wars the birthrate in the upper classes was low, and in the lower classes high: Social Class I was not reproducing itself, whereas Social Class V was more than reproducing itself. Since, at the same time, Social Class I was growing larger and Social Class V growing smaller by virtue of occupational realignment, upward social movement was promoted also by this divergence of their birthrates. On the other hand, upward movement was slowed by the relatively lower death rates in the higher classes.

A British national survey of occupational and social mobility examined the movement of men in relation to their social origins by comparing the occupational status achieved by men with that of their fathers (115). This study showed a rate of movement between the social classes that even in the second quarter of this century was no less than in the United States (2), the stereotype of a mobile society. Nevertheless, the general picture in Britain, and the United States as well, is of a rather stable social structure with a high rate of self-recruitment in the upper classes, in that their children tend also to achieve occupations of these social classes. A relatively high degree of stability also exists at the other end of the social scale among unskilled manual workers. This stability in the top and bottom social classes is reinforced through marriages between partners of the same social origin and educational level (116,117). The middle and largest category of skilled workers shows the greatest amount of movement. A person's social origin therefore plays a large part in his or her own occupational achievement. This stability prevents many children of the upper classes from "falling" and many of those of the lower classes from "rising." Upward mobility may be seen as a kind of sequential advance in Indian file: Class I is more likely to recruit from Class II than from Class III, and so on. A jump from the bottom direct to the top in one generation is a rare achievement, and the mainspring of an individual's drive to the top is often the foresight and aspirations of a grandmother.

Vertical social mobility is significant for epidemiology because mobility is a continuing process that may create biological disparities between the social classes. Individuals with special traits, it can be supposed, may be selected for upward or downward movement so that particular social groups have a predominance of certain types. These traits, either genetic or social or a combination, may be expressed in physical and social endowments, in attributes of mind or personality, and in patterns of health and disease. To interpret their social distribution, the processes of social mobility through marriage, education, and occupation must be understood.

Social movement can complicate the incidence of a disease at particular social levels. The downward drift found with chronic bronchitis (118) probably represents a simple process that can be found with any chronic disability (119). A more complicated process has been postulated for the downward drift of chronic schizophrenia, where the disorder alters fundamental patterns of behavior and relationships, as well as producing the subtle behavior changes and the economic dependence of the sick role that occur with any chronic disorder. Individuals with schizophrenia tend to drift down the occupational scale; chronic cases move into deteriorated city areas, or into the chronic wards of hospitals; others decline in status by the criterion of occupation if not by the criteria of education and residence (120). Social supports may also play a role, for the networks of people diagnosed as schizophrenic are distinctly different from those who are not (121).

Efficiency in childbearing is another characteristic linked with social movement. Marriage has always been a main channel of social ascent for women, and a study of marriages in Aberdeen in Scotland suggests that fitness for reproduction is involved in the selection of spouses (122). In a population of primiparae, representative of the city, the well favored in height were well favored in other things: they tended to have both favorable rates for prematurity and stillbirths and to have married upwards, (their husbands were higher in the occupational scale than their fathers). By contrast, stunted women tended both to have poor obstetric records and to marry downwards. The disparities in height and reproduction were probably related as much to childhood infection, nutrition, and nurture as to genetic endowment (123). In the result, women who reproduced efficiently were recruited by marriage to the higher occupational classes from the lower, while those who reproduced inefficiently remained in the lower occupational classes or married into them.

An association of upward movement with favorable obstetric rates and downward movement with poor ones will tend to make the existing social class gradient in such rates steeper. Some of this social movement may only be apparent, however, an artifact produced by the inadequacy of the Registrar General's occupational scale as a model of society. Occupations grouped within each social class show irregularities in such reproductive indices as stillbirths and infant mortality, and some occupations do better than others ranked higher in the class scale (see Chapter 6).

For example, in Britain in the 1950s the wives of textile workers in Social Class IV lost fewer infants than the wives of skilled coalminers in Social Class III (124). Social and biological selection linked with movement from one class to another might be expected therefore to correspond imperfectly with the direction of movement. Despite discrepancies, however, an underlying regularity does exist. In general, the wives of men in occupations involving rough manual labor have high rates for stillbirths and infant mortality, whereas the wives of men in occupations involving light or sedentary work have low rates. Grouping occupations in this way sometimes cuts across the Registrar General's scale, and the effect on epidemiological analysis depends in part on the structure of occupations present in a particular community. The general consistency of the Aberdeen figures, however, argues that a process of social selection and movement between the social classes contributed to the social class gradient of obstetric death rates.

Intelligence is the personal attribute most commonly thought to help individuals to achieve upward mobility, and social mobility has indeed been shown to relate to measured intelligence. In Stockholm, for example, the intelligence of men aged 24 in 1949 was related to their occupational status as compared with their fathers'. Men with high scores who had lower-class fathers had tended to move up, as measured by a three-class scale, and men with lower scores but higher-class fathers had tended to move down (125). In the Aberdeen sample of primiparae, women who had married up had the greatest proportion of high scorers and those who married down the least proportion (126). These results need to be interpreted with due caution, as we shall discuss.

Intelligence is a subtle and intangible quality compounded both of inherited and acquired elements. From the moment of birth innate ability, the genotype, is modified constantly by learning and experience, which is then incorporated into the resulting phenotype. Indeed, the modification of the genotype begins with conception; alcohol abuse by the mother and other metabolic disorders during gestation can affect the measured intelligence of children (127). Psychologists have attempted to measure the various components of phenotypic intelligence by more or less objective tests. The validity of intelligence tests is put in doubt because these components cannot yet be defined with precision, and intelligence tests necessarily select those qualities limited enough to be measured. Intelligence quotients are a fairly reliable measure of an individual's capacities for logical deduction, abstract reasoning, and general knowledge, and are widely used for this purpose. The use of twins demonstrated the greater concordance in measured intelligence of monozygotic twins compared with dizygotic twins and siblings, indicating the genetic contribution. Conversely, the testing of twins reared in different environments demonstrated the discordance in intelligence between them, indicating the environmental contribution (128). Studies of siblings, and of people of the same stock who are reared in different situations, have also indicated the environmental contribution (129,130,131).

Almost all the measurements of intelligence that are standardized in populations and widely used are related directly or indirectly to scholastic attainments, whether they rely on "verbal" tests or "performance" tests or both. Schooling and practice in the use of verbal abstract concepts seems to confer an increasing advantage in intelligence tests. Among a Swedish cohort tested at military induction and grouped according to their intelligence score at school 10 years before, those who received secondary and university education made higher scores than those of the same IQ group who had had only primary school education (132). In line with this, in the 1920s studies of canal boat and gypsy children, who could attend school only sporadically because their families plied the canals and roads of Britain, showed a correlation among the children between test scores and school attendance, and a decline in their scores with age (133). A generation later in the United States, in the poor, isolated pockets of Appalachian communities, test scores were found to decline with age in similar fashion (134,135). The results of intelligence testing are culture bound. They are not comparable, without qualification, between cultures that place unequal value on schooling and formal education. This is not to say that no real differences between tested groups exist.

The proponents of a genetic cause of the unequal distribution of measured intelligence in the social classes have long argued their case with the proponents of an environmental cause, and both have constructed theoretical models assuming modes of genetic inheritance and of selection for social movement by innate ability (136).° Studies of the inheritance of intelligence face three difficult problems: the assumption that IQ tests are valid instruments for measuring and comparing a general ability called intelligence; the extent to which population statistical methods can be used to establish inheritance (129,137); and the tendency to reify the social concept of intelligence as a unitary "thing" located in brain structure. In the last instance, the interpretations sometimes given to the yield of factor analysis are especially instructive (138). This statistical technique was invented to detect the structure of relationships latent in assemblies of data comprising many variables. It was originally applied in psychology by Charles Spearman in 1904 to devise a unilinear scale for general intelligence. Factor analysis enables one to take a matrix of correlations, say, correlations among the items included in an intelligence test, and to reduce them to more man-

---

°The debate, which was dormant, was re-ignited by revelations that two leading proponents of the genetic theory of intelligence seem to have falsified data in defense of their cause (138,139). Re-examination of photographic evidence in Goddard's 1912 study of the Kallikak family, whose features were said to indicate an inferior physical type, showed tampering with the prints; and in Sir Cyril Burt's studies of separated twins, the correlations did not change as the sample expanded over the years, a result that points to fabrication. These startling discoveries have no bearing on the merits of the argument, but they do illustrate the intensity of the ideological issues.

ageable dimensions. It achieves this reduction by creating "factors" or "components"; these mathematical entities are derived from the weights given to each item according to the strength of its correlation with the other items that are found to cluster together. Factors are constructed in a hierarchy, according to the proportion of the total variation present in the original items that they can account for; each factor accounts for successively less of the variation of the original measures. Thus, a set of highly positively correlated measures will "factor out" into relatively few components. These mathematical entities, in themselves and without supporting evidence, can claim no correspondence to physical reality.

A tendency to reification has nonetheless insinuated itself into the use of factor analysis in mental testing. Thus Spearman himself thought that g, the principal component that resolved most of the variance in the test scores he examined, represented "general ability" or IQ and thereby explained overall performance on mental tests. But to proceed from that assumption and make the case for inheritance, Spearman and his colleagues introduced a further assumption. They proposed that the measure represented an actual physical entity called mental energy. They thus imputed biological reality to a mathematical abstraction. Subsequent analyses in this vein have offered substitutes for the physical substrate Spearman postulated for g but have kept intact the notion that it is an entity that must correspond to something inheritable in brain structure.

There is no necessary reason why a social construct such as intelligence need be a discrete entity. Equally valid mathematical analyses have been devised to show many distinct "factors" at work, each of which can be interpreted as representing specific competencies. The decision in either case is a pragmatic one. It depends upon the social uses to which test scores are put.

Whatever effects innate ability may have on the social mobility of individuals, genetic theories cannot by themselves account for the observed class distribution of low tested intelligence. A concentration of low scores in the lower social classes has always been reported since methods of measuring intelligence were devised and generally applied. This finding is consistent whatever standard is used, whether by comparing results of intelligence tests applied to national or local samples, or by comparing the degree of educational backwardness and mental subnormality manifested by children of different social classes (135,140,141). The mentally subnormal individuals in excess in the lower social classes are mainly those with IQs in the borderland between "normal" and "pathological" levels, that is, with scores between 60 and 80 approximately. Individuals who score within this range and appear otherwise healthy have been regarded as falling at the lower limit of "normal" (142).

In a Lancashire study of educational subnormality, those *without* detectable clinical lesions in the subnormal IQ range were all drawn from lower-class families (143). They must be distinguished from individuals *with* detectable lesions of organic disorders who make low scores (who are much more evenly distributed between the social classes). Thus, none of those ascertained from the small category of "aspirant" families with some indication of upward mobility were clinically "normal," and most had signs of neurological lesions. This unequal distribution of those without detectable lesions was not a result of the selective ascertainment of lower-class children from the total population of backward children. In large populations, screened through the fallible records of school health examinations, an occasional child in the higher social classes had a subnormal IQ and no recorded handicap, but nonetheless the relative risk in schools of high social standing compared with schools of low standing was 15 to 1 (see Table 8.1).

These findings were confirmed in a subsequent study of 104 mentally subnormal children aged from 8 to 10 and culled from a complete birth cohort in Aberdeen (144). No social class gradient was found for those children with clear evidence of neurological damage and IQs below 50. Those with central nervous system damage and IQs above 50, however, were overrepresented in the lower social classes. Apparently, biological insult was exacerbated by adverse social environment. As in the Lancashire study, there was a considerable preponderance in the lowest social classes of children in the mildly subnormal range with no sign of neurological impairment. In Aberdeen too, there was a complete absence, in the families of nonmanual (I-IIIa) and journeyman/artisan (IIIb) occupations, of those children with IQs of 60 or higher and no neurological damage (see Table 8.2). Children with mild subnormality and no detectable damage tended to live in large families crowded into poor housing, and had siblings with lower IQs than children in comparable families without a mentally subnormal child.

It follows that the excess of low intelligence in the lowest social classes as a population can be ascribed in large part to cultural background and environmental adversity, not to innate lack of ability. In each social class the limits of measured intelligence in physiologically normal people are determined by the material and social environment, and the lower limit is set even lower under poor environmental conditions. Susceptible individuals in the lower classes, presumably those with poor innate ability, descend into the subnormal range of intelligence quotients because of their unfavorable environment. These individuals suffer from mental retardation in a precise sense, not from permanent mental deficiency for, unlike individuals with brain

Table 8.1 Referral for investigation of backwardness by I.Q., clinical state, and social standing of schools, in Salford, England (1955–59). Average annual rates per 1000 schoolchildren 7–10 years of age

	Social standing of schools					
	Low	Low average	High average	High	All schools	Relative risk low/high
Average annual school population	5501	11,261	1974	750	19,488	
Average annual rates						
All referrals for backwardness	10	10	7	4	9	2.5
All I.Q. 50–79	4.3	3.0	2.8	0.5	3.3	8.6
I.Q. 50–79 with recorded lesions	0.5	0.3	0.3	0.26	0.4	1.9
I.Q. 50–79 clinically normal only	3.8	2.7	2.5	0.26	2.9	14.6

Source: Stein, Z. A., and Susser, M. W. (1969). Mild mental subnormality: social and epidemiological studies, in *Social Psychiatry, Res. Publ. Ass. Nerv. Ment. Dis.*, 47, The Association for Research in Nervous and Mental Disease, Baltimore, Md.

Table 8.2 Social class distribution of mentally subnormal children by IQ and presence or absence of central nervous system damage

Social class	IQ <50 CNS damage	IQ ≥50 CNS damage	IQ ≥50 No CNS damage
I–IIIa	7 (1.03)[a]	1 (0.14)	0 (0)
IIIb	4 (0.74)	6 (1.01)	3 (0.27)
IIIc	6 (1.28)	4 (0.78)	12 (1.22)
IV	3 (0.97)	2 (0.60)	14 (2.20)
V	3 (1.03)	12 (3.80)	19 (3.10)
Total	23	25	48

[a]Ratio of actual number/expected number.

Source: Adapted from Birch, H. G., Richardson, S. A., Baird, D., Horobin, G., and Illsley, R. (1970) *Mental Subnormality in the Community: A Clinical and Epidemiological Study*, Baltimore.

injuries, they may improve their rank on intelligence test scores in later years (142). They therefore have the prospect of a degree of recovery. The tendency towards delayed maturation among individuals living under poor conditions (145) has been observed for other developmental processes, for instance, physical growth, sexual maturation, and control over the bladder sphincter in sleep (146).

The effects of adverse environment on tested mental performance have been well documented in studies on migrants in the United States. Measured intelligence in black migrants from southern cities had a "dose-response" type of relationship to exposure to the environment of northern cities, even though this environment was far inferior to that of middle-class whites (147). Children born in the North had the highest scores, the most recent migrants the lowest. In the southern cities, the school records of children who migrated compared with those who remained yielded no evidence that self-selection of the migrants could have produced the results.

These were cross-sectional studies, and a possible doubt remained about the effect of changes over time, if the performance of each age-group were to be followed longitudinally. In further longitudinal studies a replication of the results was obtained. Among black children in Philadelphia who had reached the 12th grade, cohorts were defined by grade of entry to the Philadelphia schools. Their test performance was followed over the nine years or less they had taken to pass through the schools (148). On entry to the Philadelphia schools, children from the South had much the same average scores, whatever their age at entry, but for every year spent in Philadelphia their scores more closely approached those of the native-born children (see Table 8.3).

A variety of studies affirm that intelligence test scores, including the low ranges of special medical interest, vary systematically with environment (135). Thus, institutional environments handicap development, and intimate affective relations with adults promote it. Even in a special institutional environment the development of infants with Down's syndrome admitted within a few months of birth was inferior to that of a comparison group kept at home (149). To some degree this handicap can be

Table 8.3   Mean I.Qs. of cohorts of native and migrant black children, by grade at first entry to Philadelphia schools, in successive grades[a]

Group[c]	1A[b]	2B	4B	6B	9A
Philadelphia-born who attended kindergarten (N = 212)	96.7	95.9	97.2	97.5	96.6
Philadelphia-born who did not attend kindergarten (N = 424)	92.1	93.4	94.7	94.0	93.7
Southern-born entering Philadelphia school system in grades:					
1A (N = 182)	86.5	89.3	91.8	93.3	92.8
1A − 2B (N = 109)		86.7	88.6	90.9	90.5
3A − 4B (N = 199)			86.3	87.2	89.4
5A − 6B (N = 221)				88.2	90.2
7A − 9A (N = 219)					87.4

[a]Philadelphia Tests of Mental and Verbal Ability.

[b]A refers to first half of school year, B to second half.

[c]Out of a total of 1234 migrants, 304 were excluded for missing tests (292) or attending kindergarten (12). 326 Philadelphia-born children were excluded for missing one or more tests.

Source: adapted from E. S. Lee (1951), Negro intelligence and selective migration: a Philadelphia test of the Klineberg hypothesis, *Amer. sociol. Rev.,* 16, 227–33; as cited in Stein, Z. A., and Susser, M. W. (1970) The mutability of intelligence and the epidemiology of mild mental retardation, *Rev. Educ. Res.,* 40, 29–67.

overcome. Homeless infants of subnormal development, removed from an Iowa institution to the personal care of subnormal girls in another institution and then adopted, were followed through 30 years. They achieved intelligence scores and social and work adjustment that were normal and far superior to a comparison group who had not been removed from the institution and adopted (150). While cogent questions have been raised about the comparability of the original reference group in the Iowa study, similar results have been obtained since. In another study, mentally subnormal children from a traditional large London institution for mental deficiency were removed to a smaller one designed to give a homelike atmosphere. The new environment stimulated their intellectual and social development compared with those left in the large institution (151).

Planned programs of mental stimulation have been shown to accelerate the intellectual development of mildly retarded preschool children, especially those without discernible organic lesions, whether or not they have been placed in institutions (152). Schooling produces a similar effect in children living in poverty and in a deprived cultural environment. Thus, children in Appalachian communities two generations ago showed a discernible mental spurt at the age of school entry (134). In the Headstart program of the late 1960s aimed to give deprived preschool children a few weeks' start in schooling, participants had a mental spurt, but this did not keep them ahead of the children who went straight into school without benefit of Headstart, for they too then had an equal spurt (153). The spontaneous improvement made by mildly retarded persons in adolescence and young adulthood, noted above, also points to the possibility of recovery from retardation.

The environmental elements that give rise to the mutability of measured intelligence within and between groups have not been isolated. It is not known whether the important causes are the cognitive and affective content of the culture, or the structure of social relationships. Studies of the past decade do rule out malnutrition as the cause of permanent cognitive deficits—malnutrition seems most likely to depress cognition in young children because of the illness that accompanies it, and not after recovery. Any long-term effects cannot be separated from those of the adverse social environment in which it occurs (154). Well-controlled experiments sustained over a period of years among young children reared in deprived communities—whether in Cali, Colombia, or in Milwaukee—have demonstrated substantial gains in IQ in response to programs of social and intellectual stimulation combined with good nutrition (155). That infants raised in enriched institutional residences show no evidence of cognitive retardation at five years of age suggests also that, whatever the necessary factors are, they can be provided in the absence of a normal familial environment (131).

It can be said, too, that the adverse impact of all the suspect elements has diminished in industrial societies as economic production has increased. A prediction, made on the basis of a hypothesis of environmental determinants of intelligence, can only be that the mean level should have improved with time. In an earlier era a genetic hypothesis led to the contrary prediction that the mean level of intelligence should decline. Since measured intelligence had a declining gradient with social class, and since the lower social classes produced more children than the higher, the psychologists of the time expected mean intelligence in the population to decline with time. This hypothesis was tested in two national surveys in Scotland that used identical IQ tests on all 11-year-old children in 1932 and 1947. The result contradicted the expectation of those who launched the study: they found a rise in the mean scores and a decline in the proportion of low scores (156). Data from England, Sweden, and Appalachia all support the result (135,157). Although some geneticists have countered that the failure of the prediction was owed to the lesser fertility of mentally retarded persons, this applies in the main to those few with moderate or severe retardation, and cannot explain the results for a population.

These results do not deny that selection for social mobility by measured intelligence could have a part in producing the disparity in intelligence scores observed between the social classes. Indeed, one American study estimated, from a model of intergenerational mobility built on a number of more or less sound assumptions, that disparities between a son's measured intelligence and a father's occupation could account for 60 per cent of the son's mobility (158). However, the achievement of social mobility by individuals does not depend solely on their intelligence and other personal attributes, for the social system sets up barriers between the classes that cannot be overcome by these attributes alone. Education and specialized skills are essential to the individual who wishes to "get ahead" in industrial societies, and higher social and financial rewards follow (159). The formal system of higher education through school and university is therefore a channel for social mobility, though one that operates also to reinforce the existing class structure. Hence, once open it is kept open through successive generations, so that educational opportunities are not the same for social groups regardless of intellectual ability (160,161). Other societal modes of testing and selecting also operate to provide social groups with unequal capacity and opportunity for social mobility. Functional associations shift individuals from one social position to another (e.g., the Armed Forces, churches, political parties, trade unions, and employers' federations). The institutionalized means whereby society tests and selects individuals and then distributes them into different social levels are complicated in themselves and intricately related to one another.

Family and school combine to furnish children with the foundations of character and their general intellectual level. This early training sets a limit to adult achievement, both in occupation and in social life generally. As children enter the phase of secondary education, formal training becomes more diverse, and at this time selection for special training begins. The social function of education is to inculcate the knowledge and behavior that will enable children to take their place as adults in society (see Chapter 11). The educational system therefore has a dual purpose, first, to train all children in the fundamentals of their culture, and, second, to select some for special training. Continuity between the generations in occupation and culture is thereby preserved, but at the same time education must cater for the discontinuities of a changing society. Individual children may be selected to fill new occupations and enjoy a mode of life quite different from that of their parents. Neither continuity nor discontinuity, however, is independent of the education, the occupation, and the social standing of a child's parents; parental attributes facilitate both these processes. Those whose careers are discontinuous with those of parents tend to leave their communities and go to work elsewhere; the most successful children are siphoned off by the educational system. Parental occupation usually determines the kind of home and neighborhood in which children are reared, and the schools they attend. The values they learn from parents and peers determine attitudes towards schooling, as well as capacity to succeed in it. Teachers have middle-class values, whatever their social origin, and foster and encourage middle-class traits and attitudes, and for this reason many working-class children withdraw from school. Hence a conflict in values between home and school may hinder the working-class child.

In Britain, two distinct educational systems, the independent private ("public") schools and the state-supported schools, further stratify the population; indeed, the social classes can almost be defined in terms of these educational systems. Both function to preserve continuity between parents and children and also to create discontinuities between them. A child from the lowest social classes can achieve a higher social position than his or her parents through success in the state school system; conversely, a child of a family that has achieved a high social position can maintain this position through the private system. Although it was estimated that only 2.6 per cent of children attended "public" schools, their social significance has been quite out of proportion to the small numbers, for these schools have continued to educate many people prominent in business, the professions, and government (162).

In many industrial societies competition for higher education has become severe. People have come to realize the crucial part of education in providing social opportunity. But the chances of success are linked to the father's occupation, the family's social standing, and parental education. The higher the family ranks in these matters, the better the chances of obtaining a higher education. In the United States as elsewhere, social processes operate to train and select children for their future social class positions (161,163). The discrimination in education between social classes rests on subtle effects of values, norms, and expectations. An experiment in California schools showed how the expectations of teachers, and the educational attainments and measured intelligence of children, could feed back into each other (164). The teachers were told that certain of their pupils, randomly chosen by the experimenters, were "late bloomers" and could be expected to improve markedly in schooling and intelligence. A follow-up based on objective tests showed that these randomly chosen children had indeed fulfilled the expectations, instilled into their teachers by the experimenters, of accelerated development and heightened achievement. The results stand despite severe criticism.

This experiment is no less relevant in England, where "streaming" in primary schools (and, in the past, entry to grammar schools, the academic secondary schools of the state system) theoretically rests only on the child's capacity judged by objective tests. Teachers in primary schools tend to underestimate the ability of lower-class children and to overestimate that of their middle- and upper-class counterparts, when compared to objective ratings by test scores (165). Children of unskilled manual workers gained relatively few grammar school places, while children of professional workers gained many. Moreover, placement was not always a step towards occupational mobility between children and their parents, for working-class pupils have tended to leave school earlier than middle-class ones. The influence of parental social class further emerged in the later achievements of children who performed equally well on leaving primary for secondary schools. Middle-class children tended to come out at the top at the end of their school careers, even if ranked low at entry, whereas working-class children tended to come out at the bottom, even if ranked high at entry. Thus many working-class children fell far short of their potential achievements (135,163,166) (see also Chapter 11).

We repeat that the selection process for social mobility through the educational or other channels is not a matter of any single attribute such as intelligence or diligence, or Protestant rectitude, or ruthless striving. Social class and culture, as well as health and disability, enter into the process. The connection between measured intelligence and social mobility can be only partial, as in Aberdeen and Stockholm. To the question with which this discussion began, namely the connection between innate intelligence and social mobility, there is no certain answer.

Social mobility, however, plainly has both biological and social significance in maintaining heterogeneity within human populations. In this chapter we have discussed a few of the ways in which the process of mobility influences people. In the broad view, it provides a means for diffusing both genetic and cultural traits, and so for enriching the diversity of human beings and their modes of life. Through the conjunction of the unfamiliar and the diverse, social mobility stimulates new forms of social and psychological adaptation. To the degree that it destroys parochialism, tempers chauvinism, and fosters a sense of the relativity of human values and moral systems, it is an instrument that may contribute to human survival. To the degree that social mobility creates momentum towards new power concentrated in the hands of those who control specialized knowledge and technology, it is an instrument that facilitates new forms of social stratification, and a source of conflict between the social classes that are thus created.

References

1. **Sorokin, P.** (1927). *Social Mobility*, New York.
   Ginsberg, M. (1932). *Studies in Sociology*, London.
2. **Lipset, S.,** and **Bendix, R.** (1959). *Social Mobility in Industrial Society*, London.
   Featherman, D. L., and **Hauser, R. M.** (1978). *Opportunity and Change*, New York.
   McRoberts, H. A., and **Selbee, K.** (1981). Trends in occupational mobility in Canada and the United States: A comparison, *Amer. Sociol. Rev., 46,* 406–21.
3. **Flugel, J. C.** (1930). *The Psychology of Clothes*, London.
   Laver, J. (1949). *Style in Costume*, London.
4. **Kark, S. L.** (1949). The social pathology of syphilis in Africans, *S. Afr. Med. J., 23,* 77–84.
   Sax, S. (1951). *Public Health Aspects of Syphilis among the Bantu people of the Union of South Africa*, M.D. thesis, University of Witwatersrand, Johannesburg.
5. **Douglas, J. W. B.,** and **Blomfield, J. M.** (1958). *Children under Five*, London.
6. **Gordon, L.** (1976). *Woman's Body, Woman's Right: A Social History of Birth Control in America*, New York.
   National Center for Health Statistics. (1982). *Trends in Contraceptive Practice: United States, 1965–76*, Series 23, No. 10, Hyattsville, Md.
7. **Kasl, S.** (1977). Contributions of social epidemiology to studies in psychosomatic medicine, *Adv. Psychosom. Med., 9,* 160–223.
8. **Lazarsfeld, P. F., Berelson, B.,** and **Gaudet, H.** (1948). *The People's Choice*, New York.
   Lenski, G. E. (1954). Status crystallization: Non-vertical dimension of social status, *Amer. Sociol. Rev., 19,* 405–13.
9. **Jackson, E. F.** (1962). Status consistency and symptoms of stress, *Amer. Sociol. Rev., 27,* 469–80.
10. **Lindemann, E.** (1960). Psychosocial factors as stress or agents, in *Stress and Psychiatric Disorder*, ed. Tanner, J. M., Oxford.
    Caplan, G. (1961). *An Approach to Community Mental Health*, London.
11. **Hinkle, L. E.,** and **Wolfe, H. G.** (1957). Health and the social environment: Experimental investigations, in *Explorations in Social Psychiatry*, ed. Leighton, A. H., Clausen, J. A., and Wilson, R. N., London. pp. 105–37.
    Hinkle, L. E., Redmont, R., Plummer, N., and **Wolfe, H. G.** (1960). An examination of the relation between symptoms, disability, and serious illness, in two homogeneous groups of men and women, *Amer. J. Publ. Hlth. 50,* 1327–36.
12. **Brown, G. W.,** and **Birley, J. L. T.** (1968). Crises and life changes and the onset of schizophrenia, *J. Hlth. Soc. Behav. 9,* 203–14.
    Brown, G. W., and **Harris, T.** (1978). *Social Origins of Depression: A Study of Psychiatric Disorders in Women*, New York.
13. **Halliday, J. L.** (1948). *Psychosocial Medicine*, London.
14. **Susser, M.** (1968). *Community Psychiatry: Epidemiologic and Social Themes*, New York.
15. **Mechanic, D.** (1976). Stress, illness and illness behavior, *J. Human Stress, 2,* 2–6.

16. **Graham, S.** (1974). The sociological approach to epidemiology, *Amer. J. Publ. Hlth.*, *64*, 1046–49.

    Neugarten, B. L., and **Datan, N.** (1974). The middle years, in *American Handbook of Psychiatry*, vol. 1, ed. Arieti, S., New York, pp. 592–608.

17. **Erikson, E. H.** (1950). *Childhood and Society*, New York.

18. **Lee, J. A. H.** (1957). An association between social circumstances and appendicitis in young people, *Brit. Med. J.*, 1, 1217–19.

    Robins, L. N. (1966). *Deviant Children Grown Up: A Sociological and Psychiatric Study of Sociopathic Personality*, Baltimore.

    Robins, L. N., and **Murphy, G. E.** (1967). Drug use in a normal population of young Negro men, *Amer. J. Publ. Hlth.*, 57, 1580–96.

    Josephson, E. (1969). Violence and the health of youth, in *VD-The Challenge to Man: A Report on VD Research Priorities*, Amer. Soc. Hlth. Ass., pp. 24–37.

    Boyd, J. T., Doll, R., Hill, A. B., and **Sissoons, H. A.** (1969). Mortality from primary tumours of bone in England and Wales 1961–63, *Brit. J. Prev. Soc. Med.*, *23*, 12–22.

    Morris, J. N. (1975). *Uses of Epidemiology*, 3rd ed., Edinburgh.

    Waldron, I., and **Eyer, J.** (1975). Socio-economic causes of the recent rise in death rates for 15–24 year olds, *Soc. Sci. Med.*, *9*, 383–96.

19. **Knupfer, G., Clark, W.,** and **Room, R.** (1966). The mental health of the unmarried, *Amer. J. Psychiat.*, *122*, 841–51.

20. **Tetlow, C.** (1955). Psychoses of childbearing, *J. Ment. Sci.*, *101*, 629–39.

    Thomas, C. L., and **Gordon, J. E.** (1959). Psychosis after childbirth, *Amer. J. Med. Sci.*, *238*, 363–88.

    Seager, C. P. (1960). A controlled study of postpartum mental illness, *J. Ment. Sci.*, *106*, 214–30.

    Paffenbarger, R. S., Steinmetz, C. M., Pooler, B. G., and **Hyde, R. T.** (1961). The picture puzzle of the postpartum psychosis, *J. Chron. Dis.*, *13*, 161–73.

    Pugh, T. F., Jerath, B. K., Schmidt, W. M., and **Reed, R. B.** (1963). Rates of mental disease related to childbearing, *New Eng. J. Med.*, *268*, 1224–28.

    Tod, E. D. M. (1964). Puerperal depression: A prospective epidemiological study, *Lancet*, *2*, 1264–66.

    Pitt, B. (1968). Atypical depression following childbirth, *Brit. J. Psychiatry*, *114*, 1325–35.

    Kendell, R. E., Wainwright, S., Hailey, A., and **Shannon, B.** (1976). The influence of childbirth on psychiatric morbidity, *Psychol. Medicine*, *6*, 297–302.

    Paykel, E. S., Emms, E. M., Fletcher, J., and **Rassaby, E. S.** (1980). Life events and social support in puerperal depression, *Brit. J. Psychiat.*, *136*, 329–46.

    Kendell, R. E., Mcguire, R. J., Connor, Y., and **Cox, J. L.** (1981). Mood changes in the first three weeks after childbirth, *J. Affective Disorders*, *3*, 317–26.

    Cox, J. L., Connor, Y., and **Kendell, R. E.** (1982). Prospective study of the psychiatric disorders of childbirth, *Brit. J. Psychiat.*, *140*, 111–17.

21. **Thernstrom, S.** (1972). *Poverty and Progress: Social Mobility in a Nineteenth Century City*, New York.

    Sennett, R., and **Cobb, J.** (1976). *The Hidden Injuries of Class*, New York.

22. **Langner, T. S.,** and **Michael, S. T.** (1963). *Life Stress and Mental Health*, New York.

23. **Kleiner, R. J.,** and **Parker, S.** (1963). Goal-striving, social status, and mental disorder: A research review, *Amer. Sociol. Rev.*, *28*, 189–203.

    Kleiner, R. J., and **Parker, S.** (1965). Goal-striving and psychosomatic symptoms in a migrant and non-migrant population, in *Mobility and Mental Health*, ed. Kantor, M. B., Springfield, Ill., pp. 78–85.

24. **Hyman, H.** (1953). The value systems of different classes, in *Class, Status, and Power: A Reader in Social Stratification*, eds. Bendix, R., and Lipset, S. M., Glencoe, Ill., pp. 426–42.

    Hoggart, R. (1957). *The Uses of Literacy*, Fairhaven, N.J.

25. **Merton, R. K.** (1957). *Social Theory and Social Structure*, rev. ed., New York.

26. **Havighurst, R. J.** (1957). The leisure activities of the middle aged, *Amer. J. Sociol.*, 63, 152–62.

    Ryan, W. (1981). *Equality*, New York.

27. **Ruesch, J., Harris, R. E., Christiansen, C., Loeb, M. B., Dewees, S.,** and **Jacobson, A.** (1948). *Duodenal Ulcer: A Socio-Psychological Study of Naval Enlisted Personnel and Civilians*, Berkeley.

    Ellis, E. (1952). Social psychological correlates of upward social mobility among unmarried career women, *Amer. Sociol. Rev.*, 17, 558–63.

    Hollingshead, A. B., Ellis, R., and **Kirby, E.** (1954).Social mobility and mental illness, *Amer. Sociol. Rev.*, 19, 577–84.

    Myers, J. K., and **Roberts, B. H.** (1959). *Family and Class Dynamics in Mental Illness*, New York.

28. **Wardwell, W. I., Hyman, M. M.,** and **Bahnson, C. B.** (1968). Socio-environmental antecedents to coronary heart disease in 87 white males, *Soc. Sci. Med.*, 2, 165–83.

29. **Syme, S. L., Borhani, N. O.,** and **Buechley, R. W.** (1965). Cultural mobility and coronary heart disease in an urban area, *Amer. J. Epidem.*, 82, 334–6.

    Syme, S. L., Hyman, M. M., and **Enterline, P. E.** (1965). Cultural mobility and the occurrence of coronary heart disease, *J. Hlth. Hum. Behav.*, 6, 178–89.

30. **Lehman, E. W., Schulman, J.,** and **Hinkle, L. E.** (1967). Coronary deaths and organizational mobility, *Arch. Environ. Hlth.*, 15, 455–61.

31. **Wardwell, W. I.,** and **Bahnson, C. B.** (1973). Behavioral variables and myocardial infarction in the Southeastern Connecticut Health Study, *J. Chron. Dis.*, 26, 447–461.

32. **Wan, T.** (1971). Status stress and morbidity: A sociological investigation of selected categories of work-limiting chronic conditions, *J. Chron. Dis.*, 24, 453–68.

33. **Hinkle, L. E., Jr., Whitney, L. H., Lehman, E. W., Dunn, J., Benjamin, B., King, R., Plakun, A.,** and **Flehinger, B.** (1968). Occupation, education, and coronary heart disease, *Science, 161*, 238–46.

34. **Zohman, B. L.** (1973). Emotional factors in coronary disease, *Geriatrics, 28*, 110–119.

    House, J. S. (1974). Occupational stress and coronary heart disease: A review and theoretical integration, *J. Hlth. Soc. Behav.*, 15, 12–27.

    Jenkins, C. D. (1971). Psychologic and social precusors of coronary disease, *New Engl. J. Med.* 284, 244–255, 307–317.

35. **Susser, M.** (1967). Causes of peptic ulcer. A selective epidemiologic review, *J. Chron. Dis.*, 20, 435–56.

    Pflanz, M. (1971). Epidemiological and socio-cultural factors in the etiology of duodenal ulcer, *Adv. Psychosom. Med.*, 6, 121–51.

36. **Form, W. H.** (1973). Auto workers and their machines: A study of work, factory and job dissatisfaction in four countries, *Social Forces 52*, 1–15.

    French, J. R. P., Jr. (1974). Person-role fit, in *Occupational Stress*, ed. McLean, A., Springfield, Ill., pp. 70–79.

    Strauss, G. (1974). Is there a blue-collar revolt against work? in *Work and the Quality of Life*, Cambridge, Mass., pp. 40–69.

37. **Lockwood, D.** (1958). *The Blackcoated Worker*, London.

38. **Blalock, H. M.** (1967). Status and consistency: Integration and structural effects, *Amer. Sociol. Rev.*, 32, 790–801.

Jackson, E. F., and Curtis, R. F. (1972). Effects of vertical mobility and status inconsistency: A body of negative evidence, *Amer. Sociol. Rev.*, 37, 701–13.

39. Abramson, J. H. (1966). Emotional disorder, status inconsistency and migration, *Milbank Mem. Fd. Quart.*, 44, 23–48.

40. Cobb, S., and Kasl S. V. (1966). The epidemiology of rheumatoid arthritis, *Amer. J. Publ. Hlth.*, 56, 1657–63.

41. Haynes, S. G., Eaker, E. D., and Feinleib, M. (1983). Spouse behavior and coronary heart diseases in men: prospective results from the Framingham Heart Study. I. Concordance of risk factors and the relationship of psychosocial status to coronary incidence, *Am. J. Epidem.*, 118, 1–22.
Suarez, L., and Barrett-Connor, E. (1984). Is an educated wife hazardous to your health? *Am. J. Epidem.*, 119, 244–49.

42. Tyhurst, J. S. (1957). The role of transition states, including disasters, in mental illness, in *Symposium on Preventive and Social Psychiatry*, Washington, D.C., pp. 149–69.

43. Richardson, I. M. (1956). Retirement: A socio-medical study of 244 men, *Scot. Med. J.*, 1, 381–91.
Ekerdt, D. J., Baden, L., Bossé, R., and Dibbs, E. (1983). The effect of retirement on physical health, *Amer. J. Pub. Hlth.*, 73, 779–83.
Ekerdt, D. J., Bossé, R., and Goldie, C. (1983). The effect of retirement on somatic complaints, *J. Psychosom. Res.*, 27, 61–67.

44. Lindemann, E. (1944). Symptomatology and management of acute grief, *Amer. J. Psychiat.*, 101, 141–48.

45. Susser, M. W. (1981). Widowhood, a situational life stress or a stressful life event?, *Amer. J. Publ. Hlth.* 71, 793–95.

46. Anonymous (1903). Assortative mating in man, *Biometrika*, 2, 481–98.

47. Ciocco, A. (1940). On the mortality in husband and wives, *Human Biology*, 12, 508–31.

48. Kraus, A. S. and Lilienfeld, A. M. (1959). Some epidemiological aspects of the high mortality rate in the young widowed group, *J. Chron. Dis.*, 10, 207–17.

49. MacMahon, B., and Pugh, T. F. (1965). Suicide in the widowed, *Amer. J. Epidem.*, 81, 23–31.

50. Parkes, C. M. (1964). Recent bereavement as a cause of mental illness, *Brit. J. Psychiat.*, 110, 198–204.

51. Stein, Z., and Susser, M. (1969). Widowhood and mental illness, *Brit. J. Prev. Soc. Med.*, 23, 106–10.

52. Bowlby, J., Ainsworth, M., Boston, M., and Rosenbluth, D. (1956). Effects of mother-child separation: A follow-up study, *Brit. J. Med. Psychol.*, 19, 211–47.
Rutter, M., and Madge, N. (1976). *Cycles of Disadvantage*, London.

53. Stein, Z. A., and Susser, M. W. (1966). Nocturnal enuresis as a phenomenon of institutions, *Develop. Med. Child. Neurol.*, 8, 677–85.

54. Stein, Z. A., and Susser, M. W. (1965). Sociomedical study of enuresis among delinquent boys, *Brit. J. Prev. Soc. Med.*, 19, 174–81.

55. Gregory, I. (1965). Anterospective data following childhood loss of a parent, *Arch. Gen. Psychiat.*, 13, 99–109.
Greer, S., and Gunn, J. C. (1966). Attempted suicide from inact and broken parental homes, *Brit. Med. J.*, 2, 1355–57.

56. Wardwell, W. I., Hyman, M. M., and Bahnson, C. B. (1964). Stress and coronary heart disease in three field studies, *J. Chron. Dis.*, 17, 73–84.
Syme, S. L., Hyman, M. M., and Enterline, P. E. (1964). Some social and cultural factors associated with the occurrence of coronary heart disease, *J. Chron. Dis.*, 17, 277–89.

57. **Murphy, H. B.** (1961). Social change and mental health, *Milbank Mem. Fd. Quart., 39*, 385–445.

Sydiaha, D., Lafave, H. G. and **Rootman, I.** (1969). I. Ethnic groups within communities: A comparative study of the expression and definition of mental illness, *Psychiat. Quart., 43*, 131–46.

Struening, E. L., Rabkin, J. G., and **Peck, H. B.** (1969). Migration and ethnic membership in relation to social problems, in *Behavior in New Environments*, ed., Brody, E., Beverly Hills, pp. 217–47.

58. **Thomas, W. I.,** and **Znaniecki, F.** (1927). *The Polish Peasant in Europe and America*, New York.

Malinowski, B. (1945). *The Dynamics of Culture Change*, London.

Little, K. L. (1948). *Negroes in Britain*, London.

Ruesch, J., Jacobson, A., and **Loeb, M. L.** (1948). Acculturation and illness, *Psychological Monographs: General and Applied, 62*, 1–40.

Anastasi, A., and **Foley, J. P.** (1949). *Differential Psychology*, New York.

Kluckhohn, C., and **Murray, H. A.** (1949). *Personality in Nature, Society and Culture*, London.

Hallowell, A. I. (1950). Values, acculturation and mental health, *Amer. J. Orthopsychiat., 20*, 732–43.

Kardiner, A., and **Ovesey, L.** (1951). *The Mark of Oppression*, New York.

Richmond, A. H. (1954). *Colour Prejudice in Britain*, London.

Collins, S. (1957). *Coloured Minorities in Britain*, London.

Banton, M. (1959). *White and Coloured: The Behaviour of British People Towards Coloured Immigrants*, London.

Sanua, V. D. (1959). Differences in personality adjustment among different generations of American Jews and non-Jews, in *Culture and Mental Health*, ed. Opler, M. K., New York.

Barnouw, V. (1973). *Culture and Personality*, rev. ed., Homewood, Ill.

59. **Fox, R.** (1978). *So Far Disordered in Mind: Insanity in California 1870–1930*, Berkeley.

60. **Ødegaard, Ø.** (1932). Emigration and insanity, *Acta. Psychiat.* (Kbh), Suppl. 4.

61. **Malzberg, B.,** and **Lee, E. S.** (1956). *Migration and Mental Disease*, New York.

Lazarus, J., Locke, B. Z., and **Thomas, O. S.** (1963). Migration differentials in mental disease: State patterns in first admissions to mental hospitals for all disorders and for schizophrenia in New York, Ohio, and California as of 1950, *Milbank Mem. Fd. Quart., 41*, 25–42.

62. **Allers, R.** (1920). Uber psychogene storungen in sprachfremder umgebung, *Z. Ges. Neurol. Psychiat., 60*, 281.

Frost, I. (1938). Home-sickness and immigrant psychosis, *J. Ment. Sci., 84*, 801–47.

Kino, F. F. (1951). Aliens' paranoid reaction, *J. Ment. Sci., 97*, 589–94.

63. **Prior, I.** (1977). Migration and physical illness, *Adv. Psychosomatic Med., 9* 105–31.

64. **Jaco, E. G.** (1959). Mental health of Spanish Americans in Texas, in *Culture and Mental Health*, ed. Opler, M. K., New York.

Taylor, Lord, and **Chave, S. P. W.** (1964). *Mental Health and Environment*, London.

Hare, E. H., and **Shaw, G. K.** (1965). A study in family health, *Brit. J. Psychiat., 111*, 461–72.

Dohrenwend, B. P. (1983). The epidemiology of mental disorder, in *Handbook of Health, Health Care, and the Health Professions*, ed. Mechanic, D., New York, pp. 157–94.

65. Saszewski, J., and Haenszel, W. (1961). Cancer mortality among Polish-born in the United States, *J. Nat. Cancer Inst.*, 35, 291–97.

Gordon, T. (1967). Further mortality experience among Japanese Americans, *Publ. Hlth. Rep.* (Wash.), 82, 973–84.

Haenszel, W., and Kurihara, M. (1968). Studies of Japanese migrants. I. Mortality from cancer and other disease among Japanese in the United States, *J. Nat. Cancer Inst.*, 40, 43–68.

Higgs, R. (1979). Cycles and trends of mortality in 18 large American cities, 1871–1900, *Explorations in Economic History*, 16, 381–408.

66. Marmot, M. G., and Syme, S. L. (1976). Acculturation and coronary heart disease in Japanese-Americans, *Amer. J. Epidem.*, 104, 225–47.

67. Eastcot, D. F. (1956). The epidemiology of lung cancer in New Zealand, *Lancet*, 2, 37–39.

Dean, G. (1959). Lung cancer among white Southern Africans, *Brit. Med. J.*, 2, 582–7.

68. Poskanzer, D. C., Schapira, K., and Miller, H. (1963). Multiple sclerosis and poliomyelitis, *Lancet*, 2, 917–21.

Poskanzer, D. C. (1965). Tonsillectomy and multiple sclerosis, *Lancet*, 2, 1264–66.

Visscher, B. R., Detels, R., Coulson, A. H,. Malmgren, R. M., and Dudley, J. P. (1977). Latitude, migration and the prevalence of multiple sclerosis, *Amer. J. Epidem.*, 106, 470–75.

Detels, R., Myers, L. W., Ellison, G. W., Visscher, B. R., Malmgren, R. M., Madden, D. L., and Sever, J. L. (1978). Changes in immune response during relapses in MS patients, *Neurology*, 31, 492–95.

Kurtzke, J. F., and Hyllested, K. (1979). Multiple sclerosis in the Faroe Islands: I. Clinical and epidemiological features, *Ann. Neurol.*, 5, 6–21.

Kurtzke, J. F., Beebe, G. W., and Norman, J. E., Jr. (1979). Epidemiology of multiple sclerosis in U.S. veterans. I. Race, sex and geographic distribution, *Neurology*, 29, 1228–35.

Kurtzke, J. F. (1980). Epidemiologic contributions to multiple sclerosis: An overview, *Neurology*, 30, No. 7, Part 2, 361–79.

69. Cassel, J. C., and Tyroler, H. A. (1961). Epidemiological studies of culture change. I. Health status and recency of industrialization, *Arch. Environm. Hlth.*, 3, 31–39.

70. Gampel, B., Slome, C., Scotch, N. A., and Abramson, J. (1962). Urbanization and hypertension among Zulu adults, *J. Chron. Dis.*, 15, 67–70.

Scotch, N. A. (1963). Sociocultural factors in the epidemiology of Zulu hypertension, *Amer. J. Publ. Hlth.*, 53, 1205–13.

71. Henry, J. P., and Cassel, J. C. (1969). Psychosocial factors in essential hypertension: Recent epidemiologic and animal experimental evidence, *Amer. J. Epidem*, 90, 171–200.

72. Cassel, J. C. (1975). Studies of hypertension in migrants, in *Epidemiology and Control of Hypertension*, ed. Paul, O., Miami, pp. 41–58.

73. Stahl, S. M., Grim, C. E., Donald, C., and Neikerk, H. J. (1975). A model for the social sciences and medicine: The case for hypertension, *Soc. Sci. Med.*, 9, 31–38.

Ostfeld, A. M., and D'Atri, D. A. (1977). Rapid sociocultural change and high blood pressure, *Adv. Psychosom. Med.*, 9, 20–37.

74. Hawkins, N. G., Davies, R., and Holmes, T. H. (1957). Evidence of psychosocial factors in the development of pulmonary tuberculosis, *Am. Rev. Tuberc. Pulmon. Dis.*, 75, 768–80.

Jaco, E. (1970). Mental illness in response to stress, in *Social Stress*, eds. Levine, S. and Scotch N., Chicago, pp. 210–27.

Levi, L., ed. (1971). *Society, Stress and Disease*, London.

Dohrenwend, B. S., and Dohrenwend, B. P., eds. (1974). *Stressful Life Events*, New York.

French, V. R. P., Jr., Rodgers, W. and Cobb, S. (1974). Adjustment as person-environment fit, in *Coping and Adaptation*, ed. Coelho, G. V., Hamburg, D. A., and Adams, J. E., New York pp. 316–333.

75. Rubin, R., Gunderson, E., and Arthur, R. (1971). Life stress and illness patterns in the U. S. Navy. V. Prior life change and illness onset in a battleship's crew, *J. Psychosom. Res., 15,* 89–94.

Rahe, R. H., Floistad, I., Bergan, T., Ringdal, R., Gerhardt, R., Gunderson, E. K., and Arthur, R. J. (1974). A model for life changes and illness research, *Arch. Gen. Psychiat., 31,* 172–77.

Paykel, E. S. (1974). Life stress and psychiatric disorder: Application of the clinical approach, in *Stressful Life Events*, ed. Dohrenwend, B. S., and Dohrenwend, B. P., New York pp. 135–49.

Myers, J. K., Lindenthal, J. J., and Pepper, M. P. (1974). Social class, life events and psychiatric symptoms: A longitudinal study, in *Stressful Life Events*, ed. Dohrenwend, B. S., and Dohrenwend, B. P., New York pp. 191–205.

Bramwell, S. T., Masuda, M., Wagner, N. N., and Holmes, T. H. (1975). Psychosocial factors in athletic injuries, *J. Human Stress, 1,* 6–20.

76. Brown, G. W. (1974). Meaning, measurement, and stress of life events, in *Stressful Life Events*, ed. Dohrenwend, B. S., and Dohrenwend, B. P., New York, pp. 217–43.

77. Theorell, T. (1974). Life events before and after the onset of a premature myocardial infarction, in *Stressful Life Events*, ed. Dohrenwend, B. S., and Dohrenwend, B. P., New York, pp. 101–17.

78. Michaux, W. W., Gansereit, K. H., McCabe, O. L., and Kurland, A. M. (1967). The psychopathology and measurements of environmental stress, *Comm. Ment. Hlth. J., 3,* 358–72.

Kagan, A., and Levi, L. (1974). Health and environment-psychosocial stimuli: A review, *Soc. Sci. Med., 8,* 225–41.

79. Rabkin, J. G., and Struening, E. L. (1976). Social change, stress, and illness: A selective literature review, *Psychoanalysis and Contemporary Science, 5,* 573–624.

Dohrenwend, B. S., and Dohrenwend, B. P., ed. (1981). *Stressful Life Events and Their Contexts*, New York.

Susser, M. (1981). The epidemiology of life stress, *Psycholog. Med., 11,* 1–8.

80. Kasl, S. V. (1972). Physical and mental health effects of involuntary relocation and institutionalization on the elderly: A review, *Amer. J. Publ. Hlth., 62,* 377–84.

Kasl, S. V. (1976). Effects of housing on mental and physical health, in *Housing in the Seventies. Working Papers. I. National Housing Policy Review,* U.S. Department of Housing and Urban Development, Washington, D.C., pp. 286–304.

81. Antonovsky, A. (1974). Conceptual and methodological problems in the study of resistance resources and stressful life events, in *Stressful Life Events*, ed. Dohrenwend, B. S., and Dohrenwend, B. P., pp. 245–58, New York.

Hudgens, R. W. (1974). Personal catastrophe and depression, in *Stressful Life Events*, ed. Dohrenwend, B. S., and Dohrenwend, B. P., New York, pp. 119–34.

Mason, J. (1975). A historical view of the stress field, *J. Human Stress, 1,* 6–12.

82. **Wolf, S.,** and **Ripley, H.** (1947). Reactions among Allied prisoners of war subjected to three years of imprisonment and torture by the Japanese, *Amer. J. Psychiat., 104,* 180–93.

Hinkle, L., and **Wolff, H. G.** (1957). Health and the social environment: Environmental investigations, in *Explorations in Social Psychiatry,* ed. Leighton, A., Clausen, J., and Wilson, R., New York, pp. 105–37.

83. **Lazarus, R. S.** (1971). The concepts of stress and disease, in *Society, Stress and Disease,* vol. 1, ed., Levi, L., London, pp. 53–58.

Mechanic, D. (1978). *Medical Sociology,* 2nd edition, New York.

Antonovsky, A. (1979). *Health, Stress and Coping,* San Francisco.

84. **Brown, G. W., Birley, J. L. T.,** and **Wing, J. K.** (1972). Influence of family life on the course of schizophrenic disorders: A replication, *Brit. J. Psychiat., 121,* 241–58.

85. **Kaplan, B. H., Cassel, J. C.,** and **Gore, S.** (1977). Social support and health, *Medical Care,* 15, suppl. 5, pp. 47–50.

86. **Thoits, P. A.** (1982). Conceptual, methodological, and theoretical problems in studying support as a buffer against life stress, *J. Hlth. Soc. Behav., 23,* 145–59.

87. **Caplan, G.** (1974). *Support Systems and Community Mental Health,* New York.

Cassel, J. (1976). The contribution of the social environment to host resistance, *Amer. J. Epidem., 104,* 107–23.

Cobb, S. (1976). Social support as a moderator of life stress, *Psychosom. Med., 38,* 300–14.

Liem, R. and **Liem, J.** (1978). Social class and mental health reconsidered: The role of economic stress and social support, *J. Hlth. Soc. Behav.* 19, 139–56.

Caplan, R. D. (1979). Social support, person-environment fit and coping, in *Mental Health and the Economy,* ed. Ferman, L., and Gordis, J., Kalamazoo, Mich. pp. 89–137.

88. **Lowenthal, M. F.,** and **Haven, C.** (1968). Interaction and adaptation: Intimacy as a critical variable, *Amer. Sociol. Rev., 33,* 20–30.

Brown, G. W., Bhrolchain, M. N., and **Harris, T.** (1975). Social class and psychiatric disturbance among women in an urban population, *Sociology, 9,* 225–54.

Myers, J. K., Lindenthal, J. J., and **Pepper, M. P.** (1975). Life events, social integration and psychiatric symptomatology, *J. Hlth. Soc. Behav., 16,* 421–27.

Cobb, S., and **Kasl, S. V.** (1977). Termination: The consequences of job loss, Department of Health, Education and Welfare, (NIOSH Publication) No. 77–224, Cincinnati.

Dean, A., Lin, N., and **Ensel, W. M.** (1980). The epidemiological significance of social support systems in depression, in *Research in Community and Mental Health,* vol. 2, Greenwich.

Turner, R. J. (1981). Social support as a contingency in psychological well-being, *J. Hlth. Soc. Behav., 22,* 357–67.

89. **House, J. S.** (1981). *Work Stress and Social Support,* Reading, Mass.

90. **Pearlin, L., Lieberman, M. A., Menaghan, E. G.,** and **Mullan, J. T.** (1981). The stress process, *J. Hlth. Soc. Behav.* 22, 337–56.

91. **Andrews, G., Tennant, C., Hewson, D. M.,** and **Vaillant, G. E.** (1978). Life event stress, social support, coping style, and risk of psychological impairment, *J. Nerv. Ment. Dis., 166,* 307–16.

Lin, N., Simeone, R. S., Ensel, W.M., and **Kuo, W.** (1979). Social support, stressful life events, and illness: A model and an empirical test, *J. Hlth. Soc. Behav., 20,* 108–19.

92. **Gersten, J. C., Langner, T. S., Eisenberg, J. G.,** and **Simcha-Fagan, O.** (1977). An evaluation of the etiologic role of stressful life-change events in psychological disorders, *J. Hlth. Soc. Behav.*, *18*, 228–44.

93. **LaRocca, J. M., House, J. S.,** and **French, J. P.** (1980). Social support, occupational stress and health, *J. Hlth. Soc. Behav.*, *21*, 202–18.

94. **Kasl, S. V.** (1984). When to welcome a new measure, *Amer. J. Publ. Hlth.*, *74*, 106–8.

95. **Holmes, T. H.,** and **Rahe, R. H.** (1967). The social readjustment rating scale, *J. Psychosom. Res.*, *11*, 213–18.

96. **Cassel, J.** (1970). Physical illness in response to stress, in *Social Stress*, ed. Scotch, N., and Levine, S., pp. 189–209, Chicago.
    Gersten, J. C., Langer, T. S., Eisenberg, J. G., and **Orzek, L.** (1974). Child behavior and life events: Undesirable change or change per se?, in *Stressful Life Events*, ed. Dohrenwend, B. S., and Dohrenwend, B. P., New York, pp. 159–170.
    Vinokur, A. and **Selzer, M. L.** (1975). Desirable versus undesirable life events: Their relationship to stress and mental distress, *J. Pers. Soc. Psychol.*, *32*, 329–37.
    Mueller, D. P., Edwards, D. W., and **Yarvis, R. M.** (1977). Stressful life events and psychiatric symptomatology: Change or undesirability, *J. Hlth. Soc. Behav.*, *18*, 307–17.
    Ross, C. E. and **Mirowsky, J.** (1979). A comparison of life-event-weighting schemes: Change, undesirability, and effect-proportional indices, *J. Hlth. Soc. Behav.*, *20*, 166–77.
    Thoits, P. A. (1981). Undesirable life events and psychophysiological distress: A problem of operational confounding, *Amer. Sociol. Rev.*, *46*, 97–109.

97. **Kanner, A. D., Coyne, J. C., Schaefer, C.,** and **Lazarus, R. S.** (1981). Comparison of two modes of stress measurement: Daily hassles and uplifts versus major life events, *J. Behav. Med.*, *4*, 1–39.

98. **Paykel, E. S., Myers, J. K., Dienelt, M. N., Klerman, G. L., Lindenthal, J. J.,** and **Pepper, M. P.** (1969). Life events and depression: A controlled study, *Arch. of Gen. Psychiat*, *21*, 753–60.

99. **Levitsky, D. A.** and **Barnes, R. H.** (1970). Effects of early malnutrition on the reaction of adult rats to aversive stimuli, *Nature*, *225*, 468–69.
    Zimmerman, K. R., Strobel, D. A., Steere, P., and **Geist, K. R.** (1975). Behaviour and malnutrition in the rhesus monkey, *Primate Behavior*, *4*, 241.

100. **Cobb, S.** (1974). A model for life events and their consequences, in *Stressful Life Events*, ed. Dohrenwend, B. S., and Dohrenwend, B. P., New York, pp. 151–56.

101. **Tennant, C.** and **Bebbington, P.** (1978). The social causation of depression: A critique of Brown and his colleagues, *Psychol. Med.*, *8*, 565–75.
     Shapiro, M. B. (1979). The Social Origins of Depression by G. W. Brown and T. Harris: Its methodological philosophy, *Behav. Res. Ther.*, *17*, 597–603.

102. **Brown, G. W.,** and **Harris, T.** (1978). Social origins of depression: A reply, *Psychological Medicine*, *8*, 577–88.
     Brown, G. W., and **Harris, T.** (1979). The sin of subjectivism: A reply to Shapiro, *Behav. Res. Ther.*, *17*, 605–13.

103. **Neugebauer, R. N.** (1980). The reliability of life event reports, in *Stressful Life Events and Their Contexts*, ed. Dohrenwend, B. P., and Dohrenwend, B. S., New York, pp. 85–107.
     Neugebauer, R. (1983). Reliability of life event interviews with outpatient schizophrenics, *Arch. Gen. Psychiat.*, *40*, 378–83.

104. Spitzer, R. L., Endicott, J. and Robins, E. (1975). Clinical criteria for psychiatric diagnoses and DSM-III, *Amer. J. Psychiat.*, *132*, 1187–92.

Wing, J. K., Cooper, J. E., and Sartorius, N. (1974). *Measurement and Classification of Psychiatric Symptoms*, Cambridge, Mass.

Weissman, M., Sholomskas, D., Pottenger, M., Prusoff, B., and Locke, B. Z. (1977). Assessing depressive symptoms in five psychiatric populations: A validation study, *Amer. J. Epidem.*, *106*, 203–14.

Robins, L. N., Helzer, J. E., Croughan, J., and Ratcliff, K. S. (1981). National Institute of Mental Health Diagnostic Interview Schedule: History, characteristics and validity, *Arch. Gen. Psychiat.*, *38*, 381–89.

Robins, L. N., Helzer, J. E., Ratcliff, K. S., and Seyfried, W. (1982). Validity of the Diagnostic Interview Schedule, version II, DSM-III Diagnoses, *Psychol. Med.*, *12*, 855–70.

105. Srole, L., Langner, T. S., Michael, S. T., Opler, M. K., and Rennie, T. M. C. (1962). *Mental Health in the Metropolis: The Midtown Manhattan Study*, New York.

106. Leighton, D. C., Harding, J. S., Macklin, D. B., MacMillan, N. M., and Leighton, A. H. (1963). *The Stirling County Study of Psychiatric Disorder and Socio-Cultural Environment*, vol. 3: *The Character of Danger: Psychiatric Symptoms in Selected Communities*, New York.

107. MacMahon, B., and Pugh, T. F. (1970). *Epidemiology: Principles and Methods*, Boston.

Fleiss, J. L. (1973). *Statistical Methods for Rates and Proportions*, New York.

Ibrahim, M. A. ed. (1979). The case-control study: Consensus and controversy, *J. Chron. Dis.*, *32*, 1–190.

Stolley, P. D., and Schlesselman, J. J. (1982). Planning and conducting a study, in *Case-Control Studies: Design, Conduct, Analysis*, ed. Schlesselman, J. J., New York, pp. 69–104.

Breslow, N. E., and Day, N. E. (1980). *Statistical Methods in Cancer Research*. Vol. I. *The Analysis of Case-Control Studies*, Lyon.

108. Neel, J. V., and Schull, W. J. (1956). *The Effects of Exposure to the Atomic Bombs on Pregnancy Determination in Hiroshima and Nagasaki*, Washington, D.C.

109. Stein, Z., Susser, M., Saenger, G., and Marolla, F. (1975). *Famine and Human Development: Studies of the Dutch Hunger Winter of 1944/45*, New York.

110. Vaillant, G. E. (1979). Natural history of male psychologic health: Effects of mental health on physical health, *New Eng. J. Med.*, *301*, 1249–54.

111. Berkman, L. F., and Syme, S. L. (1979). Social networks, host resistance, and mortality: A nine year follow-up study of Alameda County residents, *Amer. J. Epi.*, *109*, 186–204.

112. Raphael, B. (1977). Preventive intervention with the recently bereaved, *Arch. Gen. Psychiat.*, *34*, 1450–1454.

113. Central Statistical Office (1982). *Social Trends*, *12*, H.M.S.O., London.

114. Central Statistical Office (1982). *Annual Abstract of Statistics*, H.M.S.O., London.

115. Glass, D. V., ed. (1954). *Social Mobility in Britain*, London.

116. Berent, J. (1954). Social mobility and marriage, in *Social Mobility in Britain*, ed. Glass, D. V., London.

117. Zeitlin, M. (1974). Corporate ownership and control: The large corporation and the capitalist class, *Amer. J. Sociol.*, *79*, 1073–119.

118. Meadows, S. H. (1961). Social class migration and chronic bronchitis. A study of male hospital patients in the London area, *Brit. J. Prev. Soc. Med. 15*, 171–76.

119. **Larover, P. S.** (1958). Chronic illness and socio-economic status, in *Patients, Physicians and Illness*, ed. Jaco, E. G., Glenco, Ill., pp. 37–49.
Croog, S., Levine, S., and **Lurie, Z.** (1968). The heart patient and the recovery process, *Soc. Sci. Med., 2,* 111–64.

120. **Goldberg, E. M.,** and **Morrison, S. L.** (1963). Schizophrenia and social class, *Brit. J. Psychiat., 109,* 785–802.
Dunham, H. W. (1965). *Community and Schizophrenia: An Epidemiological Analysis,* Detroit.

121. **Hammer, M., Makiesky-Barrow, S.,** and **Gutwirth, L.** (1978). Social networks and schizophrenia, *Schizophrenia Bulletin 4,* 522–45.
Mueller, D. P. (1980). Social networks: A promising direction for research on the relationship of the social environment to psychiatric disorder, *Soc. Sci. Med., 14A,* 147–61.

122. **Illsley, R.** (1955). Social class selection and class differences in relation to still births and infant deaths, *Brit. Med. J., 2,* 1520–24.
Illsley, R. (1980). *Professional or Public Health: Sociology in Health and Medicine,* London.

123. **Baird, D.** (1945). The influence of social and economic factors on stillbirths and neonatal deaths, *J. Obstet. Gynaec. Brit. Emp., 52,* 339–66.
Baird, D. (1977). Epidemiologic patterns over time, in *The Epidemiology of Prematurity*, ed., Reed, D. M. and Stanley, F. J., Baltimore, pp. 5–15.

124. **Heady, J. A.** (1959). Occupation and mortality: Filial mortality, *Brit. J. Industr. Med., 16,* 70–73.

125. **Boalt, G.** (1954). Social mobility in Stockholm: A pilot investigation, in *Transactions of the Second World Congress of Sociology,* vol. 2, p. 67.

126. **Scott, E. M., Illsley, R.,** and **Thomson, A. M.** (1956). A psychological investigation of primigravidae. II. Maternal social class, age, physique and intelligence, *J. Obstet. Gynaec. Brit. Emp., 63,* 338–43.

127. **Neugut, R.** (1981). Epidemiological appraisal of the literature on the fetal alcohol syndrome in humans, *Early Hum. Dev., 5,* 411–29.

128. **Newman, H. H., Freeman, F. N.,** and **Holzinger, K. J.** (1937). *Twins: A Study of Heredity and Environment,* London.
Shields, J. (1958). Twins brought up apart, *Eugen. Rev., 50,* 113–23.
Vanderberg, S. G., and **Johnson, R. L.** (1966). *Further Evidence on the Relation Between Age of Separation and Similarity in I.Q. among Pairs of Separated Identical Twins,* Research Report No. 18, Twin Study, University of Louisville School of Medicine, Ky.

129. **Loehlin, J. C., Lindzey, G.,** and **Spuhler, J. N.** (1975). *Race Differences in Intelligence,* San Francisco.

130. **Eyferth, K. L.** (1961). Lerstungen verscheider Grupen von Vestzunfskind-Intelligenztest fur kinder (HAWK), *Archiv fur die Gesante Psychologie, 113,* 222–41.

131. **Tizard, B., Cooperman, O., Joseph, A.,** and **Tizard, J.** (1972). Environmental effects on language development: A study of young children in long-stay residential nurseries, *Child Dev., 43,* 337–58.
Tizard, B., and **Rees, J.** (1974). A comparison of the effects of adoption, restoration to the natural mother, and continued institutionalization on the cognitive development of four-year-old children, *Child Dev., 45,* 92–99.

132. **Husen, T.** (1951). The influence of schooling upon I.Q., in *Studies in Individual Differences*, ed. Jenkins, J. J., and Patterson, D. G., New York, pp. 677–93.

133. **Gordon, H.** (1923). *Mental Health and Scholastic Tests among Retarded Children*, Educ. Pamphlet No. 44, Board of Education, London.
134. **Wheeler, L. R.** (1942). A comparative study of the intelligence of East Tennessee mountain children, *J. Educ. Psychol.*, 33, 321–34.
135. **Stein, Z. A.,** and **Susser, M. W.** (1970). The mutability of intelligence and the epidemiology of mild mental retardation, *Rev. Educ. Res.*, 40, 29–67.
136. **Burt, C.,** and **Howard, M.** (1956). The multifactorial theory of inheritance and its application to intelligence, *Brit. J. Statist. Psychol.*, 8, 95–129.
       Conway, J. (1958). The inheritance of intelligence and its social implications, *Brit. J. Statist. Psychol.*, 11, 171–90.
       Halsey, A. H. (1958). Genetics, social structure and intelligence, *Brit. J. Sociol.*, 9, 15–28.
       Jensen, A. R., (1969). How much can we boost I.Q. and scholastic achievement?, *Harvard Educ. Rev.*, 39, 1–123.
137. **Feldman, M. W.,** and **Lewontin, R. C.** (1975). The heritability hang-up, *Science*, 190, 1163–68.
138. **Gould, S. J.** (1981). *The Mismeasure of Man*, New York.
139. **Kamin, L. J.** (1974). *The Science and Politics of IQ*, Hillsdale, N.J.
       Hearnshaw, L. S. (1979). *Cyril Burt, Psychologist*, London.
140. **Scottish Council for Research in Education** (1953). *Social Implications of the 1947 Scottish Mental Survey*, 35, London.
141. **Wood Report** (1929). *Report of the Mental Deficiency Committee*, H.M.S.O., London.
142. **Lewis, E. O.** (1933). Types of mental deficiency and their social significance, *J. Ment. Sci.*, 79, 298–304.
       Penrose, L. S. (1949). *The Biology of Mental Defect*, London.
143. **Stein, Z. A.,** and **Susser, M. W.** (1960). Families of dull children: Parts II, III and IV, *J. Ment. Sci.*, 106, 1296–319.
       Stein, Z. A., and **Susser, M. W.** (1969). Mild mental subnormality: Social and epidemiological studies, in *Social Psychiatry*, ed. Redlich, J., *Res. Publ. Ass. Nerv. Ment. Dis.*, 47, 62–85.
144. **Birch, H. G., Richardson, S. A., Baird, D., Horobin, G.,** and **Illsley, R.** (1970). *Mental Subnormality in the Community: A Clinical and Epidemiological Study*, Baltimore.
145. **Clarke, A. D. B., Clarke, A. M.,** and **Reiman, S.** (1958). Cognitive and social changes in the feeble-minded: Three further studies, *Brit. J. Psychol.*, 49, 144–57.
146. **Tanner, J. M.** (1955. *Growth at Adolescence*, Oxford.
       Stein, Z. A., and **Susser, M. W.** (1967). The social dimensions of a symptom, *Soc. Sci. Med.*, 1, 183–201.
147. **Klineberg, O.** (1938). *Negro Intelligence and Selective Migration*, New York.
148. **Lee, E. J.** (1951). Negro intelligence and selective migration: A Philadelphia test of the Klineberg hypothesis, *Amer. Soc. Rev.*, 16, 227–373.
149. **Stedman, D. J.,** and **Eichorn, D. H.** (1964). A comparison of the growth and development of institutionalized and home-reared mongoloids during infancy and early childhood, *Amer. J. Ment. Defic.*, 69, 391–401.
150. **Skeels, H. M.** (1966). Adult status of children with contrasting early life experiences, *Monogr. Soc. Res. Child Dev.*, 51, No. 3.
151. **Lyle, J. G.** (1959). The effect of an institution environment upon the verbal development of institutional children: I. Verbal intelligence, *J. Ment. Defic. Res.*, 3, 122–28.
       Lyle, J. G. (1960). The effect of an institution environment upon the verbal develop-

ment of insitutional children: II. Speech and language and III. The Brooklands residential family unit, *J. Ment. Defic.*, *4*, 1–13, 14–23.

Tizard, J. (1964). *Community Services for the Mentally Handicapped*, London.

152. Kirk, S. A. (1958). *Early Education of the Mentally Retarded*, Urbana, Ill.

153. **Westinghouse Learning Corporation** (1969). *The Impact of Headstart: An Evaluation of the Effects of Headstart Experience on Children's Cognitive and Affective Development*, Preliminary Report, Ohio University, Columbus, Ohio.

154. **Susser, M.** (1981). Prenatal nutrition, birthweight, and psychological development: an overview of experiments, quasi-experiments, and natural experiments in the past decade, *Amer. J. Clin. Nutr.*, *34*, 784–803.

   Susser, M. (1984). Causal thinking in practice, *Pediatrics*, *74*, 842–49.

155. **Garber, H. L.** (1975). Intervention in infancy: A developmental approach, in *The Mentally Retarded and Society: A Social Science Perspective*, ed. Begab, M. J., and Richardson, S. A., Baltimore, pp. 287–304.

   McKay, H., Sinisterra, L., McKay, A., Gomez, H., and **Lloreda, P.** (1978). Improving cognitive ability in chronically deprived children, *Science*, 200, 270–78.

156. **Scottish Council For Research In Education** (1949). *The Trend of Scottish Intelligence: A Comparison of the 1947 and 1932 Surveys of the Intelligence of Eleven-year-old Pupils*, London.

157. **Emmett, W. G.** (1950). The trend of intelligence in certain districts of England, *Population Studies*, 3, 324–37.

158. **Anderson, C. A., Brown, J. C.,** and **Bowman, M. A.** (1952). Intelligence and occupational mobility, *J. Pol. Econ.*, *40*, 218.

159. **Sewell, W. H.,** and **Shah, V. P.** (1969). Social class, parental encouragement, and educational aspirations, *Amer. J. Sociol.*, 73, 559–72.

160. **Floud, J., Halsey, A. H.,** and **Martin, F. M.** (1956). *Social Class and Educational Opportunity*, London.

161. **Katz, M.** (1968). *The Irony of Early School Reform*, Cambridge, Mass.

   Greer, C. (1972). *The Great School Legend*, New York.

   Bowles, S., and **Gintis, H.** (1976). *Schooling in Capitalist America*, New York.

162. **Floud, J.** (1954). The educational experience of the adult population of England and Wales as of July 1949, in *Social Mobility in Britain*, ed. Glass, D. V., London.

   Public Schools Commission, *First Report* (1968). Department of Education and Science, H.M.S.O., London.

   Boyd, D. (1973). *Elites and Their Education*, Slough.

163. **Hollingshead, A. B.** (1949). *Elmtown's Youth*, London.

   Warner, W. L., Havighurst, R. J., and **Loeb, M.** (1950). *Who Shall Be Educated?*, London.

   Jencks, C. S. (1972). *Inequality: A Reassessment of the Effects of Family and Schooling in America*, New York.

   Yamaguchi, K. (1983). The structure of intergenerational occupational mobility: Generality and specificity in resources, channels and barriers, *Amer. J. Soc.*, 88, 718–45.

164. **Rosenthal, R.,** and **Jacobson, L.** (1968). *Pygmalion in the Classroom*, New York.

165. **Barker Lunn, J. C.** (1970). *Streaming in the Primary School*, Slough.

166. **Himmelweit, H.** (1954). Social status and secondary education since the 1944 Act: Some data for London, in *Social Mobility in Britain*, ed. Glass, D. V., London.

   Department of Education and Science (1978). *School Population in the 1980s*, Report on Education, 92, London.

9

The family in health and disease: concepts and methods

The family is the reproductive nucleus of society, a fundamental social institution whose primary and essential task is to socialize "the stream of newborn barbarians" so that they may take their place in life as mature and independent adults. From the moment a child is born, the family governs the early experience that permeates the course of physical and mental development. Every society, from nomads to city dwellers, has the institutions of marriage and family. Through the family human beings maintain physical continuity by reproduction, and social and cultural continuity by training and education. The family regulates both the status and behavior of the immature individual among relatives, and mediates that person's relations with other members of society (1).

Biologically, the family endows the individual with a complement of genes, and every individual is the combined product of the interaction between genetical inheritance, family experience, and the broader social environment. In inherited conditions such as achondroplasia, or Huntington's chorea, or fragilitas ossium, the genes impose an unmistakable shape on the patient's life as well as on his physique. In a condition like diabetes, the effects are sometimes equally important, if less obvious; diabetic parents may produce diabetic children, and in addition uncontrolled diabetes in the mother poses risks of maldevelopment and of disordered growth in the offspring from around the time of conception through the whole period of gestation. Inheritance is not, however, the sole cause of diabetes, for inheritance and environment interact; viral infection plays a part in the juvenile onset form, but especially in individuals with a genetic susceptibility indicated by the histocompatibility antigen complex (2). In the adult onset form of the disease, twin studies indicate a stronger genetic component, but family diet and mode of life still play their part as, for instance, in the obese type of diabetic, or in those forms that have begun to appear among Africans who are newly adapting themselves to urban life, or in Melanesian islanders who have migrated to the New Zealand mainland (3).

The health of a child is bound up with the family's internal and external environment even before it is born, and the fetus in the womb can be harmed or helped by the health, nutrition, and behavior of the mother. Starvation of a mother can give rise, depending on the stage of gestation, to infants born prematurely and of low birthweight, with attendant high risks of mortality and damage to the nervous system (4). Her unborn child can be damaged by maternal infections like rubella, toxoplasmosis, cytomegalovirus, herpes, and syphilis, or by the reaction of a mother's (Rh) antibodies to the fetal blood, as well as by maternal metabolic imbalance produced by diabetes and other disorders. Maternal smoking during pregnancy slows fetal growth, slightly shortens the period of gestation, and reduces the chances of survival to live birth at term; it may just possibly retard postnatal mental development. The drinking of alcohol also increases fetal loss through miscarriage, and heavy drinking may lead to the malformed facies and retarded mental development of the fetal alcohol syndrome. The unwitting ingestion of heavy metals, the taking of therapeutic drugs, and the abuse of narcotics all may exact a toll in pregnancy (5). The process of birth itself can maim a child. Subsequent experiences in infancy, in the quality of feeding and methods of training, for instance, further influence development, physique, stature, and personality.

The household members of a biological family share a pool of genes and a common environment as well as common modes of thought and behavior, and together these decide their susceptibility to disease. In relation to infection, the family can be seen as a kind of trellis over which the organisms spread. The ease with which infection spreads depends on the family's material and social environment, which includes housing, heating, sanitation, and diet. A house that is damp and overcrowded encourages streptococcal infections and their sequelae such as rheumatic fever and nephritis, and a house that is dry and spacious obstructs their spread. Tuberculosis also flourishes under the same conditions. Its spread illustrates the interaction between genetic susceptibility and physical environment. Although it is classically a social disease of poverty, genetic susceptibility appears in the greater concordance for tuberculous infection found in identical twins than in nonidentical twins, a concordance that extends even to the organs affected by the disease (6). Rheumatic fever behaves in much the same way. Although the disease occurs in similar poor conditions, its manifestations are concordant in type both in affected twins and sibs (7). Some families provide a more or less efficient trellis for the spread of virus of poliomyelitis, for there appear to be "hot" families who are good disseminators of virus and "cold" families who are poor disseminators (8). These characteristics are likely to be determined by a social and physical environment that provides different chances of acquiring natural immunity against virus infection, with the better-off at highest risk of paralytic disease (see Chapter 6).

It is not only infective agents that pass between members of a family. Parents may transmit cultural perceptions and behavioral norms to their children and, if these are distorted, create deviant behavior and failures of adaptation among them (9). Husbands, wives, and their children may interact in a manner that may be sufficient to generate common neuroses and psychosomatic disorders in the family. As we have noted elsewhere with duodenal ulcer, rheumatoid arthritis, and hypertension, however, hard evidence is hard to come by (10).

The relations of members of a family with persons outside the family also contribute to the state of their health. Infections such as the childhood exanthemata and those of the upper respiratory tract are acquired from external contacts. Small children who consort with others most often introduce the common infections, and the larger the number of children, the more frequently the infections occur. The risk of exposure to this kind of infection depends on the age and number of the children, and on the social class and the mode of life of their parents. Children from small, uncrowded families typical of the higher classes are especially liable to these infections when they are of school age; in the larger families of the working class, children still in the preschool stages are more liable to suffer. Infants from many higher-class families are brought up in relative isolation, and make their first regular contacts with other children late, thus incurring frequent exposure to infection only when they go to school. In contrast, children from working-class families are accustomed from infancy to play with others outside the home, and run the more serious risks of infection at early ages. In all classes, however, family behavior must accommodate to changing economic and social circumstances. Consequently epidemic patterns are not static. For instance, the rapidly enlarging numbers of infants of working mothers exposed to others in daycare facilities have altered the sources, types, and frequency of family infection in many urban centers (11). These factors affect both the prognosis and the efficiency of preventive measures, and are of some practical importance both to health officers and to doctors responsible for the care of individual patients.

Efficient prevention of many infectious diseases requires that the family be regarded as a unit with shared environment. Meningococcal meningitis in epidemic form is typically a disease of military recruits and children; when thrown together in barracks up to 90 per cent of men may carry the organism, although few succumb. It can also appear in more insidious epidemic form within a social network. Symptomless carriers of the organism spread the infection and the proportion of carriers is raised not only among case contacts, but among all members of the network. Thus, one study of a network, in which three young cousins were attacked successively, found a carrier rate of 44 per cent among the first degree relatives of the cases, of 20 per cent among all the members of the network who had contact with cases at the relevant period, and of only 3 per cent in a control population (12). Where there is tuberculosis or whooping cough in the home, a newborn child taken from a maternity hospital is exposed to a high risk of death. Tuberculosis tends to spread through a community by way of families. Treatment aimed at containing this disease may be fruitless unless it is followed up by tracing the individual's chain of contacts through the family into the community. In countries where tuberculosis remains a major killer among the infections, clinics and mass x-ray units cannot wholly succeed in their object of prevention when they deal only with cases discovered among patients who approach them for examination, for the greatest concentration of cases is often to be found among those people who do not submit themselves for examination (see Chapter 3). A means of reaching such cases is through the family—for instance, by subjecting young children to routine tuberculin tests. A positive result at that age gives notice of contact within a narrow range of persons, probably within one family. The family thus provides opportunities for controlling infection as well as for spreading it. Tuberculosis is only one example, but similar principles apply to syphilis or scabies, typhoid, or dysentery.

With time many of these diseases have become less important, but as they declined a great residue of chronic degenerative and psychiatric conditions appeared behind them. Some of these have a well-established familial incidence, for instance, ischemic heart disease, hypertension, rheumatoid arthritis, diabetes, gout, and peptic ulcer. Among psychiatric conditions, manic-depressive psychosis, schizophrenia, psychoneurosis, alcoholism, sociopathy, and some forms of mental deficiency all have a familial incidence; in most the nature or extent of the contributions of heredity and family environment have still to be established.

As long as the means of prevention and specific cures for these chronic conditions are lacking, they present primarily a problem of long-term management, in which family support is a crucial element. Symptoms and sickness do not occur in isolation from other family events. Short-term observations based on diaries kept by low-income families show that the frequency of problems of different kinds and degrees is interconnected. The frequency of symptoms and uptake of medical care, high or low, were accompanied by corresponding rates of acute upsetting events, and of crises and chronic stress (13).

Separating heredity and environment

In theory, no trait can be uninfluenced by heredity, but neither can it be uninfluenced by environment. The environmental influence is both current and past (14); evolutionary adaptation is in all species a profound expression of their interaction with past environments. On this historical scale, and at this macrolevel of organization, the contributions of heredity and environment are inextricable. Yet, at the quotidian level of research in the health sciences, it remains critical to achieve discrimination between genetic and environmental factors; each type of factor leads to different strategies in the search for causes, and in prevention and intervention.

The recurrence of any trait or disease within a family immediately raises the question of a genetic effect. As we shall see, family recurrence is only one kind among several indicators of genetic effects. Nor can such an observation, even if repeated in other families, do more than raise the index of suspicion. Once the suspicion of familial aggregation has been raised, a *first* step must be to establish it as fact.

Familial aggregation is demonstrated by the excessive frequency of a trait or disorder within families as compared with the population at large. With a quantifiable trait, the correlations between family members must be greater than among unrelated individuals drawn from the same population. With a discrete trait or disorder, multiple cases within families must be found more often than would occur by chance from the population distribution. In a cohort approach, individuals with a family history of a trait or a disorder (the "exposure") are identified and followed: they must be at higher risk of developing the condition than is a comparison group without a family history. In a case-control approach, individuals already affected by a trait or disorder are identified: the risk must be higher in relatives of the *probands*, the index cases with the disorder under study, than in the relatives of an unaffected comparison group (controls).

In both approaches, age-adjustments need to be made to ensure comparable periods of observation (accomplished by life-table methods that take account of person-years of exposure). In addition, the case-control design presents difficulties peculiar to itself. In strict analogy with other uses of the design, affected relatives are treated as attributes of the case or the control. Estimates of risk should thus compare the proportion of cases and controls with affected relatives and not the proportions affected among the relatives of cases and controls. Adjustments should also be made for the number as well as the age of relatives. If the disorder affects fertility, then the risk of a case having affected sibs will be understated because the parent will have produced fewer children, and the risk of having an affected parent will be understated because fewer such parents will exist in the population at large (15). Cohort studies with longitudinal follow-up are not affected in the same way, because an affected parent is identified at the outset, but reduced fertility may add to the characteristic problem in such designs of finding a large enough sample and may bias that sample towards less severe forms of the disorder.

One way of dealing with the limits a case-control approach places on the efficient use of all the available information about affected relatives is to construct an historical cohort design around the cases and controls. Cases and controls themselves are excluded from the analysis, and the risk of the disorder in their relatives is compared. This is done by reconstructing the complete experience of the respective case and control families by going back to the formation of their respective nuclear families. The risk of developing the disorder from the time of birth in each is estimated from longitudinal life-tables that take into account the period over which each family member is at risk. (Representativeness is as for a case-control and not a cohort study, with irrecoverable attrition of cases that do not survive to the point of recruitment.)

Ascertainment bias is especially a risk in the case-control design. A family with two affected members has a greater chance of being ascertained than a family with only one. In addition, a rare case or attribute, or affected twin pairs, or families with several cases of one disorder, are likely to attract special interest that leads to selective ascertainment. Hence a condition will appear to cluster more frequently in families with an affected member than among controls. Geneticists have devised various formulae for adjusting rates, depending on the manner of selective ascertainment (16). The intrusion of ascertainment bias is less likely when cases are detected either in cross-sectional population surveys, and are thereby representative, and least likely in a prospective cohort design.

Once the first step of establishing the fact of familial aggregation is accomplished, a *second* and more difficult step is to separate genetic and environmental effects. Familial aggregation is a universal starting signal for the investigations of human geneticists. At the outset, however, investigators must entertain environmental hypotheses with equal seriousness. The need for neutrality is made plain by the familial recurrence of acute infectious disease, which epidemiologists measure by secondary attack rates—and which at most have a minor genetic component. Such chronic and insidious infectious diseases as tuberculosis and leprosy are transmitted most easily within the intimacies of families and have high rates of familial aggregation—here too in ordinary circumstances the genetic component, while present, is not major. Deficiency and toxic disorders may also be familial: syndromes of severe childhood malnutrition, or endemic goitre, aggregate in families who share dietary deficiencies; contaminated food characteristically will poison families, and so too will contaminated water from wells or tanks.

To accomplish the separation of genetic and environmental effects, then, the epidemiologist searches for strong indicators of each type of effect. A tabulation of indicators in relation to families yields four classes. Although, as might be expected, most indicators of genetic effects depend on family recurrence, some do not. Some indicators of environmental effects also depend on family recurrence, although most do not. We shall first consider these four classes of indicator. Next we shall consider the separation of genetic and environmental effects by design: ultimately, planned research is needed to arrive at well-founded estimates of the role of heredity and experience in a given disorder. The available designs include twin studies, fixed clusters of relatives of varying degrees of relatedness, and studies based on offspring reared away from their biological parents.

Indicators of genetic effects in the presence of family recurrence

Once familial recurrence is established for a condition of unknown cause, the usual question a geneticist poses is whether or not the distribution within families fits any of the Mendelian models for single genes. The question is determined from the *segregation* of genetic traits, which is their distribution among relatives. Distributions are analyzed using expected values derived from Mendelian assumptions, that is, whether genes are dominant or recessive, autosomal or sex linked. *Segregation analysis* compares the observed occurrence of a phenotypic trait or disorder, among relatives of different degree, to the occurrence expected on the assumptions of alternative genetic and nongenetic models (17,18). The fit of various models can be tested by two approaches. One approach takes series of nuclear families containing at least one affected member, provided numbers are large enough to yield the necessary statistical power. A second approach is to test genetic models within the pedigrees of large extended families. Segregation analysis with large pedigrees has illuminated the powerful genetic component found in subsets of certain diseases, for example, breast cancer (19).

With a rare dominant gene, on the Mendelian model, one parent and on average half the offspring should be affected. With a rare recessive gene, neither parent but on average a quarter of the offspring should be affected, and the frequency of consanguinity in the parents of affected offspring will be raised. A familial distribution of cases close to the expectation of a given model gives a strong presumption of a single gene effect: for instance, a dominant single gene as in Huntington's chorea; a recessive gene as in sickle cell disease; a sex-linked recessive gene as with hemophilia.

Expected distributions can be modified by the fertility and ascertainment biases mentioned above, and also by attrition, by questionable paternity, by heterogeneity, and by penetrance. A high rate of *attrition* before the age at which the condition usually becomes manifest might result in selective survival of gene carriers. For instance, at or after implantation about 30 per cent of conceptions are lost through spontaneous abortion, but of recognized pregnancies about 15 per cent are lost, so that a large proportion cannot be enumerated in counts of familial recurrence. Again, in certain malarial areas in Africa where infant mortality is high, carriers of the sickle cell trait, who are resistant to malaria, are more prevalent at older ages than during infancy, presumably because a larger proportion of infants without the trait did not survive attacks of malaria (see pp. 21–22). *Paternity* can seldom be established with the same certainty as maternity, and it cannot be taken for granted that pater and genitor are the same. In Tecumseh, Michigan, matched blood samples of parents and children indicated a nonpaternity rate of 4 per cent (20). This rate can be expected to vary with cultures, prevailing adult sex ratios, and circumstances like war and migration. *Heterogeneity* also causes departures from expected distributions. Multiple genetic forms of a condition (as with multiple dystrophies or clotting disorders) as well as both genetic and nongenetic forms (as with club foot), may coexist in the population.

Finally, geneticists have invented the concept of *penetrance* to account for departures from genetic models. The assumption is that the genetic component, the inherited *genotype*, may not be expressed as the manifest trait or *phenotype* of the individual observed. The concept of penetrance may be used also to describe the way in which a factor modifies the expression of a gene as, say, age does for Huntington's chorea. For epidemiologists, however, such areas of darkness become the hunting ground for possible environmental causes.

Most often, segregation analysis does no more than confirm observations of strong familial aggregations such as are found with Huntington's chorea. The presumption of genetic transmission becomes virtually certain, if there is *linkage* between two distinct manifestations, as between a genetic trait and a disorder. Linkage defines the close location on the chromosome of different genes (here, for trait and for disorder), and can be inferred from the patterns of concurrence of the two manifestations within families. The concurrence of a genetic trait and a disorder in a family pedigree may indicate the narrowly defined location of the two genes on a particular chromosome— as researchers have attempted to show for an association within families of color blindness with bipolar manic-depressive disorder (21). The history of this particular attempt also shows that the demonstration of linkage is difficult. Linkage studies of the transmission from parent to child of the genes for the histocompatibility immune complex of human leucocyte antigens (HLA) together with depressive disorder have proved controversial (22). One study suggests that susceptibility to depressive disorder may be determined by genes at multiple loci, one of which is HLA linked. With the number of genetic markers currently known, the prior probability of finding linkage between a trait and a marker locus is low. Recombinant DNA techniques are expected to raise the probability rapidly.

A compilation of all known single gene effects lists more than 5000 dominants and recessives (23). Even with attributions of gross effects to major genes, however, the possibility of confounding remains a hazard. Kuru is only the most recent and dramatic illustration of a disease owed to a specific external agent that was at first misattributed to genetic transmission (24). In another cautionary demonstration some 25 years ago, the then current genetic model for the transmission of diabetes through a recessive gene was tested by fitting the same model equally well to the chance of admission to the medical school at Buffalo, New York (25). The most confirmed hereditarians will agree that this chance is more likely to reflect cultural than genetic transmission.

A lack of statistical power is a common feature of genetic models. In large part, the problem resides in the rarity of genetic effects of large magnitudes despite the large list of known single major gene disorders. It is also in part a problem of imprecise measurement which suppresses strong effects. Even in the face of a high risk of disease in genetically susceptible individuals, familial aggregation is bound to be rendered less striking if the disease also affects persons not genetically susceptible (as must often be the case, say, with virulent infections); if not all relatives are genetically susceptible (as is necessarily the case on any Mendelian model); and if the unaffected comparison group contains genetically susceptible as well as nonsusceptible individuals (as in any sizable population it most certainly will).

Traits and conditions which run in families for the most part fit no clearcut Mendelian mode of transmission. In such instances, the danger of confounding genetic and environmental causes is much greater. Attributes like measured intelligence and blood pressure, and most cases of disorders like ischemic heart disease, epilepsy, mature-onset (noninsulin dependent) diabetes and breast cancer are of this kind. The causes underlying many such distributions are likely to be multifactorial. Some geneticists—although not epidemiologists—have tended to use this term as a synonym for polygenic, that is, arising from multiple genes acting together. Even where a geneticist's usage refers strictly to multiple genes with multifactorial disorders, both genetic and environmental factors are likely to contribute and to interact. Indeed, the disorders themselves are often heterogeneous, and include subsets in which different sets of causal factors predominate (26).

The initial assumptions of polygenic inheritance are quantitative, and derive from Francis Galton's concepts and techniques of correlation. The initial assumptions of single-gene inheritance are qualitative and derive from Gregor Mendel. (These assumptions do not exclude the possibility of graded effects produced by single genes, or of apparently qualitative threshold effects produced by multiple genes.) Ronald Fisher—in a classic paper which co-opted into the same framework the then antagonistic theories of Mendelian genetics espoused by William Bateson on the one side, and the Galtonian genetics together with Darwinian evolution espoused by Karl Pearson on the other—provided the first mathematical model for polygenic inheritance (27). The model made use of the variation in the distribution of traits among relatives of differing degree, and of the correlations of those traits among them; Fisher invented the "analysis of variance" and applied it to continuous variables to explain the contribution of inheritance.

Following on this work and using the same basic assumptions, Fisher and others devised measures of "heritability" that provide estimates of the genetic and environmental components of a particular trait or disorder (28). Multiple regression analysis, based on the quantitative deviations of the trait or disorder from the mean for different types of relative, is used to partition the observed variation. Refinements of this approach make use of the variations in genetic distance between related individuals, including half-sibs and cousins (29). Path analysis and other multivariate statistical models applied to such data permit the more rigorous testing of genetic/environmental models for their fit with observed familial distributions. Environmental factors, family environment and cultural transmission are included in the more developed forms of the models (30).

The effects of multiple genes are always interwoven with those of a pervasive environment. In matters as slippery as the allocation of weights to genes and environment, no mathematical model will suffice in the absence of research designs that might definitively separate the effects of genes and environment. The assumptions of the models are vital. Three similar analyses of the contribution of heredity and environment to measured intelligence, for example, used the same data and yet obtained sharply different results; these differences were traced in the main to differing assumptions (31). One tendency of the equations is to overestimate heritability because, on the assumptions of the genetic model, expected genetic variation but not environmental variation can be well specified from the known degrees of relatedness among individuals. Environmental exposures either go unmeasured or are weakly measured. Thus, the residue of the unmeasured effects of shared environment tend to be assigned to genetic variation. Yet the observed variation is in the phenotype, the sole manifest outcome of genotype exposed to environment, and its assignment to genotype rests on assumption. Although some analytic models do include indices of environmental exposures, imprecision in the measures of factors difficult to measure is likely to suppress the full effect.

Furthermore, the distributions of genotypes and of environments that determine the results of an analysis are likely to vary from population to population. This means that multiple regression estimates of heritability will vary likewise, and that any given estimate from such an equation is local and specific to a given population until proved otherwise. This fact may underlie the problems of accuracy and precision that emerged in hundreds of simulated computer trials that tested five estimators of heritability using different size random samples of specified relatives drawn from an artifactual population (32). In this population the true level of heritability was set beforehand. Estimators of heritability proved to have a low degree of reliability in approximating to the true known level of heritability. The estimators were not very accurate, and almost always overestimated heritability. The more the environment was shared, among relatives included in the model, the greater was the overestimate. The estimates were also not precise, in that confidence intervals were wide.

In addition, the method of heritability estimates fails to cope with either biological *interaction*, or with confounding that arises from *covariation* between genotype and environment. Genotypes interact with their environments and alter them, and environment in turn may alter the manifestation of a genotype. Confounding through covariation arises when genotypes select certain environments, as conversely in natural selection the environment favors certain genotypes by facilitating their survival. Yet heritability estimates assume independence between genotype and environment. The estimates also generally ignore the interaction between genes (in the forms of dominance and epistasis) and in this case may underestimate the effects of genes: indeed, the basic procedures of the analysis of variance (or its derivative methods like multiple regression) in partitioning the heritable and environmental contributions to phenotypic variation have been seriously challenged (33).

To summarize, the challenge rests on three main issues. First, it can be argued that a subtle tautology is inherent in the method. The total variation in a manifestation is the sum of genetic and environmental variances. The variation shared by individuals of different degrees of relatedness from an assumed "genotypic" mean is assigned to the genotype. The residue is assigned to environment. The genotypic variance is in fact variation from the observed or phenotypic mean, and includes any shared environmental variance that has not been removed by design or analysis. The assumption that the variation is genetic thus leads to the tautological assertion that it is genetic, regardless of its true origin. Second, it is a fallacy to interpret estimates of heritability in a local population as if they were generally valid. The estimates will differ across populations according to the distribution of environmental and genetic factors in those populations. Third, interaction and confounding are everpresent problems that are generally not subject to analytic control. As a result, the assumption of independence between genotype and environment is likely to be violated.

Indicators of genetic effects in the absence of family recurrence

Although intra-familial patterns are the first resort in seeking genetic effects in a disorder, genetic effects can also be identified by associations quite aside from recurrence within families. Thus *biological markers* of known genetic origin may vary consistently with a disorder. With duodenal ulcer, for example, there is an excess of individuals with blood group O, and also of those who do not secrete blood group antigens in the saliva. Similarly, characteristic patterns of the histocompatibility immune complex exhibited by human leukocyte antigens (HLA) are being discovered in association with a growing number of diseases. The presence of patterned associations indicates a gene for the associated disease located in the HLA region of the chromosomes and, it follows, supports a strong presumption of genetic predisposition.

Such associations, however, are no less subject to confounding and to mistaken inferences of causality than any other, and require the same rigorous testing (2). The complex of genetic predisposition and environmental precipitating causes is well illustrated in juvenile-onset (insulin-dependent) diabetes. This disorder occurs in association with particular HLA patterns. Associations have been found between HLA and disease or less convincingly, between the HLA shared by members of affected families. The genetic factor marked by these patterns is not enough to induce the disease, since monozygous twins are often discordant for juvenile-onset diabetes. Recent evidence implicates virus infections—coxsackie B virus or perhaps other types of virus infection—as the necessary environmental precipitant (34).

Endogamous target groups aid the discovery of genetic effects—especially recessive genes which require a homozygous pair to produce a recognizable phenotype. Endogamy may be intra-familial and consanguineous—uncles marry nieces in societies of South India; cousins marry in the Middle East. It may also be extra-familial and occur within marriage *isolates.* These are social groups whose boundaries are limited, either geographically as with many island populations, or socially as with many minority religions. Residential stability in any community is likely to cause genetic traits to cluster.

With endogamy the origin of an aberrant gene may be in "genetic drift" (a matter of its chance propagation in a small population), or in a "founder effect" (as with the porphyrias and hyperlipidemias common among Afrikaners descended from early Dutch settlers in South Africa). Sewall Wright devised a coefficient of inbreeding, and defined it as "the departure, from the amount of homozygosis under random mating, towards complete homozygosis" (35). In a large population consanguineous mating will make the main nonrandom contribution to the coefficient, but the smaller and more stable the isolate, the more will a random element contribute to inbreeding. In a small population, the random contribution will be present even in the face of exogamy (36). Such a "genetic bottleneck" can account for the frequency of certain rare conditions in marriage isolates. For instance, the Cayman Islanders exhibit several unusual syndromes, Ashkenazi Jews from Central Europe and the shtetls of the Baltic suffer an excess of Tay-Sachs and other diseases, and the Amish communities in the United States too have their special disorders, such as dwarfism (37).

Naturally, marriage isolates also have distinctive cultures and behavioral forms, and these too play their part in producing special configurations of disease. Culture is assuredly a main source of several unusual features of mental disorder among the Old Order Amish of Pennsylvania. No cases of drug abuse, alcoholism, or sociopathy were discovered in 12,000 people over a five-year period. Major depression accounted for an unusual 71 percent of all cases of recognized mental disorder, without the usual predominance of females (38). Among Seventh Day Adventists in California and Mormons in Utah, the low frequency of risk factors and the concordant low mortality for coronary heart disease and lung cancer indicate the absence of particular environmental hazards (39). Isolates are therefore target groups for epidemiologists in search of environmental causes as well as for geneticists. Ambitious studies of communities in which pedigrees can be traced for a century or more and linked by computer—among Icelanders, the Mormons of Utah, the Mexican-Americans of San Antonio, the French Canadians of Quebec—have been launched with the object of identifying both genetic and environmental factors (40).

Indicators of environmental effects in the presence of family recurrence

Where environmental and genetic effects are confounded, environmental effects in turn can be identified by discovering contributory variables that go far to exclude a genetic origin because of their special character. Just as with the two classes of genetic indicators discussed above, one class of environmental indicators is connected with familial aggregation, and a second class is not. To tease out indicators of environmental effects in the presence of family recurrence is to seek the converse of genetic indicators. Environmental indicators rely on disease clusters in families that do not conform with Mendelian models but do conform with the behaviour of factors of environmental origin such as infection and chemical or physical exposure.

Clustering in time of the onset of disease within families is one such pattern (14). For acute communicable disease this mundane phenomenon is well known to all; for chronic disease it takes on new significance. Time clustering may be seen in relation to the onset of disease among sibs or among parents and children, as with Hodgkins disease; such a cluster can be inferred from a pattern of disease onset more strongly related to calendar time or period than to age. Conversely, a pattern of disease onset more strongly related to age than to calendar time or period goes against an environmental effect. Subtle fallacies must be guarded against by the analyst who uses this method. Affected pairs gathered over a restricted time period (as is usual) while unrestricted in age (as is also usual), are likely to give rise to the false appearance of a time cluster (41). The pairs must necessarily arise within the restricted observation period, while they may be of any age. Time clustering may also be seen in the concentration of congenital defects among successive births, such as has been reported for tracheoesophageal and for neural tube defects (42), or in the contiguity of the birth orders that carry the highest risk for a disorder.

Clustering among family members of a single sex (14) is less conclusive than time clustering. Such *sex clustering* may indicate, besides environmental effects, either sex-linked genetic effects or constitutional gender effects. In the case of kuru, the fact that the disease did not conform with Mendelian inheritance became apparent from the unusual sex distribution. While the children affected were of both sexes, as expected from a Mendelian model, among adults on the contrary the disease was confined to women (24).

The interplay of shared family experience and degrees of genetic relatedness points to the role of the environment—a *cohabitational effect*—when traits or diseases are shared in the same or greater degree both by genetically unrelated and by related members. Members of family households live together, but comprise both genetically related and unrelated individuals. Typically spouses are genetically unrelated, and typically parents and children and sibships are genetically related. Simultaneous comparisons of the similarities between genetically unrelated and related persons living together are controlled for current domestic environment. If the similarities between spouses are as great as the similarities between genetically related individuals living together—parents and offspring, or sibships—the effects are likely to be owed to a cohabitational effect (43). If the similarities between genetically unrelated persons are less than those between persons who are so related, then the presumption of a genetic factor is stronger.

Confounding must still be guarded against. Spouses may resemble each other not because they live together, but because social and cultural forces promote *assortative mating*. The shared characteristics of spouses at marriage may in turn be either genetic or environmental. Sibs may resemble each other more than parental couples do for several reasons over and above their genetic relatedness: their exposure to family environment differs in content from that of spouses since parents and children are of different generations; unlike spouses sibs may be of the same gender; and the

Table 9.1 Comparison of blood and urinary similarities in older siblings and younger spouses (numbers and correlations)

Variable	Young husband-wife pairs[a]		Sub-adult sibling pairs[b]	
	N	r	N	r
Vitamin A	62	0.60	283	0.46
Vitamin C	69	0.46	314	0.53
Riboflavin	68	0.15	322	0.14
Thiamine	48	0.06	219	0.06
Hemoglobin	122	0.11	538	0.33

[a]By age of husband, 17.5–24.5 years.

[b]By age of older sibling, 16.5–18.5 years.

Source: Garn, S. M., Cole, P. E., and Bailey, S. M. (1979). Living together as a factor in family-line resemblances, *Human Biology, 51,* 565–587.

shared experience of sibs occurs at earlier ages than for spouses and susceptibility varies with age. Useful discrimination may be provided by taking account of duration of exposure to common environment. Thus, when measures of neurosis between spouses were observed to converge with increasing duration of marriage, the likelihood was strengthened that some form of shared experience underlay the change, that is, a neurotic person seemed to induce or transmit neurosis to the spouse. Similar convergence between spouses has been observed if inconsistently with blood pressure in marriages of long duration, as well as with fatness measured by subcutaneous skinfolds (43,44). Table 9.1 shows that a community sample of young spouses (with a short period of cohabitation) and sibling pairs of similar ages (with lifelong cohabitation) have much the same correlations for a number of nutritional indices in blood and urine. This implies that genetic factors, shared by siblings but not by spouses, made a lesser contribution to the correlation than current environmental factors shared alike by sibs or by spouses. Genetically unrelated members of a household are not confined to spouses. Adopted children are an obvious case; half-sibs, too, are not related to their step-parents. Table 9.2 shows, in the same community, that as biological siblings grow older, the correlations of cholesterol values among them converge on the correlations among adoptive siblings and become indistinguishable from them.

Table 9.2 Sibling similarities in cholesterol (numbers and correlations)

Age group	Biological siblings		Adoptive siblings	
	N	r	N	r
5–9	242	0.50	22	0.29
10–14	914	0.38	90	0.25
15–18	746	0.28	70	0.23
Total	1902	0.36[a]	182	0.25[a]

[a]Mean *r* from mean *z* — transform of *r*, Techumseh Community Health Study.

Source: Garn, S. M., Cole, P. E., and Bailey, S. M. (1979). Living together as a factor in family-line resemblances, *Human Biology, 51,* 565–587.

Maternal or *vertical transmission* to offspring (without any linkage to their sex) also excludes regular Mendelian inheritance. Besides the occurrence of this mode with the prenatal transmission of infections such as syphilis, toxoplasmosis, cytomegalovirus, and rubella, it has seemed the likely mode in some noninfectious diseases, as well as in the indolent infection of leprosy. When the onset is at birth, the condition must take origin in factors that are specific to the biology and experiences of the mother, for instance, an intrauterine factor. Another possible origin of a condition seen at birth is in the cytoplasm and mitochondria of the maternal ova, since sperm carry nuclear material but not these cellular elements. When maternal transmission is seen with conditions of later onset, lactation, feeding and maternal behavior also enter into the potential causal calculus.

With regard to the familial occurrence of epilepsy, the best available data point to a pattern of maternal transmission. The children of mothers with epilepsy have been found to be at much higher risk of epilepsy than the children of fathers with epilepsy. A Mendelian theory, whether of single or multiple genes, cannot account for the pattern (45). In pyloric stenosis of infancy, likewise, the offspring of affected women are at three times higher risk than those of affected men (46). In this disorder, however, an alternative genetic explanation has been offered.

Unlike epilepsy in which there is no notable imbalance in the sex ratio, in pyloric stenosis a four to fivefold preponderance of male infants is found. To explain imbalance of this kind, a theory of polygenic inheritance proposes that the penetrance of the genes among the less affected sex—here females—is lower; in other words, the threshold dose that must be reached before the condition will be expressed is higher (47). The differing threshold for each sex, it is surmised, unbalances the sex distribution. Given a dose equal to males, females would then less often manifest the disorder. When, affected by the necessary heavy dose, they do manifest the disorder, they would more often transmit it than would affected males. Males would more often manifest the disorder than females but, affected by a lighter genetic dose, would less often transmit it. In addition, female relatives of an index case are less likely to manifest the condition, and male relatives more likely.

When put to the test of mathematical modelling, this theory of polygenic inheritance does not conform with observed familial distributions of pyloric stenosis. The model of a major gene effect with varying penetrance could not be rejected, but neither did it satisfactorily explain the higher than expected risk in offspring as compared with the siblings of affected women. The investigators preferred a theory of maternal transmission, as with epilepsy above. Concordance among dizygous twins, higher than expected from incidence among siblings, suggested that the source was intrauterine (48).

Indicators of environmental effects in the absence of family recurrence

To consider next environmental indicators not connected with familial aggregation, the need scarcely arises in acute or massive episodes as with epidemic infections, seasonal fluctuations, or smog disasters. In most chronic disease epidemiology, by contrast, much of the time genetic and environmental effects are confounded.

Perhaps the most frequently used environmental indicators are *secular trends,* that is, population changes over time. For example, the rapid secular trend of increasing height among the Japanese after the Second World War virtually excludes a genetic explanation for the trend, despite the known hereditary component in individual height first established by Galton (27). In essence, the effects of environmental change are observed with the genetic components held constant.

Migrants afford another target group in which the effects of environmental change can be observed with the genetic component of the population held constant (49). Frequencies of disease that remain stable in a migrating group point to the possibility of genetic factors, but do not in themselves give more support to genetic than to environmental factors. A migrating group that sustains endogamy in breeding is likely to sustain other cultural forms brought from the homeland that influence health. However, rates in endogamous migrants that depart from those of the home population over one, two, and three generations, and shift towards those of the host population as assimilation to a new culture proceeds, are near to conclusive indicators of environmental effects (see Chapter 8, pp. 324ff). Naturally, powerful biases can arise from the self and social selection for factors that differentiate migrants from home and host populations—for example, social class, occupation, marital state, sex, personality, intelligence—and these must be controlled.

The genesis of studies of the environment in classical times followed on the recognition of epidemic disease, which in essence is *clustering in time and place.* Likewise, the underlying idea of the first statistical method devised to detect such clustering solely from numerator data—applied first to esophageal anomalies and then to leukemias—was that its discovery would indicate the presence of an environmental effect (42). While the method has been refined and supplemented by others, its yield of clusters has on the whole been meager and sometimes inconsistent. Possibly the approaches are insufficiently sensitive, or possibly the phenomenon of clustering itself is not a common or general one.

Family variables unconnected with recurrence can also shed light on environmental factors. *Family size* associations are useful if not conclusive indicators. Adult height declines with increasing family size. A family size effect is consistent with the well-founded view of height as an index of the physical and biological environment during growth. Improbable as are most postulates of a genetic basis for individual family size, however, heredity cannot be decisively excluded. Thus confounding could arise because the fertility of groups or individuals could be associated with their genetic constitution. For instance, with both schizophrenia and mental retardation, reduced fertility is a consequence of the disorder and, in turn, the disorder could be genetic.

On the other hand, for *birth order* one can scarcely conceive of a genetic basis on any reasonable grounds. In the same large population, measured intelligence, like height, was found to decline with increasing family size. Unlike height, test scores were also linked with birth order. This additional association with birth order leads to a conclusive inference of environmental effect, and suggests that the developing mind requires something more than the nutritional adequacy and physical health that suffice for height. The association of measured intelligence with family size suggests the influence of familial microculture, but cannot alone support the inference. But the declining gradient of measured intelligence with increasing birth order—with family size controlled—can scarcely be anything but environmental (50). The analysis of birth order without controls and in incomplete families, it should be noted, can be a misleading enterprise and requires care (see pp. 486ff).

Separating genetic and environmental effects by design

When familial patterns are compatible with either genetic or environmental models, analysis and mathematical modeling can seldom yield solutions that are conclusive, however plausible they may appear to be. Resort must then be had to the separation of genetic and environmental effects by design. Prerequisities for decisive approaches are two. First, both the genetic risk and the environmental exposure of the individuals comprising the population must be specified. Second, either individuals of the same degree of genetic relationship must have different environmental experience (as with separated twins or half-sibs), or individuals genetically unrelated must have similar environmental experience (as with cohabiting sibships including both adopted and natural offspring).

Twin studies

Twin studies offer one approach to a design for separating genetic from environmental factors. Rather more than a century ago, Francis Galton and others raised the hope that biologists could separate heritable from environmental factors by comparing the degree of similarity of monozygous (MZ) twins developed from a single ovum with that of dizygous (DZ) twins developed from separate ova (51). Later, after Mendel's work was understood, came the realization that monozygous twins had an identical set of genes while dizygous twins, like other siblings, shared on average only one-half of their genes. Twins also share developmental experience more closely than do other siblings, however, and the effect of shared experience on their attributes is confounded with the effect of their shared genes. A well-known model neutralizes the confounding variable, whether it is shared experience or shared genes.

$$\text{Shared genes} \longrightarrow \text{concordant inherited attributes}$$

Therefore,

(a) MZ twins more concordant than DZ twins and sibs;
(b) DZ twins and sibs equally concordant.

But,

$$\text{Shared experience} \longrightarrow \text{concordant acquired attributes}$$

In sum, therefore,

(a) MZ twins more concordant than DZ twins, or equally concordant;
(b) DZ twins more concordant than sibs.

Thus,

MZ $-$ DZ = genetic effect (MZ and DZ share experience to the same degree, and environmental effects cancel out);

DZ $-$ Sibs = environmental effect (DZ and sibs share the same number of genes, and genetic effects cancel out).

These comparisons take advantage of a matched design provided by nature. The confounding variables, either shared experience or shared genes, are converted into uncontrolled variables equally distributed between the different types of twins. With a dichotomous variable, these relationships are tested by the rates of concordance for the variable among pairs. With continuous variables, relationships are tested by the amount of variance shared by pairs and derived from the correlations between them; this approach is complex and tangled in controversy (52).

The equal distribution of experience among monozygous pairs is not as easily achieved as this model suggests (53). After fertilization, the precise forms taken by a pair may be affected, for instance, by the stage of cell division and growth at which a particular zygote splits into two. After implantation, two-thirds of monozygous twins share a single chorion and placental circulation, and because of imbalance in their shared blood supply, they may differ more than dizygous twins in their intra-uterine experience and in birthweight. After birth, the degree of concordance in the experience of monozygous and dizygous twins is likely to be reversed. Monozygous twins may resemble each other so closely that difficulties in maintaining their separate identities may lead to joint mental disturbance.° The assumption that monozygous and dizygous twins have equally similar environments has seemed more or less defensible to different investigators who have addressed the problem (54). In a series of twin pairs, developmental measures exhibited a tendency to converge in monozygous twins as they grew older, and to diverge in dizygous twins. While the difference in trends could result from the gradual expression of genetic endowment (55), the difference is no less likely to be the result of different socialization experiences of the two twin types.

In comparing monozygous with dizygous twins, therefore, confounding by shared experience cannot be assumed to be distributed equally between the members of either type of twin pair and thus to cancel out entirely. This uncertainty diminishes somewhat the value of twin studies in demonstrating genetic effects. By contrast, the degree of genetic confounding in twin studies in precisely known. This precision enhances the value of twin pairs, and of monozygous pairs especially, in studies of environmental effects. Discordance between individual members of pairs of monozygous twins can be attributed to environment, for their genetic attributes are matched and wholly neutralized.

Elaborations of twin studies have been attempted in order to yield a wider range

---

° The possibility of such disturbance, indeed, has been advanced as a factor that could have confounded the apparent genetic concordance of MZ twins for schizophrenia. However, the raised rate of schizophrenia among MZ twins expected on this hypothesis has not been found.

of degrees of relatedness. One innovation has been to follow the offspring of monozygous twins and to construct comparisons among the twins, their spouses, and their children (56). Such a design includes a number of unusual genetic relationships and paths of transmission. For example, the offspring are socially cousins but genetically half-siblings. The design brings its own problems. Because numbers are necessarily small, only common characteristics can be studied. Moreover, environmental exposure remains unmeasured, and must still be inferred from the variation that remains unexplained. A study of this kind found that serum cholesterol levels among the offspring appear to be dependent on maternal levels; another obtained the same result for verbal intelligence. Where there is no sex imbalance to suggest linkage to the X chromosome, associations between mothers and children to the exclusion of fathers do not support a genetic cause present before conception and acting in Mendelian fashion. They point either to an origin in maternal cells outside the nucleus (as was discussed above) or to a prenatal or postnatal origin and an environmental source.

Fixed clusters

Fixed clusters less closely related than twins have also been used to separate genetic and environmental effects. In one design referred to above, the variation of a trait such as birthweight among individuals of varying degrees of relatedness served to indicate the potential genetic component. None was found although, once again, the environmental component was inferred and not measured by design (29). The *family set design* is an elaboration of this approach. The design preordains the composition of the related and unrelated persons in the survey sample. Each kindred provides the same set of relatives as specified in the design. Preferably, the family sets are studied under more than one set of environmental conditions. In theory, such sampling makes possible the examination of environmental variation with genetic variation controlled and, conversely, of genetic variation with environment controlled (57).

Thus the family set design might begin with individuals identified in surveys of populations living under distinctive environmental conditions. In the example of a study of blood pressure, blacks were surveyed in two Detroit communities, a depressed and a better-off city area. To be included in the study, each proband had to have a specified set of relatives—in the original design, a sibling, cousins, a spouse and an unrelated control. The spouse yields an index of familial environment, the control of extra-familial environment. Exclusion of a parental generation avoids the intrusion of confounding between parents and children as a result of change in attributes between generations over time.

On the environmental side, blood pressure levels were distinctly higher under conditions of urban stress and deprivation. The population samples are necessarily selective and unrepresentative of the communities from which they are drawn, however, because of the family membership criteria for eligibility to enter the study; those with the requisite set of relatives are favored for entry. On the genetic side, as discussed above (32), the design seemed not to yield sufficient statistical power to make the estimates of heritability stable and reliable. In practice, the family set design has proved difficult to analyze and interpret and it is still undergoing development. The use of path models is a promising avenue that may increase the precision of statistical analysis.

Separately reared family members

The best hope of separating effects into genetic and environmental components is in the observation of members of nuclear families separated and reared under different conditions.

Separated twin pairs. Among separated monozygous twins, since the pair has identical inheritance, there is high potential for measuring the impact of disparate environments. With some allowances, the differences between members of a pair are bound to be environmental and, depending on the extent to which their environments are truly different, their similarities are likely to be mainly genetic. Although subjects are hard to come by, studies of separated twins began more than half a century ago (58) and were used to examine the genetic and environmental contribution in a variety of outcomes, including tuberculosis and other disorders. Another series of studies of separated twins aimed particularly at separating the genetic and environmental components of measured intelligence.° One innovation in these studies was the attempt to measure directly the cultural differences in the environments of the separated monozygous twins (59). Unfortunately, the examiner was probably not blind to the identity of the subjects, and therefore liable to bias.† Even were that not so, we have noted that because of the crudeness and imprecision of such measures, especially in comparison with the precise genetic estimates assigned to relatives, a tendency to underestimate environmental contributions is built in.

Indeed, studies of twins demand care and caution. When twins are adopted or fostered, they come from and enter unusual environments that are likely to be correlated with each other. Selectivity is a feature of most twin studies of any kind; an excess of monozygous and of female pairs tends to be recruited as volunteers. Misclassification introduces one more hazard common in epidemiology but exaggerated in assigning concordance in twin studies (62). Even a low error rate in classification is liable to produce a high proportion misclassified in any subset that comprises only a small fraction of the total population under study. Small subsets of discordant twins are prone to arise where the discordance with reference to some factor is low, and especially with monozygous pairs since they are less in discord than dizygous pairs. Misclassification of concordant pairs as discordant, among a small number of truly discordant pairs, could have a marked effect. Under these conditions, the effect of misclassifying concordance as discordance on an environmental factor, say, smoking, is to suppress the association of the factor with a disease under study, and to

---

°Sir Cyril Burt's twin studies have since become notorious (60). He enlarged the numbers of separated pairs through the years without giving evidence of actual accretion of new cases; against all expectations, the values of certain of the key correlation co-efficients changed not at all as the sample grew larger (59, 61).

†In fact, the intelligence tests and scores were not given blind either, and were liable to the same bias.

strengthen the inference that heredity is involved. Nevertheless, most of the discordance between the individual members of monozygous twin pairs validly determined can safely be ascribed to environment in the womb and after birth.

Half-sibs. The study of related individuals who are reared separately from their biological families is in practice more difficult to accomplish with twins than with half-siblings, or with siblings adopted or fostered out of the family. Within and across families, half-sibs reared by natural mothers—singly or with stepfathers—can be compared with half-sibs reared by natural fathers and stepmothers. Half-sibships can also be compared with full sibships. One such study of maternal half-sibships and full sibships found no differences between them in recurrence risks for several anomalies (63). If there is sufficient statistical power, such results leave no room for a paternal contribution to genetic variation, and indicate a maternal effect. The cause might be an environmental factor during pregnancy or before or, if genetic, involves a mode of transmission which departs from the regular Mendelian single gene model. A more discriminating design, while difficult to achieve, would include paternal half-sibs as well, and thereby provide environmental as well as genetic variation.

Institutionalization. A more common set of strategies, where problems of confidentiality can be overcome, is to study individuals who have been either institutionalized, fostered, or adopted and thereby separated from their biological parents. Studies of unrelated children institutionalized from an early age in different settings can demonstrate environmental effects. It is true that confounding, because of the selection of children with particular attributes for particular settings, is a hazard of all such studies. Nonetheless, studies of offspring separated from their families and placed in a variety of settings have yielded convincing evidence of environmental effects on such developmental outcomes as measured intelligence, behavior disturbances, and sphincter control. For each of these aspects of development, markedly adverse outcomes have been found for children placed in large institutions and children's homes as compared with fostering and adoption (64).

Adoption. The studies of institutional placements cited above, which examined unrelated individuals, could pay no regard to genetic effects. To demonstrate inheritance, related individuals must be included. To this end several approaches have been devised. Designs for adoption studies can be viewed in epidemiological terms. *Cohort* studies begin with natural parents whose children have been adopted. Parents with the disorder of interest and controls without it are first identified. Concordance for the disorder is sought in the frequency of its occurrence in the adopted-away natural offspring of each set of parents. *Case-control* studies begin with adoptees. Affected and control adoptees are identified, and concordance for the disorder is sought in the frequency of its occurrence in the natural parents and sibs of each set of adoptees. Either cohort or case-control designs may be used with so-called *cross-fostering* studies to yield environmental effects; in these, concordance for the disorder between adoptive parents and their adoptive children is compared with controls. The contribution of natural parents with the disorder to the outcome in adopted children can also be taken into account and controlled.

The vexed issue of heredity and environment in measured intelligence was addressed by several early adoption studies (65). The scope of inquiry has broadened over the years to include other dependent variables. In a pioneer effort to determine the extent of genetic transmission of schizophrenia from parent to child, a historical cohort design was used. Maternal schizophrenia was the exposure and schizophrenia in the adopted-away offspring was the outcome. From among children placed within three days of birth in state institutions in Oregon, those with schizophrenic mothers were selected for follow-up and compared with a group whose mothers were not known to be schizophrenic. A distinct excess of schizophrenia was found in the offspring separated from schizophrenic mothers (66). The follow-up diagnostic interviews in this study, however, seem to have been done with knowledge of the status of probands and controls, although two raters contributed independent evaluations.

Subsequent studies of schizophrenia aimed to test this result; the investigators used a Danish national adoption register and linked it with a national register of all admissions to psychiatric hospitals. One approach, again through a cohort design, identified all those natural parents of adoptees admitted to psychiatric hospitals with psychosis and compared the frequency of schizophrenia in their adopted-away offspring with the frequency in the offspring of a control group who had no record of admission. In this instance, too, the rate of schizophrenialike disorder was greater in the offspring of parents designated psychotic (67). A typical problem with cohort studies, we have noted, is the large sample needed to confer the necessary statistical power to study a rare condition; lack of power, and hence of statistical significance, rendered the results inconclusive.

Power was probably further reduced by the diversified diagnostic categories included in the study for parents (selected from those with manic-depressive as well as schizophrenic disorders entered in the national psychiatric register), and offspring at follow-up (not only definite schizophrenia, of which there were very few, but a whole range of psychiatric symptoms elicited on interview and classified as schizophrenic spectrum disorders). At the same time, these data yielded a result that could be taken as evidence for an environmental familial effect in schizophrenia. A psychologist is said to have distinguished, blind and with complete accuracy, the Rorschach tests of parents whose children were not schizophrenic (68). However, the direction of effect could as well be that of children on parents as parents on children. Again, numbers were small.

In another carefully executed approach a case-control design was used. Adoptees with a record of psychiatric admission were identified, and matched with adoptees who had no record of admission. The frequency of schizophrenia and "schizophrenia spectrum disorders" in their natural parents, sibs, and half-sibs was then compared (69). The contrast between all the relatives of schizophrenic adoptees and their controls suggested a striking genetic effect. Prevalence of the schizophrenia spectrum in all relatives of schizophrenic adoptees was 21.4 per cent. In all relatives of controls it was 10.9 per cent, indicating a twofold risk.

Yet these results are not entirely conclusive and have been strongly criticized and defended (70). The three main problems of the study reside in the relatively small numbers available for the study of a disease that is not common in its severe form; in the type and rigor of the analysis used; and in the apparent incoherence of the distributions among biological relatives.

First, the statistical power of the study was limited by the availability of adoptees. It was also limited by the infrequency among probands and relatives of hospital admissions for schizophrenia, which were the data provided by the national psychiatric register. In order to improve statistical power by increasing the number affected, relatives were followed and interviewed by a psychiatrist who was blind to their status in relation to cases and controls. Although no active case of schizophrenia was discovered on interview, a substantial increase in the numbers affected was achieved by the inclusion of three diagnoses—uncertain schizophrenia, schizoid personality, and inadequate personality—under the rubric of "schizophrenia spectrum disorders." Affected relatives of probands more than doubled in numbers, with the chief increment in half-sibs and in parents. For controls, only fathers showed a comparable increment. The expansion of diagnostic categories in this way is problematic in that it risks suppressing a true relationship by introducing heterogeneity. It risks producing a spurious relationship only if there was potential bias as, for instance, were the psychiatric interviewer not to have been absolutely blind to the case and control status of the relatives.

Second, the form of the analysis used in the study is questionable, and the control for confounding quite inadequate. In a case-control approach, the appropriate measure is the odds ratio, an estimate of risk for which the denominators are the numbers of cases and controls respectively. Naturally, these risk ratios should be adjusted for disparities in family size, age, age of onset, and sex, all of which might markedly influence the frequencies of observed disorder among the relatives of the comparison groups. For example, parents have a greater chance than offspring of being diagnosed because of longer exposure with greater age. Again, in this instance biological parents of schizophrenic adoptees may have had a lesser chance of being diagnosed because of the five suicides among them. The necessary data to make statistical adjustments have not been reported. Since numbers of cases and controls in each class of relatives are remarkably similar, their comparability may in fact be high. In order to make a comparison of the type attempted by the investigators, the case-control design must be converted into an historical cohort design; as described above, the relatives of cases and controls are each constituted as a cohort, and each individual (excluding cases and controls) is followed in a life-table analysis through the appropriate years of experience until the onset of disorder.

The third problem resides in the actual results of the study. These are presented in a restructured analysis in Table 9.3. In the case-control analysis in Table 9.3A, family size is dealt with by counting family units; a family is counted affected if any one member of a given class of relative is affected. In families taken as units, a significant difference is seen only if "uncertain schizophrenia" is included. Among classes of relatives, the risk of schizophrenia or schizophrenia spectrum disorders for all half-sibs (by far the largest category), and paternal half-sibs in particular, was statistically sig-

Table 9.3 A. *Case-control Analysis.* "Schizophrenia"[a] in biological relatives of adoptees with schizophrenia (cases) and in relatives of adoptees without schizophrenia (controls): numbers, odds ratios, and confidence intervals in parentheses. Odds ratios for each class of relatives calculated from the proportions of 33 case and 34 control families with at least one affected relative of each type.

Relatives (N cases, controls)	Definite schizophrenia in relative — Register and interview			Definite plus uncertain schizophrenia in relatives — Register only			Definite plus uncertain schizophrenia in relatives — Register and interview		
	cases	controls	Odds ratios	cases	controls	Odds ratios	cases	controls	Odds ratios
Mother (33,34)	2	1	2.1 (0.2–24.7)	1	1	—	5	1	5.9 (0.7–53.5)
Father (33,34)	1	1	1.0 (0.06–17.2)	1	1	1.0 (0.6–17.2)	3	3	1.03 (0.2–5.5)
Either parent (66,68)	3	2	1.6 (0.3–10.3)	2	1	2.1 (0.2–24.7)	8	3+	3.3 (0.8–13.8)
Full sibs (3,5)	1	1	1.0 (0.06–17.2)	—	1	—	1	1	1.0 (0.6–17.2)
Maternal half-sibs (41,40)	2	—	—	2	—	—	5	1	5.9 (0.7–53.5)
Paternal half-sibs (63,64)	5	1	5.9 (0.7–53.5)	4	—	—	10	2	**5.7** (1.4–34.8)
Any half-sibs (104,104)	7	1	8.9 (1.0–76.8)	4	—	—	13	3	**6.7** (1.7–26.6)
Any first degree (69,70)	3	2	1.60 (0.3–10.3)	1	1	1.03 (.06–17.2)	8	3	3.3 (0.8–13.8)
Any family mbrs (173,174)	8	3	3.3 (0.8–13.8)	6	1	7.3 (0.8–64.7)	17	4	**7.8** (2.3–27.7)

B. *Historical cohort analysis.* Odds ratios for each class of relatives calculated from the proportion of the total number affected (definite + uncertain schizophrenia) within the class. Number of relatives in each class in parenthesis.

Relatives	Adoptee — Schiz.	Adoptee — Control	Odds ratios
Mother	5 (33)	1 (33)	5.71 (0.6–52.9)
Father	3 (33)	3 (32)	0.97 (0.2–5.2)
Either parent	8 (66)[b]	3 (65)	2.85 (0.7–11.2)
Full sibs	1 (3)	1 (5)	2.00 (0.1–51.6)
Maternal half sibs	6 (41)	1 (40)	6.70 (0.8–59.3)
Paternal half sibs	14 (63)	2 (64)	**8.86** (1.9–40.8)
Any half sibs	20 (104)	3 (104)	**8.03** (2.3–27.9)
Any first degree	9 (69)	5 (70)	1.95 (0.6–6.2)

[a] "Schizophrenia" diagnosed in adoptees from psychiatric register, in relatives both from psychiatric register and on "blind" psychiatric interview.

[b] Mother definite and father uncertain for same control: father omitted from cell.

Source: Data abstracted from Kety, S., Rosenthal, D., Wender, P.H., Schulsinger, F. and Jacobsen B. (1975). Mental illness in the biological and adoptive families of adoptive individuals who have become schizophrenic: A preliminary report based on psychiatric interviewing, in *Genetic Research in Psychiatry*, ed., Fieve, R. R., Rosenthal, D., and Brill, H., Baltimore, pp. 147–165. (Bold-faced numbers are statistically significant.)

nificant. An anomaly is seen in the distribution of schizophrenialike cases among relatives of schizophrenia index cases which did not follow the pattern dictated by their
genetic distance from each other. The risk of half-sibs was actually higher than that
of biological parents (the only first-degree relatives of adoptees available in any numbers). Mothers had a sixfold but not significant risk, and the risk of schizophrenia in
fathers was not raised at all. In the historical cohort analysis in Table 9.3B, only the
differences for all half-sibs, and for paternal half-sibs, are significant.

These inconsistencies could all be owed to lack of statistical power; the wide confidence intervals allow the possibility of consistency appearing with larger numbers
in other classes of relatives. Another explanation for the incompatibility of the results
with genetic expectations in this case-control design is that the lesser fertility of
affected parents—schizophrenia is known to inhibit fertility—leads to a deficit of sibs
with affected parents, as well as to a deficit of affected parents themselves (15). Misinformation about paternity might also add confusion. The natural families of adoptees tend to be characterized by an excess of broken families and multiple liaisons of
the parents, as witness the large proportion of half-sibs compared with full sibs.

In any event, the most legitimate comparison in the available data is that of "definite schizophrenia" in mothers (which is inconclusive for lack of numbers) and, next,
that of "definite and uncertain schizophrenia" in mothers (in which the high risk has
wide confidence intervals and is not statistically significant). The comparison, which
takes each family with all its members as a single unit, shows a similar relative risk
but is statistically significant only for definite plus uncertain schizophrenia in relatives.
The similarity of the numbers in each class of relatives for cases and controls lends
plausibility to this result for all relatives combined, even in the absence of adjustments
for potential confounding. It would be more convincing still if the lower but raised
risk for all first-degree relatives were statistically significant. The study provides no
notion of a mode of inheritance. Certainly there remains room for the operation of
environmental factors. A path analysis based on the concordance for schizophrenia
among pairs of relatives of varying genetic distance, for instance, found statistically
significant evidence for both genetic and cultural transmission (71).

Other disorders, such as criminality and alcoholism, have been examined through
the lens of the same Danish adoption register. With criminality, a restructured case-
control analysis of the published data (Table 9.4) shows that both a genetic and an
environmental causal model are required to explain the results (72). Cases were adoptees with a criminal record, controls adoptees without a record. The two groups are
similar in age and social background. Criminality in the natural fathers of adoptees
with criminal records occurred about twice as often as in natural fathers of control
adoptees. In a test of cross-fostering, however, a higher frequency of criminality in
the adoptive fathers of criminal adoptees applied even more strongly than for natural
fathers. This result suggests almost equal effects of heredity and environment. (That
natural fathers were criminal about three times as often as adoptive fathers reflects
only the nature of the fathers whose children were adopted.) In a third comparison,
of a control population of children living with their natural parents, the risk of criminality in the natural fathers of delinquent children was much the same, and fell
between that of the natural and adoptive fathers of adopted-away delinquent chil-

Table 9.4 Case-control Analysis: Criminality[a]

	Fathers of Adoptees		(c) Fathers of nonadopted "controls"
	(a) Biological	(b) Adoptive	
Probands			
Crime	80 (164)	39 (180)	21 (100)
No crime	147 (473)	51 (554)	67 (706)
Odds ratios	2.1	2.7	2.5
(conf. int.)	(1.4–3.0)	(1.7–4.3)	(1.5–4.4)

[a]Criminality in fathers of criminal offspring (cases) and non-criminal offspring (controls) in (a) *biological* fathers of adoptees, (b) *adoptive* fathers of adoptees and (c) *biological* fathers of non-adopted "controls": Numbers of offspring (with numbers of offspring at risk in parenthesis), odds ratios, and confidence intervals.

Source: Data abstracted from Hutchings, B., and Mednick, S. (1975). Registered criminality in the adoptive and biological parents of registered male criminal adoptees in *Genetic Studies of Criminality and Psychopathology*, ed., R. R. Fieve, D. Rosenthal, H. Brill, pp. 105–116.

dren; they did not show the higher frequency to be expected from the combined influences of rearing and heredity. The report of this Danish register study does not provide the needed data for age-adjustment, although there are no obvious signs of disparity in cases and controls. The report mentions social matching as an acknowledged aim of the adoption procedures. Conceivably, such selection bias might explain some of these results, which do not fit a simple explanation of hereditary effects, either alone or jointly with the effects of rearing.

Alcoholism was studied using a cohort design (73). Male offspring of a cohort of hospitalized alcoholics, separated from the parent by six weeks of age, were followed and compared with the adoptive offspring of two groups of controls without a history of alcoholism (one group from the register of psychiatric admissions, and a second without such admissions). The risk of alcoholism in the offspring of alcoholics was about fourfold that of the combined control group. The age and social distribution of the groups are similar, and unlikely to account for a difference of this order. A restructured analysis is shown in Table 9.5. Moderate drinking, problem drinking, and heavy drinking did not differ significantly in the offspring of alcoholics and of controls. Thus,

Table 9.5 Cohort Analysis: Drinking habits of male adoptees at follow-up.[a]

Adopted-away offspring	Alcoholic N = 55	Nonalcoholic N = 78	Relative risk (conf. limits)
Alcoholic ever	10	4	3.54 (1.17–10.6)
Problem drinker	5	11	0.64 (0.24–1.74)
Heavy drinker	12	28	0.61 (0.34–1.09)
Moderate drinker	28	35	1.13 (0.79–1.62)

[a]Relative risks and 95% confidence intervals of adoptees with one alcoholic biological parent compared with adoptees with no alcoholic biological parent.

Source: Adapted from Goodwin, D. W., Schulsinger, F., Hermansen, L., Guze, S. B., and Winokur, G. (1973). Alcohol problems in adoptees raised apart from biological parents, *Arch. Gen. Psych.*, 28, 238–43.

any genetic predisposition to alcoholism applies not to the level of alcohol consumption of the majority, but to that minority who manifest the clinical diagnostic entity of alcoholism.

Studies of adoptive placements, it is plain, must be interpreted with care. For example, in neither of the case-control approaches (schizophrenia and criminality) were the published data sufficient for the control of confounding. Recently, sophisticated analytic techniques capable of controlling multiple variables have been used in adoption studies. In particular, a maximum likelihood approach has been applied to the study of the relationships of blood pressure in adoptees and their families (74).

Problems of design must still be coped with. In most adoption procedures, the adopting family undergoes careful evaluation and screening. As a result, confounding is always a possibility; a child from a given social background is quite likely to be adopted into a setting similar to his or her family of origin. Such bias may be difficult to discover in retrospect; although the reports on criminality and alcoholism mention the likelihood of social matching, other reports from the Danish registry are silent on the point. Further, the picture of the child's genetic background and of its early social experience is often incomplete. Since a great many children adopted at birth are born out of wedlock, the father's genetic contribution is more likely than usual to be unknown. Early social experience can be quite varied, and many involve a disturbed family life and many different placements—with relatives, in children's homes, and in foster homes. Thus, previous experience and especially age at adoption require strict control. The adoption itself may be a stressful experience with its own consequences.

Multiple settings

With the multifactorial hypotheses needed to explain the types of disorder under discussion, any attempt to separate environment and heredity is difficult. Our discussion has emphasized that studies of separated relatives are vulnerable to bias. Yet, unlike most other strategies, they are not inherently confounded, and hence they offer the best available means for this purpose. Some of the research designs so far considered are able to deal with most biological relationships. However, each is confined to a limited set of social types of family rearing. The many variations in family structure that could alter family resemblances and confound results go uncontrolled. In eliciting patterns of cultural transmission, too, the utility of these variations—so much more common and accessible than separated twins or adoptees—goes unexploited. For instance, it has been noted that among whites in the United States, the fact that more married men than women live with their parents-in-law (53 per cent vs. 39 per cent at the 1970 census), and conversely more married women than men live with their parents, could account for greater resemblance of offspring to maternal than paternal relatives and confound direct maternal effects (75).

Recent analytic approaches have tried to build into path analysis models some realities of the social variations in family structure culled from observational studies of general populations. In analyses of United States populations, seven forms of rearing patterns° have proved sufficient to describe the great part of the range observed (75). This analytic model still remains bound to single populations or their equivalents, however, since external comparison requires that the mean values for genetic and environmental factors in each population are the same, regardless of the distribution of types of family in that population. As always in epidemiology and other population sciences, therefore, no single analysis permits confident interpretation until consistent results are found across several varied replications (76). Further, individuals with natural parents who display the social, behavioral, and biological traits under study may be selected for rearing in settings that engender those traits. This danger to inference cannot be removed by any analytic model, however sophisticated, and must be guarded against by tight design and rigorous causal thinking.

The elementary family

Although the significance of the family in matters of health and the occurrence and treatment of disease is generally appreciated, the definition of "the family" is often vague and confused. Domestic groups vary in composition from one society to another, and relations within the family in industrial society vary by social class and place of residence. In its simplest form, the family consists of a husband and wife and their nonadult children, the *elementary family* of two generations. This unit is variously described also as the *nuclear, immediate,* or *simple* family. The elementary family usually forms the nucleus of the more extensive domestic groups observed in some societies. It is therefore regarded as a basic unit of social structure (77). Yet the notion of family, like that of social class and other institutions of society, is a construct shaped by expectations and imbued with values. Actual arrangements may not conform with ideal or expected norms. The distribution of households expresses actual norms. The family's primary purpose in society is to create and rear new members of society, although the union of a couple and the raising of children may subserve many other social and personal purposes.

In industrial societies the elementary family usually lives in a separate household. This type of household is the dominant unit in all residential aggregates, whatever their size and social composition. In the United States, 98 per cent of married couples live in their own households (78). The residential isolation of the elementary family is a distinctive feature of the social system of developed economies, an adaptation to the demands of industrialization. In many societies, extended families sustain larger households. In Britain or the United States a century ago, the household might comprise kin, lodgers, and servants in addition to the nuclear family. The distribution of household types in Britain today is illustrated in Table 9.6.

° The rearing patterns are: (1) biological parents only; (2) biological parent and step-parent; (3) biological parents and grandparents; (4) biological parents, uncles, and aunts; (5) biological parents and older sibs; (6) biological parents and unrelated foster parents; (7) monozygous twins and their spouses. Allowance is made for varying durations of exposure to each type of setting, as well as for differences in the nongenetic influence of natural and step-parents, and in the phenotypic correlation between mates (assortative mating). This correlation may differ between stable and unstable marriages for some behavioral traits.

Table 9.6 Household types in England and Wales

Household types	%
Married couple with children	
Single breadwinner	20
Two earners	20
Married couple, no children	27
One-parent family household	8
One-person household	
Over retirement age	15
Under retirement age	6
Two or more people, not a family	3
Two or more families	1
	100

Source: Rapoport, R. N. and Rapoport, R. (1982). British families in transition, in ed., Rapoport, R. N., Fogarty, M. P. and Rapoport, R., *Families in Britain*, London, p. 478.

The family can be considered as a system of social relationships based on distinctions of age and sex in which each individual member occupies a particular position or status that governs the individual's behavior towards other members of the family, and theirs towards the individual. The *structure* of the family comprises the related statuses of its members, which evolve as the family develops. The *culture* of the family is implicit in its shared values and goals, and in the expectations of appropriate behavior for the changing statuses and roles of which it is composed. Although this microculture is unique to the family, it reflects and shares the macroculture that surrounds it and is brought in by various members. Family relationships, with their rights and duties and obligations, are regulated and controlled by the society of which the family is a basic institution. The regulating laws and customs are not immutable, but are modified to suit changing productive, social, and political needs. Society exerts a pervasive influence on the family apart from this direct control and regulation.

Thus, the general quality of social and family life in industrial societies has been transformed during the present century through the productive and technological changes described in an earlier chapter. Working hours are shorter, work less laborious, and expectations are higher, both in respect to the span of life and to standards of living. The size of families has been reduced in all social classes through the widespread availability and use of effective methods of birth control, and in consequence of the changing modes of production. Legislation has altered the legal status of wives and mothers and given them greater equality with husbands and fathers (see p. 427) with consequent changes in their social and familial status and roles. All this has emancipated married women from the burden of constant childbearing. Mothers of these smaller families increasingly take up paid employment so that in many families the father is no longer the sole breadwinner. This is not to say that women have not contributed meaningfully to production at almost all times and places.

The behavior of all family members is influenced by these economic changes. The behavior expected of mothers and fathers and children varies at every social level in industrial society, and even within any one level; familial roles are not everywhere consistent. Certain norms are legally enforceable, for these are based on fundamental values concerning the physical and moral safety of children and the care that parents are expected to provide. Within these legal limits great variation in behavior is observed; deviance from norms is relative. As norms of behavior are flexible, it is possible for an individual family to display idiosyncratic behavior without seriously disturbing either the personalities of the children or their social adjustment. But if a family's behavior transgresses the accepted rules of others, sanctions may be applied. If the transgression is serious, as when parents are cruel to their children, these sanctions may be legal, and the parents punished. If the transgression is minor and offends customary values but not legal norms, as when a mother is slovenly or idle or a father drunken and abusive, the sanctions invoked may be informal and exercised by relatives or neighbors. Legal and customary sanctions are both important in regulating family relationships. The deviant behavior of so-called "multiproblem families" is often such that they transgress many of the norms of child care and attract the attention both of neighbors and of social agencies such as school attendance officers, child welfare officers, and the police (79). The variability of norms and of sanctions that can be deployed to ensure conformance with them can frustrate the efforts made by doctors, practitioners, or social workers to resolve family difficulties, for they sometimes inappropriately apply their own particular standards to the situation. The adjustment of family difficulties needs to be related to the norms appropriate to the family's social environment.

The elementary family comes into existence with the birth of the first child and continues to grow through the birth of others. Most adult persons therefore belong to two elementary families, to their *family of origin* (sometimes described as the family of *upbringing* or *orientation*) as son and brother or as daughter and sister, and to their *family of procreation* as husband and father or as wife and mother (80). These connections between a number of elementary families through a common member form the basis of the *kinship system*, that is, the total set of relationships between persons that arise through common descent and marriage.

Every family undergoes a process of growth and dissolution that begins with marriage and ends with the death of the spouses, and its place in society is taken by another unit of the same kind. This process is general, but circumstances may interrupt and modify the normal course of development. A household may expand to include persons other than the members of an elementary family; in many places newlywed couples in working-class districts live with a relative until they can achieve an independent household, and dependent relatives are also taken in by established families. The majority of these arrangements are temporary, for independent households are preferred. Shared households often involve an element of strain.

We shall discuss the elementary family of two generations in its social context. Aspects of family life that have a practical bearing for the health professions have been chosen as the subjects of subsequent chapters: first, marriage and conjugal relations; second, the primary function of the family in rearing and educating children; and, third, the family as a source of material and social support for its older members.

We begin by setting out an analytic structure through which to view the process of family growth, dissolution, and replacement.

The cycle of family development

Every elementary family has a history of development, a cycle of successive phases whose bounds are set in the first place by the limits of the human constitution and in the second by the social definition of roles (81). Biological factors such as the fertility and life-span of individuals and the rate of physical maturation of children, and social factors such as the legal definition of adulthood, divide this developmental cycle in our society into phases with distinctive physiological and social characteristics. Adulthood is always defined by criteria external to the family, for society lays down the age of independence, the legal rights of men and women, the age at which marriage is permitted, and political and social responsibilities. These external forces help to determine the length and duration of each developmental phase. No single social entity can be described as *the* family. A variety of family forms answers to the varying demands of the socioeconomic environment. For the health professional, the phase of the family cycle of a patient as well as the functioning of other family members must guide intervention at times of crisis and acute illness, or in relieving the burden of chronic illness. Several phases can be usefully distinguished:

> The *phase of expansion* begins with marriage and continues until the youngest child achieves adult status (see Chapter 11). This phase therefore includes the period of fertility of the parents and the period of physical and social maturation of the children. Its duration depends on the length of the period of fertility and the time taken for the youngest child to reach adult status, some 16 to 21 years, depending on when the child marries or leaves home.
>
> The *phase of dispersion* begins when the first child achieves adult status and the legal freedom to leave home if he or she chooses. It continues until all children have done so and left home. Hence, this phase does not necessarily begin with the eldest child, for a younger one, through marriage for example, may achieve adult status first. In families with more than one child, therefore, the phase of dispersion begins before the completion of the phase of expansion, and this phase may be prolonged if children continue to live with their parents after reaching adulthood.
>
> The *phase of independence* begins when all the children have become adult and have left their parent's home, and the parents again live alone.
>
> The *phase of replacement* begins when the parents retire from their major life roles, and ends with their death.

These phases of the family cycle do not represent exclusive and rigid stages in the family's development; each phase grows out of its predecessor and overlaps it; they are useful devices for observing the time factor in family development. Each phase represents a particular state of familial relations and successive phases can coexist.

The duration of each phase in a family's history is determined by a number of factors. For a given family some of these are intrinsic: the age of the wife at marriage, the extent of her fertile period, the family's state of health, and the age and conditions of retirement. Others are external. Expectations of life, degree of fertility, rates of physical growth of children, and exposure to the risk of disease and death are all influenced by the supply of food, the adequacy of shelter, the occupations of the couple, and the quality of sanitary measures and medical care.

During the past century the relative duration of the phases has altered. The most striking change is the decline in predominance of the phase of expansion. This phase may extend in duration from the 20 years that elapse between the birth and marriage of a single child to the whole span of fecundity of women, that is, that period of some 30 years or more in which they are capable of conceiving children. Fecundity has been extended because the onset of puberty in girls is earlier and because maternal mortality has been considerably reduced.

This increment in fecundity has been accompanied by a decrease in actual fertility. Although it is possible that the average age of menopause has been somewhat deferred, women bear fewer children and confine their childbearing within a shorter period than in the past. In Britain, by 1945, 80 per cent of the children born into marriages of completed fertility were born within the first 10 years of marriage. Similarly, in the United States, the usual span of childbearing years has become only about half as long as it was two generations ago. The average mother whose family reached completion in 1890 had borne 5.4 children, with an estimated interval of 10 years between marriage and the birth of the last child. The mother had not given birth to her last child until she was on average about 32 years old. In 1940, the last of three children was born when the mother was on average about 27 years old. Those women who had married and had reached the end of their reproductive period (45 to 47 years old) by 1952 had borne an average of 2.35 children. It is estimated that approximately half the women had borne their last child by the time they were 26 years old. The present median length of time between marriage and the birth of the last child is probably close to six years.

The reduction in family size has therefore come about through confining reproduction to a limited span of time early in marriage (82). It follows that a wife now 30 years of age whose fertile period is completed will be involved in phases of different duration and with different demands from those experienced by her mother. A woman with a large family typical of the nineteenth century may have a daughter already married while she herself is still nursing an infant. In large families the phases of expansion and dispersion may well intrude into the time of retirement of the parents so that a phase of independence can never develop. In families in which the parents married late in life, the phases of expansion and dispersion may similarly be prolonged into retirement.

The duration of phases in contemporary families also differs from one social class to another. In Britain, wives of unskilled and semiskilled manual workers have married earlier, begun bearing children sooner, and completed their families later, than have the higher occupational classes. The manual workers' families have therefore been larger, and the duration of the phase of expansion consequently longer, thereby limiting the duration of the independent phase, although this limitation would have been modified in part by the fact that they tend to marry younger. Hence, the sooner a wife completes her fertile period within the phase of expansion, the longer will be the phase of independence before the couple retire (83).

The extended duration of the phase of independence is a new aspect of the family developmental cycle, and has particular importance in its relation to the conjugal familial and social roles of married women. The emergence and extension of the phase of independence was a consequence of earlier age at marriage, smaller families, and increased longevity. Even in the first decades of this century in Britain and the United States, multiparity and high maternal death rates tended to ensure the predominance of the phase of expansion, with the dispersion of the children soon followed by the death of the mother. In peasant societies where the effects of multiparity and high death rates are even more marked, replacement quickly follows dispersion.

When the phase of independence succeeds dispersion, the children have by definition reached adulthood and legal independence, and their parents are no longer formally responsible for them. In many families in this phase, all the children have left home, so that the couple lives alone, with the prospect of a span of anything up to 20 years of active life before retirement. While an adult child may continue to reside with the parents, he or she is legally independent; the ties that hold parents and children together in the phase of independence are those of descent and affection, although they also may be economic in that the child may be supporting the parents or the parents supporting a university student. Many wives in this phase of independence, as well as in the phase of dispersion, join the work force or engage in some social activity outside the home.

The change in longevity has also prolonged the phase of replacement, and incidentally created the growing social problem of the care of the very old, which is principally a problem of the care of old women. In 1981 there were in the United States over 3 million more women than men who were 75 years and over. The number of such women has grown from slightly over 2 million in 1950 to over 6 million in 1981. In England and Wales in 1981 there were 736,000 more women than men who were 75 years and over. This phase of replacement is for many a period of economic dependency, and in this phase the relation of people to their offspring is of importance in their medical and social care (see pp. 537ff).

Although elementary families everywhere reproduce similar units through the cycle of development, the process of replacement is not everywhere the same. In industrial societies, occupational and social mobility complicate the process of replacement. In those societies where land and offices are inherited, the system of ordering succession guarantees that the place of the original family in the social structure is taken by another unit of the same kind. Both processes of replacement may be observed in Britain. Among the landowning classes, particularly when a title is attached to property, the place of the family in the social structure may persist despite the death of an incumbent. The family of the heir assumes the social position and responsibilities of the predecessor's family; the incumbents change, but the social position in the structure remains the same. The form of replacement is similar to that described as *positional succession* in tribal societies where kinship determines the inheritance of property and offices (84). Since the great majority of families in industrial society do not own land or fixed property, replacement is controlled by the occupational and social needs of the external society, expressed in the institutions, customs, norms, and values through which the social heritage is transmitted from one generation to the next.

In the course of the cycle of family development, relations between the family members, between husband and wife, parents and children, brothers and sisters, and eventually grandchildren are subject to change and adjustment. Each phase obliges the family members to assume new statuses and roles: the young wife becomes a mother, the older wife becomes a grandmother, siblings become uncles and aunts, and so on. In an earlier chapter we discussed the impact of such transitions for individuals. For families, the transition from one phase to another, and the assumption of new statuses, are critical episodes often accompanied by ritual or ceremonial observance, for instance, at the birth of a first child or at the first marriage among the children. These may have a public character if the family concerned happens to hold a position of economic or social influence (85).

In Japan, the transition from the status of family head to the role of a retired, elderly gentleman was marked by the institution of *inkyo-sei* in which the head of the family who was no longer able to work the land was retired, with his wife, to a small house just behind the main family house. There he and his wife would live out their remaining days performing small chores with actual control of the household residing in the eldest son. In Ireland, the transition of the small farmer into retirement occurs in much the same fashion (although in a more recent period the form of the transition has been observed to be negotiable and less rigidly prescribed by tradition). As spouses grow old and as they and their children assume new statuses and roles, other persons in families related to them by kinship and marriage in turn have new roles to play. The intermeshing of families in different phases of the developmental cycle creates networks of extra-familial kin and determines the nature of the relationships between them, and thereby the possibilities of social interaction and support (86).

Families may deviate from the characteristic developmental cycle of contemporary small families. Single-parent households may originate with women who do not marry, or with the separation, or divorce, or death of one or other parent. A single parent may choose or be obliged to perform the roles of both parents, but some roles—and certainly one or other of the two parental role models—must be lacking. In the worst circumstances, foster-parents or an institution may have to substitute for missing parents. Other common types of deviation are at the two extremes of size: large families and childless families. One-child families can no longer be considered deviant from the norm. Some families deliberately postpone childbearing, perhaps because a wife wishes to work, or because a husband works away from home or because they are compelled to live in lodgings, or because of medical and psychological disorders, or among couples with professional occupations while they consolidate their careers, or simply because children are not desired. A marked trend towards deferring childbearing was evident in the United States in the 1970s and early 1980s. The effect of such a *period of abeyance* in a family of normal size will be to defer the end of the phase of expansion and to restrict the phase of independence. Childless couples, of course, are in permanent abeyance.

Since the limitation of family size became widespread, the large family has become a potential sign of nonconformity with reproductive and social norms. Noncontracepting religious communities such as the Hutterites and the Amish still produce large families. In Britain only 1 per cent of the marriages contracted in 1925 had 10 or more children; 18 per cent of the marriages contracted in 1870–1879 had this many. The large family was a unique feature of industrial society when relative plenty and increasing control of the environment cooperated with high fertility and survival rates to produce a considerable proportion of large families in the population.

In contemporary industrial society the large family tends to be at an overall economic and social disadvantage. Even in the first decades after the Second World War in Britain, children from large families, both in the working-class and in the middle-class, showed relative nutritional deprivation, which may indicate that they had gone short of essential nutrients in the crucial years of growth. Moreover, most family dwellings have no more than four or five rooms, and a large family sooner or later results in overcrowding (87). The health of a mother who bears and rears many children is likely to suffer from the heavy demands made on her, quite apart from the strain of managing a large household under contemporary conditions. Her reproductive efficiency is also likely to decline over the years. Women of high parity are more liable to suffer from iron deficiency anemia and gynecological disorders such as prolapse and cancer of the cervix uteri and peripartum heart failure. They also have high miscarriage and stillbirth rates, and an exponential increase of chromosome anomalies, especially trisomies and Down's syndrome (trisomy 21) in particular. The children of mothers with large families suffer more deaths from respiratory infections and from accidents, particularly when the mother is young, and they also have lower measured intelligence than children from small families.

Multiproblem families have also tended to be large families. These families suffer characteristic difficulties, which involve them with a host of social agencies in the search for social support: welfare and social services, children's and health services, general practitioners and hospitals. For these families the phase of expansion is generally the most difficult, because the mother has to rear several small children at the same time. If there are also economic difficulties, the health, both physical and mental, of the whole family may suffer. During this phase, direct help from agencies may enable the family to maintain an independent existence until the time arrives when the older children become wage earners. The phase of dispersion lifts some of the load from the mother. The parents of a large family, particularly when they are poor as most of them are, can seldom achieve the phase of independence.

At the other extreme, some married couples do not complete every phase of the developmental cycle, although most must do so in order to sustain the social structure. In Britain the number of couples without children has doubled since 1900, from 8 to 16 per cent in 1977. These figures are almost equivalent in the United States, where the number of women who have never borne a child in 1980 constituted about 18.8 per cent of all women from ages 15 to 44 who had married (87).

There is evidence that childlessness will rise sharply in the succeeding cohorts of younger women. Most of this increase in childless families must have been voluntary, for medical causes of childlessness such as chronic salpingitis, tuberculosis, puerperal infection, and reproductive loss including infant death became less common through most of this century. This fecundity could have been offset to some extent by the greater proportion of marriages in the population, which might therefore include more infertile couples. In recent decades, however, gonorrhea while treatable has steadily increased in frequency especially among the young, and resulting chronic infections may be reducing the fecundity of younger generations. The rising frequency of ectopic pregnancies is probably related to such infections, at least in part (87).

The one-child family could also be considered as deviating from the norm at most past times and places, if not now in Britain or the United States. In a Dutch birth cohort of the 1940s, where "only children" were relatively uncommon, they did well on intelligence tests but not as well as the first born of two; on scores for psychological well-being and for mental impairment, however, they did worse than all other family sizes and birth orders (88). One-child families tend to have had an exceptionally long *period of abeyance*, that is, a delay between marriage and the birth of the first child, and in recent marriages the length of this period appears to be unrelated to social class differences. This suggests that the factors which defer the phase of expansion are common to all one-child families and cut across class divisions. Some one-child families have a history of repeated spontaneous abortions. In previous generations, the clinical impression was that the limitation of offspring in the spouses was frequently associated with psychological disturbances. Psychoneurosis in either parent, and an underlying fear of further pregnancies in the mother, often resulted in conscious limitation of pregnancies. In some families, the birth of an abnormal child makes them chary of risking further pregnancies. Infrequent intercourse, too, can limit the birth of further children, as well as sexual disabilities such as impotence or vaginismus. One per cent of the couples in one sample of marriages involving one "neurotic" spouse were found to have had no acts of sexual intercourse whatsoever (89). Norms for sexual behavior, marriage, and childbearing have greatly altered the pattern of family limitation. Aside from deliberate choice, other factors may be the death or desertion of a spouse, or a medical cause outside the control of the couple (e.g., an incapacitating organic or psychiatric illness that is liable to limit the number of children). In contemporary Britain and the United States, probably the most frequent circumstance that produces a one-child family is the single-parent household, most often a woman separated or divorced or one who has chosen not to marry.

The family in context

To grasp fully the significance of the dynamics of family structure, families must be seen in societal context. Economy, demography, social institutions, and cultural values shape family forms, and are in turn shaped by them. These reciprocal shaping forces are made evident by comparisons of the functions of kinship between contemporary tribal, peasant, and transitional societies on the one side with industrialized societies on the other.

In many tribal societies, formal obligations penetrate deep into the kin network. The family and its kin extensions serve as an economic unit to mobilize labor, as a political unit that defines the position and power of its members in society, and as a social unit for procreation, childbearing, and the maintenance of social norms. In peasant and feudal societies that confer property rights, family and kin become the vehicles for the accumulation and conservation of property.

In the industrialized world, in contrast with kinship societies in which genealogies are prime determinants of individual social position, status, and roles, genealogies are shallow. Formal kinship obligations scarcely extend beyond the bonds of the nuclear family. Position in the social class structure influences family norms and functions, which in turn influence the socialization and the economic and social opportunities and careers of its members, but these are indirect and informal influences through which the family may be said to become a vehicle of social control. The prime and explicit functions of the industrialized family are reduced to procreation, childbearing, and the maintenance of norms.

In these domains, however, the independent contribution of family structure and microculture remains a powerful one. The tenacity of family microculture was well illustrated by a study in Poland. Cognitive performance was tested in a complete cohort of Warsaw school children born 25 years after the city, razed in the Nazi retreat before the Soviet forces in 1945, had been rebuilt under a socialist regime. Social policies had largely succeeded in equalizing the distribution of housing and the access of all classes to schools and to medical and cultural facilities. Family culture and position in the social structure were measured by parental education and occupation respectively. When cognitive measures were related to these family measures, the social class gradient in performance so familiar in Western countries was in these children hardly less evident (90). Social equalization had failed to override the influence of family culture.

While the tenacious influence of families on individual development is evident, the nature and effect of that influence is shifting and uncertain. The continuing transformation of the economy, the social and economic structure, and the culture of industrial societies is reflected even in the most durable institutions, including families. In the period of rapid industrialization in the nineteenth century, it has been argued, the new location of work in the factories separated women and children from the workplace, and assigned to women the specialized tasks of the household (91). This separation exaggerated their nurturant roles as managers of both domesticity and personal relations, as described by Talcott Parsons and many others since. Biology sets limits to choices about childbearing and child rearing in the absence of effective contraception and artificial infant feeding, but the economy sets limits to opportunities for female work and careers, and male authority and power has set limits to the female choice of roles. Thus family roles are no less bound by time and place than Sigmund Freud's Oedipal typology derived from the families of late nineteenth century Vienna.

Modern families and households are diverse in composition and in norms of behavior as they have been in the past. What is new is that societal norms of expectation about family life incorporate the diversity. In the United States, for example, the courts have recognized among unmarried couples a variety of informal household arrangements through which couples can incur contractual legal obligations to each other. A plurality of norms have thus acquired legitimacy in the dominant value system. These are sustained—in the face of attempts by conservative forces to assert the primacy of "traditional" family values through the political process—by social and economic forces; the gradual acquisition by women of greater economic and social independence is unlikely to prove reversible. The diversity of norms allows a diversity of choices in the formation of households; family arrangements are open to negotiation, and few women any longer accord the male head of the household the automatic right to impose his will (92).

Economic development and resultant changes in norms of behavior can be expected to proceed asynchronously in relation to change in general value systems, in social institutions such as law and religion, and in social organizations. Strains are predictable as the adaptation of values and societal forms to the particulars of actual behavior lags. Mundane problems illustrate the point. Churches continue to base their voluntary efforts on a much depleted workforce of female volunteers; schools notify only mothers of events for parents, when as many as a quarter of the children may have fathers who are not in the same home.

Succeeding chapters will provide an extended illustration of the impact of society on the structure and function of families. The reciprocal impact of family structure on society at large is perhaps not as obvious. Nonetheless, diverse social phenomena are rooted in such familial forces as property inheritance, realized family size, obligations to kin, and economic survival during periods of industrial transition. Modes of impartible property inheritance among peasant farmers, for instance, have been seen to contribute to heavy migration both in current and historical situations. In rural Ireland, a farmer designated one son to inherit the farm; once the decision was known, the remaining brothers had to fend for themselves to found a family, and migrated to towns and cities, often beyond the shores of Ireland to England or the United States (86). Among the pastoral Boers of South Africa in the late eighteenth and early nineteenth centuries, inheritance was by primogeniture. The land was dry, the grazing was thin, and the farms vast in consequence. A driving force of the steady expansion of the Boers into the hinterland (culminating in the Great Trek after the British freed the slaves in 1832) and their violent confrontations with the pastoral Bantu was the need of younger sons to take new land to establish their own households (93).

The relations between family size, population density, hunger, and mortality have been matters of scientific concern ever since the work of Malthus, which evolved over a period of more than 30 years from the first through the seventh edition of his *Essay on Population* (94). In India over the past three decades, government efforts to encourage birth control, because of the looming threat of uncontrolled population increase, for a long time made no detectable impact. For peasant farmers tied to the land, the more sons to till the land the better; to restrict births in the face of the high odds of death in infancy could only reduce the number of sons (95).

In the terms of economics, it can be said that the demand for children depends on their utility, their cost, and the economic means of the parents. There is some historical evidence from Europe on this score, as well as for the Malthusian corollary of the so-called *positive check* on excessive population. That is, mortality increases as numbers outrun economic production and food supplies—or at least outrun the ability of the poor to command available food supplies (96). Certainly, as we have noted, increasing family size is associated with higher morbidity and mortality, especially among the poor.

Historical evidence from Europe also suggests the operation, as economic circumstances worsen, of the Malthusian *preventive check* on population—namely, deferral of the age of marriage (97). In France, fertility decline among the nobility in the eighteenth century—the earliest in Europe—is thought by some to have inspired by diffusion the decline in fertility among the bourgeoisie and then the lower classes. "To live like a nobleman was the aim of the bourgeois and to live like a bourgeois the aim of the lower classes" (98).

Obligations to kin that inhere in one form of social organization, and that persist when that form undergoes change, often impose constraints on the new social forms and impede the change. A Mambwe tribesman who migrated to the town in Northern Rhodesia (now Zambia) and successfully engaged in commerce, say, as a storekeeper, might easily be ruined by the necessity to provide support for those kinsmen who asked for it (99). In Imperial India, the British Raj constructed a civil service that came close to realizing Weber's ideal form of a bureaucracy: in a strict hierarchy of authority, order was maintained by formal relations, merit recognized by senior officers' earned promotion, and moves of officials at prescribed intervals prevented the development of informal local ties that might obstruct the just exercise of the formal functions of the agency. Independent India inherited this civil service, but the new state was mercantile, with persisting remnants of feudal-type landownership and peasantry. The traditional norms of Indian society were in conflict with the bureaucratic norms of independent India introduced by the British. Although the administrations of central and state governments retained their bureaucratic form, the many officials who were elected to political power adapted the form to meet their persisting family obligations. Especially in appointments and promotions and the granting of dispensations, a politician might—quite legitimately by traditional norms and values—allow kinship to override merit (100).

A now classic case study of the Lancashire cotton industry in the late eighteenth and nineteenth century makes a strong argument for the family as a force in political change (101). The increasing division of labor and the specialization of roles in the mills—the new organizations for manufacture—eventually put severe pressure on the traditional internal family organization of roles and relationships. At first, when men went into factories, "typically the skilled spinner was allowed by his master to hire his own assistants and typically, he hired his wife, children, or nephews, and appointed sons and nephews to the trade. . . . So within the anonymous city and the impersonal factory an anchor of tradition persisted; and the working-class family, at least in this section of the industry, was not under pressure to relinquish a significant portion of its tradition of apprenticeship and economic cooperation" (102). Later, technical change brought larger mills, threatened unemployment, and undermined the family apprenticeship system and the ability of working parents to supervise their children. These threats to the family led, it is postulated, to the emergence of the conflict around the issue of child labor, to the concurrent agitation in the factories, and to utopian movements and demands for a return to an idealized social order.

This interpretation has its critics (102,103), like all societal interpretation, and historical interpretation in particular. Alternative hypotheses have been offered for this as well as for other long-established views. The traditional view of the evolution of the family throughout history rests in part on an analogy, namely, the contrast between the extended families in the contemporary preindustrial world and the nuclear families of the industrial world. It was held that only when capitalism replaced the familial obligations between kin with the contractual obligations between employers and wage earners did the nuclear family appear in its contemporary form and acquire its typically powerful affective ties. From the historical demography of recent decades, especially in England, it is argued to the contrary that the nuclear family has been the core element of society from the seventeenth century and even from medieval times (104). Likewise, the emergence of romantic love as a driving force in marriage in place of contractual arrangements to ensure property rights or economic survival, it is now supposed, long preceded the industrial revolution. The emergence of sentiment in family relations in place of roles strictly ruled by economic need too has been traced back to earlier centuries (105,106).

These remain questions for scholarly argument. That over the past century there have been dramatic changes cannot be gainsaid. Family size has declined sharply; the status and the rights of wives have been strengthened and those of husbands and fathers weakened; the durability of the formal structure of families, and the average duration of the familial relationships members will sustain have been much reduced; the scope of family relationships is less all-embracing as schools and other agencies divert them away from the family; and, finally, the content of relationships has become progressively more individuated.

In the following chapters we aim to outline the ways in which, in the families of the developed world, procreation, growth, and socialization proceed through the successive phases of the family cycle.

References

1. **Radcliffe-Brown, A. R.**, and **Ford, C. D.** (1950). *African Systems of Kinship and Marriage*, London.
2. **Kaslow, R.**, and **Shaw, S.** (1981). The role of histocompatibility antigens (HLA) in infection, *Epidemiology Review*, 3, 90–114.
3. **Newburgh, L. H.**, and **Conn, J. W.** (1939). A new interpretation of hyperglycemia in obese middle aged persons, *J. Amer. Med. Assn.*, 112, 7–11.
   Seftel, H. C., and **Schultz, E.** (1961). Diabetes mellitus in the urbanized Johannesburg African, *S. Afr. Med. J.*, 35, 66–71.
   Stanhope, J. M., and **Prior, I. A. M.** (1980). The Tokelau Island migrant study: Prevalence and incidence of diabetes mellitus, *New Zeal. Med. J.*, 92, 417–21.

4. **Antonov, A. N.** (1947.) Children born during siege of Leningrad in 1942, *J. Pediat.*, *30*, 250–59.

   Smith, C. A. (1947). Effect of wartime starvation in Holland upon pregnancy and its products, *Amer. J. Obstet. Gynec.*, *53*, 599–608.

   Stein, Z., Susser, M., Saenger, G., and **Marolla, F.** (1975). *Famine and Human Development*, New York.

5. **Leck, I.** (1977). Correlations of malformation frequency with environmental and genetic attributes in man, in *Handbook of Teratology*, vol. III, ed. Wilson, J. G., and Fraser, F. C., New York, pp. 243–378.

   Strobino, B., Kline, J., and **Stein, Z.** (1978). Chemical and physical exposures of parents: Effects on human reproduction and offspring, *Early Human Development*, *1*, 371–399.

   Kalter, H., and **Warkany, J.** (1983). Congenital malformations: Etiological factors and their role in prevention, *New Eng. J. Med.*, *308*, 424–31, 491–97.

   Stein, Z. A., Kline, J., and **Kharrazi, M.** (1984). Epidemiology and teratology, in *Issues and Reviews in Teratology*, ed., Kalter, H., New York, pp. 23–66.

6. **Newman, N. H., Freeman, F. N.,** and **Holzinger, K. H.** (1937). *Twins: A Study of Heredity and Environment*, Chicago.

   Stein, L. (1950). A study of respiratory tuberculosis in relation to housing conditions in Edinburgh. I. The pre-war period, *Brit. J. Soc. Med.*, *4*, 143–69.

7. **Spagnulo, M.,** and **Taranta A.** (1968). Rheumatic fever in siblings: Similarity of its clinical manifestations, *New Eng. J. Med.*, *278*, 183–8.

8. **Dick, G. W. A.** (1959). Epidemiology of poliomyelitis, *Brit. Med. J.*, *1*, 618–19.

9. **Lidz, R. W.,** and **Lidz, T.** (1949). The family environment of schizophrenic patients, *Amer. J. Psychiat.*, *106*, 332–45.

   Spiegel, J. P. (1957). The resolution of role conflict within the family, *Psychiat.*, *20*, 1–16.

   Wynne, L. C., Ryckoff, I., Day, J., and **Hirsch, S.** (1958). Pseudomutuality in the family relations of schizophrenics, *Psychiat.*, *21*, 105–11.

   Bateson, G., Jackson, D. D., Haley, J., and **Weakland, J. H.** (1963). A note on the double-bind, 1962, *Family Process*, *2*, 165–61.

10. **Goldberg, E. M.** (1958). *Family Influences and Psychosomatic Illness*, London.

    Cobb, S., and **Kasl, S. V.** (1966). The epidemiology of rheumatoid arthritis, *Amer. J. Publ. Hlth.*, *56*, 1657–63.

    Winklestein, W., Kantor, S., Ibrahim, M. D., and **Sackett, D. L.** (1966). Familial aggregation of blood pressure, *J. Amer. Med. Assn.*, *195*, 848–50.

11. **Lidwell, O. M.,** and **Sommerville, T.** (1951). Observations on the incidence and distribution of the common cold in a rural community during 1948–49, *J. Hyg. (London)*, *49*, 365–81.

    Badger, G. F., Dingle, J. H., Feller, A. E., Hodges, R. G., Jordan, W. S., and **Rammelkamp, C. H.** (1953). A study of illness in a group of Cleveland families. II. Incidence of common respiratory diseases. III. Introduction of respiratory infections into families, *Amer. J. Hyg.*, *58*, 31–40, 41–6.

    Cruikshank, R. (1958). A survey of respiratory illness in a sample of families in London, in *Recent Studies in Epidemiology*, ed. Pemberton J., and Willard H., London.

    Fox, J. P. (1974). Family based epidemiologic studies, *Amer. J. Epi.*, *99*, 165–79.

12. **Greenfield, S.,** and **Feldman, H. A.** (1967). Familial carriers and meningococcal menigitis, *New Eng. J. Med.*, *277*, 497–502.

13. **Alpert, J. J., Kosa, J.,** and **Haggerty, R. J.** (1967). A month of illness and health care among low-income families, *Pub. Hlth. Rep. (Wash.)*, *82*, 705–13.

Haggerty, R. J., Roghman, K. J., and Pless, I. B. (1975). *Child Health and the Community*, New York.

14. MacMahon, B. (1978). Epidemiologic approaches to family resemblance, in *Genetic Epidemiology*, ed. Morton, N. E., and Chung, C. S., New York, pp. 3–12.

15. Risch, N. (1983). Estimating morbidity risks in relatives: The effect of reduced fertility, *Behavior Genetics, 13*, 441–51.

16. Fisher, R. A. (1934). The effect of methods of ascertainment upon the estimation of frequencies, *Ann. Eugen. Lond., 6*, 13–25.
    Cannings, C., and Thompson, E. A. (1977). Ascertainment in the sequential sampling of pedigrees, *Clin. Genet., 12*, 208–12.

17. Elston, R. C. (1980). Segregation analysis, in *Current Developments in Anthropological Genetics VI*, ed. Mielke, J. H., and Cranford, M. H., New York, pp. 327–54.

18. Morton, N. E., and Rao, D. C. (1978). Quantitative inheritance in man, *Yrbk. Phys. Anthropol., 21*, 12–41.

19. King, M-C., Go, R. C. P., Elston, R. C., Lynch, H. T., and Petrakis, N. L. (1980). Allele increasing susceptibility to human breast cancer may be linked to the glutamate-pyruvate transaminase locus, *Science, 208*, 406–08.

20. Sing, C. F., Schreffler, D. C., Noel, J. V., and Napier, J. A. (1971). Studies on genetic selection in a completely ascertained causcasian population. II. Family analyses of caucasian blood group systems, *Amer. J. Hum. Genet., 23*, 164–98.

21. Mendlewicz, J., Fleiss, J. L., and Fieve, R. R. (1975). Linkage studies in affective disorders: Xg blood group and manic-depressive illness, in *Genetic Research in Psychiatry*, ed., Fieve, R. R., Rosenthal, D., and Brill, M., Baltimore, pp. 219–32.

22. Targum, S. D., Gershon, E. S., Van Eerdewagh, M., and Rogentine, N. (1978). Human leukocyte antigen system not closely linked to or associated with bipolar manic-depressive illness, *Biol. Psychiat., 14*, 615–36.
    James, N. M., Smouse, P. E., Carroll, B. J., and Haines, R. F. (1980). Affective illness and HLA frequencies: No compelling association, *Neuropsychobiology, 6*, 208–16.
    Weitkamp. L. R., Stancer, H. C., Persad, E., Flood, C., and Guttormsen, S. (1981). Depressive disorders and HLA: A gene on chromosome 6 that can affect behavior, *New Eng. J. Med., 305*, 1301–6.

23. McKusick, V. A. (1978). *Mendelian Inheritance in Man*, 5th edition, Baltimore.

24. Gajdusek, D. C., and Zigas, V. (1957) Degenerative disease of the central nervous system in New Guinea: The endemic occurrence of "Kuru" in the native population, *New Eng. J. of Med., 257*, 974–78.
    Harper, P. S. (1977). Mendelian inheritance or transmissible agent? The lesson of Kuru and the Australia antigen, *J. Med. Gen. 14*, 389–98.
    Lindenbaum, S. (1979). *Kuru Sorcery: Disease and Danger in the New Guinea Highlands*, Palo Alto, California.

25. Lilienfeld, A. M. (1959). A methodological problem in testing a recessive genetic hypothesis in human disease, *Amer. J. Pub. Hlth., 49*, 199–204.

26. Edwards, J. H. (1969). Familial predisposition in man, *Brit. Med. Bull., 25*, 58–64.

27. Galton, F. (1889). *Natural Inheritance*, London.
    Fisher, R. A. (1918). The correlation between relatives on the supposition of Mendelian inheritance, *Trans. Roy. Soc. (Edinburgh), 52*, 399–433.

28. Falconer, D. S. (1965). The inheritance of liability to certain diseases estimated from the incidence among relatives, *Ann. Hum. Genet., 29*, 51–76.

29. Morton, N. E. (1955). The inheritance of human birth weight, *Ann. Hum. Genet., 20*, 125–134.

Morton, N. E. (1975). Analysis of family resemblance and group differences, *Soc. Biol.*, 22, 111–16.

30. Wright, S. (1978). The application of path analysis to etiology, in *Genetic Epidemiology*, ed. Morton, N. E., and Chung, C. S., New York, pp. 13–51.

Cloninger, C. R., Rao, D. C., Rice, J., Reich, T., and Morton, N. E. (1983). A defense of path analysis in genetic epidemiology, *Amer. J. Hum. Genet*, 35, 733–56.

Karlin, S., Cameron, E. C., and Chakraborty, R. (1983). Path analysis in genetic epidemiology: A critique, *Amer. J. Hum. Genet.* 35, 694–732.

Wright, S. (1983). On "Path analysis in genetic epidemiology: A critique." *Amer. J. Hum. Genet.*, 35, 757–68.

31. Loehlin, J. C. (1978). Heredity-environment analyses of Jencks's I.Q. Correlations, *Behavior Genetics*, 8, 415–436.

32. Rodriguez, A. (1976). A Monte Carlo simulation of the "Family Set" approach to estimate heritability, Unpublished Ph.D. dissertation, University of Texas.

33. Lewontin, R. C. (1974). The analysis of variance and the analysis of causes, *Amer. J. Hum. Genet.* 26, 400–11.

Murphy, E. A. (1979). Quantitative genetics: A critique, *Soc. Biol.*, 26, 126–41.

34. Craighead, J. E. (1978). Current views on the etiology of insulin-dependent diabetes mellitus, *New Eng. J. Med.*, 299, 1439–45.

Yoon, J. W., Austin, M., Onideram, T., and Notkins, A. (1979). Isolation of a virus from the pancraeas of a child with diabetic ketoacidosis, *New Eng. J. Med.*, 300, 1173–79.

Gamble, D. R. (1980). The epidemiology of insulin dependent diabetes, with particular reference to the relationship of virus infection to its etiology, *Epi. Rev.*, 2, 49–70.

Kobberling, J., and Tattersall, R., ed. (1982) *The Genetics of Diabetes Mellitus. Proceedings of the Serona Symposia*, vol. 47, London/New York.

35. Wright, S. (1922). Coefficients of inbreeding and relationship, *American Naturalist*, 56, 330–38.

36. Hajnal, J. (1963). Concepts of random mating and the frequency of consanguineous marriages, *Proc. Roy. Stat. Soc., Part B*, 159, 125–77.

Allen, G. (1965). Random and non-random in-breeding, *Eugenics Quarterly*, 12, 181–98.

37. Goldschmidt, E. (1963). *The Genetics of Migrant and Isolate Populations*, Baltimore.

McKusick, V. A., Eldridge, R., Stetler, J. A., and Egeland, J. A. (1964). Dwarfism in the Amish, *Trans. Assn. Amer. Phys.*, 77, 151–8.

Ward, R. H. (1972). The genetic structure of a tribal population, the Yanomamo Indians, *Ann. Hum. Genet.*, 36, 21–43.

Mourant, A. E., Kopec, A. C., and Domaniewska-Sobczak, K. (1978) *The Genetics of the Jews*, Oxford.

Motulsky, A., and Goodman, A., (1978) *Genetic Diseases among Ashkenazi Jews*, New York.

38. Egeland, J. A., and Hostetter, A. M. (1983). Amish study, I: Affective disorders among the Amish, 1976–80, *Amer. J. Psychiat.*, 140, 56–71.

39. Lyon, J. L., Wetzler, H. P., Gardner, J. W., Klauber, M. R., and Williams, R. R. (1979). Cardiovascular mortality in Mormons and non-Mormons in Utah, 1969–71, *Amer. J. Epi.*, 108, 357–66.

Phillips, R. L., Kuzma, J. W., Beeson, W. L., and Lotz, T. (1980). Influence of selection versus lifestyle on rate of fatal cancer and cardiovascular disease among Seventh-day Adventists, *Amer. J. Epi.*, 112, 296–314.

40. **Sing, C. F.,** and **Skolnick, M.,** ed. (1979). *The Genetic Analysis of Common Diseases,* New York.

41. **Mantel, N.,** and **Blot, W. J.** (1976). Is Hodgkin's disease infectious? Discussion of an epidemiologic method used to impute that, *J. Nat. Can. Inst., 56,* 413–14.

42. **Knox, G.** (1959). Secular pattern of congenital oesophageal atresia, *Brit. J. Soc. Prev. Med., 13,* 222–25.

   Khoury, M. J., Erickson, J. D., and **James, L. M.,** (1982). Etiologic heterogeneity of neural tube defects: clues from epidemiology, *Amer. J. Epi, 115,* 538–48.

43. **Garn, S. M., Cole, P. E.,** and **Bailey, S. M.** (1979). Living together as a factor in family-line resemblances, *Human Biology, 51,* 565–587.

44. **Kreitman, N.** (1964). The patient's spouse, *Brit. J. Psychiat., 110,* 159–73.

   Suarez, L., Criqui, M. H., and **Barrett-Connor, E.** (1983). Spouse concordance for systolic and diastolic blood pressure, *Amer. J. Epi., 118,* 345–51.

45. **Neugebauer, R.,** and **Susser, M. W.** (1979). Epilepsy: Some epidemiological aspects, *Psychol. Med., 9,* 207–15.

   Annegers, J. F., Hauser, W. A., and **Anderson, V. E.** (1982). Risk of seizures among relatives of patients with epilepsy: Families in a defined population, in *Genetic Basis of the Epilepsies,* ed. Anderson, V. E., Hauser, W. A., Perry, J. K., and Sing, C. F., New York, pp. 151–60.

   Ottman, R., Hauser, W. A., and **Susser, M. W.** (forthcoming) Maternal transmission of epilepsy.

46. **McKeown, T., MacMahon, B.,** and **Record, R.** (1951). The incidence of congential pyloric stenosis related to birth rank and maternal age, *Ann. Genet., 16,* 249–59.

47. **Carter, C. O.** (1961). The inheritance of congenital pyloric stenosis, *Brit. Med. Bull., 17,* 251–54.

48. **Kidd, K. K.,** and **Spence, M. M.** (1976). Genetic analysis of pyloric stenosis suggesting a specific maternal effect, *J. Med. Genet., 13,* 290–94.

49. **Haenzel, W.,** and **Kurihara, M.** (1968). Studies of Japanese migrants: I. Mortality from cancer and other diseases among Japanese of the United States, *J. Nat. Can. Inst., 40,* 43–68.

50. **Belmont, L.,** and **Marolla, F.** (1973). Birth order, family size, and intelligence, *Science, 182,* 1096–1101.

   Belmont, L., Stein, Z. A., and **Susser, M. W.** (1975). Comparison of the associations of birth order with intelligence test score and height *Nature, 255,* 54–56.

51. **Spath, J.** (1860). Studien ubër Zwillinge, *Ztschr. d. k. k. Gesellsch. d. Aerzte zu Wein, 16,* 225–41.

   Galton, F. (1875). The history of twins as a criterion of the relative powers of nature and nurture, *Fraser's Magazine, 12,* 566–76.

52. **Neel, J. V.,** and **Schull, W. J.** (1954). *Human Heredity,* Chicago.

   Cavalli-Sforza, L. L., and **Bodmer, W. F.** (1971). *The Genetics of Human Populations,* San Francisco.

   Allen, G., and **Hrubec, Z.** (1979). Twin concordance: A more general model, *Acta Genet. Med. Gemellol., 28,* 3–13.

53. **Price, B.** (1950). Primary biases in twins studies: A review of prenatal and natal difference-producing factors in monozygotic pairs, *Amer. J. Hum. Genet., 2,* 293–352.

   Scarr, S. (1982). Environmental bias in twin studies, *Social Biology, 29,* 221–9.

54. **Cohen, D. J., Dibble, E., Grawe, J. M,** and **Pollin, W.** (1975). Reliably separating identical from fraternal twins, *Arch. Gen. Psychiat., 32,* 1371–5.

Scarr, S., and Carter-Saltzman, L (1979). Twin method: Defence of a critical assumption, *Behavior Genetics*, 9, 527–42.

55. Wilson, R. S., Brown, A. M., and Matheny, A. P. (1971). Emergence and persistence of behavioral differences in twins, *Child Development*, 42, 1381–98.

56. Nance, W. E., Corey, L. A., and Boughman, J. A. (1978). Monozygotic twin sibships: A new design for genetic and epidemiologic research, in *Genetic Epidemiology*, ed. Morton, N. E., and Chung, C. S., New York, pp. 87–114.

Christian, J. C., and Kang, K. W. (1977). Maternal influences on plasma cholesterol variation, *Amer. J. Hum. Genet.*, 20, 462–67.

Rose, R. J., Boughman, J. N., Cover, L. A., Nance, E. W., Christian, J. C., and Kang, K. W. (1980). Data from kinships of monozygotic twins indicate maternal effects on verbal intelligence, *Nature, 283*, 375–77.

57. Cobb, S., Harburg, E., Tabor, J., Hunt, P., Kasl, S. V., and Schull, W. J. (1969). The intrafamilial transmission of rheumatoid arthritis, I. Design of the study, *J. Chron. Dis.*, 22, 195–202.

Charkraborty, R., and Schull, W. J. (1979). Fixed cluster designs in human genetic studies: Interpretation and usefulness, In *The Genetic Analysis of Common Diseases*, ed. Sing, C. F., and Skolnick, M., New York, pp. 343–61.

58. Newman, M. J., Freeman, F. N., and Holzinger, K. J. (1937). *Twins: A Study of Heredity and Environment*, Chicago.

59. Burt, C. (1966). The genetic determination of differences in intelligence, *Brit. Psychol.*, 57, 137–153.

60. Kamin, L. (1974). *The Science and Politics of IQ*, Potomac, Maryland.

Dorfman, D. D. (1978). The Cyril Burt question: New findings, *Science, 201*, 1177–86.

Gould, S. J. (1981). *The Mismeasure of Man*, New York.

61. Burt, C. (1955). The evidence for the concept of intelligence, *Brit. J. Educ. Psychol.*, 25, 158–77.

Burt, C. (1958). The inheritance of mental ability, *Amer. Psychol.*, 1–15.

62. Lykken, D. T., Tellegen, A. and DeRubeis, R. (1980). Volunteer bias in twin research: The rule of two-thirds, *Social Biology*, 25, 1–9.

Friedman, G. D. (1977). A potential pitfall in studying trait discordance in twins, *Amer. J. Epi.*, 15, 291–95.

63. Myrianthopoulos, N. C. (1978). An approach to the investigations of maternal factors in congenital malformations, in *Genetic Epidemiology*, ed. Morton, N. E., and Chung, C. S., pp. 363–79.

64. Skodak, M., and Skeels, H. M. (1945). A follow-up study of children in adoptive homes, *J. Genet. Psychol.*, 66, 21–58.

Stein, Z. A. and Susser, M. W. (1967). The social dimensions of a symptom: A sociomedical study of enuresis, *Soc. Sci. Med.* 1, 183–201.

Tizard, B. (1977) *Adoption: A Second Chance*, London.

65. Burk, B. S. (1928). The relative influence of nature and nurture upon mental development: A comparative study of foster parent-foster child resemblance and true parent-true child resemblance, *27th Yearbook of the National Society for the Study of Education, Part I*, 219–316.

Freeman, F. N., Holzinger, K. J., and Mitchell, B. C. (1928). The influence of environment on the intelligence, school achievement and conduct of foster children, *27th Yearbook of the National Society for the Study of Education, Part I*: 103–217.

Leaky, A. M. (1935). Nature and Intelligence, *Genetic Psychology Monographs*, 17, 236–308.

66. **Heston, L. L.** (1966). Psychiatric disorders in foster home-reared children of schizophrenic mothers, *Brit. J. Psychiat., 112,* 819–25.

67. **Rosenthal, D., Wender, P. H., Kety, S. S., Schulsinger, F.,** and **Welner, J.** (1971). The adopted-away offspring of schizophrenics, *Amer. J. Psychiat., 128,* 307–11.

68. **Wynne, L. C., Singer, M. T.,** and **Toohey, M.** (1976). Communication of the adoptive parents of schizophrenics, in *Schizophrenia 75: Psychotherapy, Family Studies, Research,* ed. Uøvstad, V. and Ugelstad, E., Oslo.
   Lidz, T. Blatt, S., and **Cook, B.** (1981). Critique of the Danish-American studies of the adopted away offspring of schizophrenic parents, *Amer. J. Psychiat., 138,* 1063–68.

69. **Kety, S. S., Rosenthal, D., Wender, P. H., Schulsinger, F.,** and **Jacobsen, B.** (1975). Mental illness in the biological and adoptive families of individuals who have become schizophrenic: A preliminary report based on psychiatric interviews, in *Genetic Research in Psychiatry,* ed. Fieve, R. R., and Rosenthal, D., Baltimore, pp. 147–56.

70. **Benjamin, L.** (1976). A reconsideration of the Kety and associates study of genetic factors in the tranmission of schizophrenia, *Amer. J. Psychiat., 133,* 1129–33.
   Gottesman, I. I., and **Shields, J.** (1976). A critical review of recent adoption, twin, and family studies, *Schizophr. Bulle., 2,* 360–400.
   Kessler, S. (1976). Progress and regress in the research of the genetics of schizophr., *Schizophr. Bull., 2,* 434–38.
   Kety, S. (1978). Heredity and environment, in *Schizophrenia: Science and Practice,* ed. Shershow, J. C., Cambridge.
   Lidz, T., and **Blatt, S.** (1983). Critique of the Danish-American studies of the biological and adoptive relatives of adoptees who became schizophrenic, *Amer. J. Psychiat., 140,* 426–35.

71. **Kidd, K. K.,** and **Cavalli-Sforza, L. L.** (1973). An analysis of the genetics of schizophrenia, *Social Biology, 29,* 276–87.
   Rao, D. C., Morton, N. E., Gottesman, I. I., and **Lew, R.** (1981). Path analysis of qualitative data on pairs of relatives: Application to schizophrenia, *Hum. Hered., 31,* 325–33.

72. **Hutchings, B.,** and **Mednick, S. A.** (1975). Registered criminality in the adoptive and biological parents of registered male criminal adoptees, in *Genetic Research in Psychiatry,* ed. Fieve, R., and Rosenthal, D., Baltimore, pp. 105–16.

73. **Goodwin, D. W., Schulsinger, F., Hermansen, L., Guze, S. B.,** and **Winokur, G.** (1973). Alcohol problems in adoptees raised apart from biological parents, *Arch. Gen. Psychiat., 28,* 238–43.

74. **Moll, P. P.,** and **Sing, C. F.** (1979). Sampling strategies for the analysis of quantitative traits, in *Workshop on the Genetic Analysis of Common Diseases: Applications to Predictive Factors in Coronary Disease,* ed. Sing, C. F., and Skolnick, M., New York.
   Annest, J. L., Sing, C. F., Biron, P., and **Mongeau, J-G.** (1979) (1983). Familial aggregation of blood pressure and weight in adoptive families, Parts I, II, and III, *Amer. J. Epi., 110,* 479–503; *117,* 492–506.

75. **Cloninger, C. R., Rice, J., Reich, T.** (1979). Multifactorial inheritance with cultural transmission and assortative mating. III. Family structure: Analysis of separation experiments, *Amer. J. Hum. Genet., 31,* 366–88.

76. **Susser, M.** (1973). *Causal Thinking in the Health Sciences: Concepts and Strategies in Epidemiology,* New York.

77. **Linton, R.** (1936). *The Study of Man,* New York.
   Firth, R. (1938). *Human Types,* London.
   Murdock, G. P. (1949). *Social Structure,* New York.

Radcliffe-Brown, A. R., and Forde, C. D. (1950). *African Systems of Kinship and Marriage*, London.

Hill, R. (1966). Contemporary developments in family theory, *J. Marr. Fam.*, 38, 10–26.

78. U.S. Bureau of the Census (1980). *Census of Population, Vol. 1, General Population Characteristics*, Washington, D.C.

79. Brockington, C. F. (1948). Problem families, *Med. Offr.*, 77, 75.

Blacker, C. P. (1952). *Problem Families: Five Enquires*, London.

Brown, G. E. Ed. (1968). *The Multi-Problem Dilemma*, Metuchen, N.J.

80. Parsons, T. (1951). *The Social System*, Glencoe, Ill.

81. Fortes, M (1958). The developmental cycle in domestic groups, Introduction to *Cambridge Papers* in *Social Anthropology*, ed. Goody, J., Cambridge.

82. Glass, D. V., and Grebenik, E. (1954). *The Trend and Pattern of Fertility in Great Britain, A Report of the Family Census, 1946*, Papers of the Royal Commission on Population, Vol. VI, Parts I and II, H.M.S.O., London.

Glick, P. C., and Parke, R., Jr. (1965). New approaches in studying the life-cycle of the family, *Demography*, 2, 187–202.

83. Titmuss, R. (1958). *Essays on the Welfare State*, London.

Department of Scientific and Industrial Research (1960). *Woman, Wife and Worker, Problems of Progress in Industry*, No. 10, H.M.S.O., London.

84. Richards, A. I. (1934). Mother-right among the Central Bantu, in *Essays Presented to C. G. Seligman*, ed. Evans-Pritchard, E. E., London.

85. van Gennep, G. A. (1960; first pub. 1909). *The Rites of Passage*, trans. Vizedom, M. B., and Caffee, G. L., London.

86. Arensberg, C. M., and Kimball, S. T. (1948). *Family and Community in Ireland*, Cambridge, Mass.

Hannan, D., and Katsiaouni, L. (1977). *Traditional Families: From Culturally Prescribed to Negotiated Roles in Farm Families*, Dublin.

87. Office of Population Censuses and Surveys (1977). *Demographic Review*, Series DR No. 1, H.M.S.O., London.

U.S. Bureau of the Census and Dept. of Commerce (1982). *Statistical Abstract, 1982–83*, Washington, D.C.

Pratt, W. F., and Mosher, W. D. (1983). *Reproductive Impairment Among Married Couples: United States*, National Center for Health Statistics, Washington, D.C.

88. Belmont, L., Wittes, J., and Stein, Z. (1980). The only child syndrome: Myth or reality, *Human Functioning in Longitudinal Perspective: Studies of Natural and Psychopathic Populations*, ed. Sells, S. B., Crandall, R., Roff, M., Strauss, J. S., and Pollin, W., Baltimore, pp. 251–62.

89. Slater, E., and Woodside, M. (1951). *Patterns of Marriage*, London.

90. Firkowska, A., Ostrowska, A., Sokolowska, M., Stein, Z., Susser, M., and Wald, I. (1978). Cognitive development and social policy, *Science*, 200, 1357–62.

91. Zaretsky, E. (1976). *Capitalism, the Family and Personal Life*, London.

92. Rapoport, R. N., Fogarty, M. P., and Rapoport, R., ed. (1982). *Families in Britain*, London.

93. Walker, E. A. (1968). *History of South Africa*, London.

94. Malthus, T. (1926, orig. publ. 1798). *Eassy on Population*, London.

95. Mamdami, M. (1973). *The Myth of Population Control: Family, Caste, and Class in an Indian Village*, New York.

White, B. (1973). Demand for labor and population growth in colonial Java, *Human Ecology*, 1, 217–36.

Harris, M. (1975). *Culture, People, Nature*, 2nd edition, New York.

96. LeRoy-Ladurie, E. (1966). *The Peasants of Languedoc*, Paris.

Weber, E. (1976). *Peasants into Frenchmen*, Stanford.

97. Wrigley, E. A. and Schofield, R. S. (1981) *The Population History of England: 1541–1871*, Cambridge, Mass.

Wrigley, E. A. (1983). The growth of population in eighteenth century England: A conumdrum resolved, *Past and Present*, 98, 121–50.

98. Dupaquier, J., Reinhard, M. and Armengaud, A. (1968). *Histoire Général des la Population Mondiale*, 3rd edition, Paris.

Dupaquier, J. (1979). *La Population Français aux 17ième et 18 ième siècles*, Paris.

99. Watson, W. (1958). *Tribal Cohesion in a Money Economy. A Study of the Mambwe People of Northern Rhodesia*, Manchester.

100. Randolph, L. E., and Randolph, S. (1974). *The Modernity of Tradition: Political Development in India*, New York.

101. Smelser, N. J. (1959). *Social Change in the Industrial Revolution: An Application of Theory to the Lancashire Cotton Industry, 1770–1840*, New York.

102. Anderson, M. (1976). Sociological history and the working-class family, *Social History*, 3, 318–34.

103. Thompson, E. P. (1963). *The Making of the English Working Class*, New York.

Foster, J. (1974). *Class Struggle and the Industrial Revolution*, London.

104. Laslett, P. (1984). *The World We Have Lost*, 3rd ed., London.

Medick, H. (1976). The proto-industrial family economy: The structural function of household and family during the transition from peasant society to industrial capitalism, *Social History*, 3, 291–315.

105. Stone, L. (1979). *The Family, Sex and Marriage in England 1500–1800*, London.

Goody, J. (1983). *The Development of the Family and Marriage in Europe*, Cambridge.

106. Shorter, E. (1975). *The Making of the Modern Family*, New York.

Soliday, G. L. (1980). *History of Family and Kinship: A Select International Bibliography*, New York.

10

Mating and marriage

Marriage is a vehicle at one and the same time for a biological and a social process. Biologically, it is the principal distributor of genes in populations, and socially it is the institutionalized means whereby new members are introduced into the social system. The manner in which people meet and marry is therefore of primary biological and social importance. In order to chart the distribution of genes among humans, study of the biological mechanisms that govern the transmission of inherited characters must be supplemented by study of social mechanisms, and the survival of offspring must also be taken into account.

Mendel discovered the key to individual variation in populations when he described the laws of genetic transmission through the mating of male and female, each carrying its own combination of genes. This discovery illuminated Darwin's hypothesis that the evolution of humans depended on natural selection and the survival of the fittest, for it showed how fitness could be transmitted. Darwinian fitness has been interpreted in more than one way. In the current consensus, it means fitness for reproduction, so that the favored female bears the most surviving offspring, while the favored male fertilizes such females (1). Thus, among mammals, "fit females" are those that are efficient in conceiving, bearing, and rearing progeny, and "fit males" are those that are virile, fertile, and strong or attractive enough to command mates.

These generalizations cannot be simply applied to human beings, as sometimes they have been. Once human social organization appears, the physical qualities that ensure fitness, or adaptive value, are modified by the demands of society. The social system controls the chances of sexual reproduction by individuals as much as does the quality of their personal attributes. Similar considerations may apply to certain social animals. The essential distinction here is between the concept of mating, a biological union, and the concept of marriage, a social union. Beasts mate, but humans marry.

Marriage is one of the oldest institutions of human society and may be defined as a union between a man and a woman such that the children borne by the woman are recognized as the legitimate offspring of both spouses (2). Social anthropologists have yet to find a society without the institution of marriage. The distinction between mating and marrying applies to the most primitive human groups, as shown in the almost universal prohibition of incest. There is no physiological bar to incest, but in virtually all societies incest is forbidden and punished; sons are forbidden to marry their mothers, brothers their sisters, and fathers their daughters.

A part of every social system is a set of rules that prohibit marriage between certain persons related by descent. This is the rule of *exogamy*, and in some systems it is extended so that a man is forbidden to marry among a group of women more distantly related than his mother, sisters, or daughters. The rule of exogamy gives recognition to the kinship bond between the man and his female relatives as an institution of society, and as a corollary forces him to choose a wife from some other group, thereby producing a social tie and a common interest in the marriage and children. *Endogamy* is the rule whereby the choice of a spouse is circumscribed within a certain group, as in a caste system. This term is sometimes used loosely to describe an observed tendency for people to marry within certain social categories, for instance, class endogamy.

Psychological mechanisms such as the Oedipus complex may deter incest, although they do not prevent it from occurring. These responses are likely to be acquired; society enforces the ban. In unusual circumstances in a few societies the incest prohibition has been relaxed. This exemption was believed to obtain only for certain persons from families with quasidivine status to whom the rules for ordinary mortals do not apply—Cleopatra is said to have been the product of some twenty-six successive sibling marriages. The idea that incest is permitted only to godlike rulers must be abandoned, however, in the face of documented historical research that shows sibling unions to have been common in Egypt during the rule of several Roman emperors in the early centuries of the Common Era (3). Incestuous marriage could be a biological disadvantage. In experimental animals inbred strains show less vigor than hybrids in growth, fertility, and longevity. Among humans, the results of small studies suggest that incestuous matings have adverse effects on the offspring in terms of mortality, severe mental deficiency, and some congenital anomalies (4). These are plausible genetic consequences. Although incest tends to occur in aberrant social circumstances and ascertainment bias is certainly present—dramatic instances with serious consequences are always more likely to be reported—the effects have seemed worse than would be expected in almost any social group. Mating of sibs seemed to occur in less socially aberrant circumstances than mating of parents and child, but the children of either type of union were at an equal disadvantage.

Incest is an extreme form of consanguineous union. Studies of other forms of consanguinity such as cousin and uncle-niece unions, which yield larger numbers, have not conclusively shown adverse effects aside from the higher risks for acquiring double recessive genes for abnormalities such as phenylketonuria, Tay-Sachs disease, and fibrocystic disease (5). Work on cousin-union consanguinity has been carried out in the Japanese cities of Nagasaki, Hiroshima, and Kure, under the aegis of the Atomic Bomb Casualty Commission. Small effects associated with inbreeding were found on stillbirths and child mortality, on the secondary sex ratio, and on certain congenital malformations. Later studies, however, have not always repeated the early results, for instance, on the sex ratio and on mortality, and investigations of additional effects have proved negative (6).

Extraneous social factors are difficult to exclude in studies of consanguinity; marriage behavior is characteristic of particular social groups. Thus, in Japan consanguineous marriage is common but it increases with declining social class, and so too do such measures of the possible outcome of consanguinity as child mortality and mental deficiency. In a polygynous Nigerian community, men assume a traditional obligation to take a relative as wife in addition to nonrelatives, thus affording a study design with close control of social factors. In this study, consanguinity was associated with a history of excess reproductive loss, but such other variables crucial in reproduction as maternal age and parity were not controlled (7). Where consanguinity has been studied in homogeneous social groups, measures of the outcome variables have usually been unsatisfactory. In the tiny island isolate of Tristan da Cunha in the South Atlantic, for instance, the total genealogy has been traced, but estimates of intelligence levels associated with inbreeding were entirely subjective (8). In the Middle East, consanguineous marriages are common, and pregnancies seem to result in a higher than expected frequency of choriocarcinoma, a rare malignant tumor of pregnancy connected with the fetus (9). One speculation is that the choriocarcinoma, like normal fetal parts, is a form of homotransplant, and that its growth is less hindered by immunological response of the mother because of greater genetic compatibility of fetus and mother in consanguineous marriages.

Fitness for reproduction and genetic attributes are thus modified by social forces. In some tribal gerontocracies the older men command the power and prestige to monopolize young women, and to prevent the more virile younger men from marrying them. The position of these older men depends on their accumulated experience. Wisdom can only come with age, for in nonliterate societies the minds of living people are the sole repositories of knowledge. The power of the older men is further enhanced by successive inheritances from their elders who die, and in most tribal societies that have polygynous marriage, the husbands are usually distinctly older than their wives (10). The exclusion of the young men from sexual access to young women is seldom absolute, however, for access can be achieved by means other than marriage, and is even condoned in some cultures. This makes difficulties for the human geneticist who wishes to trace individual heredity. In all societies it is often impossible to distinguish the *genitor*, or biological father, from the *pater*, or legal father. The *pater* may play both roles, but it would be unwise to assume that he always does so (see Chapter 9). (Among the Tokelau in the South Pacific, geneticists receive some aid from the ritual obligation placed upon a mother as she gives birth to shout aloud the name of the genitor.) Indeed, human genealogies refer not only to the descent of persons but also to the inheritance of property, or power, and consequently may be subject to manipulation. Genealogies may be revised or created to legitimize the positions of incumbents who hold property or power (11).

Medical advances in contemporary industrial society have greatly improved the capacity to reproduce. For instance, the low risk of the modern Caesarean section has allowed many women with narrow pelvic bones to have children and thus transmit the genes—assuming they exist—for this particular bone structure. The favorable or unfavorable effects of this transmission on the future population cannot be predicted, for if those theories have any substance that postulate a connection between body type, personality attributes, and predisposition to disease (12), other characteristics may well be linked with this bony structure, and be transmitted with it.

Medical and social advances have also improved the chances of children surviving, and this may have a selective effect on the transmission of certain genes in the population. The sickle cell gene found in some African peoples provides a striking example (see Chapter 1). Where there is no malaria, the reproductive advantage conferred by the sickle cell trait in a malarial environment evidently disappears; it is usually lethal for the homozygous individual in childhood or youth, and the heterozygous individual has lost the biological advantage over those without the trait. The incidence of the sickle cell trait is reported to decline among those Africans who have migrated to areas free from malaria. The frequency of the trait among North American blacks whose ancestors left Africa many generations ago is lower than might be expected, even when an allowance is made for admixture with races who do not carry the gene (13). When economic and social policies and health programs eventually rid Africa of malaria, and thereby allow children without the sickle cell trait a better chance of survival, the incidence of the sickle cell trait is thus likely to decline, and to bring about a change in the gene frequency in the population.

Similar selective processes have been invoked to explain the distribution of such other genetic traits as glucose-6-phosphate deficiency and a variety of abnormal hemoglobins (14). Populations with these conditions, which in the past may have done them more good than harm, have become subject to new and adverse forms of selective pressure. Since large populations have been exposed to drugs, deficiencies of such enzymes have been found to predispose individuals to acute adverse drug reactions, as in the acute hemolytic anemia precipitated by sulphonamides, and by primaquine prophylaxis for malaria. Carriers of porphyria genes who unwittingly take sulphonamides and barbiturates are similarly subject to acute porphyric crises; other individuals collapse when exposed to the anaesthetic succinylcholine for minor surgical procedures.

Biological and social selection are interconnected, and together are responsible for the distribution of human attributes in different societies. These forces are no less relevant within our own complex society, and their mode of operation and interaction can only be grasped through an understanding of the processes that control the social and geographical movements of individuals and families and the selection of spouses.

Assortative mating

In our society the choice of a spouse is such a private individual matter, involving so many considerations, that at first sight the process appears to lack all system and regularity. Nevertheless, the choice is not haphazard and takes place within limits both of geographic and social space. In the first place, selection must occur among persons who are in contact, for all potential husbands in society cannot meet all potential wives. Moreover, the choices of most people are affected by religious, educational, and social distinctions that act as deterrents to otherwise possible marriages, and some close relatives are forbidden to marry by legal constraint. On the other hand, these same social barriers tend to foster marriages between persons with similar characteristics, such as a common religion, comparable standards of education, and equality of social standing. First considered in the study of biological traits, the process is known as assortative mating (15).

In England and Wales, a national sample of marriages from all social levels demonstrated the high incidence of assortative mating (16). For the purpose of this study, the two associated criteria of educational level and occupations of fathers of the brides and grooms were used. Similarities in social origin and education between husbands and wives were greatest at the extreme ends of the social scale, being most marked among persons with fathers of professional, high administrative, managerial, and executive occupations, and among persons with fathers of unskilled manual occupations. "Class endogamy," although less than before, still persists in developed societies. As with occupational mobility, the least rigidity and the greatest movement occur among the categories of skilled manual and routine clerical workers. More women than men tend to marry "above them" *(hypergamy);* marriage is a channel whereby women, in particular, have achieved upward social mobility, while they have had less access to the occupational channels used by men. Education appears to be more important in the choice of spouses than social origin; educational attainment diminishes social distance. This tendency is most evident among persons with a university or professional education. In the United States, women at either end of the social spectrum, but not in the middle classes, are more mobile than men in both upward and downward directions (17).

The decline in "class endogamy" supports evidence from many societies of an expansion in size of *marriage isolates,* the term used to describe those areas or groupings within which marriages are more likely to occur than between one area or group and another (18). In physiological terms, humanity as a whole forms one great potential marriage isolate, for any two human beings of reproductive age and of opposite sex anywhere in the world are potentially capable of meeting and mating to produce offspring.

Humanity is divided into many marriage isolates by barriers of race, geography, language, social class, religion, and culture that effectively militate against intermarriage. Nevertheless, the growing ease and speed of travel and the spread of industrialism throughout the world have brought about a great increase in the geographical and social mobility of individuals, and hence in the frequency with which intermarriage occurs between isolates. One sample of local marriage records in a group of rural parishes in Hertfordshire in Britain showed a fall of about 50 per cent over the last century in the extent to which both partners in a marriage gave a place of residence in the same parish or in one immediately contiguous (19). Similar changes have been recorded elsewhere, and studies in Sweden and France showed that one effect was a decline in the number of marriages of related persons (18,20). These developments have helped to expand the proportion of married persons in the population, to reduce "class endogamy" and probably class solidarity, and also to reshuffle genetic characteristics. This last consequence of the breakdown of isolates has long been obvious in the increase in interracial marriages (21).

Residential stability in any community is likely to cause a clustering of genetic traits. In a previous chapter we noted that in a large population, consanguineous mating will make the main nonrandom contribution to the coefficient of inbreeding, but that the smaller and more stable the isolate, the more a random element will contribute to inbreeding: hence the frequency of certain rare inherited conditions that require homozygosity for recessive genes in endogamous groups or sects (22). Extreme concordance between marriage partners probably reinforces the physical and social homogeneity of such groups. With regard to marriages, concordance is likely to enhance their stability just as, conversely, divorce is relatively frequent among spouses of discordant ethnic and religious groups.

Migration into large urban isolates from rural areas and smaller towns is common feature in the history of developed and industrializing societies. This flow is encouraged by the upward social mobility of settled urban manual workers and their children, who are then replaced by the incoming strangers (23). The continuous upward social movement observed in cities has arisen partly from economic expansion and the more complex division of labor, for in cities there are more jobs that require skill or specialization than in smaller communities, and partly from the lower fertility rates found in city populations and in the higher occupational classes. If the mobile individuals are selected for special traits like high intelligence, pleasing personality, or physical beauty, the areas that are losing population might be thought to contain an increasingly homogeneous residuum with fewer of these traits. This does not seem to apply to Scotland, at least in the matter of measured intelligence, for in the national study of intelligence there, the advantage of city-dwellers was found to be slight in spite of an advantage among migrants from country to city. Studies of Southern migrant black children in New York City in the 1930s and later in Philadelphia also found no evidence of their selection by intelligence (24). Even in residentially stable groups, the degree of commingling tends to prevent the formation of inbred populations with a relatively limited pool of genes. Only 25 per cent of all unskilled manual workers in a national survey in Britain had fathers in the same occupational class, and another 45 per cent had fathers who were either skilled manual or routine nonmanual workers (25). These data make implausible the view of some theorists on the social class distribution of intelligence, who have held that the lowest classes comprise an increasingly homogeneous residuum in respect of intelligence (26). Individuals constantly percolate into contiguous social strata, although the general flow has been upwards.

Patterns of geographical and social movement therefore have obvious import for theories concerning the distribution of such graded characteristics as intelligence and blood pressure, or of specific traits determined by a single gene, or of illnesses with a particular social distribution. Whether these movements help to select particular traits or are sufficient to alter frequencies among particular social groups remains to be established (see Chapters 8 and 9).

Common physical and psychological characteristics, in addition to common social origin and background, play a part in the selection of spouses. Spouses have been found to resemble each other in such attributes as temperament, in attitudes and interests, in intelligence quotients, and also in height and in eye and hair color (27). One study of married couples suggests that neurotic characteristics, too, may have a part to play in selection and that neurotics may select each other (28). This is consistent with psychological theories of "neurotic marriage," in which individuals with exaggerated emotional needs (dependence or dominance, for example) may seek to satisfy these needs in marriage, and in which such satisfactions may be reciprocal between the spouses (29). But common characteristics among spouses can be explained as readily by their shared environment and continuous interaction as by conscious or unconscious social selection. Neurosis can arise equally from interaction between spouses and from reaction to a marital situation, as we discussed in Chapter 9 (30).

The effects of marital state

The similarity in social and personal characteristics of spouses appears also in the mortality of widowed persons, especially at young ages, which are higher than those of their married or single peers both in Britain and the United States (see Figure 10.1). Among widows and widowers in the United States, certain causes of morbidity and death have been found to be especially associated with the cause of death in the spouse, for instance, pneumonia and vascular diseases of the heart and central nervous system (31). These associations can be interpreted in three ways: first, that before

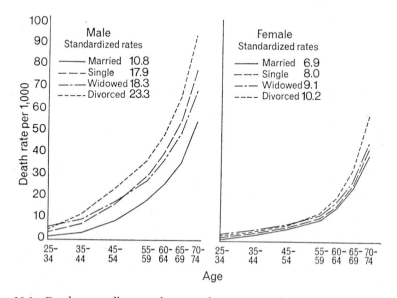

Figure 10.1 Death rates, all causes, by marital status, United States, (1949–1951). *Source:* Berkson, J. (1962). Mortality and marital status: Reflections on the derivation of etiology from statistics, *Amer. J. Pub. Hlth.*, 52, 1318–29.

marriage there is a "mutual selection of poor risk mates"; second, that after marriage both spouses shared similar unfavorable environments, that is, both were exposed to the same nutrition, infections, and other risks; and third, that after the end of the marriage, the survivor was affected by the material, social, and psychological consequences of bereavement. Whichever of these relationships obtains will markedly affect the plausibility of hypotheses; for instance, that lack of domestic care led to increased deaths from pneumonia, that taking to alcohol led to deaths from cirrhosis and promiscuity to syphilis, or that social isolation led to deaths from suicide, accidents, and tuberculosis. The issues are difficult, and studies stretching over more than a century leave much unanswered (32,33).

Difficulties of distinguishing cause and effect, similar to those found with widowhood, obtain in most analyses of health disorders and marital state. In general, married people tend to have the most favorable health experience, whether the measure used is overall survival, or death from a large array of specific causes, or the frequency of peptic ulcer, or the frequency of mental disorders. At the other extreme, divorced and separated persons tend to have the least favorable health experience. The pattern is found not only for mortality, but for acute and chronic sickness, disability, and institutionalization for care (34,35) (see Table 10.1). Some of the difficulties in determining cause and effect arise from the nature of the index selected to measure health experience. For example, prevalence rates do not indicate the order in time of the changing circumstances of marital state and the onset of disorder. Incidence rates based on entry to services give a better view of time relations, but are biased by social selection; fewer married persons than the single, divorced, and separated are admitted to public facilities such as mental and chronic hospitals. Persons using these facilities often do not have the resources to exercise choice among different forms of care. Where people do have the resources to exercise choice, as in the United States with those admitted to nursing homes, more married persons use the facilities than the single, separated, or divorced (36).

In *relative mortality ratios*, the denominator is usually the mortality rate of the married, and the numerator a mortality rate for some other marital state at the same ages; such ratios indicated the higher risk for younger age-groups among the widowed, mentioned above. Calculation of *excess risk* is an index of comparison that looks to the arithemetic difference between group rates, as of the widowed over the married. This method applied to the same data gave a result of increasing disadvantage with age for the widowed, as compared with the married, because of the much larger number of widows found at older ages (37).

Problems of indices are compounded by problems surrounding the validity of the available data. Because without distinction among them manifold causes of death show a consistent gradient running from married through single and divorced, systematic error must be treated seriously as a cause of such regularity (38). Matching of death records against census records show the data to compare well and be reliable, except for some of the special categories in question. Census undercounts of the divorced and of young widowers confirmed the suspicion of recording errors, and were similar in type both in Britain and the United States (39). Two other sources of confusion include the inflation of rates of disorder by the higher average age of wid-

Table 10.1 Marital state and health disorders: age standardized prevalence rates by sex for the population 17 years and older in the United States

	Total	Single	Married	Widowed	Divorced
Acute conditions (1972–1973)					
a. All reported[a]					
Male	143.4	151.4	140.2	136.3	135.6
Female	174.8	170.8	167.7	164.3	216.3
b. Days of bed disability					
Male	2.2	1.9	2.2	3.4	3.3
Female	2.7	2.6	2.6	3.2	2.9
Limiting chronic conditions (1972–1973)[b]					
a. Causing any limitation in activity					
Male	18.8	21.6	17.9	23.4	25.5
Female	16.6	16.1	15.1	22.9	22.3
b. Causing limitation in major activity					
Male	14.7	17.3	13.9	19.2	21.2
Female	12.7	11.5	11.6	18.3	16.6
Complete work disability (1970)					
Male	3.7	7.6	2.8	8.5	7.9
Female	5.0	5.6	4.3	8.3	7.8
Institutionalization (1970)[c]					
Male	156	621	56	349	538
Female	115	380	34	148	161

[a] Number of conditions per 100 persons per year.

[b] Percentage affected.

[c] Per 10,000

Source: Abstracted from Verbrugge, L. M. (1979) Marital status and health, *Journal of Marriage and the Family, 41,* 267–85.

owers as compared with the married of the same age-group, and the selection of the healthy for marriage and remarriage, thereby leaving a residuum of the unhealthy among the single, the widowed, and the divorced.

The main questions of interpretation, however, are to separate selection for one or other marital state from reaction to it. Two problems make this difficult: first, it is necessary to establish accurately both the affected population and the denominator population from which the affected persons are drawn; second, it is necessary to establish the order in time of the condition under study and the marital state. Since marriage is an achieved status, the denominator of the married is subject to transitions in the course of the life-arc. At the earliest nubile ages the single predominate, but the population is in a state of rapid flux, and in the twenties the married become the larger, "normal" reference population. As age increases, the single are whittled down to a self-selected and socially selected residual group whose social and personal attributes are not the same as those of young single people. Concurrently with the growth of the married population, the categories of the divorced and the remarried form and increase in size. Divorced people have a higher rate of marriage than the single (although once they remarry, they have a higher rate of divorce than the once-married); and the characteristics of the estimated one-in-seven who remain divorced cannot be taken as representative of all divorces. In later life the widowed grow in numbers, until towards the end of life they become the larger population.

Age, therefore, must be controlled with precision in the analysis of marital status with any age-related condition. The often-used standardization procedures can confuse results. The social and personal attributes of the various age-groups of the same marital status clearly differ in matters other than age, and to cast them together, as is done in standardization, offers opportunities for confounding factors. As noted above, even age-specific comparisons may not adequately control age. In those age-groups at which rapid transitions take place, the extremes of an age-group may be biased: thus, in the third decade, the single cluster in the early twenties, while in the eighth decade, the widowed can be expected to cluster in the late seventies.

It has therefore proved no easy task to discover the causes of many striking variations of health disorders with marital state. In mental disorders, marital state emerges as a powerful factor that can outweigh even so basic an attribute as sex. The risk of entry to psychiatric treatment, for instance, rises in a gradient from the married, through the single, the widowed, and the divorced. Because many people without spouses lack social support and mental hospitals provide social support, these rates could be more an index of response to a social than to a psychological strain, but the results also hold outside the hospitals. The highest rates are found among single men and divorced persons of both sexes, and the main diagnostic categories among them are schizophrenia and the sociopathies (or personality disorders or psychopathies). Either reaction or selection could underlie these distributions (40).

Schizophrenia and psychopathies could be seen as a reaction to the single state. Prolonged bachelorhood tends to be socially deviant and carries social and psychological penalties. But single men with "abnormal personalities" at the outset, in a 10-year follow-up, were reported to have married less often than expected (41). This result supports a clinical impression of incompatibility between the demands of marriage and the "schizophrenic personality." Mental disorder has obvious repercussions on marital state. Many schizophrenic persons have not married because their sickness has stigmatized them, or because incarceration in mental hospitals denied them the opportunity. Conversely, patients chronically handicapped by mental disorder who live in the community have a higher rate of divorce and separation than those confined in hospitals—the apparent consequence of the chronic disorder (42).

Reaction may be important in forms of mental disturbance generated by intimate marital relationships with spouses who are mentally disturbed. The extreme case is *folie à deux*, a condition in which couples achieve a bizarre accommodation through sharing delusions and psychotic disorders of thought. Mental illness has been recognized more often among both spouses, and the diagnoses were more often concordant, than would be expected to occur by chance (43). With this result, the recognition and treatment of mental disorder in one spouse could have facilitated recognition and treatment in the other. But the fact noted above—that where one spouse has been a neurotic patient, emotional disturbance mutual to married couples rises in frequency with the duration of marriage—provides grounds for the argument for reaction.

Reaction and selection are equally difficult to sort out in studies on a variety of other conditions. Thus, in Alfred Kinsey's pioneering study, the prevalence of homosexual practices rose with age among unmarried men (44). This could have been related to the social and psychological circumstances of bachelorhood, or to the personality of those who remained bachelors by choice or inadvertently. The same questions can be put about the higher risk of perforation of duodenal ulcer carried by single men.

In the field of mental illness, more convincing evidence for reaction to marital conditions comes from those studies of the status transition into widowhood that have paid attention to the ordering of the associated events in time. Thus, entry into psychiatric care for the first time is more frequent than expected in the general population during the period immediately following bereavement (45). Since many diagnoses were affected, bereavement appears to act as a precipitating factor. Immunity, indicated by lymphocyte function, has also been found to be depressed in the widowed some six weeks after the death of a spouse (46). Cohort studies of mortality in widowers, and a matched control study of suicide among the widowed, have also demonstrated higher rates of death in the period soon after bereavement than in later periods (47). The sexes appear to be unequally affected by widowhood; cohort studies of mortality in widows have failed to demonstrate raised mortality in the interval after bereavement (48).

In the study of some other health disorders, marital state has proved a convenient and productive indicator of associated styles of life and behavior. In an earlier chapter we discussed some intricacies of the relationships of rheumatoid arthritis to the structure and emotional content of marital relationships (see p. 321). These studies followed observations of the statistical relationships of rheumatoid arthritis, obesity, and accidents with terminated marriage in males (49). Ramazzini, in his classic work on occupational disease published in 1700, related the high prevalence of breast cancer he observed among nuns to celibacy (50). Later studies of the relations of the extremes of celibacy and infertility found among nuns to breast cancer confirmed his observations. This line of observation has led during recent decades to strong hypotheses about the effect of the sex hormones on the incidence and course of breast cancer (see Chapters 3 and 6) (51).

With cancer of the neck of the uterus the lesser susceptibility of single women cast suspicion on a coital factor (see Chapter 3). With cancers of the body of the uterus and the ovary, as well as with cancer of the breast, the greater susceptibility of single women cast suspicion on hormonal factors related to reproduction (52,53). Subsequent studies have related some of these cancers to the varying hormonal states that occur with natural and artificial menopause, and have strengthened and elaborated the etiological hypotheses. Thus, risk factors for breast cancer include early menarche and a late beginning in childbearing. During the 1970s, cancers of the endometrium lining the body of the uterus were widely induced by the use of heavy doses of estrogens for the treatment and prevention of disorders connected with the menopause (53,54).

The prevalence of marriage

Marriage is so closely bound up with other economic and social relations that an observed change in marital behavior, for instance a change in the ages at which people marry, can only be interpreted against the interplay of many other social factors.

Table 10.2 Percentages of men and women never married: selected age-groups for several countries

		Men		Women	
		20–24	45–49	20–24	45–49
Ireland	1979	81.6	24.2	66.3	14.8
Sweden	1981	95.0	12.8	84.8	7.1
Chile	1979	73.6	11.6	54.2	12.8
France	1980	74.3	10.8	51.4	7.3
United States	1982	72.0	5.4	53.4	4.1
United Kingdom	1981	74.8	8.9	53.7	5.7
India	1971	50.2	2.9	9.1	0.4
Japan	1980	91.5	3.1	77.7	4.4

Source: United Nations (1984). *Demographic Yearbook,* 1982, Special Topic: Marriage and Divorce Statistics, Table 24; and United Nations (1979). *Demographic Yearbook, Historical Supplement,* Table 11, New York.

The prevalence of marriage varies greatly between societies (see Table 10.2). Economic and social changes affect conjugal and familial relationships, and in turn such changes as age at marriage have repercussions throughout society. Moreover, the patterns of conjugal and familial behavior differ in particular social contexts, and these influence the developmental cycles of individual families, with consequent effects on society as a whole. For instance, the age at which couples marry affects the likelihood of a stable union; the earlier the marriage the less stable it is likely to be. Age at marriage also affects the subsequent period of dispersion in the family's developmental cycle. Should a couple marry late, they will be well into middle age before their children begin to marry. Before all their children have married and left them, they may have reached old age, when material and physical resources are at a minimum (see Table 10.3). The immediate medical significance of a bride's age is largely that it affects her liability to certain disorders. Older brides, for instance, have a lower chance than younger ones of incurring cancer of the cervix uteri, probably because

Table 10.3 Median age of wife at selected stages of the life cycle of the American family, 1890–1970

Stages of family life cycle	Median age of wife				
	1890	1910	1930	1950	1970
First marriage	22.0	21.2	21.4	20.1	21.2
Birth of last child	31.9	32.0	32.0	26.1	29.6
Marriage of last child	55.3	54.8	53.2	47.6	52.3
Death of one spouse	53.3	59.6	63.7	61.4	65.2

Source: Glick, P.C. (1955). The life cycle of the family, in *Marriage and Family Living,* Vol. 17, table 1, p. 4, National Council on Family Relations, Minneapolis; Glick, P. C. (1977). Updating the life cycle of the family, *Journal of Marriage and the Family, 39,* 5–12.

of later and less exposure to coitus and the associated factors. On the other hand, we have noted above that the later a bride has her first child, the higher is her liability to breast cancer (54).

In reproduction, the rise in absolute numbers of teenage pregnancies has aroused much medical and social concern. Biologically, the very young mother during gestation may compete with the nutrient needs of the growing fetus she is carrying, and some evidence supports the hypothesis that the effects may be adverse: very young mothers have an excess of premature infants. In the later teens young women are efficient in childbearing, and adverse effects arise chiefly from the adverse environment common to many young mothers. In the same way, the major effects of postnatal experience on the child of a young mother, as measured in terms of cognitive development, must be attributed not to the age of the mother alone, but to the social disadvantage associated with most teenage pregnancies. The isolated effect of maternal age on the mental performance of the child is only slight, and it is also linear; it increases year by year, with no effect special to teenagers (55). By contrast, elderly primiparae have been notorious for increased risks of prolonged and difficult labor and higher perinatal death rates (although the best modern obstetrics has largely eliminated this risk). They also have an increased risk, like all older mothers, of conception with the chromosomal anomaly trisomy 21, and consequently of Down's syndrome births in that third of such conceptions which survive to term (see Figure 10.2). In the mid-thirties, concurrent with a sharp rise in the frequency of all trisomies, maternal ability to sustain even a chromosomally normal conception to term declines and the spontaneous abortion rate for such conceptions rises almost as sharply (56). Older women have long been shown to have high risks of perinatal mortality in contrast with the favorable postnatal development of their children. They are also more likely to bear dizygous twins (57). If an older bride has many children—an uncommon occurrence in Britain today, but not in rural Ireland, for instance—convergence of late childbearing with high parity can be expected to multiply these risks. The greater risks apply mainly to women who bear children well over the age of 30, however, and these are only a small minority.

Age at marriage reflects social norms, and is related to the education, occupation, and social origin of couples. The size of the age differences between spouses also reflects social norms. Men have predominantly married women younger as well as less educated than themselves, a balance that has helped sustain male conjugal authority. The age difference has been narrowing during the course of the past century, as conjugal relations also have shifted towards greater equality (58). Education is a major factor in age at marriage: the more educated the later the marriage. In the United States the influence of occupation and career seems to be secondary to that of education. In Britain, occupation makes a strong contribution. Professional people tend to marry at a later age than manual workers, and farmers tend to marry later still. The age at which farmers and their wives marry today, however, can only be considered "late" in relation to the age at which their contemporaries of other occupations marry.

During the better part of this century, the trend was towards earlier marriage among people of all social origins. Of brides marrying for the first time in 1935 in

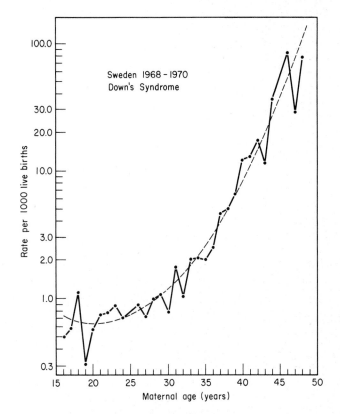

Figure 10.2 Rates of Down's syndrome per 1000 live births by maternal age. The bold line indicates observed rates; the broken line indicates values derived from the third-degree exponential equation in the 16–49 age range. Maternal ages are those at last birthday at time of delivery. *Source:* E.B. Hook, and A. Lindsjö, (1978). Down syndrome in live births by single year maternal age interval in a Swedish study: Comparison with results from a New York State study, *Amer. J. Hum. Genet., 30,* 19–27.

Britain, about 57 per cent were under 25 years of age, and in 1955 nearly one-third were under 21 years of age (59). By 1971, one man in ten and one woman in three married before the age of 20, a trend most marked in the less skilled classes. Forty per cent who married unskilled manual workers, and 4 per cent who married professionals, were teenagers (60). In the United States, between 1890 and 1970 the median age of marriages dropped from 22.0 years to 20.8 years for women, and from 26.1 to 23.2 years for men (61). This trend towards earlier marriage, and the concurrent trend towards staying longer at school, helped produce the phenomenon of the married student, and even the married schoolchild.

In recent years, the trend towards early marriage has reversed itself both in Britain and the United States. Table 10.4 shows the decline in the proportion of men and women married by age 25 in the United States between 1960 and 1975. Over the past decade the trend for women to defer marriage and childbearing is striking, particu-

Table 10.4 Percentage of the population never married, by age

	Women		Men	
Age	1960	1975	1960	1975
18	75.6	83.7	94.6	96.8
20	46.0	59.1	75.8	80.1
22	25.6	38.1	51.6	61.9
25	13.1	20.0	27.9	31.2

Source: Adapted from Sweet, J. A. (1977). Demography and the family *Ann. Rev. Sociol.*, 3, 371.

larly among the highly educated (62). The forces contributing to these trends in age at marriage are complex. They include the relative availability of male and female spouses; economic insecurity; education and preparation for career; the greater economic independence of women; their greater control over premarital fertility; and the change in ideology and norms about marriage. The so-called "new home economics model" interprets age at marriage and at childbearing as a manifestation of the relative earnings of young men, the potential earnings of young women, and the costs of their diversion to childrearing (63).

Many young persons marry before the husband has completed his training, whether in professional or skilled work, and the couple depend on the wife's earnings to balance their budget. These couples marry with no intention of starting a family immediately, and a period of abeyance ensues before the first child is born and the family enters its phase of expansion. In Britain this period of abeyance steadily increased during this century; its duration is connected with the husband's occupation and the family's social standing. The period is longer in small families than in large ones. In nonmanual workers' families, the median interval between marriage and first birth grew from 16.5 months among couples married in the year 1900–1909 to 22 months among the couples married between 1930–1934. During the same period, the

Table 10.5 Women married by age 30 who were still childless after two and three years of current marriage by the social class of their husbands, England and Wales (percentages).

	Duration of marriage (exact years)					
	A. Two years			B. Three years		
Social class of	Period of marriage			Period of marriage		
husband	1960–1964	1965–1968	1969–1971	1960–1964	1965–1968	1969–1971
Non-manual	55	59	68	38	43	49
Manual	40	40	44	27	25	30
All	46	48	54	31	32	37

Source: Adapted from Pearce, D., and Britton, M. (1977). The decline in births: Some socio-economic aspects, *Population Trends*, 7, 9–14.

interval in manual workers' families grew from 13.9 to 16.5 months. These trends continue, with the social differences persisting (see Table 10.5). In the United States, similar trends are expressed in the increase in childlessness for white women of the same age in successive cohorts, who are either voluntarily deferring childbearing, or perhaps choosing not to have children at all. Indeed, the birthrate has declined from a peak of 25.3 in 1957 to a rate of 15.5 per 1000 in 1983. Nonwhites have had a different pattern peaking in 1946 at 38.4, and declining to 21.6 in 1981. Rates of childlessness, probably involuntary, were high in cohorts earlier in this century, and are now declining (61,64).

On the other hand, a large number of young women are already pregnant when they marry and, indeed, their pregnancies accelerate marriage (60,64,65). In Britain, the proportion has declined sharply in recent years, especially in the higher social classes (see Table 10.6). Presumably women, having acquired better control over their own fertility, more often exercise it to bear children at a time that best suits them. Conversely, those young wives who are pregnant when they marry are often wholly dependent on the husband's earnings, or on support from relatives. In Britain few young couples conform with the Victorian ideal and delay marriage until they can achieve an independent home of their own; most, particularly those from the working-class, have been prepared to share a home, either in lodgings or with their relatives, until such time as they can achieve one of their own. In the United States, the pattern is different. While 9 per cent of all couples were without their own home at the peak of the housing shortage after the Second World War. In the 1970s this percentage declined, although it may again be rising.

The tendency to marry younger increased the prevalence of marriage in the population of industrial societies. In the United States in the year 1900, two out of three women in the total population had been married at some time in their lives; in 1963, this had increased to four out of five women. In 1963 only 8 per cent of the males and 6 per cent of the females were still single at the age of 40. These were peaks in the prevalence of marriage. Since then, as noted above, the rate of marriage has declined to the low levels prevalent at the end of the Great Depression of the 1930s. In 1960 the proportion of women aged 20 to 24 years who were still single reached the low level of 28 per cent; the average woman married at 20 years. By 1974 the proportion had jumped to 40 per cent, and the average woman married at 21 years (65).

Table 10.6   Percentage of all first births premaritally conceived, by social class of the father, 1970 and 1976, England and Wales

Year	Social class of father			
	I & II	III (non-manual)	III (manual)	IV & V
1970	13	18	28	37
1976	7	10	19	27

Source: Adapted from Office of Population Censuses and Surveys (1976). Birth Statistics, Series FM 1, H.M.S.O., London, Table 11.2.

The popularity of marriage—the prevalence or proportion married in the population as a whole—has been maintained by a number of factors in the face of the declining rate of marriage in the past decade. The changing demographic structure of populations dictates that marriage rates and patterns of mate selection cannot remain stable for long. Both the numbers of eligible males and nubile females and their age distributions and personal and social characteristics change as rates of birth and survival change. Changes in rates of marriage, in ages at marriage, and in acceptability of marriage partners follow demographic opportunity (66). Because of the alteration in the age-structure of the population during this century, there is now a greater proportion of marriageable adults, while at the time the sex ratio among them has moved towards equality. Throughout the past century, women outnumbered men in the reproductive age-group, that is, between the ages of 15 and 44, but this excess of women has fallen over the years. In Britain in 1870, for instance, there were 10 per cent more women than men of reproductive age, whereas by 1951 this excess amounted to only 3 per cent (59). In the 1960s, for the first time, improved survival allowed the excess of males at birth to persist into adulthood. By 1975, the male excess persisted into middle age (60).

Such shifts in the adult sex ratio are bound to have repercussions on courtship, marriage, and sex relations generally. Moreover, persons of both sexes and from all social classes now enjoy greater opportunities to meet and marry. To illustrate, the root of the Victorian problem of "redundant women" lay in the great number of spinsters deprived of the chance to marry. Mortality and emigration reduced the number of marriageable men more than women, and social, ethnic, and geographic factors circumscribed choice. Problems of imbalance of the sexes arise at different times within different social groups, and are adapted to in different ways. In the United States, the high frequency of single mothers and female headed families among lower-class blacks is in part a matter of the numerical deficiency of males. A demographic "marriage squeeze" may result in deferred or less frequent marriage, or in the choice of spouses outside the usual age ranges (66).

The rising chances of marriage may well have an uneven impact on the various types of person who have medical disabilities that are likely to restrict their entry into marriage (67). Physical handicaps and chronic diseases have acted to diminish marriage chances, but owing to the overall greater chance of marriage, more handicapped people are likely to marry. Some of the social institutions devised to help handicapped people, such as social clubs, also enable them to meet each other and so promote marriages within the group. In conditions such as diabetes and mental deficiency, these trends have raised fears of increasing their incidence because of the genetic component in their etiology (68). Concern might be justified with recessive genes of high penetrance that accounted for much of the variance in a disorder; in diabetes at least these circumstances have not been shown to hold. Persons suffering from schizophrenia are a special case. Their reduced expectation of marriage is more likely to persist than in other chronic disabilities because of the disorder of personality that causes the afflicted persons to withdraw from society and to select an occupation and mode of life conducive to social isolation.

The overall rate of admissions to hospitals and institutions is affected by the prevalence of marriage (see Table 10.1). To some extent the preponderance of unmarried persons found in institutions may be connected, in the younger age-groups, with types of sickness that have a selective impact on the unmarried; this results both in higher admission rates and in seclusion from relationships that lead to marriage. But much of this preponderance is caused by the dependence upon others of the sick and the old, and the relative lack of social support available to them. In contemporary society the elementary family is the critical resource. Widows, for instance, turn to their children for help far more often than they do to other kin (69). The availability of spouses and families with children, resulting from the larger number of marriages, strengthens family support for such dependent persons.

At the same time, marriages are likely to be put under strain by the obligations to provide this social support for dependents. In a selected population these relationships can be expressed statistically by a *dependency ratio*, which is the ratio of dependent to independent persons defined in various ways, for instance, the ratio of old, or young and old together, to the productive age-groups in between (70). In individual families this ratio becomes more favorable in the phase of expansion as the average number of children declines. It becomes less favorable in the phase of replacement as a smaller number of children is available to join in the support of aged parents and as parents live longer.

Divorce

The greater popularity of marriage increases the chances of divorce through exposure to the risk, and the divorce rates have risen both in Britain and the United States. There has also been an absolute increase. Changes in divorce laws—which like all major legislation express social and political movements—have had a powerful effect on trends. In Britain, civil divorce first became available in 1857, but before the Second World War the grounds were restricted and the costs were high. Divorce rates increased as the law was liberalized. After the Divorce Reform Act of 1969 in England and Wales, the divorce rate (per 1000 married population) doubled—from 6 to 11.8—between 1971 and 1982. Currently, in 60 percent of divorces, children under the age of 16 are involved. In the U. S. the crude divorce rate was 2.6 in 1950, 3.5 in 1970 and 5.2 per 1000 in 1980 (64,71,72).

However, the analysis of divorce rates is beset with difficulties. Problems of comparability and standardization at once arise when comparisons are drawn between societies, or over time. Even between states in the United States, the legal grounds for divorce vary greatly and so, too, have their divorce rates and the divorce-seeking population they attracted or repelled. Published figures usually deal with marriages and not with individuals. In every population, especially where divorce is permitted, there are more marriages than couples. Two people may have several marriages between them; in polygamous societies one person may be a partner in several simultaneous marriages. A further difficulty lies in choosing a suitable denominator for the divorced population, for whereas numerators taken from registration data (and gathered over time) are usually accurate, denominators taken from census questionnaires (at a point in time) are less so. An accurate rate might best be calculated from completed cohorts of marriages in which the union has come to an end, but such data are not easily collected, nor always relevant to a changing current situation. A denominator based on uncompleted unions can be biased in many ways, particularly because the potential risk of divorce must vary with the frequency and the duration of marriage; these characteristics of marriages change as ages at marriage and death change. The longer a marriage lasts, the more opportunity there is for divorce: "divorce is replacing the undertaker."

In Britain the prevalence of divorce rose from 0.05 per 1000 existing marriages in 1914 to 2.6 in 1951 and 11.8 in 1981. In the United States divorce rates rose from 1.2 per 1000 existing marriages in 1860 to 4.0 in 1900 to 8.7 in 1940; then, after a peak in the aftermath of the Second World War, and a stable rate of about 10 per 1000 through the 1950s, the rate rose sharply from the mid-1960s to reach 22.8 in 1979 (see Figure 10.3, Table 10.7). In the United States a reasonable estimate of the proportion of a marriage cohort of the early 1970s divorcing is about two out of five (i.e., between 40 and 45 per cent); about one out of five marriages contracted in 1972 in the United States ended in divorce by 1977 (72). This indicates disillusionment with specific marriages and by no means with marriage in general. A great and increasing proportion of divorced persons in Britain and the United States remarry (three-fourths

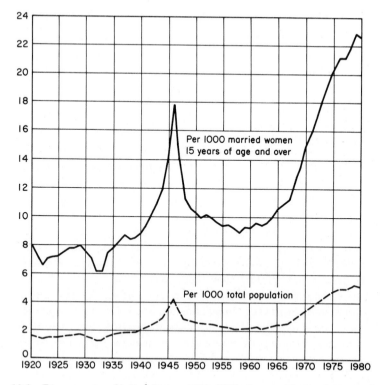

Figure 10.3 Divorce rates: United States, 1920–1980. *Source:* National Center for Health Statistics (1983). *Monthly Vital Statistics Report*, vol. 32, No. 3, Supplement, p. 1.

Table 10.7 Proportions (per 1000) of birth cohorts who had divorced by selected ages in England and Wales

Cohort[a]	Age (exact years)			
	25	30	40	50
Males				
1926	3	17	49	93
1936	2	20	100	
1946	8	68		
1952	21			
Females				
1926	9	29	58	95
1936	7	31	103	
1946	20	95		
1952	43			

[a]This represents an approximation to the year of birth of each generation.

Source: Adapted from Nissel, M. (1982). Families and social changes since the Second World War, in *Families in Britain*, ed., Rapoport, R. N., Fogarty, M. P., and Rapoport, R., London, p. 108.

of the women and five-sixths of the men), and the evidence suggests that most people who dissolve their marriages do so with the intention of remarriage. As we noted above, the rate of marriage for divorced persons is higher than for their single or widowed age-peers. In a sense, the contemporary adult population is "permanently available" for marriage, whether or not they are married (73,74).

Divorce rates in the United States are higher than anywhere else. These high rates do not necessarily indicate that marriage is less "successful" than in countries like Spain, where divorce is illegal. In 1975, 84 per cent of all families were married couples, and in these families seven out of eight husbands were in their first marriage. Indeed, despite the higher chances of divorce in the subsequent marriages of divorced persons, the divorce of unhappy couples is succeeded by as good a chance of a marriage rated satisfactory by the partners as are first marriages (75,76). The failure of a marriage sometimes rests with the marital aptitude of one partner, in which case the other partner might do well a second time; or the failure may rest with incompatibility and poor "teamwork" generated by the interaction unique to the particular couple, in which case both partners might do well a second time.

Simple measurements of the complex phenomenon of marriage happiness are difficult but feasible to obtain. In selected studies as many as 60 to 85 per cent of couples rate themselves as "very happy," and usually less than 5 per cent as "not too happy" (77). Several studies of remarriage after divorce have obtained similar results (75,76). Some people with poor marital aptitude seem to be "divorce prone," and others do not remarry; their removal from the universe of married people doubtless improves the average level of happiness and adjustment. One study estimated that about one-third of divorcées had repeated divorces (76). Persons who are divorce prone compound the divorce rates. Their pattern of marriage has been called "sequential polygamy" or "serial monogamy."

Within societies, the rates of divorce vary with age at marriage, the duration and fertility of marriage, social class and education, homogamy or the concordance of couples in age, health, and ethnic group, the stability of the parental marriage, and other factors (78). For example, in Britain today, the younger and less educated the bride, the greater her risk of divorce (See Table 10.8). In the early 1970s, the proportion of divorcing couples who were childless (childlessness included couples who had surviving children of 16 years or more) ranged around 40 per cent. Thus dependent children are involved in about 60 per cent of divorces. The trend towards a greater frequency of divorce after fewer years of marriage may cause this proportion to decline, since the interval from marriage to first birth has been on the rise. In the United States, the rates of divorce have been highest among teenagers and decline with age; black couples differ from this pattern, and divorce among them reaches a peak in the late twenties and then declines. Divorce occurs predominantly in the earlier years of marriage; about one-third of all divorces occur in the first 5 years, and almost two-thirds in the first 10 years. As in Britain in the 1960s, about 40 per cent of all dissolved marriages were childless. Both the proportion and the number of children involved in divorces have risen proportionately with the steep rise in divorce rates (see Figure 10.4). By 1974, only 25 per cent of dissolved marriages were childless (79).

As the number of children involved in divorces has increased, so the single-parent family unit has emerged on an increasing scale. In Great Britain in 1976, 750,000 one-parent families existed and comprised 6.3 per cent of all households. They included more than a million children, and about one-tenth of all families with children. Only one out of eight such parents was a father. Two-thirds of one-parent families were the consequences of marriage break-up. Thus, of the 660,000 female-headed households, 415,000 were separated or divorced, 115,000 widowed, and 130,000 single (80). In the United States in 1981, nearly 1.2 million children joined the ranks of those living with a currently divorced mother or father; this brings the total to over 5 million, or 9 per cent of all children under 18. Between 1970 and 1982, the number of single-parent households in the United States doubled, to reach 6.5 million. Currently, 13.7 million children live with one parent—half of all black children and one-sixth of all white children. In 90 per cent of all cases, the parent is the mother. Although divorce or separation remains the usual antecedent of single-parent households, in recent years the number of never-married mothers has grown mark-

Table 10.8   Divorce per 100 marriages of up to 15 years duration by age of woman at marriage

	Under 20	20–24	25–29	30–34
	33	19	13	11

Source: Office of Population Censuses and Surveys (1978). *Demographic Review*, Series DR. no. 1, H.M.S.O., London, p. 61.

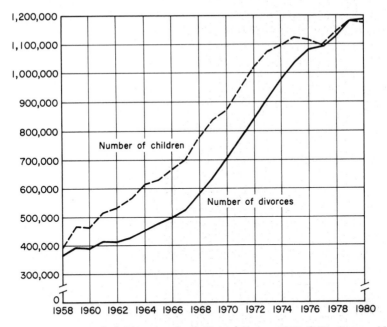

Figure 10.4 Divorces and children involved: United States, 1958–1980. *Source:* National Center for Health Statistics (1983). *Monthly Vital Statistics Report,* vol. 32, No. 3, Supplement, p. 2.

edly, from 527,000 in 1970 to 1.8 million in 1981; they now account for 16 percent of all children living with mother only (81).

We can anticipate characteristic difficulties: social, psychological, and medical, among broken families (see pp. 452–456). The extent of this problem should not be exaggerated, however, despite the number of persons involved. The decline in birth and death rates that has altered the age-structure of the population during this century has also preserved existing couples and, because women have superior chances of survival, has cut the proportion of widows in the middle ranges of life while producing more widows in the older age-range. Thus in 1982 some 75 per cent of young Americans under 18 years of age lived with both parents, and the facts point to the essential stability of marriages, especially of those contracted after the woman has passed her teens (81). As noted above, the proportion of mothers who do not marry and form single-parent households more than doubled in the 1970s. They are concentrated among the poor in black ghettos. In 1982, such households constituted 47 per cent of all families living below the poverty level, and 70 per cent of all poor black families.

Such statistics should not be crudely interpreted. The majority of black families cleave to the United States norm of the complete nuclear family. Poor housing in urban black ghettos, high rates of unemployment among males, and their deficient number relative to women ensure the dependency of women with children on welfare. For women in such circumstances, marriage often carries no advantage even when they have a steady relationship with a man; welfare is not paid where there is "a man in the house." Many adopt a domestic economy that rests on a form of social exchange between networks of female kin and friends who provide the emergency supports essential to family survival and childrearing. The female kin of a father often maintain a proprietary interest in his child; and even if he is separated from his child, he too may continue his interest and support (82).

In the broad picture, these adaptations are societal rather than racial or ethnic. "Black matriarchy" is largely a demographic notion, and indicates that a large number of black households are headed by a woman who is a single parent. Yet this is a function of a socioeconomic situation: in southern states of the United States over the last three decades, for instance, the *proportionate* increase of white and black female-headed households of the same social class was equivalent. Matriarchy also denotes a form of social relations, that is, authority and influence of the mother in family affairs, and here survey data on decision-making within families point to no remarkable differences between whites and blacks of the same social classes (83).

Conjugal roles

Marriage is bound up with legitimacy, property, and inheritance, and in most societies it has been a union that, unlike other contracts, cannot be terminated by agreement. The forms and conventions of marriage in each society are entangled in a web of legal, customary, and religious rules and regulations. Even within the United Kingdom the legal requirements for marriage differ among Scotland and England and Wales; in the United States they differ among the 50 states. Other industrial societies each have their own conventions. The web of law and custom interwoven with the marital bond subjects the individual relations between spouses to control by external forces. The relationship is not the private concern the marriage partners may believe it to be. Marriage is the institutional relationship that ensures physical and social reproduction; each marriage becomes the concern of the whole society, as represented by the state or church. Every marriage also involves the family of origin of each spouse through the relationship of in-laws, and both families of origin have an equal interest in the offspring of the new union (84).

The personal attributes of marriage partners are therefore not the sole determinants of their conjugal behavior. Customary expectations of behavior, the structure of social networks, and the occupations of both spouses enter into the relationship. Their relations with each other must adapt also to the new duties and obligations that arise in successive phases of the developmental cycle of the family they have founded. Further adaptation is required to the form of the institution of marriage in our society. This evolution is connected with changes in the social status and activities of women. Conjugal roles are one aspect of the general division of labor in society, and they are related to productive and economic activities as well as to reproduction (85).

In preindustrial Britain, as in contemporary preindustrial societies, the conjugal roles of men and women were kept distinct. The distinctions were believed to inhere in the "nature" of male and female. The wife was a housekeeper and breeder of children and the husband the provider for the family. In contemporary tribal societies that observe this segregation of roles, the activities monopolized by one sex are often forbidden to the other. Taboos on persons of one sex performing the duties of the other are one mode of enforcing conformity with these rules. Some African peoples who use both the axe and the hoe in cultivation forbid women to use the axe; this rule has had serious consequences when many of the men are withdrawn from the tribe as migrant laborers (86). The productive cycle cannot then be completed, and certain decisions that are the husband's prerogative cannot be made. In his absence, a mother of even a desperately ill child may not be able to accept a doctor's urging to admit her child to a hospital.

Women in the early nineteenth century were excluded by law from certain forms of industrial and other employment, sometimes on humane grounds as in coal mining, but sometimes to control competition with men in a society where unemployment was a constant threat. At that time, many of the tasks performed by men were physically arduous and unsuited to women. However, machines have reduced the importance of physical strength in many occupations, and other new occupations exist that were unknown in the past and have no traditional alliance with one sex (87). The physical differences between the sexes are therefore less important in the division of labor. Only men were strong enough to pilot the first airplanes, but in jet aircraft servomechanisms render physical strength unnecessary.

The rapid development of productive and economic resources transformed the traditional roles of women. In the middle of the nineteenth century, common law regarded husband and wife as one person, and society vested the husband with complete authority over his wife and children, who were treated as his inferiors and dependents. Thereafter, legislation curtailed the husband's authority and improved the position of the wife. Wives gradually acquired the right to their own property, as well as further legal rights in relation to husband and children.

During this same period, the rights of children to be protected from the cruelty or neglect of their parents have been continuously extended, and at present the community, acting through the state, can withdraw children from their families if they appear to be in need of care and protection (88). The contemporary family is distinguished by the legal equality of husband and wife and by limitations on the authority parents have over their children, who now possess enforceable rights against their parents.

The legal improvements in the marital status of women accompanied other changes in their social position, such as the right to vote and to take up work formerly monopolized by men. Cheap and effective methods of birth control liberated women from the burden of constant childbearing and allowed them to emerge as rivals to men in the productive and economic spheres. Men and women have also changed their expectations of marriage. Romantic love has come to be thought a necessary foundation for marriage, and the union is expected to provide equal satisfactions for both partners. These ideas helped create a demand for the legal dissolution of marriages that do not fulfill these expectations. In recent years consensual unions, other experiments in cohabitation without benefit of marriage, and single-parent households have become more acceptable modes in higher as well as lower social classes. Such nonlegal unions, however, are often the preliminary to marriage; *de facto*, marriage can be said to continue as before (see Tables 10.9, 10.10).

The social advance of women appears in the kind of work they do as well as in

Table 10.9 Percentages of women married, and living with men outside of marriage, by age: Denmark, France, Great Britain, Norway, and the United States, 1975–1978.

Country and year	Age					
	Total	<20	20–24	25–29	30–34	35–44
Denmark (1975)						
Married	70	7	38	78	82	91
Cohabiting	12	23	30	10	5	4
France (1978)						
Married	79	u[a]	56.7	79.8	85.1	88.2
Cohabiting	5	u	10.4	5.6	4.2	1.8
Great Britain (1976)						
Married	70	8.5	49.0	81.0	87.0	
Cohabiting	2	0.5	2.3	3.0	2.0	
Norway (1977)						
Married	71	8.4	44.8	81.3	87.4	86.6
Cohabiting	5	5.6	12.2	4.5	2.4	1.8
United States (1977)						
Married	69	8.6	46.1	70.2	75.3	77.3
Cohabiting	1	0.2	1.8	1.7	1.0	0.6

[a]u = unavailable.

Source: Leridon, H. (1981). Fertility and contraception in 12 developed countries, *Family Planning Perspectives, 13,* 93–102.

their conjugal rights. While the numbers working as domestics and in textile factories have declined, the numbers in offices and factories of other kinds have risen (89,90). Many more women have entered professions and business management. These achievements have made more of a reality, in this century, of the personal and legal rights gained by women in the last, and at no sensible cost to marriage happiness. As measured by a balanced scale of tensions and satisfactions, except when there are preschool children, marriage happiness is high among couples where the wife works by choice. It is less so where she works out of economic need (91,92).

Francis Bacon defined women as the adjuncts of men when he wrote: "Wives are young men's mistresses, companions for middle-age, and old men's nurses." While they may still perform these roles with less than full reciprocity, in many marriages they assume independent roles as wage-earners and career women. Stage in the fam-

Table 10.10 Percentages of women who have ever lived with men outside marriage, by age at the time of survey: France and Norway

Country (year)	Age					
	Total	18–19	20–24	25–29	30–34	35–44
France (1978)	14	u	23	21	14	7
Norway (1977)	24	10	35	30	20	15

Source: Leridon, H. (1981). Fertility and contraception in 12 developed countries, *Family Planning Perspectives, 13,* 93–102.

ily cycle is a determinant of women's employment outside the home (93). Most women now work before marriage, and as families have grown smaller, more and more return to work after marriage. In Britain in 1951, 21.7 per cent of women were in any kind of employment; in 1971, the proportion had doubled, to 42.2 per cent; and by 1981 more than half were estimated to be at work. In the United States in 1981 one out of three of all married women were at work (one of two among non-whites). The rate for 1900 had more than doubled by 1940, and doubled again by 1960. In 1940 married women made up less than one-third of the female work force in the United States; by the 1970s, almost two-thirds (89). Although about one-third of married women work part-time, the trend is towards working full-time. These changes have raised median family income in the United States, as the average number of paychecks per family has risen.

The modern married woman's return to nondomestic employment has profound effects on the family order. One British classification of "dual-worker families" identifies three types; a "non-career" family, in which both partners are employed in semiskilled or unskilled jobs; a "one-career" family, in which one partner has a "career" while the other holds a "non-career" job; and a dual-career family, in which both partners have careers (92,94). Married women give one or several of five main reasons for going to work: to earn; to gain social contacts; to escape domestic confinement; to establish a personal identity; to practice a skill for its intrinsic rewards. The great majority of mothers of preschool children do not work, but the proportion of mothers who do work rises steadily with the age of their children (Table 10.11). Those who remain at work throughout tend to be at social extremes, either poor and deprived or professional.

A benefit of the advance in women's status may be better mental health (95). A unique twenty year follow-up in the 1970s of the "Midtown Manhattan" prevalence survey of mental impairment of the 1950s found significant improvement in mental health measures over time. The whole of the improvement occurred among the women of the sample. Younger cohorts had less impairment than older cohorts had had at the same age. Attrition of the sample at follow-up opens this result to potential bias and some studies do not support it. Thus there was no decline of self-reported psychophysiological symptoms among women in national samples surveyed between the 1950s and 1970s (96). Yet there has been over that period a distinct convergence in the frequency of symptoms reported by men and women, which indicates at the least a relative improvement for women. The factors of marital state, number of young children, and level of education seem not to account for the improvement in women relative to men. Employment outside the home, however, does account in some degree—in an analysis of five separate surveys—for their convergence with men (97).

Yet the ability of women to exercise their rights is limited by their reproductive function, by resistance on the part of men to their entry to certain occupations, and by the persistence of traditional attitudes and values. During the period of fertility, even those wives trained for professional or other high-status occupations are often dependent economically on their husbands. In many occupations women are still struggling for equal pay. In the United States between 1962 and 1973, women kept

Table 10.11   Working mothers with children in Great Britain in 1978:
Percentage distribution by age of children

Mother's paid work	Children's age in years			
	0–2	3–4	5–9	10–15
None	79	69	52	36
Part-time	16	25	37	42
Full-time	5	6	11	22
	100	100	100	100

Source: Adapted from Nissel, M. (1982). Families and social change since the Second World War, in *Families in Britain*, ed. Rapoport, R. N., Fogarty, M. P., and Rapoport, R., London, p. 101.

pace with men in gaining access to education and occupation, but fell behind in earnings (98). Men dominate the skilled occupations, the professions, and positions of power and authority generally. Of the 2,200,000 "managers, officials, and proprietors" listed by the United States Census of 1960 as earning $10,000 a year or more, 2½ per cent were female. Seven per cent of American doctors were women. Even so, men and women are adjusting traditional attitudes and expectations where they no longer conform with new productive, social, and cultural developments. The Census data of 1980, while not strictly comparable because of shifts in listed occupational categories, indicate relative improvement for women but continuing male dominance: 7,209,661 men and 3,168,857 women were listed as "executive, administrators and managerial occupations." The average salary for men was $25,000; for women it was $12,000. Existing patterns of conjugal roles reflect the evolution of these adjustments in the various segments of contemporary society. New and traditional forms coexist, unevenly distributed across social groups.

Conjugal roles have been described as ranging between two extreme types (99). In Britain and the United States, the structure and forms of these marital relationships show regularities across the social classes and they seem typical of the extremes in those developed societies (100). At one extreme are partners with *segregated conjugal roles*, marriages in which husband and wife each have specific household tasks and familial responsibilities, and neither performs the duties of the other. They also pursue divergent leisure interests, each with companions of their own sex. At the other extreme are partners with *joint conjugal roles*, marriages in which husband and wife aim to share domestic tasks and familial responsibilities equally. They also share common leisure interests, and interact with the same persons outside the family.

The wife in segregated-role families is responsible for maintaining the home, and for cooking, shopping, and the day-to-day care of the children; in Britain she often takes responsibility for the regular payment for food, rent, municipal rates and taxes, fuel, and light (101). The wife's social network in these families is often comprised of a small number of female relatives and neighbors. The husband is responsible for providing his wife with housekeeping money and for the more arduous repairs to the home. He exercises final authority over the children, but is kept in reserve as a threat and appealed to only in the last resort; the punishment he deals out is more severe.

The husband follows his own leisure interests with male companions, who may or may not be known to his wife. The couple rarely entertains anyone at home, apart from relatives. In these segregated-role families a man is a "good" husband if he is steady and reliable and provides his wife with a regular fixed amount for housekeeping, so that she can budget properly and fulfil her conjugal role (102).

Couples with segregated roles usually have a modest estimate of the sexual satisfactions to be obtained from marriage (102, 103). Working-class women in particular see sex as an aspect of marriage perhaps less important than material security and the rearing of healthy children. In such families acknowledged sexual difficulties appear as an infrequent cause of broken marriages. The segregation of male and female roles and social activities is so marked, however, that the object of any friendship between a spouse and someone of the opposite sex is quickly assumed to be sexual.

The economic dominance of the husband in segregated-role families restricts the wife's choices. A wife with young children who finds herself unhappily married will put up with a great deal before taking the serious step of leaving the home, particularly in those industrial areas where work for unskilled married women is scarce. Unless she is willing to abandon her children, her only recourse may be to fall back on her own family of origin, and put the burden on them of supporting another family. Separation or divorce has been a last resort in intolerable circumstances, and it may be deferred until the children have grown up. In many working-class neighborhoods traditional values support modest expectations of personal happiness: woman's place is in the home and man's at work.

In some cases, where work is to be had for women but not for men, the economic dominance of men is undermined. In the ghettos of North American cities and in Hispanic-American slums, the reversal of the traditional situation appears also to undermine the stability of conjugal unions (104). As noted above, among the poorest families an unusual proportion have no man in the house, and mothers may form a succession of unstable unions with no legal ties. But in many places customary sanctions still operate to maintain segregated roles, especially where the economy allows the traditional division of labor between husband and wife to persist, as in rural Ireland, Wales, and Scotland, and in the southern United States. Even there, the mechanization of farming has changed traditional working roles, although conjugal roles may take longer to change. Where segregated roles are common, the external sanction of ridicule may sustain the traditional forms. An English working-class husband may carry out the housework and prepare the meals, and even wash the family's clothes in a time of family crisis such as illness of the wife. But he does not reveal these activities to neighbors, and so will rarely hang out washing or wheel a baby carriage.

Some American sample surveys of recent years suggest that the extreme segregated-role family is relatively uncommon. The prevalence of highly segregated roles has been in evident decline as women have taken up work outside the family, gained greater independence, and limited the extent of male prerogatives. Durkheim contended that exaggerated male and female roles and sharp divisions between men and women strengthened the bonds of marriage (105). In line with this hypothesis, rising divorce rates may reflect the decline of segregated-role marriages. In Britain the poorest classes have a rising divorce rate, and in the United States their rates exceed those of other classes (60,106). Segregated roles are not confined to the poor, however, and have been found in the marriages of even the wealthiest classes. A common pattern among the managerial classes is for husband and wife to segregate their domestic roles, but to share family decision-making and social relationships (107).

In families with joint conjugal roles, domestic and family responsibilities are shared. Both husband and wife cook, wash dishes, and undertake shopping, houskeeping duties, and day-to-day management of the children. They often have a common purse and the wife knows how much her husband earns; they have an equal voice in expenditure and in important family decisions. These couples are often self-conscious about the way they rear their children, and share the tasks of training and discipline. They also share leisure interests, and spend time together with friends of both sexes. They entertain friends at home but may be distant towards neighbors. Sexual relations are felt to be of crucial importance for the success of the marriage; each partner considers the enjoyment of the other to be almost a moral obligation. This attitude brings its own problems, for failure to achieve the high standards that are set becomes a personal failure. Sexual dissatisfactions have been found to be much more closely correlated with marital unhappiness in joint- than in segregated-role marriages (103).

The potential economic independence of the wife will play a great part in deciding how spouses perform their conjugal roles (108). Hence, both joint and segregated roles are found among working-class families and among middle-class families, but the lower economic status of women in general, and their necessary reproductive functions, make complete joint roles an ideal that can be achieved by few, as when couples have no children, or when the children are grown. Joint roles are likeliest where couples have equal education and occupational levels, especially if their occupations have high status and the wife also works. Where both partners have a professional occupation, for example, and the wife has potential economic independence, she is in a position to insist that the husband share household tasks and treat her as an equal. If the marriage is unhappy, the wife is more able to leave the home and to support herself and her children in an independent household. In the working-class, too, where both men and women can find jobs and earn relatively well—as was the case in the old textile towns of the North of England—a tendency towards joint conjugal roles has been found. Many women are far from agreeing that an equality or even a symmetry of domestic roles has been achieved (109).

Joint- and segregated-role marriages are extreme types, and most families will be intermediate, with a bias towards one or the other according to the concordance of partners in occupation and education, their external social environment, and the phase they have reached in the developmental cycle. A great variety of household and social routines exist. Hours of work obviously affect the domestic, recreational, and sexual aspects of married life. Not all men and women work on the day shift, and others may be away from home for days or weeks at a time. Spouses must therefore adjust the household routine to the necessities of employment.

In the small families now common to all social classes, the phase of independence in the cycle of family development takes on new significance to which conjugal roles must adjust. At the beginning of a marriage, husband and wife of all social classes tend to share household and leisure activities together (99). During the phase of expansion, roles are necessarily segregated to some degree by the wife's reproductive and maternal functions. Thereafter, roles may or may not become joint, according to whether the wife is able and willing to take up work outside the home, and according to the status and pay of this work in relation to that of her husband. The elements of personal choice and values may cut across these social considerations.

There are no good grounds for considering the educated ideal of joint conjugal-role marriage and its accompanying life style as more "normal" than any other. Professional judgments are liable to the traps of the sociocentric or ethnocentric predicament. Yet the distinctive conjugal roles of husbands and wives are a potential source of the differences in the mental health of married men and women. In general, married men have had lower rates of treated disorder or symptoms than married women, in particular for depression and neurosis (110). The pattern of depressive symptoms has been found to hold for marriages with a traditional division of labor, of the kind found with segregated roles. In marriages with the "nontraditional" division of labor found with joint roles, however, married men exhibited more depressive symptoms than women did (111).

Marriage and kinship

Marriage establishes the legal independence of the partners. At the same time, in industrial societies, the couple also seeks to establish an independent household. Like births and deaths, marriages disturb existing social relationships and create new ones. For the conjugal relationship at once turns families of origin into in-laws. Residential arrangements give a spatial expression to these social relationships, and through ties of descent and marriage each elementary family therefore becomes kin to a wider circle of persons. Kinship is ascribed, but not the content of the interaction in terms of kinship, which in developed societies is variable, as adults can choose in the matter. The structure and content of these relationships form a kinship system.

The type of kinship extant in any society is determined in the first place by the recognized mode of reckoning descent. "Descent" here refers to a social and not a biological relationship, for these are not necessarily conterminous. The kinship system in Britain and the United States is bilateral, in that descent is traced in both the male and female lines, although children with few exceptions take their father's name.

As each person has four grandparents, eight great-grandparents, and sixteen great-great-grandparents, which takes us back only four generations, there is a practical limit to the extent of recognized kin relationships. Rules of descent define the degrees of relationship within which marriage is forbidden, and regulate the inheritance of property. In industrial society restrictions on marrying relatives are lax, and most people are unconcerned with fixed inheritance of titles and land. As a result, few need to trace genealogies over the generations. Many do not know the maiden names and place of birth of their two grandmothers, let alone the names and places of birth of their eight great-grandparents. For that minority of persons who own much fixed property, genealogies are sometimes recorded, and their descent may be traced in theory, but usually one line only is selected and collateral lines ignored.

Consequently, the kinship system of developed societies is both shallow in depth and narrow in range. Since biologically all human beings are descended in the same way, the variability, and indeed the reality, of different kinship systems consists in the relationships between individuals that each society constrains them to recognize. Appropriate behavior is regulated by law, by social norms, and by customary usage. Industrial society has few defined and enforceable patterns of behavior for relationships other than those within the elementary family. This narrow kinship system is reflected in the paucity of terms for relatives in comparison with other societies. Terms are limited to father, mother, son, daughter, cousin, uncle, aunt, grandmother, grandfather, grandchild. The term "uncle" fails to distinguish between a father's brother and a mother's brother, and cousins are distinguished only by giving them a place according to the degree of relationship, first cousin, second cousin, and so on. The term "in-law" must suffice to describe the members of the family of origin of either spouse.

Kinship ties may be a source of conflict as well as support. This ambivalence is illustrated by the widespread avoidance customs between spouses and in-laws of the opposite sex, and between in-laws of the parental generation. These realistic arrangements recognize points of potential division within a marriage and between families. Thus a reality underlying many traditional jokes is a relationship loaded with tension between husband and mother-in-law. A married woman has dual roles, in her statuses as wife and daughter; daughter and mother may form a united front, as it were, in opposition to the husband. Hence the old jokes about "going home to mother." At the same time, a wife competes with her husband's mother for his love and support. In industrial society, these sources of conflict are implicitly recognized. Ideals of family love and harmony prevail, although they are incapable of being fully realized. The religious and moral emphasis placed on love and tolerance is society's alternate mode of containing conflict and hostility.

Tribal societies recognize and regulate by custom many areas of conflict, although they share the ideal of family harmony (112). Thus the Tallensi of West Africa have had rituals to control competition between parents and children (113). Rivalry for land, cattle, and women among the males of a family is common and accepted. In our society there are many fields of social relations external to the family, such as factories, political parties, churches, and recreational clubs, in which each person can establish an independent status. Hence, sons and fathers rarely compete directly for jobs, land, or money, and latent antagonisms are therefore not expressed in rivalry over these things. Disputes within the family relate instead to personal growth and development. These disputes are not seen as having social import outside the elementary family, and so they are not openly recognized, except by outsiders and "caretakers" of the family. The expression and resolution of disputes are different from one social class to another. In English working-class families, critical comments of parents, particularly of the mother, tend to be played down, whereas higher-class families are less hesitant in voicing their criticism, even to outsiders. In some working-class families, on the other hand, open discord is expressed in angry rows and perhaps in physical violence (114); professional families are likely to express discord less openly.

Although in industrial society only the kin ties and obligations within the elementary family have legal force, people maintain and use wider connections. These relations between extra-familial kin are primarily social: members visit one another; attend christenings, weddings, funerals, and other critical episodes in the life course; give one another mutual aid and support; and feel moral obligations towards one another. But since their kin relationships are not essential to the economic and legal systems, they can be permissive and vary widely within the same society or social group (115).

A high degree of social interaction with kin is commonly found among those families who have close-knit, contained social networks. Kinship relations outside the elementary family in industrial society satisfy needs and purposes different from those in tribal societies, where they are meshed with almost all other social relations. Extra-familial kin relationships in tribal societies have jural, political, economic, ritual, and other functions that are quite distinct from domestic relations. In some tribal societies, the largest political unit embraces a group of people, all of whom are united by recognized kinship, so that social and kinship organization are almost the same thing (116). In the *extended family*, two or more lineally related kinsfolk of the same sex, and their spouses and offspring, are all jointly subject to the same authority or single head, although each family may have a separate household. Disputes between members can be settled by submitting them to the recognized authority of the formal head (117).

In developed societies the irreducible minimum of the elementary family of two generations comprises the extent of legally enforceable relationships based on descent and kinship (118). Industrial organization, with its specialization of labor and a multitide of institutions and associations, is not compatible with a wide range of enforceable obligations of kinship outside the elementary family. The accident of birth is not supposed to determine the relations of a class society, although it may often do so. Both people and capital must be free to move, and to enter and fulfil contractual relationships.

Some households are composite and consist of three generations, while other elementary families in independent households have kinsfolk living in their neighborhood, particularly those families that have arisen from circumscribed marriages in stable communities. In composite households authority over the nonadult children remains formally in the hands of their parents. A young wife is under no legal obligation to take the advice or submit to the authority of a mother or mother-in-law in the rearing of her own children, and more likely will resent interference. Conversely, in composite households where widowed or separated parents reside with one of their married children, the parent is dependent on the child's goodwill. Divergent directions and degrees of social mobility decrease social interaction between kin and encourage dispersed, rather than contained, social networks. Among families without property, extra-familial kin relations that extend beyond the elementary family are usually centered on living parents. When these parents die, unless the adult members of an elementary family are bound together by common interest—for instance, in a title or estate, or in a business or farm—there is little to hold the adult siblings together.

Thus, the elementary family remains the basic kinship unit in developed societies, and the economic and social system is built on its reproductive functions and on the specialized work of individuals. In the absence of property, each elementary family carries within it the seeds of its own destruction. Mother, father, and children all have loyalties to different elementary families; the children to the one their parents have founded, and each parent to his or her own family of origin. As the children become adult and independent, they cease to interact with the relatives with whom their parents interacted, even if the parents are still alive, and siblings interact with each other chiefly through their parents.

Kinship is founded on the biological ties generated by mating and reproduction, and it gives these ties social expression. The social forms and the functions of the ties of marriage and descent are in large part independent of their universal biological foundation; their form and function are particular to social and economic and cultural systems. Whereas kinship has systematized political and economic import in tribal societies, it has only marginal and incidental political and economic import in industrial societies. Marriage is the social instrument through which kinship systems are maintained, and the forms, functions, and content of marriage, too, are governed by the social economic system. Social and sexual relations between men and women have fundamental significance for health and disease (119). These relations, given institutional form in courtship, marriage, and the norms for conjugal roles, are a facet of the social system. Like all other forms of social relationships, they are determinants of the configurations of health and health behavior that characterize each society.

References

1. **Dobzhansky, T.** (1959). *Evolution, Genetics and Man*, New York.
2. **Westermarck, E.** (1921). *The History of Human Marriage*, London.
   Briffault, R. (1960; first pub. 1927). *The Mothers: A Study of the Origins of Sentiments and Institutions*, abridged by Taylor, G. R., London.
   Outhwaite, R. B. (1982). *Marriage and Society; Studies in the Social History of Marriage*, New York.
   Goody, J. (1983). *The Development of the Family and Marriage in Europe*, Cambridge.
3. **Middleton, R.** (1962). Brother-sister and father-daughter marriage in ancient Egypt, *Amer. Sociol. Rev.*, 27, 603–11.
   Hopkins, K. (1980). Brother-sister marriage in Roman Egypt, *Comp. Stud. Soc. and Hist.*, 22, 303–54.
   Livingstone, F. (1980). Cultural causes of genetic change, in *Sociobiology: Beyond Nature-Nurture*, ed., Barlow, G. and Silverberg, J., Boulder, Colorado, pp. 307–40.
4. **Adams, M. S.**, and **Neel, J. V.** (1967). Children of incest, *Pediatrics*, 40, 55–62.
   Carter, C. O. (1967). Risk to offspring of incest, *Lancet*, 1, 436.
5. **Schull, W. J.** (1958). Empirical risks in consanguineous marriages: Sex ratio, malformation, and viability, *Amer. J. Hum. Genet.*, 10, 294–343.
   Schull, W. J. and **Neel, J. V.** (1966). *The Effects of Inbreeding on Japanese Children*, New York.
   Narayanan, H. S. (1981). A study of the prevalence of mental retardation in Southern India, *Intl. J. Ment. Hlth.*, 10, 28–36.

6. **Schork, M. A.** (1964). The effects of inbreeding on growth, *Amer. J. Hum. Genet., 16,* 292–300.

   Niswander, J. D., and **Chung, C. S.** (1965). The effects of inbreeding on tooth size in Japanese children, *Amer. J. Hum. Genet., 17,* 390–8.

   Schull, W. J., and **Neel, J. V.** (1966). Some further observations on the effect of inbreeding on mortality in Kure, Japan, *Amer. J. Hum. Genet., 18,* 144–52.

   Schull, W. J., Neel, J. V., and **Hashizume, A.** (1966). Some further observations on the sex ratio among infants born to survivors of the atomic bombings of Hiroshima and Nagasaki, *Amer. J. Hum. Genet., 18,* 328–38.

7. **Scott-Emaukpor, A. B.** (1974). The mutation load in an African population, I. An analysis of consanguineous marriages in Nigeria, *Amer. J. Hum. Genet., 26,* 674–82.

8. **Roberts, D. F.** (1967). Incest, inbreeding, and mental abilities, *Brit. Med. J., 4,* 336–7.

9. **Iliya, F. A., Williamson, S.,** and **Azar, H. A.** (1967). Choriocarcinoma in the Near East: Consanguinity as a possible etiologic factor, *Cancer, 20,* 144–9.

10. **Forde, C. D.** (1941). *Marriage and the Family Among the Yako in South-Eastern Nigeria,* 2nd ed., London.

    Barnes, J. A. (1951). *Marriage in a Changing Society,* Rhodes-Livingstone Papers No. 20, Cape Town.

    Fallers, L. A. (1956). *Bantu Bureaucracy,* Cambridge.

    Watson, W. (1958). *Tribal Cohesion in a Money Economy: A Study of the Mambwe People of Northern Rhodesia,* Manchester.

11. **Evans-Pritchard, E. E.** (1940). *The Nuer,* Oxford.

    Freedman, M. (1958). *Lineage Organization in South-Eastern China,* London.

    Cunnison, I. (1959). *The Luapula Peoples of Northern Rhodesia,* Manchester.

12. **Kretschmer, E.** (1925). *Physique and Character,* trans. Sprott, W. J. H., London.

    Sheldon, W. H., Stevens, S. S., and **Tucker, W. B.** (1940). *Varieties of Human Physique,* New York

    Sheldon, W. H., and **Stevens, S. S.** (1942). *The Varieties of Temperament,* New York.

13. **Allison, A. C.** (1960). Genetics, in *Medical Surveys and Clinical Trials,* ed. Witts, L. J., London.

    King, M-C., Lee, G. M., Spinner, N. B., Thomson, G., and **Wrensch, M. R.** (1984). Genetic epidemiology, *Ann. Rev. Pub. Hlth., 5,* 1–52.

14. **Harris, H.** (1969). Enzyme and protein polymorphism, *Brit. Med. Bull., 25,* 5–13.

    Cavalli-Sforza, L. L., and **Bodmer, W. F.** (1971). *The Genetics of Human Populations,* San Francisco.

15. **Jacobsohn, P.,** and **Matheny, A. R.** (1962). Mate selection in open marriage systems, *Int. J. Comp. Sociol., 3,* 98–124.

    Tharp, R. G. (1963). Psychological patterning in marriage, *Psychol. Bull., 60,* 97–117.

    Winch, R. F. (1968). Family formation, in *Int. Encycl. Soc. Sci.,* ed., Sills, D., New York, Vol. 9, pp. 1–8.

    Wolanski, N. (1974). The stature of offspring and assortative mating of parents, *Human Biology, 46,* 613–19.

16. **Berent, J.** (1954). Social mobility and marriage: A study of trends in England and Wales, in *Social Mobility in Britain,* ed. Glass, D. V., London, pp. 321–38.

17. **Glenn, N. D., Ross, A. A.,** and **Tully J. C.,** (1974). Patterns of intergenerational mobility of females through marriage, *Amer. Sociol. Rev., 39,* 683–99.

18. **Dahlberg, G.** (1948). *Mathematical Methods for Population Genetics,* New York.

19. **Pons, V.** (1955). The Social Structure of a Hertfordshire Parish, unpublished Ph.D. thesis, University of London.

20. **Sutter, J.**, and **Tabah, L.** (1951). Les notions d'isolat et de population minimum, *Population* (Paris), *3*, 481–98.
21. **Myrdal, G.** (1944). *An American Dilemma*, New York.
22. **Wright, S.** (1922). Coefficients of inbreeding and relationship, *Amer. Naturalist, 56*, 330–8.

    Hajnal, J. (1963). Concepts of random mating and the frequency of consanguineous marriages, *Proc. Roy. Soc. B., 159*, 125–77.

    McKusick, V. A., Eldridge, R., Hostetler, J. A., and **Egeland, J. A.** (1964). Dwarfism in the Amish, *Trans. Ass. Amer. Phycns., 77*, 151–68.

    Allen, G. (1965). Random and nonrandom inbreeding. *Eugen. Quart., 12*, 181–98.
23. **Lipset, S. M.,** and **Bendix, R.** (1959). *Social Mobility in Industrial Society*, London.
24. **Klineberg, O.** (1938). *Negro Intelligence and Selective Migration*, New York.

    Lee, E. J. (1951). Negro intelligence and selective migration: A Philadelphia test of the Klineberg hypothesis, *Amer. Sociol. Rev., 16*, 227–373.
25. **Glass, D. V.,** and **Hall, J. R.** (1954). Social mobility in Britain: A study of inter-generation changes in status, in *Social Mobility in Britain*, ed. Glass, D. V., London, pp. 177–259.
26. **Burt, C.,** and **Howard, M.** (1956). The multifactorial theory of inheritance and its application to intelligence, *Brit. J. Statist. Psychol., 8*, 95–129.
27. **Pearson, K.,** and **Lee, A.** (1903). On the laws of inheritance in man. I. Inheritance and physical character, *Biometrika, 2*, 357–462.

    Terman, L. M. (1938). *Psychological Factors in Marital Happiness*, New York.

    Richardson, H. M. (1939). Studies of mental resemblance between husbands and wives and between friends, *Psychol. Bull., 36*, 104.

    Burgess, E. W., and **Wallin, P.** (1943). Homogamy in social characteristics, *Amer. J. Sociol., 49*, 109–24.

    Smith, M. (1946). A research note on homogamy of marriage partners in selected physical characteristics, *Amer. Sociol. Rev., 11*, 236.

    Roberts, J. A. F. (1959). *An Introduction to Medical Genetics*, 2nd ed., London.

    Spuhler, S. N. (1968). Assortative mating with respect to physical characteristics, *Eugen. Quart., 15*, 128–40.

    Garrison, R. S., Anderson, V. E., and **Reed, S. C.** (1968). Assortative marriage, *Eugen. Quart., 15*, 113–27.

    Harrison, S. M. (1976). Assortative marriage for psychometric, personality and anthropometric variations in a group of Oxfordshire villages, *J. Biosocial Science, 8*, 145–53.
28. **Slater, E.,** and **Woodside, M.** (1951). *Patterns of Marriage*, London.
29. **Dicks, H. V.** (1953). Clinical studies in marriage and the family: A symposium on methods, *Brit. J. Med. Psychol., 26*, 181–96.

    Pincus, L., ed. (1960). *Marriage: Studies in Emotional Conflict and Growth*, London.
30. **Kreitman, N.** (1964). The patient's spouse, *Brit. J. Psychiat., 110*, 159–73.
31. **Kraus, A. S.,** and **Lilienfeld, A. M.** (1959). Some epidemiologic aspects of the high mortality rate in the young widowed group, *J. Chron. Dis., 10*, 207–17.
32. **Chen, E.,** and **Cobb, S.** (1960). Family structure in relation to health and disease: A review of the literature, *J. Chron. Dis., 12*, 544–67.

    Myers, R. J. (1963). An instance of the pitfalls prevalent in graveyard research, *Biometrics, 19*, 638–650.
33. **Susser, M.** (1981). Widowhood: A situational life stress or a stressful life event?, *Amer. J. Publ. Hlth., 71*, 793–5.

34. **Registrar General** (1936). *Decennial Supplement for England and Wales, 1931*, Part 1, H.M.S.O., London, 12.

    Ciocco, A. (1940). On the mortality of husbands and wives, *Hum. Biol., 12*, 508–31.

    Shurtleff, D. (1956). Mortality among the married, *J. Amer. Geriat. Soc., 4*, 654–66.

    Weir, R. D. (1960). Perforated peptic ulcer in north-east Scotland, *Scot. Med. J., 5*, 257–64.

    Weiss, N. S. (1973). Marital status and risk factors for coronary heart disease: U.S. health examination survey of adults, *Brit. J. Prev. Soc. Med., 27*, 41–43.

    Verbrugge, Lois, M. (1979). Marital status and health, *J. Marr. Fam., 41*, 267–85.

    Berkman, L. F., and **Breslow, L.** (1983). *Health and Ways of Living: The Alameda County Study*, New York.

35. **Malzberg, B.** (1940). *Social and Biological Aspects of Mental Disease*, Utica, New York.

    Adler, L. M. (1953). The relationship of marital status to incidence of, and recovery from, mental illness, *Social Forces, 32*, 185–94.

    Ødegaard, Ø. (1953). Marriage and mental health, *Acta Psychiat. Scand.*, Suppl., *80*, 153–60.

    Norris, V. (1959). *Mental Illness in London*, Maudsley Monograph No. 6, London.

    Pugh, T. F., and **MacMahon, B.** (1962). *Epidemiological Findings in United States Mental Hospital Data*, Boston.

    Thomas, D. S., and **Locke, B. Z.** (1963). Marital status, education, and occupational differentials in mental disease, *Milbank Mem. Fd. Quart., 41*, 145–60.

    Kramer, M. (1966). *Some Implications of Trends in the Usage of Psychiatric Facilities for Community Mental Health Programs and Related Research*, Public Health Service Publication, No. 1434, Washington, D.C.

    Adelstein, A. M., Downham, D. Y., Stein, Z. A., and **Susser, M.** (1968). The epidemiology of mental illness in an English city: Inceptions recognized by Salford psychiatric services, *Soc. Psychiat., 3*, 47–59.

36. **Morgan, R.** (1964). Marital status and living arrangements before admission to nursing and personal care homes, *Vital and Health Statistics*, Series 21, No. 17, U.S. Department of Health Education and Welfare, Public Health Service, Washington, D.C.

37. **Sheps, M. C.** (1961). Marriage and mortality, *Amer. J. Publ. Hlth., 51*, 547–55.

38. **Berkson, J.** (1962). Mortality and marital status, *Amer. J. Publ. Hlth., 52*, 1318–29.

39. **Hambright, T. Z.** (1960). Comparability of marital status, race, nativity, and country of origin on the death certificate and matching census record, *Vital and Health Statistics*, Series 2, No. 34, U.S. Department of Health, Education and Welfare, Public Health Service, Washington, D.C.

40. **Susser, M.** (1968). *Community Psychiatry: Epidemiologic and Social Themes*, New York.

    Bachrach, L. L. (1975). *Marital Status and Mental Disorder: An Analytical Review*, Washington, D.C.

    Brown, G. W., and **Harris, T.** (1978). *Social Origins of Depression: A Study of Psychiatric Disorder in Women*, New York.

    Kessler, R. C., and **Essex, M.** (1982). Marital status and depression: The importance of coping resources, *Social Forces, 61*, 484–507.

    Cleary, P. D., and **Mechanic, D.** (1983). Sex differences in psychological distress among married people, *J. Hlth. Soc. Behav., 24*, 111–21.

    Gove, W. R., Hughes, M., and **Style, C. B.** (1983). Does marriage have positive effects on the psychological well-being of the individual? *J. Hlth. Soc. Behav., 24*, 122–31.

41. **Essen-Möller, E.** (1961). A current field study in the mental disorders in Sweden, in *Comparative Epidemiology of the Mental Disorders*, ed. Hoch, P. H., and Zubin, J., New York.

42. **Susser, M. W., Stein, Z. A., Mountney, G. H.,** and **Freeman, H. L.** (1970). Chronic disability following on mental illness in an English city. Part II. The location of patients in hospitals and community, *Soc. Psychiat.*, 5, 69–76.

43. **Penrose, L. S.** (1944). Mental illness in husband and wife: A contribution to the study of assortative mating in man, *Psychiat. Quart.*, Suppl., *18*, 161–6.
    Gregory, I. (1950). Husbands and wives admitted to a mental hospital, *J. Ment. Sci.*, *105*, 457–62.

44. **Kinsey, A. C., Pomeroy, W. B.,** and **Martin, C. E.** (1948). *Sexual Behavior in the Human Male*, Philadelphia.

45. **Stein, Z. A., Susser, M. W.** (1969). Widowhood and mental illness, *Brit. J. Prev. Soc. Med.*, *23*, 106–10.

46. **Bartrop, R. W., Lazarus, L., Luckhurst, E., Kiloh, L. G.,** and **Penny, R.** (1977). Depressed lymphocyte function after bereavement, *Lancet*, *1*, 834–46.

47. **Young, M., Benjamin, B.,** and **Wallis, C.** (1963). The mortality of widows, *Lancet*, *2*, 454–6.
    MacMahon, B., and **Pugh, T. F.** (1965). Suicide in the widowed, *Amer. J. Epidem.*, *81*, 23–31.

48. **Cox, P. R.,** and **Ford, J. R.** (1964). The mortality of widows shortly after widowhood, *Lancet*, *1*, 163–4.
    Helsing, K. J., Szklo, M., and **Comstock, G. W.** (1981). Factors associated with mortality after widowhood, *Amer. J. Publ. Hlth.*, *71*, 802–809.

49. **Cobb, S.,** and **Kasl, S. V.** (1966). The epidemiology of rheumatoid arthritis, *Amer. J. Publ. Hlth.*, *56*, 1657–63.

50. **Ramazzini, B.** (1940; first pub. 1700). *Diseases of Workers*, trans. by Wright, W. C., Chicago.

51. **Rigoni-Stern** (1842). Fatti statistici relativi alle mallattie cancerose, *Gior. Servire. Progr. Path. Terap.*, *2*, 507–17.
    Gagnon, F. (1950). Contribution to the study of the etiology and prevention of cancer of the cervix of the uterus, *Amer. J. Obstet. Gynec.*, *60*, 516–22.
    Logan, W. P. D. (1953). Marriage and childbearing in relation to cancer of the breast and uterus, *Lancet*, *2*, 1199–202.
    Taylor, R. S., Carroll, B. E., and **Lloyd, J. W.** (1959). Mortality among women in 3 Catholic religious orders with special reference to cancers, *Cancer*, *12*, 1207–25.
    Fraumeni, J. F., Jr., Lloyd, J. W., Smith, E. M., and **Wagoner, J. K.** (1968). Cancer mortality among nuns: Role of marital status in etiology of neoplastic disease in women, *J. Nat. Cancer Inst.*, *42*, 455–68.

52. **Lilienfeld, A. M.** (1956). The relationship of cancer of the female breast to artificial menopause and marital status, *Cancer*, *9*, 927–34.
    Damon, A. (1960). Host factors in cancer of the breast and uterine cervix and corpus, *J. Nat. Cancer Inst.*, *24*, 483–516.
    Kelsey, J. L. (1979). A review of the epidemiology of human breast cancer, *Epidemiol. Rev.*, *1*, 74–109.
    MacMahon, B. (1979). Oestrogens in the genesis of endometrial and breast cancer, *INSERM*, *83*, 81–92.

53. **Weiss, N. S.** (1975). Risks and benefits of estrogen use, *New Eng. J. Med.*, *293*, 1200–2.

Kelsey, J. L. (1981). Epidemiological studies of the role of estrogens in the etiology of breast cancer, *Banbury Report*, 8, 215–28.

54. MacMahon, B., and Yuasa, S. (1970). Lactation and reproductive histories of breast cancer patients in Tokyo, Japan, *Bull. Wld. Hlth. Org.*, 42, 185–94.

55. Cohen, P., Belmont, L., Dryfoos, J., Stein, Z., and Zayac, S. (1980). The effects of teenage motherhood and maternal age on offspring intelligence, *Social Biology*, 27, 138–154.

Stein, Z. A. (1985). A woman's age, *Amer. J. Epi.*, 121, 327–42.

56. Penrose, L. S. (1949). *The Biology of Mental Defect*, London.

Stein, Z., Kline, J., Susser, E., Shrout, P., Warburton, D., and Susser, M. W., (1980). Maternal age and spontaneous abortion, in *Human Embryonic and Fetal Death*, ed. Potter, I. H., and Hook, E. B., New York, pp. 107–27.

57. Morris, J. N., Heady, J. A., and Daly, C. (1955). Social and biological factors in infant mortality, *Lancet*, 1, 343–9, 395–7, 445–8, 499–502, 544–9.

Bulmer, M. G. (1959). The effect of parental age, parity, and duration on the twinning rate, *Ann. Hum. Genet.*, 23, 454–8.

McCormick, M. C., Shapiro, S., and Starfield, B. (1984). High-risk young mothers: Infant mortality and morbidity in four areas in the United States, 1973–1978, *Amer. J. Pub. Hlth.*, 74, 18–23.

58. Presser, H. B. (1975). Age differences between spouses: Trends, patterns and social implications, *Amer. Behav. Sci.*, 19, 190–205.

59. Glass, D. V., and Grebenik, E. (1954). *The Trend and Pattern of Fertility in Great Britain, A Report on the Family Census of 1946*, Papers of the Royal Commission on Population, Vol. VI, Parts I and II, H.M.S.O., London.

60. Office of Population Censuses and Surveys (1978). *Demographic Review: A Report on Population in Great Britain*, Series DR No. 1, H.M.S.O., London.

61. Keyfitz, N., and Fleiger, W. (1968). *World Population: An Analysis of Vital Data*, Chicago.

Carter, S., and Glick, P. (1970). *Marriage and Divorce*, Cambridge, Mass.

Muhsam, H. V. (1974). The marriage squeeze, *Demography*, 11, 291–99.

Poston, L, and Gotard, E. (1976). Trends in childlessness in the United States, 1910–75, *Social Biology*, 24, 212–224.

U.S. Bureau of the Census (1976). *Historical Statistics of the United States: Colonial Times to the Present*, Washington, D.C.

U.S. Department of Health and Human Services (1982). *Health, U.S.A., 1982*, Department of Health and Human Services Publication No. (PHS) 83-1232, Hyattsville, Md.

Jackson, B. (1982). Single parent families, in *Families in Britain*, ed., Rapoport, R. N., Fogarty, M. P. and Rapoport, R., London, pp. 159–79.

National Center for Health Statistics (1984). *Monthly Vital Statistics Report*, Vol. 32, No. 13.

62. Bayer, A. E. (1969). Marriage plans and educational aspirations, *Amer. J. Sociol.* 75, 239–44.

Sweet, J. A. (1977). Demography and the family, *Ann. Rev. Sociol.*, 3, 363–405.

63. Willis, R. J. (1973). A new approach to the economic theory of fertility behavior, *J. Pol.. Econ.*, 81, (supplement), 514–69.

Ermisch, J. (1982). Investigations into the causes of postwar fertility swings, in *Population Change and Social Planning*, ed. Eversley, D. and Kollmann, W., London, pp 141–55.

64. **U.S. Dept. of Commerce and Bureau of the Census** (1984). *Statistical Abstract 1984,* Washington, D.C.

65. **U.S. Bureau of the Census** (1976). Household and family characteristics: March 1975, *Curr. Popul. Rep.,* Ser. P-20, No. 291, Washington, D.C.
    U.S. Bureau of the Census (1976). Marital status and living arrangements: March 1975, *Curr. Popul. Rep.,* Ser. P-20, No. 287, Washington, D.C.
    U.S. Bureau of the Census (1976). Fertility history and prospects of American women: June 1975. *Curr. Popul. Rep.,* Ser. P-20, No. 288, Washington, D.C.
    U.S. Bureau of the Census (1976). Number, timing and duration of marriages and divorces in the United States: June 1975, *Curr. Popul. Rep.,* Ser., P-20, No. 297, Washington, D.C.

66. **Coale, A. J.** (1971). Age patterns of marriage, *Population Studies,* 25, 193–214.
    Matras, J. (1973). *Population and Societies,* Englewood Cliffs, N.J.

67. **Ødegaard, Ø.** (1946). Marriage and mental disease: A study in social psychopathology, *J. Ment. Sci.,* 92, 35–59.
    Ødegaard, Ø. (1953). New data on marriage and mental disease, *J. Ment.* Sci., 99, 778–85.
    Sunby, P. (1959). Occupation and insanity, *Acta Psychiat. Scand.,* Suppl. *106.*

68. **Edwards, J. H.** (1969). Should diabetics marry?, *Lancet, 1,,* 1045–7.

69. **Townsend, P.** (1957). *The Family Life of Old People,* London.
    Lopata, H.Z. (1978). Contributions of extended families to the support systems of metropolitan area widows: Limitations of the modified kin network, *J. Marr. Fam.,* 2, 355–64.

70. **Bogue, D.** (1969). *Principles of Demography,* New York.

71. **Office of Population and Surveys** (1983). *Population Trends,* 32, H.M.S.O., London.

72. **Schoen, R.,** and **Nelson, V. E.** (1974). Marriage, divorce, and mortality: A life table analysis, *Demography,* 11, 267–90.
    Preston, S. H. (1975). Estimating the proportion of American marriages that end in divorce, *Sociol. Methods Res.,* 3, 435–60.

73. **Farber, B.** (1964). *Family Organization and Interaction,* San Francisco.
    Central Statistical Office (1977). *Social Trends,* No. 8, H.M.S.O., London.

74. **National Center of Health Statistics** (1980). National estimates of marriage dissolution and survivorship: United States, *Vital and Health Statistics,* Series 3, No. 19.

75. **Locke, H. J.,** and **Klausner, W. J.** (1948). Marital adjustment of divorced persons in subsequent marriages, *Sociol. Soc. Res.,* 33, 97–101.
    Locke, H. J. (1951). *Predicting Adjustment in Marriage: Comparison of a Divorced and a Happily Married Group,* New York.

76. **Bernard, J.** (1956). *Remarriage, A Study of Marriage,* New York.
    Glick, P., and **Norton A. J.** (1973). Perspectives on the recent upturn in divorce and remarriage, *Demography,* 10, 301–14.

77. **Orden, S. R.,** and **Bradburn, N. M.** (1968) Dimensions of marriage happiness, *Amer. J. Sociol.,* 73, 715–31.

78. **Bumpass, L. L.** and **Sweet, J. A.** (1975). Background and early marital factors in marital disruption, *CDE Work. Pap. 75–31,* Cent. Demogr. Ecol., Univ. of Wisconsin, Madison.

79. **Central Statistical Office** (1979). *Social Trends,* No. 9, H.M.S.O., London.
    U.S. Department of Commerce and Bureau of the Census (1980). *Social Indicators,* III, Washington, D.C.
    Eversley, D. and **Bonnerjea, L.** (1982). Social change and indicators of diversity, in *Families in Britain,* ed. Rapoport, R. N., Fogarty, M. P., and Rapoport, R., London, pp. 75–94.

80. **Finer, M.** (1974). *Report of the Committee on One-Parent Families*, H.M.S.O., London.
    Macintyre, S. (1979). Some issues in the study of pregnancy careers, *Soc. Rev.*, 27, 755–72.
81. **U. S. Bureau of the Census** (1982). Marital status and living arrangements, *Curr. Pop. Rep.*, Series P-20, No. 372.
    U. S. Department of Commerce and Bureau of the Census (1983). Population profile of the United States: 1982, *Curr. Pop. Rep.*, Series P-23, No. 130.
    National Center for Health Statistics (1984). Advance report of final divorce statistics, 1981, *Monthly Vital Statistics Report*, Vol. 32, No. 9, Supplement (2).
82. **Stack, C.** (1974). *All Our Kin: Strategies for Survival in a Black Community*, New York.
83. **Hyman, H. H.**, and **Reed, J. S.** (1969). Black matriarchy reconsidered; evidence from secondary analysis of sample surveys, *Public Opinion Quarterly*, 33, 346–53.
    Scanzoni, J. H. (1971). *The Black Family in Modern Society*, Boston.
    Jackson, J. J. (1973). Family organization and ideology, in *Comparative Studies of Blacks and Whites in the United States*, ed. Miller, K. S. and Dreger, R. M. pp. 408–47.
    Dobbins, M. P. and **Mulligan, J.** (1980). Black matriarchy: Transforming a myth of racism into a class model, *J. Comp. Fam. Stud.*, 11, 195–217.
84. **Radcliffe-Brown, A. R.** (1952). *Structure and Function in Primitive Society*, London.
    Weitzman, L. J. (1981). *The Marriage Contract: Spouses, Lovers, and the Law*, New York.
85. **Blood, R. O. Jr.** and **Hamblin, R. L.** (1958). The effect of the wife's employment on the family power structure, *Social Forces*, 36, 347–52.
    Blood, R. O. Jr., and **Wolfe, D. M.** (1960). *Husbands and Wives: The Dynamics of Married Living*, Glencoe, Ill.
    Aronoff, J., and **Crano, W. D.** (1975). A re-examination of the cross-cultural principles of task segregation and sex role differentiation in the family, *Amer. Sociol. Rev.*, 40, 12–20.
    Nag, M. (1975). Sociocultural patterns, family cycle and fertility, in *Population Debate: Dimensions and Perspectives, 11*, New York, pp. 289–312.
    Oppenheimer, V. K. (1977). The sociology of women's economic role in the family, *Amer. Sociol. Rev. 42*, 387–406.
    Kuhn, A., and **Wolpe, A-M.** ed. (1978). *Feminism and Materialism*, London.
86. **Richards, A. I.** (1939). *Land, Labour, and Diet in Northern Rhodesia*, London.
    Schapera, I. (1947). *Migrant Labour and Tribal Life: A Study of Conditions in the Bechuanaland Protectorate*, London.
    Peters, D. U. (1950). *Land Usage in Serenje District*, Rhodes-Livingstone Papers, No. 19, London.
    Gulliver, P. H. (1955). *Labour Migration in a Rural Economy*, East African Institute of Social Research, Kampala.
    Watson, W. (1958). *Tribal Cohesion in a Money Eoconmy: A Study of the Mambwe People of Northern Rhodesia*, Manchester.
87. **Caplow, T.** (1954). *The Sociology of Work*, Minneapolis.
    Cantor, M., and **Laurie, B.** ed. (1977). *Class, Sex and the Woman Worker*, Westport, Conn.
88. **Lee, B. H.** (1974). *Divorce Law Reform in England*, London.
    Mays, J. B., and **Forder, A.** ed. (1983). *Penelope Hall's Social Services of England and Wales*, 10th edition, London.

89. **Bureau of Labor Statistics** (1982). *Labor Force Statistics Derived from the Current Population Survey: A Databook,* Washington D.C.
90. **Central Statistical Office** (1982). *Social Trends,* H.M.S.O., London.
91. **Wright, J. D.** (1970). Are working wives really more satisfied? *J. Marr. Fam., 40,* 301–13.
    Gove, W. R. and **Geerken, M. R.** (1977). The effect of children and employment on the mental health of married men and women, *Social Forces, 50,* 66–76.
92. **Gowler, D.** and **Legge, K.** (1982). Dual-worker families, in *Families in Britain,* ed. Rapoport, R. N., Fogarty, M. P., and Rapoport, R., London, pp. 138–158.
93. **Waite, L. J.** (1980). Working wives and the family life cycle, *Amer. J. Sociol., 86,* 272–94.
94. **Rapoport, R.** and **Rapoport, R. N.** (1971). *Dual Career Families* Harmondsworth.
95. **Srole, L.,** and **Fischer, A. K.** (1980). The Midtown Manhattan Longitudinal Study vs. 'The Mental Paradise Lost' doctrine: A controversy joined, *Arch. Gen. Psychiat., 37,* 209–21.
96. **Veroff, J., Douvan, E.,** and **Kulka, R.** (1981). *The Inner American: A Self Portait from 1957–1976,* New York.
97. **Gove, W. B.** (1972). The relationship between sex roles, marital status and mental illness, *Social Forces, 51,* 33–44.
    Kessler, R. C., and **McRae, J. A.** (1981). Trends in sex and psychological distress, *Amer. Sociol. Rev., 46,* 443–52.
    Kessler, R. C. and **McRae, J. A.** (1982). The effect of wives employment on the mental health of married men and women, *Amer. Sociol. Rev., 47,* 216–27.
98. **Featherman D. L.,** and **Hauser R. M.** (1976). Sexual inequalities and socioeconomic achievement in the United States, 1962–1973, *Amer. Sociol. Rev., 41,* 462–83.
99. **Bott, E.** (1971). *Family and Social Network,* 2nd ed., New York.
100. **Young, M., Geertz, H.** (1961). Old age in London and San Francisco: Some families compared, *Brit. J. Sociol., 12,* 124–41.
101. **Rowntree, G.** (1959). The finances of founding a family, *Scottish Journal of Political Economy, 1,* 201–32.
102. **Young, M.,** and **Willmott, P.** (1957). *Family and Kinship in East London,* London.
103. **Rainwater, L.** (1964). Marital sexuality in four cultures of poverty, *J. Marr. Fam., 26,* 457–66.
    Rainwater, L. (1966). Some aspects of lower class sexual behavior, *J. Soc. Issues, 22,* 96–108.
104. **Frazier, E. F.** (1939). *The Negro Family in the United States,* Chicago.
    Lewis, O. (1961). *The Children of Sanchez: Autobiography of a Mexican Family,* New York.
    Lewis, O. (1966). *La Vida: A Puerto Rican Family in the Culture of Poverty—San Juan and New York,* New York.
    Rainwater, L. (1966). The crucible of identity: The Negro lower class family, *Daedalus, 95,* 172–216.
    Willie, C. V. (1981). *A New Look at Black Families,* New York.
105. **Durkheim, E.** (1947). *Divison of Labour in Society,* 2nd ed., Glencoe, Ill.
106. **Plateris, A. A.** (1969). Divorce statistics analysis, *Vital and Health Statistics,* Series 21, No. 17, U.S. Department of Health Education and Welfare, Public Health Service, Washington, D.C.
    U. S. Bureau of Census (1977). Marriage, divorce, widowhood, and remarriage by family characteristics: June 1975, *Curr. Popul. Rep.,* Ser. P-20, No. 312, Washington, D. C.

Leete, R. (1979). Changing patterns of family formation and dissolution in England and Wales, 1964–76, *Studies on Medical and Population Subjects*, no. 39, H.M.S.O., London.

Dominian, J. (1982). Families in divorce, in *Families in Britain*, ed. Rapoport, R. N., Fogarty, M. P., and Rapoport, R., London, pp. 263–85.

107. **Willmott, P.,** and **Young M.** (1960). *Family and Class in a London Suburb*, London.
Young M., and **Wilmott, P.** (1973). *The Symmetrical Family*, London.

108. **Weller, R. H.** (1968). The employment of wives, dominance and fertility, *J. Marr. Fam., 30*, 437–40.

109. **Anthony, S.** (1932). *Women's Place in Industry and Home*, London.
Zweig, F. (1952). *The British Worker*, Harmondsworth.
Zweig, F. (1952). *Women's Life and Labour*, London.
Puhl, J. M., and **Puhl, R. E.** (1971). *Managers and Their Wives*, London.
Oakley, A. (1974). *The Sociology of Housework*, New York.

110. **Susser, M.** (1968). *Community Psychiatry: Epidemiologic and Social Themes* New York.
Gove, W. R. (1972). The relationship between sex roles, marital status, and mental illness, *Social Forces, 51*, 34–44.
Dohrenwend, B. P., and **Dohrenwend B. S.** (1974). Social and cultural influences on psychopathology, *Ann. Rev. Psychol., 25*, 417–52.
Bachrach, L. L. (1975). *Marital Status and Mental Disorder: An Analytical Review*, National Institute of Mental Health, Series D, No. 3, U.S. Dept. of Health, Education and Welfare, Publ. No. (ADM) 75-217.
Radlof, L. (1975). Sex differences in depression. The effects of occupation and marital status, *Sex Roles, 1*, 249–65.
Fox, J. W. (1980). Reply to Gove and Tudor's comment on sex differences in psychiatric disorders, *Amer. J. Sociol. 82*, 1336–45.

111. **Rosenfield, S.** (1980). Sex differences in depression: Do women always have higher rates? *J. Hlth. Soc. Beh., 21*, 33–42.

112. **Schapera, I.** (1940). *Married Life in an African Tribe*, London.
Evans-Pritchard, E. E. (1951). *Kinship and Marriage Among the Nuer*, Oxford.
Gluckman, M. (1955). *Custom and Conflict in Africa*, Oxford.

113. **Fortes, M.** (1949). *The Web of Kinship Among the Tallensi*, London.

114. **Kerr, M.** (1958). *The People of Ship Street*, London.
Komarovsky, M. (1964). *Blue Collar Marriage*, New York.

115. **Firth, R.** (1956). *Two Studies of Kinship in London*, London.

116. **Fortes, M.,** and **Evans-Pritchard, E. E.,** eds. (1940). *African Political Systems*, London.

117. **Srinivas, M. N.** (1952). A joint family dispute in a Mysore village, *Journal of the M.S. University of Baroda, 1*, 10–31.
Gulliver, P. H. (1955). *The Family Herds*, London.
Bailey, F. G. (1957). *Cast and the Economic Frontier*, Manchester.

118. **Parsons, T.** (1949). Age and sex in the social structure of the United States, in *Personality in Nature, Society and Culture*, ed. Kluckhohn, C., and Murray, H. A., London.

119. **Kaplan, P. H., Cassel, J. C.,** and **Gore, S.** (1977). Social support and health, *Medical Care, 15*, Supplement, 47–58.
Pilisuk, M. (1978). Kinship, social networks, social support and health, *Soc. Sci. Med., 12B*, 273–80.
Hammer, M., Gutwirth, L., and **Phillips, S. L.** (1982). Parenthood and social networks: A preliminary view, *Soc. Sci. Med., 16*, 2091–2100.

11

Infant to adult

All human infants are born with similar needs for food, safety, and comfort. These needs, together with the slow physical maturation characteristic of newborn human beings, prolong the period of infancy and total dependence on adult caretakers. Several years of partial dependency in childhood and adolescence follow infancy. These prolonged developmental stages between birth and adulthood, together with the extraordinary capacity of the human species for learning, allow time for the adaptive process of socialization. In the process of socialization, children acquire cultural knowledge, values, and motives, and they learn and adjust to the various social roles allotted to them by society. Human development, therefore, involves the simultaneous and interacting processes of physical growth and of mental and social growth, all of which are subject to both inborn and societal developmental timetables.

Physical growth in children of every society conforms to the basic curve illustrated in Figure 11.1. This pattern imposes a degree of uniformity on the stages of adjustment experienced by all children regardless of individual and cultural differences. Thus the early experiences and behavior of a British or American infant have much in common with an African one. At the same time, variations in rates of growth occur as a result of both genetic and environmental differences between populations. Season and climate, socioeconomic status, childrearing norms, nutrition, and disease, all play a part (1). For example, in the United States the fetal growth rate of blacks is more rapid than that of whites up to around 30 weeks gestation, but in late pregnancy these relative positions are reversed, so that ultimately the average birthweight of blacks is lower than that of whites. During infancy and adolescence the growth rates are again reversed and the growth of blacks accelerates relative to whites (2). A similar acceleration in growth rate occurs in early postnatal life in black populations in Africa, suggesting a possible genetic factor. However, this acceleration slows at about six months of age, probably as a result of poor environmental conditions, to below European reference standards (1).

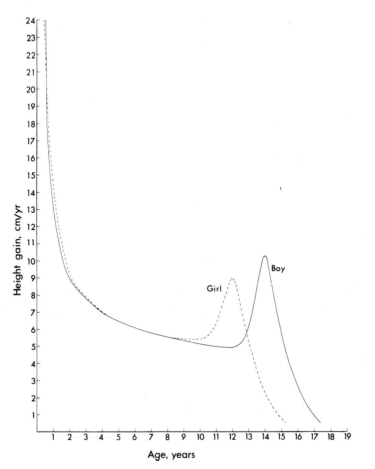

Figure 11.1 Mean growth velocity in centimeters per year of boys and girls. *Source:* Marshall, W. A. (1978). Puberty, in *Human Growth*, ed. Falkner, F., and Tanner, J. M., New York, p. 144.

Age at menarche is another developmental event that is particularly sensitive to environmental variation. Factors that favor growth, such as good nutrition, are consistently associated with earlier ages at menarche. The same is true of a light physical workload. Hence, in European countries menarche starts between two and four years earlier today than it did a century ago. Similar gaps exist in the present day between industrialized and developing countries, and between high and low income groups within societies (see Figure 11.2 and Table 11.1) (3). In industrial societies the trend toward an earlier onset of puberty is seen in both males and females. This trend, coupled with the lengthy period devoted to high level and technical education, results in a longer and less clear-cut transition from puberty to adulthood. In contrast, adolescence in many nonindustrial societies is of minimal duration and involves well-defined role changes (4).

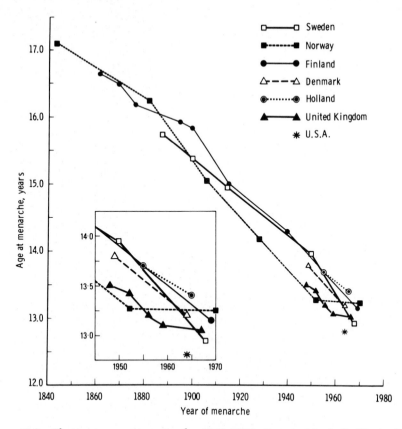

Figure 11.2 Change in age at menarche 1840–1970. *Source:* Marshall, W. A. (1978). Puberty, in *Human Growth*, ed., Falkner, F., and Tanner, J. M., New York, p. 168.

Table 11.1 Median age (in years) of menarche in well off and poor girls

Place	High income	Poor
United States (African descent)	12.6	13.0
United States (European descent)	13.0	13.5
Hongkong	12.5	13.3
Tunis	13.5	14.0
Bagdad	13.6	14.0
South Africa (Bantu urban)	13.4	14.9

Source: Adapted from Tanner, J. M., and Eveleth, P. B. (1975). Variability between populations in growth and development at puberty, in *Puberty: Biologic and Psychosocial Components*, Berenberg, S. R., ed., Leiden, The Netherlands, pp. 256–73.

Despite wide cross-cultural differences in the content of roles and in the timing of role changes, children in all societies pass through four broad stages in the process of social maturation, namely, *infancy, childhood, puberty,* and *adolescence.* The discussion in this chapter concerns the imprint of the social context on health and development during each of these stages.

Family context and human development

The family is an institution that can take on a great variety of forms (see Chapter 9). Across cultures, diverse principles of descent and marriage generate diverse forms, from the mother-children units common in the Caribbean, to the patrilineal extended family units (consisting of parents and their sons, daughters-in-law, and grandchildren) common to many other societies throughout the world. Within a single society, too, a variety of family structures is found. In the United States the nuclear family, although clearly the norm, does not describe the family context known to many children. In a study of the families of 1700 first-grade students from a poor black community in Chicago no fewer than 86 distinct family structures were identified (5). In all societies continued shifts in household composition are induced by such events as new marriage bonds, parental death or separation, or the attachment to existing households of widows, orphans, and others.

Pregnancy, birth, and the newborn infant

The particular set of familial relationships acquired at birth is a matrix that shapes the experiences and personality of each individual. This matrix differs according to family structure, and within a family it is unique for each child. For instance, an eldest child spends at least some time as an only child, while from birth the youngest confronts other siblings and older, more experienced parents. The newborn child has an immediate and active role to play. Every child imposes new demands on its caretakers and causes a reordering of the structure of existing relationships. The quality of existing relationships may also alter; new elements enter the accord between spouses after they become parents, and even sexual relations sometimes change. For the older children in the family, the newborn child is a rival for parental love and attention. The birth of a child confers new statuses on others, such as parents, siblings, grandparents, stepparents, and so on. New statuses entail new roles, and individuals are expected to adjust their behavior accordingly. The arrival of children has effects beyond the nuclear family, and extends to parental social networks. In both American and British populations, contact with adult kin has been found to increase; for nonworking mothers, however, social networks tended to grow smaller and social isolation greater (6).

Pregnancy forewarns of new relationships and generates anticipations. Each culture provides a store of traditional values and role expectations that guide preparations for the new birth. During pregnancy mothers have been found to become less directive and more understanding of their children, and to have less contact with them, than before the pregnancy (7). The tendency to limit contact is institutionalized in some cultures, and among the Newars of Nepal children are forbidden to touch a pregnant woman because of the belief that grave symptoms of malnutrition will result (8). Such customs during pregnancy can be functional; role changes forced by the birth of a new sibling are to a degree anticipated. On the other hand, abrupt role changes associated with a mother's pregnancy, such as weaning, may put her older children at risk for developmental and health problems, especially when the spacing between siblings is close. Whether there is an optimal birth interval or age at which children are least disturbed by the birth of a sibling is not clear; and, indeed, such an interval is likely to vary between societies (9). Family role transitions consequent on the birth of a new child are modified by socioeconomic resources and the amount of social support available to a family.

Should a pregnancy result in stillbirth, there will be grief for the loss. This acute life crisis is normally resolved through a process of mourning characterized by an initial stage of shock and grief; later by a stage of guilt, denial, anger, depression, and anxiety; and eventually by equilibrium. The concurrence of birth and death—two simultaneous life crises—complicates the process. Furthermore, anger, blame, and guilt are likely to be intensified when the cause of the death cannot be determined, as is true with some 70 per cent of stillbirths. Even when no cause of death can be found, however, an autopsy and an explanation of the results help allay parents' guilt and anxiety (10). There is also evidence that parents are helped to cope with a stillbirth when they are allowed to see and hold the baby at the time of birth (11). Although mothers are often encouraged to become pregnant right away, as if to replace the lost child, some authors maintain that "replacement pregnancies" interfere with the grieving process and the parents' acceptance of the next child (12,13,14). They suggest that the next pregnancy be delayed for a year or so, the time it normally takes for mourning to be fully expessed and the crisis of stillbirth to be resolved.

The social significance of an early infant death cannot but differ between a society in which the infant mortality rate is 200 or 300 per 1000, and one in which the rate is between 10 and 20 per 1000. In Britain and the United States today, *sudden infant death syndrome* is the most frequent cause of early postnatal loss after the perinatal period and, not surprisingly, this residual cause of death is under intense study. The response of parents to the loss with sudden infant death syndrome is similar to that with stillbirth (12).

Should a newborn child be markedly abnormal and survive, the crisis is more difficult to resolve (14). The initial response of parents to the knowledge of handicap in their child also mirrors the response to stillbirth, except that psychological denial may trigger a period of medical "shopping around" for a more hopeful diagnosis or the prospects of a cure (15). The eventual attainment of equilibrium entails acceptance of the handicap, adjustment to the child's special needs and limited capabilities, and coping with a stigmatized condition. The reactions associated with giving birth to an impaired infant tend to disrupt communication between parents and health care professionals, but are less likely to do so when professionals have some knowledge and understanding of parental responses normal to these circumstances.

It is in the event of a recognizably abnormal livebirth that physicians and nurses are often least prepared to deal with parents. Rarity contributes to unpreparedness.

Down's syndrome, still probably the commonest gross abnormality recognizable at birth, has a frequency of only about one in 800 total births (depending on the distribution of childbearing ages in the population). Many professionals share with society at large values that depreciate the worth of a handicapped child, especially a mentally handicapped child. These values engender an attitude of rejection that can impair professional ability to communicate with parents and effectively transmit information to them. The same values may contribute to the tendency for physicians to delay telling parents of the condition of the child until it becomes unavoidable. Yet the tendency to be vague and delay in communicating diagnoses of impairment may in fact have unintended benefits for the child. Clear and definite medical diagnoses of physical impairment given to parents have been seen to turn their attention away from the abilities of the child that remain unaffected, and to lower their expectations of the child (16). Less clear diagnosis and less definite prognoses may encourage the parents to normalize the child's development.

At the same time, retrospective studies have found that parents told early of the child's condition responded better than those told late and after delay (17). Few such retrospective studies, however, can convey the complex dynamics of the social and psychological events involved. Recollection is subject to bias, including that of the normal grieving response. The question of when to inform parents of the diagnosis is probably less important than the manner in which it is done, and specific guidelines for the "informing interview" have been drawn up (15). Eventually, in industrialized societies, parents of a severely impaired child must decide whether to place the child in an institution or to care for it themselves. Dissonance between feelings of love and responsibility for the child, concern for family functioning, and social attitudes toward handicapped people are bound to make this a difficult and painful decision.

Early socialization

For most children the family is the primary social context for learning ethical and moral attitudes, manners, and styles of behavior. This process of socialization begins in early infancy with customary methods of feeding and handling and, later, training to control bodily functions (18). As with family contexts, so with cultures caretaking methods experienced by infants vary. The contrasts between infant care in a less-developed society and in an industrial society are sharp. In a tribal or peasant society, infants are normally carried or kept close to the caretaker's side during most of the day and night, and nursing at the breast is a frequent response to crying. In industrialized societies, infants more commonly sleep in separate quarters, are commonly fed according to a schedule and are allowed to cry without immediately being fed or even soothed. In some societies children are beaten for trivial offenses, while in others they are seldom punished at all. Similarly, the age at which children are toilet trained and the rigor or leniency involved vary widely across cultures (19).

Socialization is not a unidirectional process in which the infant is a passive recipient, an asocial being assimilated and made capable of performing roles demanded by society. Even the newborn display remarkable social, cognitive, and perceptual capacities. In early and late infancy smiling, vocalizing, crying, visual references, auditory discrimination, memory, fear reactions, and imitation are all indicators of significant development.

Newborns have been shown to respond to visual signals, and it now appears that infants can recognize and remember some words repeated to them as early as two weeks of age. The behavior of one-year-old infants has been found to predict adult speech responses (20). For every individual child, temperament or idiosyncratic behavioral style enters into the socialization process (21).

Infants and children play an active role in their own socialization. This they do through their developing capacity to interact with social environments and to elicit responses from caretakers, as well as through the contribution of their temperamental dispositions to social situations (21,22) While the mother is an important agent of socialization during infancy, the whole social network of the infant participates in this process, including the father, siblings, and other caretakers and children (23). Different figures contribute to different stages and aspects of the child's socialization. A study in six cultures of the relative contributions of child-infant, child-peer, and child-parent interactions to child development derived three generalizations that held for all six cultures (24):

1. Children display nurturant behavior most often in interactions with infants.
2. Children develop sociable and aggressive behavior in their interactions with peers more than with either infants or adults.
3. Children display intimate-dependent behavior, such as touching and seeking help, most often in interactions with parents.

Single-parent homes and atypical family structure

According to census data, 18.6 per cent of all children in the United States live with only one parent, the majority with unwedded, divorced, or separated mothers. The same data indicate that 45 per cent of the children born in 1977 will live with a single parent before they reach the age of 18 (25). Absence of a father or mother figure in the home may put children at risk for various health problems. The "pediatric social illnesses" such as accidents, poisonings, failure to thrive, child abuse and neglect, and juvenile delinquency, as well as depression, respiratory disorders (bronchitis and pneumonia), gastroenteritis, and enuresis have all been found to occur disproportionately often in children of single-parent or disrupted homes (26,27,28,29,30,31).

Although single-parent status is often associated with a complex of disadvantages, so far it is demonstrably causal for few of these associated disorders. Low family income and such stressful life events as divorce, separation, imprisonment, illness, or death all confound the associations. Other factors that might mediate the effects of single parenthood include informal parent surrogates, visiting with divorced parents, age, and developmental stage. No studies have been able to control for all of these factors. In those that have controlled for some, family discord and inadequate parenting seem to add more to the risk of antisocial behavior in children than single parenthood itself (28).

Many children undoubtedly experience the active departure of a divorced parent from the household as a terrifying event and express anxiety and confusion about it for prolonged periods. Thus during the first year after divorce, deterioration in the relationship of the custodial parent with the child, and concomitantly in children's behavior, is frequent (32,33). The absence of fathers, especially when divorce is the reason, has been associated with long-term cognitive deficits in children, most markedly in quantitative skills (34). The absence of fathers as a result of marital discord is associated with disordered behavior. The effect of discord is strong enough to account almost entirely for the higher rates of antisocial behavior in boys from single-parent families. Thus where one-parent homes are headed by widowed mothers, the rates of delinquency differ little from those in two-parent homes (28,35,36). Conversely, where discord between parents is marked, delinquency is no less common in children residing with both parents than in children of divorced or separated parents. (37,38,39). Juvenile delinquency, which is largely a male phenomenon, is linked to paternal personality and behavior as well as to fathering (27,37). Antisocial traits in a father are among the strongest predictors that delinquency in a child will persist into adulthood as antisocial behavior (40). Maternal personality also has a role. One study found a threefold excess of personality disorder in the mothers of delinquent boys compared with controls (35).

In American society, divorce may affect boys and girls differently. In one longitudinal study of 48 children, all in the custody of divorced mothers, emotional and behavioral effects were more adverse and enduring in boys than girls (41). In contrast with boys, for girls no comparable association has been found between divorce and juvenile delinquency, excepting one study indicating a high frequency of drug use (29). In the preliminary results of one of the few studies to include both mothers and fathers as custodial parents, however, children living with a parent of the same gender were better adjusted than children living with a parent of the opposite gender (42). This suggests that the type of gender relationship rather than gender itself affects adjustment.

The effects of divorce on children, like that of single parenthood in general, may be the result of many factors associated with divorce either as cause or consequence, for example, inadequacy of parental roles, financial hardship, and stressful life events. Divorce and single-parent homes in American society today are so common that they can hardly be considered aberrant (25). The effects on children are surely changing as society makes adjustments to this situation, and as new norms evolve for meeting the special needs of children.

Most children raised by a single parent are brought up by their mothers. This pattern reflects the biology of reproduction as well as cultural and legal traditions that favor the mother as the parent with primary responsibility for child care. In the event of divorce, the mother usually is awarded custody of the children, while in the event of parental death, children are more likely to be put in foster care with a maternal than a paternal loss. Yet during some or all the stages of development, some children must grow up without mothers or even mother surrogates. Numerous attempts have been made to identify adverse effects of such maternal deprivation (43). Once again, however, as with single parenthood and divorce, absence of a mother is itself associated with adverse and modifying factors.

Some of these confounding factors were controlled in a series of studies that used *nocturnal enuresis* as a conveniently measured symptom likely to be sensitive to family environment; the frequency and persistence of the symptom was observed under a variety of rearing and socialization experiences (31). Enuresis can be considered as a developmental deviation in the normal process of acquiring sphincter control. While physical maturation sets the lower limits for acquiring control, social circumstances influence the likelihood of doing so. Children who attended day nurseries, in a milieu that imposed a high degree of conformity in schedules, achieved control of the bladder sooner than others. Children who stayed at home with their mothers during the first year of life achieved control a little later. Somewhat delayed in comparison were children from families that exposed them to close interaction with several adults from an early age, and to less exclusive relations with their mothers. More delayed were children whose mothers were unable to provide adequate care, usually because of the convergence of several factors, such as poor intellect, an unstable husband, large numbers of children (especially if one or more were handicapped), and poverty. The children in whom enuresis persisted into puberty, the oldest age groups, were those who had experienced total disruption of relations with their mothers.

In pubescent and adolescent boys at a residential school for delinquents, those who were enuretic had lost mothers through desertion, separation, and divorce significantly more often than those who had nocturnal sphincter control. There was no association, however, between enuresis and loss of the mother through death. This finding suggests that the disturbed relations that ordinarily surround a mother's active departure from the home may contribute more to the delay of the development of sphincter control than the maternal loss alone. A comparison between children reared in foster homes and children who remained in institutional care points in the same direction. Among children over ten years of age, the rate of enuresis was nearly five times as high in children who remained in institutions as in those who had been placed with foster parents. In this instance it may not be the fact of maternal absence in itself, but the inferior quality and intimacy of care, and the lack of opportunity to form close attachments with adults, that induce the persistence of enuresis into late childhood.

The quality of care and nurture received by children not reared by their own parents can influence their physical growth as well as their personalities, social development, and attainment in school. This effect on physical growth was demonstrated serendipitously in a nutritional experiment in Germany following the Second World War (44). The children in two orphanages, Bienenhaus and Vogelsnest, were started on identical diets. Unexpectedly, identical diets did not result in identical weight gain. At the end of the first six months the children in Bienenhaus had gained consistently less than those in Vogelsnest (Figure 11.3). For the second six months, in a predetermined cross-over design, the experimenters supplemented the original experimental diet in Vogelsnest, where children were already doing better. Those in Bienenhaus continued unsupplemented with the initial diet. Unexpectedly again, the gains in weight were reversed. The Vogelsnest children failed to maintain their previous advantage, despite their supplemented diet. The Bienenhaus children, still on the original unsupplemented diet, began to make greater gains, and at the end of the second six months had overtaken the Vogelsnest children.

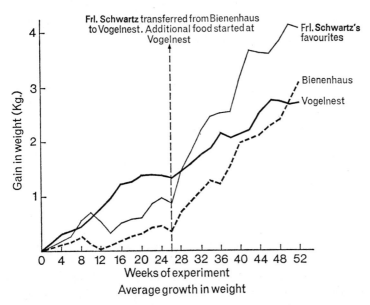

Figure 11.3   Weight gain on controlled diet over two six month periods, in children from two German orphanages after the Second World War, in relation to a particular matron. *Source:* Widdowson, E. M. (1951). Mental contentment and physical growth, *Lancet, 1,* 1316–18.

The puzzled investigators finally discovered that the matron of Bienenhaus, the strict and authoritarian Fraulein Schwartz, had been transferred to Vogelsnest at the time of the cross-over, halfway through the experiment. Throughout the experiment, it thus turned out, this same matron had been in charge of the children who did not thrive. The strict regime imposed by Fraulein Schwartz was in marked contrast to that of the matron she replaced at Bienenhaus and of the matron who succeeded her at Vogelsnest: both these matrons were kind and nurturant caretakers.

The part played by the relations of the children with the mother-substitute was clearly central. This part was further emphasized by the divergent patterns of the growth curves of eight children who were Fraulein Schwartz's "favorites." She had moved these eight children with her from Bienenhaus to Vogelsnest. Both during the first six months in Bienenhaus and the second six months in Vogelsnest, the growth of the eight favorites was superior to that of the other children with whom they lived.

In another classic study, a small group of infants who were retarded in development were removed from the impersonal care of an Iowa orphanage to the personal and intimate care of mentally retarded women in another institution. They soon attained developmental levels that made them eligible for adoption, and outstripped a matched contrast group who remained in the orphanage (see Table 11.2). The experimental group, followed through 30 years, led normal lives in the community; the contrast group led the typical lives of mentally retarded persons in institutions

Table 11.2   IQ scores[a] of an experimental group removed from an orphanage to the care of women in an institution for the mentally retarded, compared with scores of a contrast group remaining in the orphanage

	Age at start in months	Duration of experiment in months	Mean scores at start	Scores at end
Experimental group (N = 13)	$18 \cdot 3 \pm 6 \cdot 6$	$18 \cdot 9 \pm 11 \cdot 6$	$64 \cdot 3 \pm 16 \cdot 4$	$91 \cdot 8 \pm 11 \cdot 5$
Contrast group (N = 12)	$16 \cdot 6 \pm 3 \cdot 2$	$30 \cdot 7 \pm 5 \cdot 8$	$86 \cdot 7 \pm 13 \cdot 9$	$60 \cdot 5 \pm 9 \cdot 7$

[a] Kuhlmann—Binet (1922).

Source: adapted from H. M. Skeels, (1966). Adult status of children with contrasting early life experiences, *Monographs of Society for Research in Child Development, 51,* No. 3; as cited in Stein, Z. A., and Susser, M. W. (1970) The mutability of intelligence and the epidemiology of mild mental retardation, *Rev. Educ. Res, 40,* 29–67.

(45). This study has flaws in design, but subsequent accumulation of data has added conviction to its conclusions.

These studies underline the importance of the social setting for the socialization process, in particular the personal relations between those children who are admitted to institutions and the adults who care for them. As a result of such findings, efforts have been made to improve the care of children in institutions and hospitals by giving them opportunity to form and maintain lasting bonds with caretakers. Some hospitals now encourage parents to stay in hospital with their sick children. Yet we are still far from providing needed attention to the many normal and handicapped children in long-term institutions. Two-year-old children in London residential nurseries had each been cared for by an average of 24.4 adults during the preceding 20-month period, compared with 2.2 for children residing with their parents. The prevalence of psychiatric disorders in institutionalized children, which is high, increases directly with the number of caretakers encountered by the children (46). In the United States and Britain foster-parenting is encouraged as an alternative to institutionalization for children who cannot be cared for by their natural parents or adopted. Whether this system indeed offers children a more stable and enriched social environment than the institutions it is intended to replace remains to be studied.

Despite the developmental problems of children raised in families with atypical structure, by no means all such children experience inadequate care. Moreover, children reared in so-called "intact" families may experience the same kinds of developmental problems. Their source is often to be found in wider economic and social conditions as well as in disturbed family context. A pervasive example of the effects of all these forces in the less-developed countries of the world is malnutrition, a leading contributor to infant and child morbidity and mortality. In some less-developed countries one child in two, and in many not less than one in five, will die before reaching the age of five. The interaction of malnutrition and infection is widely recognized as the common underlying pathology of high rates of debility and death, but it is the interaction with poverty and cultural deprivation that underlies the developmental handicap and growth retardation associated with malnutrition. Those who survive the combined effects of chronic undernutrition and social deprivation are likely to experience intellectual impairment as well as disease (47). Poverty is the universal common denominator in the distribution of malnutrition. Ignorance on the part of caretakers and inequitable distribution of food within families are more particular contributing factors.

Mild mental retardation, specifically the "cultural-familial" syndrome for which there is no known organic etiology, is another disorder the source of which lies in environments of poverty and deficient intellectual stimulus. This can be inferred from the course of the disorder, its susceptibility to intervention, and its distribution in populations. After infancy the average mental performance of affected individuals declines until pubescence, with a parallel increase in the overall frequency of mild mental retardation between infancy and adolescence. In early adulthood there is a degree of intellectual recovery among those affected as children, as well as a decline in overall frequency of mental retardation. The familial character of the syndrome is indicated by the fact that affected children are often not seen as handicapped by other family members who, in turn, have a heightened risk of being classified as mildly retarded (48). Unlike severe mental retardation and the minority of mild cases that are rooted in organic impairment—both of which are distributed fairly evenly with a relatively slight excess among the lower social classes—the cultural-familial form is heavily concentrated in the lower social classes. Comparisons over time, although subject to reservations, indicate that mild mental retardation is likely to have declined in frequency, parallel with improvements in socioeconomic conditions. The strongest evidence that inadequate social and intellectual stimulation is the source of this disorder is provided by at least two well-designed experiments that were able to boost measured IQ substantially by means of an intensive educational program from an early age (49).

Child maltreatment encompasses a spectrum of disorders that are unequivocally rooted in a child's social environment and in inadequate caretaking. They include emotional and physical neglect, sexual abuse, and physical abuse or "battering." Of these forms of maltreatment, least is known about emotional neglect and sexual abuse. For both the damage is primarily psychological and less easily recognized by health and social agencies than physical injury. In a recent survey of nearly 800 women in an American college, 19 per cent identified themselves as having been sexually abused as children, nearly all by adult male relatives (50). Sexual abuse has been distinguished from rape in that it is usually persistent, perpetrated by an adult known to the child, and does not necessarily involve force or sexual intercourse. Clinical cases may present with nonspecific developmental and psychiatric abnormalities, venereal disease, or pregnancy (51).

Clinical sources provide the majority of data on battering and physical neglect— "the battered child syndrome." Once the condition was brought to the attention of pediatricians in the United States in the 1960s, mandatory reporting systems were instituted. Physicians and other professionals are required to report all known and suspected cases of child abuse and neglect to state authorities. The minimal estimates made from official reports have yielded rates from 1.1 to 2.6 per 1000 children under 18 years of age per year (52). Fatality rates among reported cases range from 10 to 18 per cent, but these rates are inflated by reporting bias.

Child abuse in the United States and Great Britain is reported in all socioeconomic, racial, and ethnic groups. Reported incidence is highest for children under five, though the risk of abuse remains substantial throughout childhood and adolescence. Rates have increased dramatically in recent years, but this may be owed entirely to increased awareness and efficiency of reporting. A parent of the victim, more often the mother than the father, is usually identified as the perpetrator. Although most of the literature on child abuse concerns its occurrence in Euro-American settings, it is not absent in the developing world (53,54).

Serious biases in the diagnosis and reporting of ascertained cases preclude valid inferences about the risk factors of child abuse. One source of bias is in the reluctance of physicians to assign diagnoses and file legal reports that implicitly condemn their clients—that is, the parents of their patients (26). Abused children from middle- and upper-class families treated by private physicians are said to be more likely to be misclassified as accident victims than are the abused children from lower-class families treated in public hospitals, where physician-patient rapport is often poor and mandatory reporting more stringently enforced. Hence, heightened surveillance probably contributes to the overrepresentation among reported cases of urban and lower-class children. To heal the physical wounds of child maltreatment is usually the health professional's immediate task, yet this offers only symptomatic relief for the child. For children once maltreated are at great risk for continued abuse or neglect. Adequate intervention must attend to the depleted social network of the child and parents.

Stages of development

In the remainder of this chapter we discuss the social aspects of human development in terms of the four broad stages mentioned above. These stages correspond with important changes in physical and cognitive growth, but have important social dimensions as well. The first stage, infancy, covers approximately the first two years of life; the second, childhood, covers the period between infancy and the onset of puberty; the third stage is pubescence; and the fourth, adolescence, extends from the completion of puberty until the assumption of adult status. The duration of each stage as well as the behavior considered appropriate to it differs from one society to another, partly because diet and habitat influence rates of physical development but mainly because the behavior expected from a child in each stage is socially determined. Moreover, for some children the stage of adolescence may not occur at all; this is the case for girls in some traditional societies when the preference is for them to be married in childhood and to assume the childbearing role immediately after puberty (55).

Within societies and social classes, individual children develop unevenly (56). This is self-evident in school classrooms where children of the same age vary in both the maturity of physical appearance and in the capacity to perform social roles. Children are differently endowed also in temperament and innate abilities. Social systems both encourage and limit human diversity in order to fill necessary social roles. The process of learning, from infancy onward, lies at the center of socialization. Children in societies with a simple technology learn skills primarily by undertaking practical tasks and can be largely trained by their kinsfolk. Education is continuous with other social processes. By contrast, children in industrialized societies with an extreme specialization of labor learn much outside their families. They must acquire a great deal of formal instruction in schools divorced from their other social activities. This dichotomy between informal and formal learning in different types of societies becomes less marked as schooling comes to more children in non-Westernized areas of the world.

The school system functions to meet social and economic needs. From the perspective of the society, one need is to endow all children with standardized elements of the culture such as values, morals, and formal systems of symbols (including language, mathematics, and categorization of knowledge). Another is to select individuals for training in specialized skills. For the performance in school tasks during childhood and adolescence can determine the trajectory of an individual's career.

Within and between each developmental stage outlined above are transitional phases that are unique in occurrence and meaning to a given culture. The transition between infancy and childhood for the Ainu of northeast Asia occurs with the simultaneous events of the birth of a sibling and competence in eating adult food. A Trobriand infant in Melanesia, on the other hand, becomes a child when he or she is able to walk (57). In most industrial societies entry into school marks a critical transition, one in which children must learn to work and play with a new set of strangers. In many traditional societies, the onset of puberty also marks a critical transition to a new status and is celebrated with complex rituals. Other transitions, which may or may not be formally or culturally recognized, evolve out of personal experiences such as the loss of a loved one, having one's first sexual experience or moving to a new location. All transitions can generate acquisition of new statuses and mark critical episodes in a child's development. Culture, social class, and family background are important variables in determining the nature of these transitions as well as the child's capacity to adjust to new demands and opportunities.

Infancy

During infancy, as we have noted, biological maturation imposes a similarity on the experiences and development of all children. Without nurture over a period of years no human infant can survive. Infants typically form bonds or emotional attachments to their primary caretakers during the first year of life. This bonding during infancy has been assigned a large role in later development, particularly in socialization and the ability to form lasting emotional relationships. The age at which bonding occurs has been observed to differ across cultures according to the amount of intimate contact maintained between infants and adults (22). Ugandan infants, who remain in physical contact with the mother or some other caregiver at virtually all times, have been found to express attachment behavior about four months earlier than American infants (58).

Biological maturation sets the lower limits for the acquisition of behaviors and psychological functions, but leaves room for wide variation induced by social environment and childrearing practices. During infancy, sensorimotor development reflects such influences. Social deprivation, for example, is thought to account for sensorimotor retardation in institutionalized infants (28,59). Cross-cultural studies point to the corollary, an acceleration of sensorimotor development in environments rich in social stimulation (60). Ganda infants in Uganda tend to sit, crawl, stand, walk, and vocalize much earlier than the average Western infant. The modes of rearing infants in traditional Ganda society appear to facilitate this rapid development; there is heightened physical contact, social interaction, and social stimulation, immediate gratification of basic needs, and lack of confinement. During the second year of life, a decline in the level of adult attention and social stimulation received by Ganda infants runs parallel with their scores on sensorimotor tests (58). In other cultures too, specific infant care practices appear to correspond with rates of specific aspects of development (61). Physical differences across populations, however, are also likely to contribute to some of these variations in the rate of development, and they have seldom if ever been adequately controlled in such studies.

After early infancy, human development remains malleable and susceptible to new experiences and environmental conditions (62). In the United States, measures of infant cognition begin to diverge among the social classes by the end of the first year, with infants from the middle- and upper-classes scoring higher (19,63,64). Infant cognitive scores up to these ages consist primarily of sensorimotor items and do not predict later "measured intelligence" (59). Rather, they give an indication of current central nervous system development and function. Researchers influenced by psychoanalytic theory have attempted to link early childrearing practices to adult personality and behavior (19,65,66). These efforts have proved difficult and largely unrewarding. Measures tend to be weak and nondiscriminating. In the long latent interval between infancy and adulthood, subsequent experience overwhelms early experience and, if uncontrolled, may suppress its effects.

The socialization process is continuous, however, and carries forward from infancy into the later developmental stages. The effects of socialization at such stages may be immediate, or continuously elaborated, or deferred. Both gender roles and the use of language are crucial aspects of social behavior that begin to be learned in infancy. In most societies, male and female infants are treated differently from the day they are born. In Western societies, gender roles are inculcated by dressing girls and boys according to their sex and encouraging them to play with toys thought appropriate to the domain of each sex. Boys are given toy weapons and motor vehicles while girls are given dolls and miniature homemaking items. Boys are expected to be rough, unruly, and adventurous and girls to be gentle and submissive. Comparable differences in expectations and roles occur in many non-Western societies as well (57).

Social conditioning and adoption of gender roles begins well before a functional divergence in sexual physiology can be seen to occur. Hence, the role preferred by hermaphrodites seems to depend more on social training than on physical characteristics of the body (67,68). The socialization of gender roles that begins in infancy seems to have relevance for the types of psychological problems seen in school children as well as in adults (69,70,71). Girls and women consistently express more symptoms of anxiety, fearfulness, and timidity, while in boys and men defensiveness, aggression, lack of control, and antisocial behavior are more frequent.

This is not to gainsay a biological influence in the divergent social behavior of males and females: the relative contributions of biology and socialization are still to be clarified. In captive primate populations, males and females differ markedly in modes of play, dominance, and responsiveness to infants (72). Such findings are not easily generalized to all primate species nor to those living in natural settings. In human beings, constitution and physiology may account for some of the variance in the social behavior and personality of males and females. Boys are generally more vulnerable to environment than girls. They have higher death rates, more severe handicaps, and higher rates of almost all child psychiatric conditions. At birth, for given length of gestation boys are on average larger and heavier than girls but skeletally less mature (as indicated by the joining of epiphyses). From infancy on through adulthood, males have a greater proportion of muscle tissue than females (71). In comparison to boys, girls have proportionately more body fat; they grow faster and reach puberty sooner and may outstrip boys at that stage, although in general and thereafter they are lighter and shorter.

In infancy and throughout the preschool period the predominant social environment of the child usually will be the family. In traditional societies this environment often includes members of an extended family. Traditional methods of rearing prevail and are perpetuated from generation to generation. Elderly members often play an important role in childrearing tasks and when the need arises can readily substitute for the parents.

The situation differs in modernizing societies where styles of parenting change from generation to generation. In one Lancashire industrial town, we observed differences between the rearing practices of earlier and later generations of working-class mothers who had children of the same age. The differences were most evident in their use of services. The right to health care under the National Health Service had been acquired by all a decade before, but had a visible effect only on the young mothers. They accepted and sought maternity and child health services and the guidance of doctors to a much greater degree than the older mothers.

In contrast to traditional societies, in modernizing societies parenting skills are often learned in part from the latest published text, and the grandmother is divested by professional experts of her traditional role of advisor in child care. Parenting tends to be a more individualized and isolated activity. A certain uniformity in childrearing is imposed by enduring cultural values, by the wide readership of some texts and by knowledge conveyed through other media. But recommended methods change, so that parents may bring up each of their children by different methods based on successive editions of the same book.

In modern times, as more and more women enter the paid work force, fathers participate increasingly in infant and child care activities. Another recent trend is for families with working parents to rely on group day care for infants and children. Despite popular fears about possible deleterious effects of day care, most recent investigations detect no important differences in cognitive, social, or emotional development between children who attend day care centers and those reared exclusively at home (28,59). Children in day care, however, do experience more infections.

Language. The acquisition of language, so crucial for both human evolution and individual development, begins in infancy. Language is not only the predominant human means of communication, but lies at the root of our ability to acquire and store cultural knowledge. Through language human beings build on knowledge transmitted across generations and gain control over their environments. Language plays a central role in human thought and perception, yet its precise relationship is not well understood. Thus a longstanding linguistic and anthropological formulation—the Sapir-Whorf hypothesis—gives language an instrumental role in shaping human thought and perception (73). This theory eludes empirical confirmation or disconfirmation. Critics of the concept maintain that cognitive development is primary and enables language (74). Others hold that language and cognitive development foster each other and together engender learning in a dialectical relationship (75). In small children, language ties in with development. Their use of words facilitates neuromuscular coordination and the physical manipulation of objects and situations (76).

Although the rate at which children acquire linguistic skills may vary considerably, the sequence in which they do so appears to be universal. Regardless of what language is being acquired, nominative and function words appear in children's speech months before verbs, and certain phonemes (for instance, m, n, b, p. f) are articulated correctly earlier than others (for instance, t, s, l, r, z) (77). Between 10 and 13 months, vocalizations with a recognizable linguistic function normally occur. An infant's speech is limited to single-word utterances until about 18 months, when a rapid expansion of vocabulary as well as semantic and syntactic ability appears. Children master much of their native tongue between the ages of two and five. Moreover, at five years they exhibit "code-switching," or the ability to use several speech styles appropriate for different functions and social situations (78).

Mental retardation and other developmental disorders tend to delay or retard language acquisition. When language is learned, however, it generally follows the same sequence as that seen in normal children. There is some evidence that environmental factors also influence the rate at which children acquire language. Firstborn children advance from using two-word phrases to more intelligible speech at an earlier age than later born (79). Institutionalized children, who were found to have considerably less speech directed at them than children raised in home environments, were linguistically underdeveloped at age five (80).

Social class and ethnicity have been shown not to influence the age at which children acquire language (75,79), but they do determine the particular dialect a child learns to speak. Within a single language, *dialects* represent systematic variation in language style, usage, and structure. Dialects arise as a reflection of the distinctiveness of social groups or strata (e.g., in regard to social class, age, sex, or ethnicity) and reinforce these distinctions in everyday life. Within a speech community, a particular dialect may acquire a special status for historical, political, or social reasons, usually because of its associations with dominant or privileged groups. This dialect becomes the "standard dialect," the preferred speech form in public institutions, the professions, and the educational system. Although members of a speech community often believe that the standard dialect is more logical, complex, or mellifluous, the identification of dialects as standard or nonstandard results from their association with higher social class rather than their intrinsic linguistic features. Prestige, power, and control of the education system entrench a standard dialect.

Early studies of children's dialect differences across the social classes sought a linguistic explanation for the inferior school performance of working-class children. These studies suggested that the speech of working-class families conformed to a "restricted code" that was thought to be communicatively inferior to the "elaborated code" used both in schools and in middle-class homes (81). These differences are relative, not absolute, since members of all class groups use both codes; the point is that working-class children hear and use elaborated code less frequently than middle-class children and hence are less familiar and comfortable with it. A conclusion drawn from these studies was that "the normal linguistic environment of the working class is one of relative deprivation" (82). In the United States, the findings from such studies were used to justify educational programs aimed at correcting the supposed language deficits of children from poor families. These interventions, which began in the 1960s, have been criticized for their insensitivity to linguistic differences associated with cultural background (83).

Linguistic analyses of actual verbal behavior in natural contexts show that all language varieties are equivalent in their expressive capacities. A detailed empirical analysis of American Black English, for instance, showed this dialect to be governed by highly systematized grammatical rules that differ only slightly from standard English (84). Nonetheless, because familiarity with the standard dialect is important for school performance, children from lower socioeconomic groups enter school at a disadvantage. Unlike middle- and upper-class children who experience little discrepancy between the dialect of the classroom and that of the home, children raised in lower-class homes must master a second dialect in order to succeed in the school environment. School tests assume expertise in the standard dialect. Moreover, students reared in nonstandard dialects face an additional barrier when teachers disapprove of the use of socially inferior dialects and evaluate lower-class students accordingly. Although many students do learn the standard dialect, as indicated in their adept alternation between standard and nonstandard speech depending on the social context ("code-switching"), the need to acquire and master a new dialect poses a special burden for lower-class children.

Childhood

A period of *social weaning* bridges the transition from infancy to childhood. For the first time the child is taken for prolonged periods from the direct care of its parents and submitted to the authority of strangers. Depending on the society, on the urban or rural setting, on social class and the occupations of the parents, this experience begins in daycare centers for some children as early as the first year of life, or in kindergarten and nursery schools at three or four years of age, or as late as five and six years of age in so-called infant schools. A special curriculum allows for the social immaturity of the child. For some, especially rural children, there is no transitional institution to ease the entry to school.

Schooling. During later childhood, which lasts from about the age of six until the onset of puberty, children acquire a primary education. The rate of physical growth remains steady until the spurt at puberty, and this is a time of active social development. If indeed the psychosexual latency postulated by psychoanalytic theory is a reality, perhaps this social activity can be seen as its complement. At school, children's motor freedom is gradually restricted until they learn the primary lesson of most classrooms: to sit quietly at a desk and concentrate on a task that has no immediate relevance to any of their home situations or experiences. Children thereby acquire some of the elementary skills of the culture; they begin to read, to manipulate figures, to handle new tools, to study art and music and their natural environment.

As soon as children are established in a class with others they also acquire a social life independent of their caretakers, and through group play learn to adjust to this life. They begin to transfer their interest from the family to other children of their own age, to emerge as social individuals and to understand social values. This transitional period from social infancy to childhood corresponds with an expansion of socially oriented responses. In many industrial societies, "serious" schooling does not begin until about the age of seven.

The school is the major socializing instrument of the society at large, and its socializing influence is effected only partly through formal teaching. The school is a small society that governs much of the child's life, and its influence pervades many areas of thought and feeling. In and out of the classroom the school cultivates common attitudes, generates respect for historical and existing figures of authority in the wider society, and ties children into the web of dominant values about personal morality, about political good and evil, and about national aspirations (85). In the United States the integration into the existing society of millions of European immigrants in the nineteenth and early twentieth centuries is familiar lore. In the face of strong ethnic groupings that still persist, their acculturation to American values was accomplished in the schools. This function is symbolized in the American flags that drape the platforms of school assembly halls throughout the land, and in the Oath of Allegiance that the children recite each morning. The more recent history of schooling in the United States, during the 1970s, illustrates the role of socialization in blocking the assimilation of minorities. Resistance to the attempt to integrate schools racially by court ordered busing—besides convulsing several cities and providing a leading edge for political conflicts—asserted and cultivated ethnic, religious, racial and class identities (86).

On entering school, the child is brought into contact with the wider social structure of the community. Children come to understand the significance of social prestige and social class, and of the standing and affiliations of their own families. The particular primary school a child attends is determined by family background and reflects the major social cleavages. Many children from well-to-do families enter fee-paying schools; others go to free schools; while yet others attend parochial schools. Within the two broad categories of private and public education there are further divisions representing distinctions of social origin.

This educational segregation exposes children to dissimilar experiences and training. In Britain, for example, upper middle-class boys who enter fee-paying boarding schools may be taught wholly by men in the company of other boys; girls are excluded. Their sisters attend private schools for girls only, where they are taught by women. On the other hand, working-class and many middle-class children of both sexes attend the same primary schools where they are taught together, generally by women with a minority of male teachers. At school the authority of women over children is direct and frequently exercised, but "serious" punishment and supervision more often belongs to men (87). Hence, schools reinforce and elaborate sex roles through the engendering of authority positions and the behaviors of the teachers, as well as through sex-typed instruction and toys. The degree of sex-typing has varied between social classes and with historical periods.

Children in both the private and public streams of primary education progress at this time to more formal studies, in arithmetic, reading and writing, singing, art, natural history, geography, history, and physical exercise. Much of their schoolwork is unrelated to the content of their family life, which so far has been the main source of their knowledge of adult life. Subjects are sharply divided and the periods of instruction regular and disciplined: regularity and order make a constant impression. The school situation is artifically constructed not only for pedagogy and the transmission of values, but as preparation for the social demands of adult life. In a sense, educationists construct a model situation from their perceptions of the role expectations of the society to give children practice for the situations they will confront in the adult world. The emphasis and the impact of these experiences differ between the social classes, and nowhere has this been more evident than in the matter of children's play.

Play. Play, like schooling, is a central experience of childhood. During the period of early childhood the manner in which children play is of primary importance in their social development. Pediatricians have come to recognize the therapeutic value of providing opportunities for play even in hospitals. The egocentric play of infants gradually merges into group play involving larger numbers of children and more complicated situations. The child identifies with these play-groups, and through them learns how to cooperate with others and also to compete with them, to play appropriate roles, to understand and obey social rules, and to realize her or his position in a larger world. The play-group teaches children how to discriminate between others by social criteria, and thus prepares them for the next period of development, when they will be influenced by the social standing and values of their parents and kin-groups.

The quality of play is deeply influenced by culture. In many societies "play" tends to be a simulation of adult activities, and the objects used are scaled-down versions of adult tools and utensils. In nonindustrial societies separation between the adult world and the child's world is less than that found in industrial societies, and children undertake productive tasks at a tender age. Cultures vary in the importance they place on children's play. To the eye of a British pediatrician, Ghanaian nurses seemed apathetic to the need for play in children's wards (88).

The word "play" is no less slippery than the word "class"; the *Shorter Oxford Dictionary* devotes three columns to a definition. Play is often used in a context that implies pleasure or absence of constraint, activity that is an end in itself (89). But play is not mere amusement. Freud considered that children's play reflects their wish to be like grown-up people and to act like them. Children may even repeat unpleasant experiences in play because these help them towards a more thorough mastery of the situations they enact. This "repetition compulsion" is not confined to children; adults, too, repeat both painful and pleasurable experiences in actuality or in symbol (90).

Adult constraints on the behavior of children at home and in school extend also to their play. Imposed forms of play are used as an aid to socialization, a kind of pleasant coercion; play becomes children's work. When, say, a father sings a nursery rhyme to his child, or a teacher encourages infants to dance, the lesson embraces more than the words of the rhyme or the actions of the dance. The child learns behavior appropriate to the roles of father and child, teacher and pupil, and gains a grasp of language and gesture, of authority and submission, all within a particular cultural context. These activities can be described as *pedagogic play* (91).

The social games of children help prepare them for their adult roles (92). We refer here primarily to children's social play that involves the participation of others, whether adults or children, and not to the *egocentric play* of young infants. In egocentric play children express their fantasies, wishes, and experiences in a symbolic way (93), and this takes up less and less of a child's play time as the child matures, goes to school, and learns to play in the company of others.

In schools organized games are an institutionalized form of pedagogic play. Since the nineteenth century, especially in Britain, games have been used as a method of building "character and leadership." The rules and regulations controlling organized games are made and maintained by adults. When children under the notice of critical adults play such games well, or attempt to play them well, they are learning a prime lesson in adjustment to adult demands and expectations. The social importance of these games lies in the moral and ethical training they provide and not in the acquisition and practice of skills to be used in adult life. They encourage a spirit of competition and striving for success. They also teach children to value group loyalty and teamwork, although always in a context of competition. Organized games form a direct link with the adult world, and for this reason have the prestige and power of their adult source. They help to inculcate what Piaget described as a "morality of constraint," a series of objective duties based on respect for persons in authority, and accepted in the same way as language, one of the realities imposed by the adult world (94). The morality inculcated through organized games conditions attitudes and behavior among adults. Phrases taken from games, such as "fair play," "below the belt," "it's not cricket," and so on, symbolize complex codes of behavior.

In many societies during this period children also form *play-groups* of their own. In these groups children enjoy equality of status; adults are excluded and assigned the status of aliens. These peer-groups consist of from 2 to about 12 children of all ages between 7 and 13 (95). In the play-group, children of this age have a society of their own, free of adult supervision and comment, a form of child-ruled or *pediarchic play*. The exclusion of adults is so fundamental to pediarchic play that the games are difficult to observe and record. This may be one reason why psychologists have tended to give less attention to children's play during this period than during the periods of infancy and adolescence that precede and follow it.

A central activity of these play-groups is a number of traditional games, in which the form of play is unlike the pedagogic play outlined above. The rules and regulations for pediarchic play are usually enshrined in jingles and rhymes that have been handed down from one generation of children to the next and many of them have a long pedigree (96). One game still played by British children is almost identical to a game described in the *Satyricon*, and the controlling jingle still contains corrupted Latin words. These games have no counterpart in adult life, have none of the prestige associated with organized group games, and are dismissed by adults as of no importance. Most children usually abandon them at puberty. Children themselves distinguish clearly between pediarchic and pedagogic play. Pediarchic play is often described as "street games," for the street is the only space available, outside the home or school, where such play can be observed by adults.

The play-group is usually an association of neighboring children, a selection of companions on the basis of equal status in both age and residence. This form of selection appears to be characteristic of children in many societies at this period of their development. In urban societies, a family's place of residence and its social standing are often closely related, so that the play-group becomes an extension of the home. Association in egalitarian play-groups fosters loyalties both to the kind of people to whom children conceive of themselves as belonging and to the place where they live, thus providing a foundation on which to build a growing understanding of social distinctions within a society as a whole. The conflict and rivalry so common between play-groups expresses this loyalty to place and people and translates physical separation into social distance. Adults appear to be aware of this function of the play-group. Higher-class parents and aspirant working-class parents who "look down" on their neighbors often control children's choice of companions (91), and forbid them to join in local play-groups. By so doing, they encourage their children to apply social criteria in a conscious way. In exchange for the play-group, these parents may substitute pedagogic play, for instance, by sending their children to dancing classes or to organized activities such as Scouts and Guides.

Pediarchic play-groups have important functions in socializing the child. They provide physical safety and psychological assurance, and help to establish a recognition of social rights and duties. The protective function of the play-group has been noted as particularly important in those urban areas of the United States where white and black, Jew and gentile, all lived in the same district as if in hostile encampments (95). Through play-group experience children learn to cooperate in group activity. They learn the need to keep rules, to accept various roles, and to modulate their own desires in the interests of the majority. These games help to develop an understanding of what is just or "fair"—in Piaget's term, a "morality of cooperation" that rests on mutual understanding between equals (94). Because play-groups are an association of social equals, children learn to value others in terms of their individual qualities.

The sick child. In childhood, health disorders cut across the path of normal development. Their influence can be insidious or highly visible. Infections and malnutrition in combination, and probably independently, retard growth and development, as measured by weight and height and by skeletal maturity (97,98). This influence on physical development is complemented by a parallel influence on psychological and social development.

The immediate psychological effect of a health disorder on a child depends on many factors. These include the nature, severity, and course of the disorder; the age and social situation of the child; and the location, duration, and the type of care given. The child who enters the hospital must face loneliness and separation from parents and home; strange children, some of whom will be depressed, miserable, and in pain; and frightening technical procedures, such as the induction of anesthesia and surgery, that have an unpleasant or painful aftermath.

Children exhibit a variety of responses to these circumstances (99). Young children may regress in their feeding, dressing, and toilet behavior; others try to maintain self-sufficiency. Some children see illness as punishment for "being bad" and feel guilty. Some are depressed, some hypochondriacal, some deny that they are ill, and some have fantasies about the nature of their disorders. Older children may worry about expense, missed schooling, games, and fun. When they are the objects of anxiety among parents or among nurses and physicians, this anxiety may be communicated to the child and cause agitation.

Clinical observation suggests that illness at each age takes on different psychological meanings for the sick child in the hospital. These meanings follow in rough chronological sequence (99). During infancy, separation from the parents may raise fears of the parents' desertion. Thus, infants admitted to the hospital together with their mothers did not show the regressive behavior observed in controls admitted alone in the usual fashion (100). At three years of age children may envisage mutilation and dismemberment; at five years, they have a realization and fear of death. At seven years, children feel deprived of the material things available outside, may resent being confined in the hospital, and may feel defeated. At nine years the children develop fantasies about their internal body image, the ravages of disease, and their external body image—for instance, the disfigurement and dissection of the body. At ten years, their concerns become socially oriented towards peers as a reference group; illness seems to them a disgrace that detracts from their moral prestige among them.

These observations of sick children are far from typical of the common childhood experience of sickness. They draw largely on hospital studies of children with serious chronic disease. Out of hospital and in the society of schoolchildren, the experience of serious sickness, hospital stay, or operation may enhance the child's prestige rather than detract from it. For each child under 17, the annual number of consultations with general practitioners is between four and five in the United States, but the rate of hospital admissions is less than one-tenth of the consultation rate (101). Between cultures and between generations, the frequency of disease among children, their perceptions of illness, and the readiness of adults to accord them the sick role, can be expected to vary. Values and expectations about health have changed as control over disease has been gained and as the experience of sickness among children has diminished in frequency and severity. A child in the developed world may now entirely avoid not only such dangerous infections as diptheria, whooping cough, poliomyelitis, and tuberculosis, but also the milder infections of measles, rubella, and mumps. In the United States measles is on the verge of being eliminated by a national vaccination campaign begun in 1967 (101) (see Figures 11.4 and 11.5).

Until recently, many of these diseases were seen as inescapable dangers or discomforts, necessary conditions of childhood, as they remain in the developing world. Although we have emphasized that disease, illness, and sickness are separable entities, they are closely related. The capacity to control disease, and to reduce its incidence and effects, changes both conceptions about illness and adaptations to the sick role. While the child in today's industrial society acts out the sick role less often than in the past, children are more likely to receive professional attention for minor illnesses, and parents and pediatricians will be as much concerned with the course of a child's development as with sickness.

The course of a sickness that may end in death or disability makes an extensive impact on the social life of the child and the child's family. A number of studies report increased marital discord in families with a chronically ill child (102). In pediatric encounters this impact on social relations tends to be shut out from view. The social structure of a hospital or clinic sets up a limiting frame of reference for its staff; it conditions them to perceive the technical problems of disease. Medical training almost universally reinforces the frame of reference induced by the structure of the health care setting. Special training and effort is therefore needed to enable the staff to per-

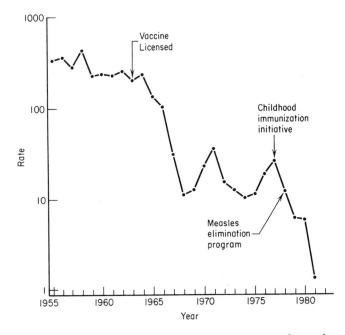

Figure 11.4 Measles (rubeola)—Reported cases per 100,000 population, by year, United States, 1955–1981. *Source:* National Center for Health Statistics (1983). *Morbidity and Mortality Weekly Report,* vol. *31,* No. 54, p. 48.

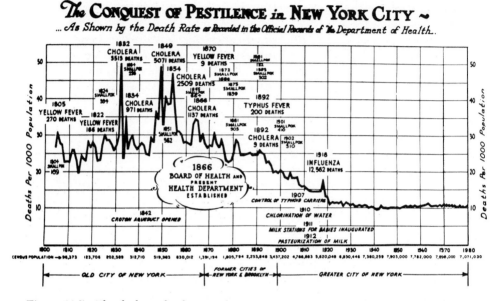

Figure 11.5 The decline of infectious disease in New York City. *Source:* New York City Department of Health (1981). *Summary of Vital Statistics 1980,* New York.

ceive the psychological problems of illness, and to empathize and deal with them. For instance, in one hospital unit that cared for children with a uniformly fatal prognosis, successful reorientation of the staff took place when parents were brought in to live with their children. The morale of the staff improved as they recognized the problems of the parents and found that they could help them (103).

Medical morale is often low in situations that seem hopeless for the patient. The dyadic patient-doctor relationship generates a need for therapeutic optimism on the part of the doctor, so that effectiveness in treatment correlates well with the desirability and prestige of specialties in medical eyes. To comprehend the full social situation of the child, however, investigations must extend beyond the hospital, for that situation involves the family and social world of the parents as much as the child.

Sickness, like disease, is a process with a natural history and course.° Disease begins with the exposure of susceptible persons to causal factors, and expresses itself more or less quickly in some primary physiological or psychological dysfunction. This primary dysfunction generates both secondary dysfunction in various bodily systems, and reactive responses that may contain and halt the disease process, although sometimes at the cost of further damage. Illness and sickness can be classed among the secondary

---

°The term *natural history* is used in epidemiology to refer to the occurrence and distribution of disease in *populations,* whereas others use it also to refer to the cause, course, and prognosis of disease in an individual. While both senses could apply here, the emphasis is on individual course and prognosis.

dysfunctions of disease (see Chapter 4); in a broader view, however, they are also reactive responses that bring outside support to the body's resistance to the disease process. Illness and sickness, like disease, each have their own natural course. For the practice of medicine the implication of natural history is that, as the process of sickness evolves, each emergent event progressively limits the possible course of the remaining sequence. Knowledge of a typical course clarifies prediction and prognosis. The study of the natural history and course of *disease* perforce extends beyond medical institutions, but even the study of *sickness* is incomplete without such extension.

One family study of poliomyelitis in children, from onset through the return home, dramatized the course of the sickness by breaking it up into stages around an acute crisis (104). Although in the developed world this disease has been quelled, families still undergo similar experiences with other diseases, and the study itself remains unique. Despite the existence of a poliomyelitis epidemic, before the onset of illness all seemed normal. In the *warning stage,* the child's slight malaise progressed until the parents recognized a cue that something more might be amiss and felt threatened. During this warning stage, each parent protected the other by not speaking openly of their own suspicions or, if the matter was discussed, one parent assumed the role of comforter to the other. In some cases, after the diagnosis was confirmed, the comforter broke down and became the comforted.

The call for the doctor ushered in a short and fearful *impact stage.* In almost all cases the doctor gave only a tentative diagnosis. Thus, exchanges between doctor and parents were veiled, qualified, and equivocal. This pattern continued through subsequent episodes of the sickness: the parents had thereby been initiated into a world where what was left unsaid was as important as what was said.

At such a time few doctors are direct. In the early stage of infection they must deal in probabilities. They are tentative because they have to avoid errors, and so protect their future relations with the family and their professional reputations. Where there is greater certainty, many doctors will seek to avoid the shock of brutal confrontation, and in justification can point to the frequent phenomenon of "denial" in patients with serious disease. Uncomfortable with the "dirty work" of conveying unpleasant information that dashes hope, family doctors may prefer to leave that duty to other more distant figures in the hospital.

Patients and parents of sick children will usually give a view of their preferences quite different from what their doctors assume (17,105). Many patients claim to prefer unhappy certainty to the anxiety of uncertainty, and ask for information so that they may absorb it and adjust to it. They withdraw confidence from the doctor who does not satisfactorily communicate with them; they may come to resent the doctors and even use them as a scapegoat for their troubles. The hospital doctors are seen as indeed distant, yet they delegate the role of giving the unpleasant information, in anonymous collusion with colleagues, no less often than the family doctor (106). The doctor in these ambivalent situations may, in fact, not be able to do right, and elicits resentment as much as thanks. The divergence between the professional and the family perceptions of the problems that surround sickness can thus lead to mutual frustration.

In the *inventory stage* there was a gradual lessening of tension during the weeks, then months, of the child's stay in hospital. With the decline of the acute crisis physicians visited the child less often, and the family received fewer telephone calls, inquiries, and gifts for the child. By the nature of the condition, recovery did not accompany the decline of outside interest in the child, who was gradually put aside in the lives of others excepting the immediate family. Doctors and nurses avoided the questions of the parents. The family, lacking feedback from physicians and still believing the child might recover, focused their attention on the routine serial tests of muscle function and on the physiotherapist's reports. This physical focus served to divert their attention from the reality of the permanent residual disability. They failed to take proper stock and were delayed in making psychological and social preparation for the return of a physically disabled child. The physicians abetted the delay, for they showed little interest in a child whose physical treatment was routine and of whom no further recovery could be expected. The parents saw this routinized care as rejection by the child's attendants. By the time the child left the hospital, most of the parents reciprocated with antagonism.

The disabled children had now to return home and take up the threads of social life. Parental accommodation to the changed role of the child was variously successful. Some parents became active in local organizations for the welfare of handicapped children; others concentrated on the individual care of their own disabled children to the extent of isolating themselves from their communities. Family adjustment clearly affected the child's adjustment. But in this study numbers were small, and the children covered a range of ages and had unequal disabilities, so that generalization is unsafe.

There was no doubt, however, that the residual physical disorders of the children raised barriers for them, as they tried to bridge the social distance created by their enforced absence from their peers. In these efforts, the severity of the disability alone was not a final determinant. Some children were able to find, within their old play-groups, new roles from which their disabilities did not disqualify them (e.g., as the scorer for the neighborhood team). Some, on the other hand, could not return to the same schools as before, nor rejoin their play-groups. Some who were thus excluded joined new circles of handicapped children; others became isolated. Thus, a major outcome of the episode for the children was the effect on social relations, and the consequences for mental and physical development that flow from these relations.

In other studies, follow-up surveys of the effects of long-term hospital stay have revealed relatively little psychiatric disturbance. Bowlby initiated a controlled study of children who spent long periods in a tuberculosis sanatorium to test the evidence for the syndrome of maternal deprivation he had described and failed to find it. Another uncontrolled follow-up of children who spent long periods in an orthopedic hospital in New York also produced little evidence of disturbance. (This institution, it must be admitted, was especially designed to cater to children's needs.) Both surveys studied older children without visible impairments and sought long-term effects on the individual psyche and not on social relationships (107). In the study of the acute crisis and aftermath of paralyzing poliomyelitis, where family and not individual adjustments were studied and impairment was permanent, the social relationships of the children did change.

Various family studies suggest that family troubles of many kinds, especially among the poor, appear as crises. Disease can be included with other troubles in a broad classification of crises because of the common social consequences. Adjustment after the crisis depends in part on the social situation and the pre-existing cohesiveness and supportiveness of the family. The situation may be righted; recovery may never be complete; the gathering of family forces provoked by the trouble may stimulate a higher level of function than before; or recurrent crises may gradually depress the customary level of family function. The difficulties of treating crises and family function in unitary terms, or even with a multiplicity of measures, should not be underestimated.

In one example in the city of New York, a teenage girl developed sudden acute abdominal pain at night. The family upheaval that followed centered around the fact that the father, a recently arrived immigrant, could not bring himself to call a doctor, and his adolescent son took it on himself to do so. The crisis of role allocation that followed disturbed the family more fundamentally, and for longer, than did the surgical emergency itself or the anxiety it provoked (108). Selected features of the sequence of events can be set out schematically:

Family member	Provoking event	Effect
Daughter	Acute appendicitis	Pain, crying, and distress
Father	Daughter's distress	Indecision, anxiety
Son	Sister's distress and father's indecision	Decision to override father's authority
Mother	Daughter's distress, father's indecision, son's assumption of authority	Devaluation of spouse
Father	Devaluation by wife and son	Marital and intergenerational strife; loss of self-esteem

The handicapped child. Handicap is a lifelong problem that can become prominent in childhood. By analogy with sickness, three components of handicap can be distinguished: organic, functional, and social. In accord with our definitions in Chapter 1, we shall term the primary organic component *impairment,* a static disorder of anatomical structure or physiological, biochemical, or molecular responses, most usually a deficit; this is the analogue (and, as in poliomyelitis, sometimes the outcome) of the process of disease. We shall term the functional component *disability,* by which is meant the limitations on performance imposed by the combination of impairment and the individual's psychological reaction to it. In this usage disability is the analogue of illness. *Handicap* is the term we shall use for the social component, the manner and degree to which the primary impairment and functional disability modify the performance of social roles and relations with others. Handicap is the analogue of the sick role, and indeed has much in common with the chronic ambulant form of the sick role (see pp. 295ff. & elsewhere).

The primary impairment of anatomical structure or psychological resources sets organic limits on what a child can do. The resulting degree of functional disability the child exhibits, however, has powerful psychological determinants; these derive from temperament, and from the incentives and reinforcements that flow from relations with others to shape a growing personality. The ultimate form of the social handicap has powerful social determinants; these derive from expectations attached to the roles the child is assigned by society, and from the manner in which the child meets those expectations or deviates from them.

Characteristic problems arise in the socialization of the handicapped child. These include the problems of dependence, of exclusion and segregation, of marginality, and of stigma and self-image. A disabled child, by the nature of the condition, is likely to be more dependent than age-peers for physical needs, and for protection from the physical and social environment. In many families these needs elicit typical attitudes and role expectations and characteristic role assignments. In a study of twin pairs, only one of whom in each pair had cerebral palsy, the roles of normal and handicapped children could be contrasted (109). In most pairs, the normal twin had many opportunities for learning about social norms and expectations, and for acquiring understanding of the environment. The handicapped twin, like a "sick" child, was denied these opportunities and kept close within the confines of the home. The normal twin was chiefly engaged in relations of equality with age-peers outside the family; the handicapped twin was chiefly engaged in dependent relations with their mothers. There was a general tendency for the families of handicapped children to split into two groupings: mother with handicapped child, and father with healthy sibs. Thus, in the care of handicapped children a conflict exists between their special needs for nurture and protection and their need for opportunities to learn the norms of social roles. Although normal social exposure may endanger the impaired child, it also enables the child to make the maximum use of residual potential, and to learn ways of overcoming impairment and functional disability.

Their families may exclude individual handicapped children from the activities of their unhandicapped age-peers to an extreme degree. In such cases the handicapped child may become the focus of all family activities, influencing parental choices of occupation and residence, and isolating the family altogether from ordinary social and community activities (110). At the group level, exclusion becomes segregation. Because it is often uneconomical to meet the special educational needs of children with severe impairments on an individual basis, these children are grouped in special schools where facilities and expertise are concentrated. This segregation reinforces the pressure towards socializing children for the special roles of the handicapped. Special schools not only set them aside, but class them as different from others who are not handicapped. An American study, for instance, showed that in the eyes of the wider society the blind have an inferior position equivalent to that of a minority ethnic group (111). This position of inferiority, felt both by the minority and the majority, often evokes unfounded and damaging stereotypes.

Some classes of handicapped people may indeed share minority values distinct from the wider society. Distinct values may be reinforced by distinct social circles. People who are congenitally deaf learn to communicate, and therefore to commingle, with each other to the exclusion of most of the rest of society. These deaf people often do not accept the attitudes of hearing persons about the undesirability of hearing impairments, and especially of perpetuating the impairment through mating and marriage. In their view a deaf person makes as desirable a mate as a hearing person; a deaf child is no less valuable than a hearing child.

The clear social separation of groups of handicapped persons from the nonhandicapped creates a social position that is marginal between the two classes. Physicians and educationists face problems of judgment in deciding whether partial or mild impairments of sight, hearing, limb, or intellect call for education in special schools. Their decisions may well affect the degree of the child's functional disabilities, and ultimately the handicapped role. The child with partial impairments suffers from a conflict of values and loyalties. In similar plight, a "coloured" person in South Africa (see pp. 80ff.) could identify with the dominant whites or the subject blacks and, before registration laws fixed race permanently, he or she might pass from one group to the other. Marginality has psychological as well as social effects. Partially sighted persons have been found to be less well-adjusted than people with unimpaired vision, and also than those who are totally blind (112). Impairments that arise late in development, like partial impairments, may lead to a marginal position and affect socialization to the handicapped role. Similarly, children who lose their hearing in their teens are often disturbed by having to attend schools for the deaf.

These disturbances have more sources than the unhappy awareness of an impaired body and the constraints imposed by functional disability. Marginality is a creation of the attitudes of society to handicap. The child itself will have absorbed society's attitudes and must reconcile them with its own view of self. Many cultures attach a stigma to handicap, the intensity of which varies with its particular form. Groups of children, asked to choose friends from pictures of children with a variety of impairments, were consistent in the average order of preference they assigned to each handicap (113,114). The unimpaired were invariably preferred, even by handicapped children. Preferences were age-specific and sex-specific: each age-group and each sex placed different values on bodily characteristics. Thus boys were more concerned about functional impairment, girls about cosmetic impairment. As is to be expected with a societal phenomenon, the degree of stigma attached to each handicap also varied between cultures, and children of different cultural backgrounds showed different orders of preference.

The stigma attached to handicap has psychological and social consequences for handicapped people (115). The stereotype may evoke emotional responses and social perceptions in the beholder that overshadow all the other attributes of the handicapped individuals. The handicap thus devalues and depreciates the person. Among professionals, the labeling of a child by a single handicap tends to divert attention from other impairments that may accompany it, as well as from abilities. The label "cerebral palsy" for instance, is held to have impeded investigation of the intellectual and sensory effects that accompany the motor defect caused by cerebral damage (116). In the presence of handicap, people without handicaps change their usual social behavior, embarrassed by the cultural stereotypes they hold, as well as by their uncertainty about the hurt their responses may cause. By so doing, they do not give the feedback that defines role expectations in normal social interaction, and they distort the socialization process imparted through such interaction. Among handicapped children, therefore, distorted feedback alone may give rise to behavior discordant with the usual modes of a culture. The possibilities of discordance are enhanced by the children's lack of social experience outside the family. For the learning of social roles and the acquisition of social understanding flows from the opportunities for a wide range of social interaction. The opportunities for normal social interaction are further restricted, because the nonhandicapped children most likely to associate with those who are handicapped may themselves tend to be isolated and to perceive the values of their age-peers less accurately than others (114). When a handicapped child is more or less integrated into a social group, however, the incongruous status may be dealt with by assigning such special roles as mascot or scapegoat.

Stigma is communicated to the "spoiled" person (117) who must somehow adjust self-image to perceptions absorbed from others (118). One writer, immobilized for years within the loving nidus of her family by the tuberculous erosion of her vertebrae, describes how as a girl she had always believed that she was a beautiful person (119). Only after she could rise from her bed did she become aware of the hunchback caused by the collapse of her vertebrae, and only after she could venture into the world did she become aware of the ugliness that others saw in her impairment. One's image of oneself is created in part by others. Handicapped people learn to anticipate reactions to their visible impairments; they develop a variety of coping mechanisms that enable them to present themselves to strangers, and to desensitize the stranger to the initial shock.

Handicaps need not be visible to attract stigma. People who acquire the label of leprosy or mental illness without the condition being visible risk being stigmatized by society. They too have learned, in the course of normal socialization, to stigmatize the condition they themselves have come to suffer from. As a result, they may delay their entry into medical care, and when they do seek care they may make a stormy adjustment to the patient role.

The fate of those severely handicapped children who cannot escape dependency is ultimately a matter of values. The depreciation of the value of handicapped persons in society at large is powerful enough to pervade the caretaking professions. A doctor's decision about a child may place the interests of others, parents or community, above those of the child, and override the Hippocratic injunction to place the patient's needs above all others. The conflicts of interest within the families attended by the doctor make some such decisions unavoidable. The burdensome prospect of years of emotional, social, and economic strain for the parents of a surviving and severely handicapped child who may neither walk, nor hear, nor speak, nor see, can hardly be overestimated.

As a result, the clash of values between those who would sustain all human life in any circumstances and those who would forbear has become prominent in political and legal domains. These clashes stem from the technical power modern medicine has acquired: failed cardiorespiratory systems can be kept going and vital nutrients can be supplied. But even in the wealthiest societies the world has ever seen, some of these decisions are guided by implicit cost-effectiveness calculations of the potential economic productivity of the handicapped child. Because of the low value placed on handicapped children, those willing to take care of them are also depreciated. The institutions to which they are consigned suffer a kind of anomie; they tend to have low prestige, to be alienated from the mainstream of society, and to be sequestered in their location (120).

Some of these utilitarian attitudes are stimulated by fears of a growing burden of handicap to be carried by the rest of society. In fact, in Britain and perhaps in other industrial societies, the total frequency of handicaps was probably in decline in the first two decades after the Second World War. Surveys of London schoolchildren showed a decrease in a majority of types of handicaps. A decrease was found in the prevalence of rheumatic heart disease, tuberculosis of bones and joints, and the motor handicaps of poliomyelitis; there was an increase only in the prevalence of cerebral palsy and severe mental retardation (121).

Prevalence, we have noted previously, is the product of duration and incidence (pp. 30ff). In developed countries, among children with impairments that lead to handicap, duration, as indicated by survival after birth, has greatly increased. At the same time, survival of very low birthweight babies who are at especially high risk of impairment and later handicap, has greatly increased. It is almost certainly this factor of survival that led to the increases noted above in the *prevalence* of cerebral palsy and mental retardation. Recent evidence suggests, however, that in the most favorable social circumstances, as in Sweden, the *incidence* of mental retardation and possibly of cerebral palsy has declined. A continuing decline will eventually be reflected in prevalence since there is an ultimate age-limit to survival (48,122). A significant increase in the incidence of impairments might be expected only under special conditions: for instance, an impairment that has a strong genetic component with dominant transmission, that in the past has generally been fatal in childhood, and that at the present time permits survival into the fertile ages. With recessive conditions like phenylketonuria in which homozygous individuals now survive and reproduce, the added incidence of homozygous cases in the population will be negligible.* Another set of special conditions might be found where environmental factors, such as radiation, chemical pollution, and drugs are on the increase and could affect the unborn fetus, and yet could allow it to survive.

In developed and less-developed countries the pattern of incidence, duration, and prevalence of impairments such as mental retardation is almost certainly different (123,124). The data from less-developed countries are too scant to support much gen-

---

*The most serious consequence of survival with phenylketonuria is not genetic. Homozygous females who become pregnant expose their offspring in utero to their own high blood level of phenylalanine, and no means has yet succeeded in protecting the fetus from serious developmental damage.

eralization. No data are available on prenatal damage, although it is a reasonable supposition that the incidence is higher. The incidence of postnatal damage to the brain is certainly greater in less-developed countries. The sources of damage include bacterial and viral meningeal infections and the encephalopathies that occur with measles, whooping cough, and electrolyte imbalance resulting from diarrheal dehydration. At the same time, in less-developed countries high incidence is offset by high death rates and short survival, especially among those already vulnerable from handicap (124). Offsetting may occur prenatally through losses by miscarriage, just as it does postnatally through losses by death.

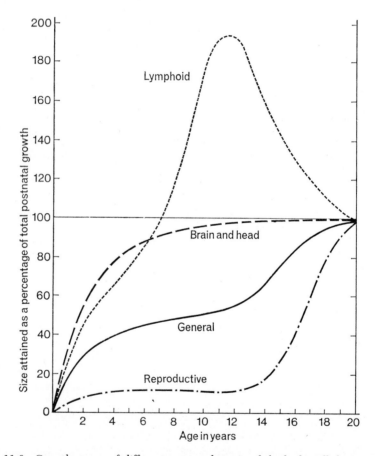

Figure 11.6 Growth curves of different parts and tissues of the body. All the curves are of size attained, and plotted as a percentage of total gain from birth to maturity (20 years), so that size at age 20 is 100 on the vertical scale. *Source:* Redrawn from Scammon, R. E. (1930). *The Measurement of Man*, Minneapolis; and in Tanner, J. M. (1962). *Growth at Adolescence*, 2nd ed., Oxford.

Pubescence

The attainment of puberty, when reproductive organs become fully functional, is marked by menstruation and ovulation in the female, and by emission of sperm in the male. Puberty is completed when the individual is able to reproduce. Pubescence, hovever, reflects the ongoing process of physiological and morphological maturation in several systems. The process includes growth and development in body size, in the gonads, reproductive organs, and secondary sex characteristics, and in the circulatory and respiratory systems. Each body system has a rate of growth in some measure independent of the rate of growth of other systems, and the combination of rates makes a unique pattern for every individual. At puberty the nervous system is almost mature, and the lymphatic system has begun to regress. There is accelerated growth of the skeleton and muscles—the "adolescent growth spurt"—and especially of the reproductive system (see Figures 11.1 and 11.6). Although each individual child has an individual pattern of growth, which includes psychological and intellectual growth, school systems tend to treat all children of the same age as developmental equals, and a minimum legal age is set at which schooling may terminate. English law arbitrarily sets the age of puberty of girls at 12 years and of boys at 14. Yet variability between individuals in rates of growth is greatest during pubescence (97,125). Figure 11.7 illustrates this variability in the age-height velocity curves of five boys during puberty. The dotted line represents the mean height of the boys at each age and shows how averaging can seriously distort the shape of the growth curve during puberty.

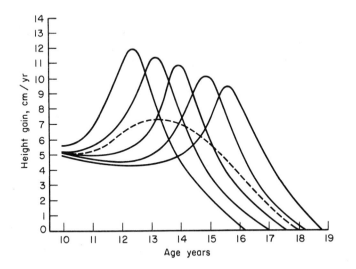

Figure 11.7 Average and individual growth velocities of five boys in centimeters per year by age. *Source:* Tanner, J., Whitehouse, R., and Takaishi, M. (1966). Standards from birth to maturity for height, weight, height velocity and weight velocity: British children, 1965, *Arch. Dis. Childh., 41,* 454–71.

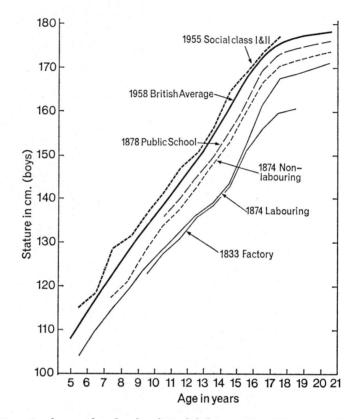

Figure 11.8   Secular trend in height of English boys, 1833–1958. *Source:* Tanner, J. M. (1962). *Growth at Adolescence,* 2nd ed., Oxford.

Despite the universality of pubertal changes, cultures differ considerably in the treatment of puberty and of pubertal children. For some, the attainment of sexual and reproductive maturity, signalled by rites of initiation and celebration, marks entry into adulthood. For others, particularly Euro-American cultures, entry into and exit from pubescence coincide more with educational than reproductive transitions. The opening of the period of pubescence at about the age of 11 or 12 is marked by the transfer from primary or junior school to secondary or high school. The end of the period at age 15 to 16 is marked by the minimum age for leaving school. In Britain, this step into pubescence is a major transition. For many children it determines the range of occupations and social roles that will be open to them in adult life. As with all transitions, psychological and social readjustment is necessary. Problems of adjustment may be reflected in the finding that, in industrial society, school "phobia"—fear of school and refusal to attend—occurs frequently in association with transfer to a higher school or class (126), while in nonindustrial societies adjustment problems may be manifested in anxiety states, hysteria, or psychosomatic disorders attributed to witchcraft.

Rates of growth vary between social groups. For growth is retarded by poor social conditions or, alternatively, stimulated by good conditions to attain its maximum potential. The impact of social conditions is evident early in life, notably during the last trimester of pregnancy. A marked social class effect on fetal growth in late pregnancy leads to high rates of low birthweight in the poorest classes, with the added risks for infant survival and development that are dependent on birthweight (127).

Among pubescent children the impact of the social and economic environment on development is marked. In British children born in the period after the Second World War, measures of height and weight showed the lower social classes to be still at a disadvantage. Height has increased and the pubertal growth spurt has appeared earlier, on average, as social conditions have improved (see Figure 11.8 and Table 11.1). This advance of maturation seems to have continued even into the relatively good conditions of the 1950s. Even in the upper classes, the records of a well-known British public school showed that the pubertal growth spurt had occurred at a younger age well into the post war period (128).

Slow growth might not affect the endpoint attained if maturity were deferred so that growth continued longer; but except where growth retardation is extreme, this does not appear to be the case. Among adults of the early postwar years in Britain, the stunted growth of the poorest classes was visible even to the naked eye. Since then there have been sizeable gains in adult stature in all social classes, yet clear differences remain in height and weight between children of different socioeconomic backgrounds (3,133,134). Skeletal maturity is likewise associated with social class according to studies conducted in a number of countries (129).

Moreover, with regard to the rate of intellectual development, there is no doubt that disparities persist between the social classes both in Britain and the United States (130). The disadvantage of children in the poorest social classes is great enough to force a large number of them below the threshold of "normality" and into the category of mild mental retardation (see pp. 337ff). Unlike physical growth, however, their intellectual growth may continue into their early adult years and bring about a degree of recovery from retardation (131).

Sexual maturation is another growth process influenced by the social environment. In this case, organic factors must intervene between social experience and physical outcome, although their nature remains obscure. Age at menarche provides one epidemiological marker of the progress of sexual maturation in girls; little is known about social and cultural differences in other aspects of sexual maturation. Over the past century, as social conditions have changed, the age at menarche has advanced by an estimated three to four months per decade (see Figure 11.2). The decline continues in many countries, although data from London and Oslo suggest a halt (97,132). The previous social class disparities observed in Britain in the age of onset of the menarche are no longer apparent, and social class differences found in other industrial countries are small (3). In markedly disparate conditions, however, differences in menarcheal age remain striking. The common attribution in the past of early sexual maturation to hot climates is now seen to be unfounded. The age at menarche is consistently late where social conditions are poor, whether the comparison is between girls in developed and developing countries, for instance, or between the poorest and the somewhat better off Xhosa girls living in the poverty of the Transkei in South Africa (see Table 11.1) (3,135).

The configuration of features associated with physical maturity cannot be attributed to a single simple cause. The scholastic and intellectual advantage of early maturers, for instance, is not founded simply in the advanced development of the brain and body (136). Among all sibship sizes in the British National Survey of Health and Development, "only" children were advanced both in sexual maturity and various measures of intellect. Sexual maturity did not explain the intellectual advantage of only children, for within the category of only children the association of maturity with intellect disappeared. Thus family size alone, or its associated factors, better explained the differences in measured intelligence between sibships. Among larger families, the pattern was irregular and still less open to simple interpretation. Although a small association of height with measured intelligence persisted in a sample controlled for age, sex, social class, and family size, this association bore no relation to sexual maturity (133). From these studies family size appears to be an antecedent factor that affects both measured intelligence and rate of maturing and explains their association. The source of the intellectual advantage of early maturers, and perhaps of some of their other attributes, must therefore be sought elsewhere than in their maturity.

The introduction of birth order as a variable helps to clarify these relationships somewhat. In an analysis of a national cohort of births examined at military induction in the Netherlands, the association of height with family size held at all levels of birth order and social class, but it did not hold for birth order with family size controlled. The association of measured intelligence, however, did hold for birth order as well as for family size. The persisting birth-order effects for test scores but not for height suggest that antecedents of adult measured intelligence are likely to stem from family environment and intrafamilial socialization. Height is an index of the physical and biological environment during growth and its persistent relationship with family size is consistent with environmental effects. The development of measured intelligence, however, evidently requires more than nutritional adequacy and good physical health (137).

At puberty, psychological and social turbulence often accompanies physiological changes. In girls regular ovulation is gradually established, attended not uncommonly by dysmenorrhea. More girls than boys of this age are admitted to the hospital and operated on for appendicitis, but the fact that fewer girls die of appendicitis may indicate that menstrual disorders affect diagnosis and inflate the number of cases among girls (138). The nature and severity of menstrual symptoms during menarche and menstruation have proved difficult to identify, for a host of methodological reasons. Women's reports of menstrual distress may reflect cultural stereotypes about menstruation as well as their actual subjective experience. Indeed, some studies based on day-to-day assessment of women's mood and activity failed to identify premenstrual or menstrual distress, even among women who retrospectively reported experiencing such changes. It remains possible that a subgroup experiences specific menstrual distress or premenstrual syndrome (139,140). The transition of the menarche may be either eased or exacerbated by the circumstances under which girls learn about the significance of pubertal changes. Girls have often been left in ignorance to obtain garbled explanations of these mysterious happenings from their peers. Some parents regard this subject as improper and not suitable for discussion with their daughters (141).

In boys, sexual activity reaches a peak at puberty (142). Sexual outlet may take the form of fantasies and dreams, masturbation, nocturnal emissions, and occasionally homosexual and heterosexual experiment. Boys have shared with girls the difficulties of inadequate sources of sexual information and of parental disapproval and lack of understanding. In Judeo-Christian cultures, attitudes towards masturbation have been intensely intolerant, resulting in strong feelings of guilt, shame, and anxiety. Among some the belief persists that masturbation causes physical and mental disorder. Traditional attitudes are rapidly changing, however. The "pluralistic ignorance" that isolated individuals from the knowledge that they shared common sexual needs and behavior has been reduced by Freud's emphasis on the fundamental contribution of sex to human behavior, by new knowledge of the norms of sexual development beginning with the work of Kinsey, and by school programs of sex education (142, 143,144).

The pubescent period is distinguished by an accelerated social differentiation, and children of different social backgrounds begin to diverge in their behavior and interests. Like physical and mental growth, social development shows greater variability at these ages than before. Previous periods engender less marked variation in development. The same broad experience of home, primary school, and play-group combines to equip children, within the limits of their personal capacities and family background, with the stock of fundamental skills, interests, attitudes, and observances that are the common elements of the culture.

Social strain characterizes each of the transitions of social maturation. Children move to new situations where they must adjust themselves to a large number of strangers; they must learn the roles and duties of their new status, submit to new expectations, and begin new lessons. In societies where children are transferred from primary or junior to secondary or high schools, they move into educational streams or tracks with curricula and interests that become increasingly specialized and divergent. Differentiation produces different categories of schoolchildren; for instance, those educated with a view to university and entry into professional or other highly skilled occupations; those who will take up skilled clerical or manual work; and those who will become semiskilled or unskilled workers.

This educational specialization is crucial to social differentiation, and in many industrial societies, takes a broadly similar form although it differs in degree. In Britain, the segregation of children in secondary schools according to educational attainment was too long an open and unchallenged tenet of the educational system and it accentuated social segregation because of the strong association of educational attainment and social class. In the United States a similar result is brought about without deliberate educational segregation by the social distribution of educational attainments, combined with the residential segregation of racial groups, ethnic groups, and social classes around local schools (86).° Educational segregation of this kind stimulates in children a consciousness of variation in social standing, and hence an awareness of the significance of social standing and prestige in the community at large. For some children it is also the first stage in the process of creating a discontinuity of occupation and culture between themselves and their parents.

The individual behavior of children reflects these distinctions of social class, for example, in the symptom of persistent nonattendance at school commonly encountered by child psychiatrists. This symptom is related to two separate disorders: school refusal or phobia, which occurs as a symptom of anxiety disorder, and truancy, which occurs as a symptom of conduct disorder. A sample of children referred to a London child psychiatric clinic for school refusal, when compared with truants and normal controls, included an unduly high proportion of children from families of Social Classes I and II, with a high prevalence of family neurosis, and a high degree of protectiveness in the mothers (126). These children were generally timid, fearful, and well behaved at school, but willful and demanding at home. They often had symptoms of anxiety, disturbances of eating and sleeping, and abdominal pain, nausea, and vomiting. The truants in this series of cases included an undue proportion from working-class families. These children tended to have suffered separations from their mothers in the first 10 years of life, with a degree of maternal rejection, and separation from fathers after the first 5 years. Many had experienced frequent changes of school. Truancy was associated with enuresis and features of conduct disorder, especially stealing, lying, and wandering from home.

Sensitivity of children to social distinctions of age, sex, and social class influences their behavior. They begin to assert a right to exercise independent choices, particularly in the style of their clothes and the use they make of their leisure. They begin to insist on their status as senior schoolchildren and look forward to the privileges of adolescence; they resent being treated as "children." Pubescent children often show amnesia for the rhymes that regulate most pediarchic games, although previously they might have used them daily. This amnesia illustrates the learning mechanisms involved in acquiring behavior appropriate to a new phase. Former modes of learned behavior must be inhibited before a new mode can be substituted (145).

The play-group gives way to other pursuits. Some are organized, like the Scouts and Guides, sports, and clubs; others are unorganized. Most children form intense friendships with two or three children of the same age and usually of the same sex, small *pal-groups* of between two and five members, who visit one another's homes and share leisure activities. In these pal-groups children find support and sympathy, mutual assistance, and criticism in their first tentative experiments with the adolescent behavior appropriate to the next stage of development to which they aspire.

Here again there are social divergences. For example, in Britain children in the academic streams, encouraged by their parents, were found to choose their friends on social distinctions that were often minute, as well as on personal qualities. These

---

°The intense political conflicts that surrounded efforts to desegregate schools racially by means of busing children out of their local areas was a pointer to the heavy social investment of local group and status affiliations.

friends might not live in the same neighborhood, although they were usually in the same educational grade. This discrimination implies a widening acquaintance with the community and a deepening awareness of social distinctions; mutual visiting introduces the children to other homes and neighborhoods and gives them other standards by which to judge their own homes and families.

At the other extreme, children in the nonacademic streams were less discriminating. They too form pal-groups, seeking their friends in their own neighborhood, often enough among former members of their play-groups. As a result, higher-class children who entered these nonacademic streams tended to find themselves isolated (146). The circumscribed loyalty to place and people fostered by the play-group is reinforced in the pal-group. The obverse of local loyalties may be hostility towards persons they consider unlike themselves. Where groups of neighborhood children carry these attitudes into the classroom, the teacher, as an outsider, may face great hostility (147).

These social divergences have their source in family life as well as in neighborhood norms and in social selection for different types of schooling. Thus observations in home settings in Britain reveal sharp class differences in verbal behavior. Middle-class children tend to be more inquisitive, to ask more questions prompted by curiosity than by disputes about control, and to receive more adequate responses from adult caretakers than working-class children. Comparable observations in classrooms show that, far from being compensated, these social class differences in children's questioning behavior are more pronounced in the school context (148,149).

Many higher-class families expect all their children to enter academic educational tracks. The goal they set for their children is a professional or equivalent career. They tend more than lower-class families to supplement the formal schooling of their children by encouraging them in such individual pursuits as bird-watching and stamp-collecting, and by fostering their interest through conversation, gifts of books and microcomputers, visits to museums and theatres, and so on. These pursuits leave less time for pediarchic play; some higher-class children may never have played traditional street games. At puberty, these children are likely to be given sex instruction by parents and to have formal contacts with the opposite sex in dancing classes and parties under adult surveillance. Emphasis on individuality and living conditions that afford a "room of one's own" encourage individuation.

In upwardly mobile families, parents tend to be anxious about school attainments, and a child's poor performance may disturb family relations. The fact that schoolchildren are in greater concord about educational goals with their mothers than with their friends does not assure harmony. The frequent geographical mobility of such families is especially poorly tolerated by pubescent children (150). Uprooting from one local culture and transfer to another seems to be a greater impedance to social integration than at any other time in childhood. Previously well-adjusted children may feel alienated, or they display a depression that resembles mourning.

At the other extreme, poor lower-class families may reap little reward from formal education and be indifferent to it. The short-term exigencies of an uncertain weekly wage do not encourage the goal-directed activity and long-term planning common in higher-class families. Shared leisure interests of the family tend to be restricted to the neighborhood, with television and spectator sports prominent. Friends are bound by affective relationships, and seldom by such pedagogic games as tennis, organized team sports, or the cultivation of intellectual and artistic pursuits. Girls are still likely to consider marriage their true career. Parents rarely give sex instruction and ignore sexual experimentation; in general the subject is taboo between parents and children. In Britain, despite the greater knowledge, permissiveness, and closer surveillance of children in the higher classes, the actual sex behavior reported by teenagers has differed little between the classes. Experience did differ somewhat by type of education, with children in academic streams having less experience (151,152).

Working-class parents are less likely than middle- or upper-class parents to expect their children to go on to college and into professional jobs for which college is required (153), yet there is an overriding social pressure towards doing so. But attitudes towards schooling are not fixed. People are influenced by their particular reference groups (154), and aspirant families can acquire new norms of expectation as a result of outside stimulus. Ambitions for children can be triggered by the success of a relative's child, or because of a parent's change of job and the extension of the family's social horizon, or even by a change of house and adjustment to the standards of new neighbors. Such changes in attitude increase the probability of clashes within the family. One parent may oppose the other, while the child is indifferent, or both parents may disparage education while the child is enthusiastic. Difference between siblings in aspirations and performance may add to the dispute.

Despite the pressures towards acquiring social mobility through education, there remain families who are positively hostile to schools. They regard schooling as an imposition that keeps children away from work or "real" life, or they resent the teachers as representatives of a dominant and alien culture. The street and neighborhood often have a greater influence on the child than does his formal education. Among the children of such families, impositions of schooling can lead to antisocial behavior or withdrawal from and rejection of the dominant cultural values imposed by the educational system.

The pubescent period is therefore one of rising family strain on the three main family relationships: between husband and wife, between parents and children, and between siblings. Husband and wife may disagree concerning their course of behavior toward the pubescent children, now more susceptible to external influences. Assertive feelings of jealousy and rivalry between siblings may focus on differences of education; the education of girls may be sacrificed to that of boys, or the education of elder children to that of younger (155).

Family size and birth order. In these conflicts the size and structure of the family is significant, for authority is exercised differently in large and small families (156). One American study found, for example, that in some large working-class families the eldest girls were often obliged to take over the discipline and daily care of younger children (157); these girls tended to resent the responsibilities of "mother surrogate." In turn, the splitting of the maternal role provoked resentment and feelings of hostility towards the eldest girl among the younger siblings.

Indeed, from beginning to end the socialization process within a family as a whole, and the experience it affords each individual child, varies with the internal structure of the family. Large families have been characteristic of some historical periods, economic forms, cultures, religious groups, and social classes, and small families characteristic of others. These macrocultures have set their stamp upon the microcultures of the typical family within them.

Large families are now most common among the poorest classes and the poorest societies, and poverty is the cause of many of their handicaps. The high prevalence of rheumatoid arthritis among large families, for instance, can probably be attributed to the high prevalence of the disease in the lower social classes. When the effort is made to hold such antecedents as social class constant, however, large families may still appear at a disadvantage. The father's income can less often be supplemented by that of a working mother, who must care for the many children. When resources are limited, the expenditure on each family member is inevitably less, just as each has less parental attention, living space, and food. Undernutrition in large families, common in the Great Depression of the 1930s, still persisted among the poor both in Britain and the United States in the 1960s (158). An indication of the economic handicap of the large family with limited resources appears in the growth of children born in 1947 and included in the British National Survey of Health and Development. Children of large sibships were shorter and only children were taller, but only in the working class (159). In a study of a large cohort of 20-year old Dutch men born in the mid-1940s, height was inversely related to family size in both the manual and nonmanual social classes (137). Close spacing of births adds to the density of the large family and is likely to compound its problems. A combination of frequent infection and undernutrition may be involved in children's growth patterns.

The social and biological consequences of high fertility are difficult to separate from those of low social class and maternal age. High parity is associated with low social class and with more advanced maternal age. All three of these factors are also associated with increased rates of low birthweight, of toxemia of pregnancy, and of perinatal deaths. Moreover, the frequency of trisomic chromosomal abnormalities is exaggerated in older mothers and greater age is the inevitable condition of women who continue childbearing. The young children of the large family are subject to more infections and a higher overall mortality. Their development of sphincter control is slow and their performance on intelligence tests and at school is inferior (133,159,160). Despite these health consequences, cultural preferences for large sibships persist in much of the underdeveloped world and undermine efforts to bring high fertility rates under control. This is particularly true in agricultural societies where infant mortality is high and each child is perceived as an economic asset to the family and a source of security for the parents in old age (161).

Birth order and parental age are structural factors obviously related to family size. Each child, according to birth rank and sex, and the number and sex of the sibs, has a unique experience within the family. In a nuclear family with several children the eldest child begins life with an exclusive relationship to young parents, whereas the youngest child has to share older parents with a number of siblings. Parents and children repeat the exeperience anew with each new arrival. Strains in the family may be greater with the novel experience of the first child than with successors. Both parents and younger children can learn from the experience of the eldest. But the gain in experience must be offset against the diminishing resilience of parents who are progressively older as they confront successive children. In poor families, birth order affects the resources available for each child. The eldest may have a comfortable infancy and a straitened adolescence, whereas the youngest may have a straitened childhood but benefit from the raised income when both parents and elder sibs go out to work. Where the family is upwardly mobile, its progress may provide increasingly higher standards of living for successive children.

The individuality and variety of experience dictated by birth order is patent. Yet because of problems of method and interpretation, few birth order effects can be accepted as securely established. To begin with, the distribution of family size in a population has a powerful effect on the prevailing frequency of birth ranks. When uncontrolled, family size may therefore give rise to statistical associations of birth rank with characteristics of individuals. One approach to controlling family size uses only the position of affected subjects within their own families. The method depends on the assumption that, in the population at large, birth order is random within each family size, and that only a manifestation linked with birth order will deviate from a random distribution (162). This method effects control for family size in completed families; it has been subject to artifactual errors where incomplete families have been studied and where cases might have been lost through death or migration before ascertainment. When unexpected, factors such as changing incidence of the disease, or patterns of reproduction altered in response to birth of an affected child, can also confound results (163). Refined methods using the same basic assumption have been devised to cope with these problems, and to control such other confounding factors as maternal age and fertility that may produce apparent associations with birth order (164).

The analysis of birth rank is further complicated when variations through time and between social groups in fertility (and hence in the number and size of families) produce distributions of birth rank among groups of families that are not random (165). Thus some reported distributions of birth ranks in schizophrenia, from which social-psychological hypotheses were derived, were in fact compatible with nonrandom distributions in the normal population (166). These nonrandom distributions were to be expected because of trends in fertility that have differed through time and between the social classes. This is not to say that significant differences in the birth order of schizophrenic patients may not exist.

We have already noted that, at the very beginning of the life-cycle, the outcomes of pregnancy and birth are affected by high parity of the mother. But toxemia of pregnancy, low birthweight, and reproductive loss vary in curvilinear manner. Rates are high with first births, and decline with subsequent births, only to rise again with high birth rank. Among infants, we have noted (p. 370) that pyloric stenosis is one condition that is strongly linked with first births (167). Among adults, eminence and achievement are linked with the first-born (168). This association, found consistently since Galton's studies of the nineteenth century, is probably secondary to the greater educational opportunities and academic achievement of the first-born. The first-born perform better at high school, and many more gain entrance to college and university (168,169). The modest advantage in measured intelligence of first-born children (170) seems alone insufficient to explain their superiority in educational achievement and eminence.

These relationships of primogeniture, and other more tenuous and inconsistent findings that link birth order with mental disorder, asthma (in the first-born), and peptic ulcer (in the last-born) (171) have set off a search for their sources in the formation of personality. Alfred Adler described the typical first-born as a "power-hungry conservative." Subsequent research has not provided data to confirm his view. It has yielded tentative connections with psychological dependence and a need for affiliation with others, with more strongly developed conscience, and with an upbringing subject to greater strictures than the later born (66,172).

Family disturbances during the pubescent period are shaped by the structure and the history of the family up to that time, and they foreshadow the dispersal of the elementary family and the eventual independence of children. The painful readjustments of roles within the family at this time reflect maturation and the child's necessary progress towards independence.

Adolescence

Adolescence is the period between puberty and the final achievement of adult status and independence. Adolescence is protracted in industrial societies, for its onset is advanced by the earlier maturation of children, and its end is deferred by the extension of education. The complexity of techniques in many fields of activity compels young people to undertake a prolonged period of training. Industrial societies are subject to rapid technical and social changes, unlike those nonindustrial societies where children more often grow up to perform the same duties as their parents, and to follow the same customs and standards of morality. Children in industrial societies have to acquire skills and observances unfamiliar to their parents. As adults they pursue different occupations and leisure interests, and they come to accept new standards, a process accentuated by social mobility. Adolescence is therefore a period when the divergences that began in the schools at puberty widen into different fields of experience. With the increased availability of education in the developing world and the rapid transformation of its economies, divergences between adolescents and parents become increasingly common there as well.

Many children leave school at the earliest legal age and at once go out to work, while others remain at school and then at university until they are well into their twenties. In other words, the period of adolescence, defined by the social criterion of status transitions, varies in duration with the educational progress of the individuals, the social class of their families, and their own ambitions and achievements. The lengthy training that the majority of adolescents undergo creates problems because of the discordance between physical, emotional, and intellectual maturation. The maturing adolescent attempts to establish an independent social existence free of parental control. Parents often resist these attempts because they fail to recognize the changing needs of young people they are accustomed to regard as children. During the prolonged dependence of children, parents—habituated to exercising authority over them and to making decisions for them—find it difficult to relinquish these functions. Like their adolescent children, parents have to learn and create norms for a relationship with their children that is evolving towards equality and independence.

During childhood the relationship between children and parents is distinctly asymmetrical. The parents exercise power and authority, and the children return deference and obedience. Most societies, if not all, have a rule that children must honor and obey their parents, as well as love them. This relationship is generalized, so that children are subordinate to adults outside the family and are expected to show them a similar deference. In school, particularly, the relationship between teacher and pupil is one of superordination and subordination, whereas the relationship between pupils is symmetrical. The continuity of society depends on one generation transmitting to the next its traditions, knowledge, skill, manners, religion, and standards of taste. This transmission is effected in part through the authority adults exercise over children (173).

Every family in a highly differentiated society does not conform to these demands. There are persons at all social levels who are opposed to relations of authority and, accordingly, to the conventional school system. When these persons are well-to-do, they often send their children to schools that aim at greater equality between teacher and pupil. Families among the poor may also repudiate the values of formal education, but are compelled to send their children to school; the children of these families may refuse to defer to their teachers. Both types of family are likely to have adolescent problems specific to themselves.

Opposition between successive generations is common. Each new generation must struggle to achieve independence, to leave the parents on whom they have been dependent for care and attention, and to take up adult status and create new families of their own. Conflict between fathers and sons is so widespread that Freud ascribed to it the origins of society (174). Unconscious psychological forces present in relations between parents and children may well intensify conflict between them at this period. For example, the reluctance to allow their children to marry shown by a few parents can be connected with their own ambivalent feelings towards sexual activity in their children, as well as with their hopes and fears for their own future and that of their children, which the marriage will inevitably affect. Moreover, the achievement of adult status by the first of their children marks the onset of a new phase in the family cycle, the phase of dispersion. Parents may regret a development that signals the end of their own reproductive powers and foreshadows the time of their replacement.

Psychological explanations thus illuminate individual cases. They are not appropriate explanations for integenerational conflict as a mass phenomenon. The conflict of interests between generations is minimized in some societies through institutions that regulate relations between the parental and filial generations, and the transmission of power and authority from one to the other. Some African societies use a system of male age-sets, with an ascending gradient of seniority, status, and privileges. When a new cohort of boys is initiated, all the existing age-sets move up one grade in progression; young warriors become full warriors, and full warriors become elders. Conflict therefore takes place between proximate age-sets, but not between fathers and sons, for the time interval between age-sets is so arranged that fathers and sons are never members of proximate age-sets. This formal arrangement reduces the conflict of interests that their society recognizes as inevitable (175,176). *Rites-de-passage* mark the transitions of status accorded each individual when his or her age-set is judged mature. These rituals of transition leave no room for doubts about the individual's proper status and roles, and similar rituals also mark the changed statuses achieved by the individual through marriage and other events in the life-arc.

Industrial society has few institutionalized means of handing over a share in economic and social power to adolescents, or of awarding adult status. In the many functional associations outside the elementary family, in employment, politics, religion, and recreation, each individual must establish a separate status. The law recognizes individual responsibility for particular activities at diverse ages. In Britain adolescents of fifteen are allowed to work, but must be maintained by parents until they are sixteen, although then they can drive motorcycles, or voluntarily enter a mental hospital. They must wait until age seventeen before they can drive cars. At eighteen they can be served with alcohol, and now they have acquired the vote, but they only become fully independent at twenty-one, when they can marry without parental consent.

In this diversity each family faces its own problems of personal growth and development, and each must find its own solutions to friction and conflict. The "crisis of identity" typical of adolescence in industrial societies has its social source in the lonely uncertainties about the nature of the adult roles the individual will be allowed to play, and about the untested capacity to make the passage from childhood dependence to adult independence (177). Each one of many adult statuses must be acquired through painful transition, each one of the many accompanying roles negotiated, learned, and adapted. Few statuses are ascribed and assured; many must be struggled for alone and achieved.

Two distinct social processes are involved. First, the primary, general processes whereby adolescents achieve adult status, during which their relationship with the parental generation changes from one of dependence and social inequality to one of independence and equality. Second, the process of adjusting the differences in behavior and standards between the generations that arise from economic, social, and cultural innovations. These innovations often lead adolescents to adopt patterns of behavior deprecated by their parents or by the wider society.

The more rapid is social change, the greater the opportunity for conflict. In recent years, a much larger number of adolescents have been able to take advantage of the enhanced access to knowledge about society that has informed higher education. Depending on the level of economic security and expectation, this knowledge tends to make a large body of young people trenchant critics of society. They see existing social and political forms and values that diverge from the ideal values professed by their elders and teachers, and that clearly hinder solutions to the crucial problems of survival facing modern civilization. Their demand for new social forms and values, in the face of the rapid desuetude of old forms, accentuates the built-in conflict between generations, and progressively shortens the time-span in which successive generations come to be separated from each other by developing distinctive cultural preferences.

Peer-groups. During adolescence external influences on young people begin to pull them out of their families. As they mature, the family becomes increasingly unable to satisfy their needs, and this process now reaches a climax. They seek the company of their peers, among whom they can establish an individual identity. In both one-sex and mixed-sex groups, they learn to accommodate their sexuality, share and sift personal experiences, and thereby develop a trust in their own judgment of people and ideas, without reference to their parents. Their social personalities are still embryonic and insecure, and peer-groups provide the opportunity to experiment in the relative security of group support (178). The resulting pressures to conform to the moral and material standards of the group appear in the uniform dress of adolescence and in the anticipation of "adult" behavior such as smoking, so often upsetting to parents (179). The parental response symbolizes the cleavage in attitudes and standards between the adolescent and the parental generation in such matters of dispute as staying out late, sexual behavior, smoking, drinking, the use of drugs, and the way time and money are spent.

The pal-groups that emerged during the pubescent period now assume social importance. The standards and behavior of these groups vary with the social standing of their families. The higher the social level, the wider the range of choice. Even among those adolescents whose relationships are contained within one limited neighborhood, the widening experience of society that results from their going out to work leads to a more varied selection of companions. Their choice of activities also differs by family social standing. Higher-class adolescents have a wide range of organized activities, from mountain-climbing to foreign travel, whereas many working-class adolescents are confined to local activity, and some may expend much energy in organizing neighborhood gangs. Yet higher-class adolescents often retain the status of pupils, being still at school or university, whereas working-class adolescents of the same age may have been out at work for some years and some, particularly girls, may have married and borne children in or out of wedlock.

One important social function of the pal-group is to provide support while individuals gain knowledge and experience of a number of members of the opposite sex. These groups protect individuals from too early an emotional involvement with one person and, through mutual criticism and advice, aid discrimination and selection. This group association precedes pairing and established courtship. In those social milieux where no formal social arrangements exist to pair off and marry maturing individuals, the pal-group forms an essential institution for learning and testing.

The loose confederations of the pal-groups of boys are rarely organized, generally come together through territorial association in cafes, at street corners and clubs, have no recognized leadership, and are usually ephemeral. They help to spread acquaintance among boys and to extend their awareness of personal as well as social distinctions. They also provide support when they meet strange groups in public places such as dancehalls. While adolescent boys spend most of their leisure time with their pal-groups, a number of these pal-groups occasionally coalesce into larger confederations. These confederations should be distinguished from gangs. Gangs have an authority structure, recognized leadership, rites of admission and other rituals, and often take to organized delinquent activity (180).

Crime is a particular problem of adolescent males (36,37,38,40,183). In Britain official statistics indicate that the incidence rates of indictable offenses among male juveniles increase sharply after childhood to peak at over 80 per 1000 by age 14. They then decline gradually but remain high through the teens. After 20, the rates fall sharply and by the thirties they dwindle to below 10 per 1000 (see Figure 11.9). The shape of this curve is similar for girls but the rates are much lower. Girls are less than one-fifth as likely as boys to appear in court for a criminal offense during the peak 14- to 17-year age interval (182). Convictions for indictable offenses represent an unknown fraction of the total number of offenses, and the incidence of conviction is influenced in different areas by the local attitudes of police, magistrates, and public, as well as variations in legal codes. Self-report surveys indicate that most adolescent boys admit to criminal behavior at some time (28). Social inferences from criminal statistics must therefore be made with caution. In cities the rates for neighborhoods of the same social class may vary from under 10 per cent to 90 per cent (184).

The validity of crime rates is further complicated by the varying definition of acceptable behavior in different social groups. Some persons tolerate behavior that is in conflict with the law, or regard it as a minor transgression, as with traffic violations. In addition, the skills and resources needed to handle social situations vary from one family to another. For example, in those families where the parents are hostile to education and indulgent to their children, treating them as though their needs and desires were the same as those of adults, the parental response to the criminal behavior of a child is often "don't get caught," rather than "it is wrong." The rejection of authority, and the morality of equality, inculcated both at home and in the play-

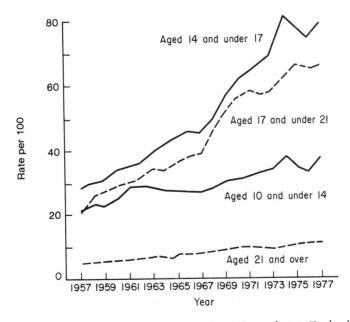

Figure 11.9   Indictable offenses over time. (Rate per 1000 population, England and Wales 1957 to 1977.) *Source:* Rutter, M. (1979). *Changing Youth in a Changing Society: Patterns of Adolescent Development and Disorder*, London, p. 120.

group, predisposes these children at adolescence to flout established authority. When apprehended for delinquent behavior, they can usually count on the sympathy of their families. These adolescents revolt less against their parents, who have tended to treat them as equals, than against society at large, which does not accord them adult status.

On the other hand, strained relations in the home or other personal difficulties are sometimes channelled into delinquent acts. Studies of delinquents suggest that a disproportionate number of them emerge from poor families, from homes with high levels of family conflict, and from families in which one or both parents have a history of antisocial behavior (28,36,37,38,181,182). The correlation between poverty and crime cannot account for the existence of higher-class crime, or for the general increase in crime rates among the young as they have developed into a relatively privileged group. Substance abuse and crimes of violence have all risen among the adolescent group. A survey of nine European countries, including Britain, showed that in the decade after the Second World War all had registered an increase in adolescent crime and delinquency accompanied by a rise in the standard of living (185). In Britain this trend has continued and at an even greater rate of increase since the late 1960s (see Figure 11.9). Several other indices of social disturbance have risen together with the rates of juvenile offenses. In the postwar period, for instance, the rates of suicide and attempted suicide among young people have risen dramatically in Britain, and in the United States suicide currently ranks as the second leading cause of death among young people (182,186,187); drug and alcohol abuse among young people is a matter of general alarm (188); and the toll of fatalities from road accidents is highest at these ages. These phenomena suggest that in contemporary industrial society there are processes at work that particularly affect adolescents of all social classes. The word "delinquency" covers a multitude of offenses, some more likely to come to notice than others. There is no single cause of delinquency.

The absorption of adolescents in their external relations can put severe strains on their family relations. Some families adjust because parents are tolerant and can restrain their anxieties, or because parental standards are undemanding so that there is a relatively small gap between norms of adults and children. Others quarrel and may make an outright break. Where training for future occupations is most prolonged, the strain is likewise prolonged; there is more time for quarrels to develop and more occasions for them.

An adolescent who fails to achieve independence because of physical handicap, or mental illness, or mental deficiency puts a heavy strain on the family. The potential obligation of the family persists throughout life, instead of being limited to the period of growth. For many families these demands exceed their psychological resources and the aid of caretaking agencies becomes essential. To the degree that social factors determine the handicapped role, they also determine the capacity for independence. A handicapped person of high education and social standing is not barred from remunerative work and can afford mechanical and domestic help. In the poorer classes such persons may need help from social agencies, and suitable places in sheltered employment; they often remain dependent on their families. On the other hand,

retarded children in higher-class families may be forced into a condition of permanent dependence because they are able to work only at low prestige jobs that are
unacceptable to their families.

Sexual behavior. The variety of norms and modes of sexual behavior in different societies, and at different times in the same societies, points to their social origin. Cross-
cultural evidence indicates considerable diversity in proscribed and prescribed sexual
behaviors; some societies have permitted great heterosexual freedom, apart from
incest, and others have permitted great homosexual freedom. Considerable diversity
appears in regard to extra- and premarital heterosexual intercourse, the acceptability
of particular sexual acts, male and female sexual styles, masturbation, and the overt
expression of childhood sexuality. Prescriptions and proscriptions are modified and
refined by considerations of age, point in the life cycle, rank and gender. For example,
in the New Guinea highlands, male homosexuality is a common feature of relations
between adolescent boys and men of an older generation. Ingestion of semen by teenage boys in the course of oral sex is considered necessary for continued growth to
adulthood. When young men attain maturity, however, heterosexuality is expected
of them. Thus specific sexual behavior that may be preferred or required at one stage
in the life cycle may differ from that required in another. Gender is an important
factor in this instance as well; no comparable lesbian experience is considered necessary for growth of girls in New Guinea (189,190).

Firm generalizations about patterns of human sexual behavior is made difficult by
scant data and questions about the reliability and representativeness of the data available. In addition, even reliable and representative data about sexual acts leave numerous questions about the subjective and cultural meaning of specific acts to those
engaging in them. Terms frequently used to categorize sexual behavior are themselves
historical and cultural products: "homosexual," "lesbian," and "heterosexual" are relatively recent, introduced in the last half of the nineteenth century by psychiatrists
and early sexologists. Although both heterosexual and homosexual behavior probably
have existed in all human societies and at all times, the way of thinking about sexuality reflected in the terms "heterosexual" and "homosexual" is particular to Euro-
American culture and cannot safely be generalized to other cultures or other times
(190,191,192,193). Though researchers might count the number of homosexual acts
among men in the New Guinea highlands and the United States, the experience of
the highland boy cannot be equated with that of the active homosexual male in American or European urban centers.

Sexual developments and behaviors that appear in puberty show continuity with
infant and childhood experience. Later forms draw on prior self-exploration of the
body and attitudes toward it, sensual and sexual contact with adults and peers, sex
play and masturbation, and the acquisition of sexual information and misinformation.
Under the influence of Freud, Western culture in the past century has moved away
from the view that children remained asexual until puberty, when sexual drives were
thought to appear in concert with physical changes of puberty; infant and child sexual
experience and interest are recognized. Paradoxically, the nineteenth century denial

of prepubertal sexuality was undercut by persistent efforts to identify and eliminate both masturbation and sex play among prepubertal children through draconian threats and punishments.

Children coming of age in a culture that prohibits and controls sexual expression may find the transition to adulthood, with new and unfamiliar sexual privileges, to be a sharp and unsettling reversal of expected behavior. Children of cultures that permit and encourage public enactment of adult sexual behavior find the transition to adult sexuality less unfamiliar and difficult. In any case, cross-cultural reports of widespread sexual activity and interest in childhood undermine the notion of sexual latency as a universal feature of child development (143,190,191). As many as half of all adults will report sex play in childhood, although the use of recall data is likely to lead to an underestimate. The physical expression of true genital sexuality, however, begins only with puberty. Sex behavior, like any other behavior, is the manifestation of innate potential modified by learning and experience. Much that is commonly attributed to instinctual drives is learned. Gonadal hormones influence erotic responsiveness, but the weight of this influence declines with the ascent of the evolutionary scale, and is least in humans. It seems to be innately determined, in a number of primate species, that males are easily exhausted by copulation while females can sustain repeated copulation without apparent difficulty. Even among nonhuman primate species, however, sexual behavior has important learned components. Without observing mature animals, younger male primates are unable to copulate. Females achieve sexual congress without apparently having to learn the act (189,192,193).

Generalizations about intrinsic differences between male and female sexuality in human beings are more difficult to make. The malleability of sexual behavior, not only across cultures but also over time within the same cultures, warns the careful observer not to assume too much. Early surveys of sexual behavior, particularly those of Kinsey, found large differences between male and female sexual behavior. Onefifth of men and only one-tenth of women reported that they had experienced orgasm through masturbation by the age of twelve. Within two years of puberty virtually all the men had had this experience. Only two-thirds of women reported ever having masturbated, and they had done so much less frequently than man (142,144). Since the 1970s, however, the gross differences between male and female sexual behavior appear to have decreased. Women engage in both masturbation and coition at earlier ages and more frequently (194,195).

Thus, although the sexual behavior of males and females is observably different, the source of many of the differences is as likely to be social as intrinsic to each sex. The available observations indicate that males early exhibit a drive to find sexual gratification for its own sake with a minimum of learning, while in females such a drive tends to appear after arousal by learning and experience. In females this drive, when it does not continue to be latent, commonly reaches a peak later in life than in males. Most males are quickly conditioned to sexual stimuli, and must learn only when and where and in what manner to act sexually. Females are seemingly more slowly conditioned to sexual stimuli, and learn through sexual experience itself how to be sexual for its own sake.

Sex is thus genitally centered for boys earlier in life than it is for girls. Typically, boys and not girls seek out heterosexual gratification and initiate physical sex activity. For adolescent girls heterosexual relations have greater social than physical content. This social content presages a heavy future investment in marriage and the family. "Lolitas" are rare and their sex behavior, as that of other young girls, is likely to express nonsexual as well as sexual motivations. Thus, the adolescent sex behavior of girls has not proved, on longitudinal study, a reliable predictor of adult sexuality (142).

The contrasting sexuality of boys and girls is mirrored in personality development. Aggressiveness in boys and dependency in girls have been found in longitudinal studies to be fairly stable elements of personality (196). At adolescence these patterns are reinforced by further training for adult sex roles. Girls learn the language of romantic love and the rituals of courtship as a preparation for marriage. By contrast adolescent boys, when they first go with girls, tend to be seeking sexual satisfaction; the social context for this behavior is prestige and manliness among their male peers. In these heterosexual exchanges boys and girls train each other in their mutual expectations. A process thus begins that modifies the sexual and social elements of heterosexual relations towards their future adult form. Girls must modify their predominantly social and role-oriented motivations to accommodate the private pleasures of physical sexuality; boys must modify their predominantly physical desires to accommodate affection and the social obligations of courtship and marriage (152,197).

It appears that the social structuring of sexuality is consistent with the structuring of other forms of social life. By no means have all societies assigned a passive role to women in the sex act. But in Western society, before recent changes, the "double standard" of sexual morality—which, if attenuated, persists—conferred privileges of sexual freedom on men, while it exacted chastity and fidelity from women. This morality has been embedded in the social and economic dominance of men, and in their legal and political powers over women. Since the double standard meshed with the asynchrony that has existed in male and female sexual expression, it has persisted through large sectors of society despite the changing positions of women. In this situation of inferiority women have been exploited as sex objects, as well as in other ways. In turn, they used sex for social rather than sexual purposes: to win a mate; to bind him in a stable union; to seal his responsibility for his offspring.

As women have achieved political emancipation and greater legal and economic equality, and as their functions in the nuclear family have narrowed, their claims for social and sexual satisfaction have altered. The mass production of contraceptives provided a technology that made it possible to enjoy and cultivate sex, detaching eroticism and sexuality from reproduction and its unwanted consequences. The sexual behavior of females in Western societies, which has begun to change, can be expected to change still further and to alter traditional relationships between men and women.

In industrial societies the social diversity of sex activity appears in social class and ethnic differences, although concentration of research on white, middle-class, and heterosexual subgroups makes generalization about other groups difficult. In Kinsey's surveys in the United States, working-class men reported premarital coitus at an earlier age and more often than those of higher social class, while higher-class men had indulged more in "heavy petting." In their later years, however, higher-class men had sustained a higher frequency of both marital and extramarital sex activity. Working-class women, too, had tended to experience coitus earlier than higher-class women, a prelude to their earlier marriages. They reportedly indulged less in both petting during courting and in foreplay during marital sex, and they less often achieved orgasm than highly educated women. In a British survey, compatible differences between the classes in petting and sex behavior have been found. On the whole, however, differences in the sexual activity of women in different social classes have been relatively slight compared to class differences among men.

These differences between men and women of high and low social class are reflected in their conjugal sex relations. In working-class marriages and in marriages with segregated conjugal roles, the frequency of sexual activity flags sooner than it does in higher-class and joint-role marriages. In an American study of a representative sample, less than a fifth of lower-class wives of segregated-role marriages reported interest and enjoyment in sex against almost two-thirds in joint-role marriages (198). Lower-class wives have tended to view sexual intercourse as something that men want, with themselves as passive recipients, while husbands have tended to view a wife's active interest in sex as a threat of infidelity (199). In the joint-role marriage, where the ideal norm is more egalitarian, couples more often cultivate mutual sexuality. On the other hand, failure to achieve the ideals prescribed by marriage and sex manuals is likely to generate guilt and frustration (200).

Sexual behavior thus reflects the social structure. Social class variations in behavior arise out of cultural attitudes; these are modified both by opportunities for the acquisition of scientific knowledge about the nature of sexuality and its control that are provided by social position and education, and by the opportunities for learning how to be sexual. Thus, an American survey of a representative national sample, and another of high-school and college students in three states, found an ethnic divergence in sex attitudes, for instance, about premarital sex, even greater than the class divergences. The difference between ethnic group norms was clearly present within the same social classes (201). The need for caution in interpretation of data is great with a subject that has been so laden with guilt and so hedged with taboos. But the consistency of results of surveys using different methods, such as structured questionnaires and depth interviews, supports the validity of the results.

The validity of the data is less clear when sex attitudes and behavior are examined for trends in time. Much of the relevant information must be drawn from age-specific analyses of cross-sectional surveys. In such analyses girls appear much more accepting of premarital sex than their mothers, whether they are American girls at college (202), or a representative sample of English girls (151). The revised norm appears to be that love or affection between partners justifies the sex act. Yet attitudes are malleable, and it is hazardous to infer that the views of middle-aged women remain the same as when they were girls. On the one hand, mothers are subject to the same pervasive cultural forces towards frankness and permissiveness about sex as are their daughters. On the other hand, elements of family structure induce countervailing forces against permissiveness: in an American study married women with children were less permissive than were married women of the same age who had no children; the first-born were less likely to approve premarital intercourse than the later born; the more daughters a father had and the more sons a mother had, the more firmly they held their attitudes about sex (202). The overall cultural trend, however, is not in doubt. It has been sufficiently powerful to relax the laws on obscenity and pornography and to alter many social taboos about sexuality. In turn, this relaxation, taking effect through the media of mass communication, mass entertainment, and mass education, has added to the momentum of the change in values about sex.

Curiously, evidence about a time trend in sexual behavior, parallel to the trend in attitudes, has proved hard to come by. Kinsey's pioneering surveys of the 1940s still provide some of the more useful data. The reports of women who had reached sexual maturity between the First World War and the time of the surveys in the early 1950s indicated no appreciable increase in premarital sex experience. On the other hand, there did seem to be an increase in women's extramarital sex experience through roughly the same period. These surveys were cross-sectional and could only make inferences about cohort changes; they relied on the recall of retrospective information, and they were unrepresentative samples of volunteers. More recent representative surveys, up to the late 1970s, yield evidence of an appreciable increase in reported premarital sex experience among young unmarried women (194,203). A British survey found that in 1971–1975 three-quarters of women marrying had had premarital sexual relations with their husbands, compared with one-third in 1956–1960.

During the past half century, several aspects of social and physical sexual behavior point to change in the direction both of increased premarital intercourse and increasing similarity between male and female sexual behavior. These indicators include the relaxation of such higher-class constraints on courting as chaperones; the growth of opportunities for privacy between young men and women created by the automobile; the greater permissiveness of parents; the spead of knowledge about contraception, and of new methods of contraception; increased access to abortion with legalization; and the increase in rates of out-of-wedlock births among the higher as well as the lower classes. Most recently, the advent and ready availability of the pill—birth control by means of the ingestion of estrogens—has enormously simplified women's control of their fertility. Rapid changes in the structure and values of industrial societies are associated with changes in sexual behavior as well as changes in moral attitudes.

Births out-of-wedlock. The frequency of births to unmarried adolescent girls varies between social classes, status groups, and cultures (204,205,207). The definition of illegitimacy is similarly variable: in the United States, unlike Britain, "illegitimacy" is determined by the legal marital status of the mother, whether or not the mother's husband was the child's biological father. Illegitimate births cannot be taken as a direct measure of the frequency of heterosexual activity outside marriage. The chances of a birth to an unmarried mother following sexual intercourse are affected by fertility and the regularity of ovulation, by standards of education, knowledge of sexual matters, the use of contraception, by the resort to abortion, and the probability of marriage. All these factors vary widely between social groups. For instance, Kinsey estimated from his samples that induced abortions terminated some 90 to 95 per cent of prenuptial pregnancies among women born between 1890 and 1930, but abortions were less frequent among blacks and lower-class women. The use of contraception, too, has had a sharp class gradient (206), although class differences are decreasing (207). The accuracy of reporting and the amount of concealment also affect the supposed distributions.

When pregnancy occurs, the reaction of the families concerned largely depends on their social environment. In many societies, premarital relations among young people are tolerated; indeed, in those Scandinavian rural communities of the past where fertility in women was highly valued, pregnancy was said to be a prerequisite for marriage. In Britain prenuptial conception among farmers' wives is still much higher than among wives of professional men or salaried employees. In some working-class districts prenuptial conception is tacitly condoned, so long as marriage intervenes before the child is born, and is often a preliminary to marriage. Each social group has a distinctive style of courting, marriage, and parenthood that is reflected in the statistics of birth and marriage. Age at marriage has been earlier in the lower social classes with a higher proportion of prenuptial conceptions, and a greater number and closer spacing of subsequent children, although demographic differences between social classes have been decreasing.

Thus the social distribution of births to unmarried mothers and of prenuptial conceptions has been similar. In a British cohort study, about 5 per cent of women in the professional and salaried classes married between 1925–1939 had prenuptial conceptions, while this percentage for the wives of manual workers was 25 per cent; for the wives of farmers it was 20 per cent, and for farmworkers' wives it was 30 per cent. Prenuptial conceptions, for the purpose of official statistics, include all births that occur within eight months of marriage. This figure, willy-nilly, included premature births of children conceived after marriage. Because premature births are most frequent in the poorest social class, prenuptial conception rates therefore overstate the social class gradient.

During the decades after the Second World War in Britain, the United States, and other industrial countries, prenuptial conceptions and births to unmarried mothers have been on the increase. An increase is apparent in the number of illegitimate births per 1000 total live births, the *illegitimacy ratio*, and in the number of births per 1000 unmarried women, the *illegitimacy rate*. The illegitimacy ratio gives a measure of the proportion of out-of-wedlock births to all births. Because the numerator varies with the size as well as with the fertility of only the unmarried female population, and the denominator with the size and fertility of both the married and the unmarried populations, this ratio gives a poor measure of behavior of unmarried women. For this purpose, it is safe only to use the illegitimacy rate.

In England and Wales the illegitimacy rate declined from a peak of 18.3 in the mid-nineteenth century to 5.5 in the 1930s. In the steep rise since then, the rate reached 28.6 in 1975, outstripping the previous highest recorded figure. In the United States national vital statistics show more than a fourfold rise, from 7.1 in 1940 to 29.6 in 1981 (204,208). Inference from prenuptial conception rates suggests that the increase had begun with the marriage cohorts at the beginning of the century, with an especially sharp rise in the cohorts married in the period immediately after the Second World War. A large increase in the rates for black mothers in the earlier period created a wide divergence from the rates for whites. Since the 1960s, however, the illegitimacy rate for black women has decreased, while that for white women has risen more sharply and somewhat narrowed the gap between them.

Changes in demographic trends, as well as changes in social attitudes about premarital intercourse, contraception, abortion, and out-of-wedlock childbearing, have contributed to current trends in the United States. The total number of out-of-wedlock births increased more than eightfold between 1940 and 1980 (204,208). Since the mid-1960s, there has been a continuing increase in the absolute number of births to unmarried women in contrast to the decline in births among married women partly as a result of the increased number of unmarried women. Thus as general fertility has fallen, out-of-wedlock births have constituted a larger proportion of all births. Despite the increase in absolute number of births to unmarried women, between 1970 and 1976 the rate of illegitimate births among them declined somewhat, only again to rise sharply over the succeeding five years. The rising trend, present in all age groups, is especially pronounced among women under 20. Thus, out-of-wedlock births are increasingly concentrated among teenage mothers, particularly in the United States (204,208). At present, teenage women comprise one-half of the unmarried female population of reproductive age (15–44 years) and are responsible for nearly one-half of all out-of-wedlock births. The rate of births for unmarried black teenagers is 66.9 per 1000 for 15–17-year-olds and 117.6 per 1000 for 18–19-year-olds—five times the rate for white teenagers in the respective age groups (204). Part of the differential between white and black mothers is a matter of the timing of marriage following a prenuptial conception. When and whether a marriage takes place depends, on the one hand, on the norms and values attached to marriage and, on the other, on the means available to realize those values. In this regard we have noted the variable use of contraception, abortion, and adoption, as well as social controls over sex relations.

Family reactions to the rarer premarital pregnancies of higher-class girls are various. Marriage was not the only solution even before the legalization of abortion. If the parents considered the potential husband to be unsuitable, the problem could be resolved by terminating the pregnancy, or having the child adopted, or by sending the girl away from home for the delivery or longer. Knowledge of birth control has long been widespread in the higher classes, although access for teenage girls was often limited, and prenuptial conception less a normal part of the course of courtship and marriage. An illegitimate birth tends to create greater emotional and social distress for the affluent family than it does economic and material distress. Such distress may be exacerbated in the case of girls who still have the status of pupils.

In these circumstances, the out-of-wedlock birth of an adolescent girl is an expression of social structure rather than psychological disturbance. Thus even in England in the 1950s, a time when a strong stigma attached to out-of-wedlock pregnancies, an intensive study of pregnant adolescent girls selected from a prenatal clinic found little in the way of psychopathological disturbance (209). Most of the girls eventually married, about half of them to putative fathers. Nevertheless, economic and material problems are likely to loom large for unmarried teenage mothers, since they are less likely to complete high school, less likely to obtain early prenatal care, and more likely to experience high rates of fetal death and to deliver low birthweight infants. Most of the disadvantage of teenage pregnancies arises as a result of the social circumstances that are conducive to them and that stem from them. Beyond puberty, obstetric risks are low. With regard to the supposedly adverse effects on the measured intelligence of offspring, once social factors are tightly controlled, no effect conditional on the teen ages could be found. A slight rise in mental performance with maternal age was entirely linear (210). The single-parent family which may be the consequence of teen-age pregnancy, however, is at a definite disadvantage in material, educational and personal assets.

When adolescents finally acquire adult status, they become independent members of society free to pursue their own interests and choose their own companions. They enter into social relationships with persons outside the family, at work, and in other fields of activity. Most of these activities take place outside the home, and more often with unrelated persons than with kinsfolk; many young people at this time of their lives use their parents' home largely as a dormitory. This independence does not usu-ally imply a break with their families of origin, but rather that their relations with parents and siblings are now based primarily on love and affection, and occasionally on economic interests, and not on legal restraints. The familial bond becomes only one of many, and the young adult adopts new roles and statuses in the pursuit of interests that compete for his or her attention and loyalty, while taking up new duties and responsibilities.

References

1. **Eveleth, P.** (1979). Population differences in growth: Environmental and genetic fac-tors, in *Human Growth, Volume 3: Neurobiology and Nutrition*, ed. Falkner, F. and Tanner, J., New York, pp. 373–84.
2. **Garn, S. M.** (1980). Human growth, *Annual Review of Anthropology*, 9, 275–92.
3. **Van Wieringen, J.** (1978). Secular growth changes, in *Human Growth, Volume 2: Post-natal Growth*, ed. Falkner, F., and Tanner, J., New York, pp. 445–74.
4. **Richards, A. I.** (1956). *Chisungu: A Girl's Initiation Ceremony among the Bemba of Northern Rhodesia*, London.
5. **Kellam, S., Ensminger, M.,** and **Turner, J.** (1977). Family structure and the mental health of children, *Arch. Gen. Psychiat.*, 34, 1012–22.
6. **Hammer, M., Gutwirth, L.,** and **Phillips, S.** (1982). Parenthood and social networks: A preliminary view, *Soc. Sci. Med. 16*, 2091–100.
7. **Baldwin, A. L.** (1947). Changes in parent behavior during pregnancy: An experiment in longitudinal analysis, *Child Development*, 8, 29–39.
8. **Nepali, G.** (1965). *The Newars*, Bombay.
9. **Black, D,** and **Sturge, C.** (1979). The young child and his siblings, in *Modern Perspec-tives in the Psychiatry of Infancy*, ed. Howells, J., New York.
10. **Drotar, D., Baskiewicz, A., Irvin, N., Kennell, J.,** and **Klaus, M.** (1975). The adapta-tion of parents to the birth of an infant with a congenital malformation: A hypothetical model, *Pediatrics, 56*, 710–17.
    Cohen, L., Zilkha, S., Middleton, J., and **O'Donnohue, N.** (1978). Perinatal mortality: Assisting parental affirmation, *Amer. J. Orthopsychiat., 48*, 727–31.

Bowlby, J. (1980). *Loss: Sadness and Depression—Attachment and Loss, Volume III*, New York.

Kirkley-Best, E., and Kellner, K. R. (1982). The forgotten grief: A review of the psychology of stillbirth, *Amer. J. Orthopsychiat.*, 52, 420–29.

11. Kennell, J., Slyter, H., and Klaus, M. (1970). The mourning responses of parents to the death of a newborn infant, *New Eng. J. Med.*, 283, 344–49.

12. Weinstein, S. E. (1978). Sudden infant death syndrome: Impact on families and a direction for change, *Amer. J. Psychiat.*, 135, 831–34.

13. Cain, A., and Cain, B. (1964). On replacing a child, *Amer. Acad. of Child Psychiat.*, 3, 443–55.

Jolly, H. (1976). Family reactions to stillbirth, *Proc. Roy. Soc. Med.*, 69, 835–37.

Rowe, J., Clyman, R., Green, C., Mikkelsen, C., Haight, J., and Ataide, L. (1978). Follow-up of families who experience a perinatal death, *Pediatrics*, 62, 166–70.

14. D'Arcy, E. (1968). Congenital defects: Mother's reactions to first information, *Brit. Med. J.*, 3, 796–98.

15. Gabel, S., and Erickson, M., eds. (1980). *Child Development and Developmental Disabilities*, Boston.

16. Richardson, S. (1969). The effects of physical disability on the socialization of a child, in *Handbook of Socialization Theory and Research*, ed. Goslin, D., New York.

Horobin, G., and Vaysey-Paun, M. (1981). Sociological perspectives, in *Brain Dysfunction in Children*, ed. Black, P., New York, pp. 221–37.

17. Drillien, C. M., and Wilkinson, E. H. (1964). Mongolism: When should parents be told?, *Brit. Med. J.*, 2, 1306–7.

Berg, J. M., Gilderdale, S., and Way, J. (1969). On telling parents of a diagnosis of mongolism, *Brit. J. Psychiat.*, 115, 1195–96.

18. McGraw, M. B. (1935). *Growth: A Study of Johnny and Jimmy*, New York.

Gesell, A., and Ilg, F. L. (1943). *Infant and Child Care in the Culture Today*, London.

Fenichel, O. (1945). *The Psychoanalytic Theory of Neurosis*, New York.

Illingworth, R. S. (1953). *The Normal Child*, London.

Piaget, J. (1956). In *Discussions on Child Development*, vols. I–IV, ed. Tanner, J. M., and Inhelder, B., London.

Tanner, J. M., and Inhelder, B. eds. (1956–1958, 1960). *Discussions on Child Development*, vols. I–IV, London.

Parsons, T., and Bales, R. F. (1956). *Family, Socialization and Interaction Process*, London

19. Whiting, J. W. H., and Child, I. L. (1953). *Child Training and Personality: A Cross-Cultural Study*, New Haven.

Leiderman, H., Tulkin, S., and Rosenfeld, A. (1977). *Culture and Infancy: Variations in the Human Experience*, New York.

20. Masters, J. C. (1981). Developmental psychology, *Ann. Rev. Psychol.*, 32, 117–51.

21. Thomas, A., Chess, S., and Birch, H. (1970). The origin of personality, *Scientific American*, 223, 102–9.

22. Lamb, M. (1978). Father-infant and mother-infant interaction in the first year of life, *Child Development*, 48, 167–81.

Minde, K., and Cohen, N. (1979). Cross-cultural approach to child psychiatry as applied to the infant and young child, in *Modern Perspectives in the Psychiatry of Infancy*, ed. Howells, J., New York, pp. 295–324.

23. Lamb, M. (1978). The development of sibling relationships in infancy: A short-term longitudinal study, *Child Development*, 49, 1189–92.

24. **Whiting, B.**, and **Whiting, J.** (1975). *Children of Six Cultures*, Cambridge, Mass.
25. **Glick, P. C.** (1979). Children of divorced parents in demographic perspective, *J. Soc. Issues, 35*, 170–82.
26. **Newberger, E. H., Reed, R. B., Daniel, J. H., Hyde, J. N.**, and **Kotelchuck, M.** (1977). Pediatric social illness: Toward an etiologic classification, *Pediatrics, 60*, 178–85.
27. **Biller, H.** (1976). The father and personality development: Paternal deprivation and sex-role development, in *The Role of the Father in Child Development*, ed. Lamb, M., New York, pp. 89–156.
28. **Rutter, M.**, and **Madge, N.** (1976). *Cycles of Disadvantage*, London.
29. **Kalter, N.** (1977). Children of divorce in an outpatient psychiatric population, *Amer. J. Orthopsychiat., 47*, 40–51.
30. **Koller, K. M.**, and **Castanos, J. N.** (1970). Family background in prison groups: A comparative study of parental deprivation, *Brit. J. Psychiat., 117*, 371–80.
    Cortes, J., and **Gatti, F.** (1972). *Delinquency and Crime: A Biopsychosocial Approach*, New York.
    Connor, W. (1972). *Defiance in Soviet Society: Crime, Delinquency and Alcoholism*, New York.
    Eisenberg, J., Langner, T., and **Gersten, J.** (1975). Differences in the behavior of welfare and non-welfare children in relation to parental characteristics, *Archiv. Behav. Sci., 48*, 3–33.
    Brown, G., Harris, T., and **Copeland, J.** (1977). Depression and loss, *Brit. J. Psychiat.. 140*, 1–18.
    Robins, L., and **Ratcliff, K.** (1979). Risk factors in the continuation of childhood antisocial behavior into adulthood, *Int. J. Ment. Hlth., 7*, 96–116.
    Wadsworth, M. (1979). *Roots of Delinquency: Infancy, Adolescence and Crime.* Oxford.
    Wadsworth, M. E. J. (1979). Delinquency prediction and its uses: The experience of a twenty-one year follow-up study. *Int. J. Ment. Hlth., 7*, 43–62.
    Fergusson, D. M., Horwood, L. J., and **Shannon, F. T.** (1981). Birth placement and childhood disadvantage, *Soc. Sci. Med., 15E*, 315–26.
31. **Stein, Z.**, and **Susser, M.** (1967). The social dimensions of a symptom: A socio-medical study of enuresis, *Soc. Sci. Med., 1*, 183–201.
32. **Wallerstein, J. S.**, and **Kelly, J. B.** (1980). Effects of divorce on the visiting father-child relationship, *Amer. J. Psychiat., 137*, 1534–39.
33. **Clingempeel, W. G.**, and **Reppucci, N. D.** (1982). Joint custody after divorce: Major issues and goals for research, *Psychol. Bull., 91*, 102–27.
34. **Shinn, M.** (1978). Father absence and children's cognitive development, *Psychol. Bull., 85*, 295–324.
35. **Andry, R. G.** (1960). *Delinquency and Parental Pathology*, London.
    Gregory, I. (1965). Anterospective data following childhood loss of a parent. I. Delinquency and high school dropout, *Arch. Gen. Psychiat., 13*, 99–109.
36. **McCord, W.**, and **McCord, J.** (1959). *Origins of Crime*, New York.
37. **West, D. J.**, and **Farington, D. P.** (1973). *Who Becomes Delinquent? Second Report of the Cambridge Study in Delinquent Development*, London.
38. **Power, M., Ash, P., Shoenberg, E.**, and **Sorey, E.** (1974). Delinquency and the family, *Brit. J. Soc. Wk., 4*, 13–38.
39. **Jenkins, R.** (1968). The varieties of children's behavioral problems and family dynamics, *Amer. J. Psychiat., 124*, 134–39.

40. **Robins, L.** (1979). Study of childhood predictors of adult outcomes: implications from longitudinal studies, in *Stress and Mental Disorder*, ed. Barret, J., New York, pp. 219–36.

41. **Hetherington, E., Cox, M.,** and **Cox, R.** (1978). The aftermath of divorce, in *Mother-Child, Father-Child Relationships*, ed. Steens, J. and Matthews, M., Washington, D.C.

42. **Levitin, T. E.** (1979). Children of divorce, *J. Soc. Issues*, 35, 1–25.

43. **Krieger, I.** (1979). Maternal and psychosocial deprivation, in *Modern Perspectives in the Psychiatry of Infancy*, ed. Howells, J., New York, pp. 142–62.

44. **Widdowson, E.** (1951). Mental contentment and physical growth, *Lancet*, 1, 1316–18.

45. **Skodak, M.,** and **Skeels, H. M.** (1945). A follow-up study of children to adoptive homes, *J. Genet. Psychol.*, 66, 21–58.
    Skeels, H. M. (1966). Adult studies of children with contrasting early life experiences, *Monogr. Soc. Res. Child. Dev.*, 51, No. 3.

46. **Tizard, J.,** and **Tizard, B.** (1971). The social development of two-year-old children in residential nurseries, in *The Origins of Social Relations*, ed., Schaffer, H. R., London, pp. 147–63.
    Wolkind, S., and **Renton, G.** (1979). Psychiatric disorders in children in long-term residential care: A follow-up study, *Brit. J. Psychiat.*, 135, 129–35.

47. **Susser, M.** (1981). Prenatal nutrition, birthweight, and psychological development: An overview of experiments, quasi-experiments, and natural experiments in the past decade, *Amer. J. Nutr.*, 34, 784–803.

48. **Wadsworth, M. E. J., Butler, N.,** and **Corner, B.,** eds. (1984). *Stress and Disability: The Long Term Problem*, Bristol.
    Stein, Z., and **Susser, M.** (1984). The epidemiology of mental retardation, in *Stress and Disability in Childhood: The Long-Term Problem*, eds., Wadsworth, M., Butler, N., and Corner, B., Bristol.

49. **Garber, H.,** and **Heber, R.** (1973). *The Milwaukee Project: Early Intervention as a Technique to Prevent Mental Retardation*, Storrs, Connecticut. University of Connecticut Technical papers.
    McKay, H., Sinisterra, L., McKay, A., Gomez, H., and **Llorda, P.** (1978). Improving cognitive ability in chronically deprived children, *Science*, 200, 270–78.

50. **Finkelhor, D.** (1979). *Sexually Victimized Children*, New York.

51. **Newberger, E.** (1982). Pediatric understanding of child abuse and neglect, in *Child Abuse*, ed. Newberger, E., Boston, pp. 137–58.

52. **Friedrich, W.** (1976). Epidemiological survey of physical child abuse, *Texas Medicine*, 72, 81–84.
    Oliver, J., Cox, J., and **Buchanan, A.** (1978). Severely ill-treated young children in Northwest Wiltshire, in *The Maltreatment of Children*, ed. Smith, S., Baltimore, pp. 121–53.
    New York State Department of Social Services (1981). *Child Protective Services*, Albany.
    U.S. Department of Justice (1981). *Source Book of Criminal Justice Statistics*, United States Government Printing Office, Washington, D.C.

53. **Bhattacharya, A.** (1966). Multiple fractures, *Bulletin of Calcutta School of Tropical Medicine*, 14, 111–12.
    Bwibo, N. (1971). Battered child syndrome, *East African Medical Journal*, 48, 56.
    Nwako, F. (1974). Child abuse in Nigeria, *Internal Journal of Surgery*, 59, 11–12, 613–15.
    Korbin, J., ed. (1981). *Child Abuse and Neglect: Cross-Cultural Perspectives*, Berkeley.

54. **Oliver, J.** (1978). The epidemiology of child abuse, in *The Maltreatment of Children*, ed. Smith, S., Baltimore, pp. 96–120.

55. **Dumont, L.** (1970). *Homo Hierarchicus: The Caste System and Its Implications*, Chicago.

56. **Scammon, R. E.** (1930). The measurement of the body in childhood, in *The Measurement of Man*, ed. Harris, A., et al., Minneapolis.
Healy, M. (1978). Statistics of growth standards, in *Human Growth: Volume 1: Principles and Prenatal Growth*, ed. Falkner, F., and Tanner, J., New York, pp. 169–82.

57. **Munroe, R.,** and **Munroe, R.** (1975). *Cross-Cultural Human Development*, Monterey, Calif.

58. **Ainsworth, M. D. S.** (1967). *Infancy in Uganda: Infant Care and the Growth of Love*, Baltimore.
Ainsworth, M. (1976). Infant development and mother infant interaction among Ganda and American families, in *Culture and Infancy: Variations in the Human Experience*, ed. Leiderman, P., Tulkin, S., and Rosenfeld, A., New York, pp. 119–50.

59. **Kagan, J., Kearsley, R.,** and **Zelazo, P.** (1978). *Infancy: Its Place in Human Development*, Cambridge, Mass.

60. **Werner, E.** (1972). Infants around the world: Cross-cultural studies of psychomotor development from birth to two years, *J. Cross-Cult. Psychol., 3*, 111–34.

61. **Brazelton, T., Robey, J.,** and **Collier, G.** (1969). Infant development in the Zinacanteco Indians of Southern Mexico, *Pediatrics, 44*, 274–93.

62. **Bronfenbrenner, U.** (1975) Is early intervention effective? In *Handbook of Evaluation Research*, Volume 2, ed. Guttentag, M. and Struening, E., Beverly Hills, 519–603.

63. **Kagan, J.** (1971). *Change and Continuity in Infancy*, New York.

64. **Deutsch, C. P.** (1973). Social class and child development in *Review of Child Development Research*, ed. Caldwell, B. M., and Ricciuti, H. M., Chicago, pp. 233–82.

65. **Kluckhohn, C.,** and **Murray, H. A.** (1949). *Personality in Nature, Society and Culture*, London.
Sewell, W. H. (1952). Infant training and personality of the child, *Amer. J. Sociol., 59*, 150–9.
Caldwell, B. M. (1964). The effects of infant care, in *Review of Child Development Research*, ed. Hoffman, M. L., and Hoffman, L. W., New York, pp. 9–88.

66. **Sears, R. S., Maccoby, E. E.,** and **Levin, H.** (1957). *Patterns of Child Rearing*, New York.

67. **Ellis, A.** (1945). The sexual psychology of human hermaprodites, *Psychosom. Med., 7*, 108–25.

68. **Money, J.,** and **Erhardt, A.** (1972). *Man and Woman, Boy and Girl: The Differentation and Dimorphism of Gender Indentity from Conception to Maturity*, Baltimore.

69. **Kagan, J.,** and **Wright, J.,** eds. (1963). *Basic Cognitive Processess in Children*, Lafayette, Indiana.

70. **Sarason, S. B., Davidson, K. S., Lighthall, F., Waite, R. R.,** and **Reubush, B. K.** (1960). *Anxiety in Elementary School Children*, London.
Dohrenwend, B. P., and **Dohrenwend, B. S.** (1976). Sex differences in psychiatric disorders, *Amer. J. Sociol., 81*, 1447–54.
Gould, M., Wunsch-Hitzig, R., and **Dohrenwend, B.** (1980). Formulation of hypotheses about the prevalence, treatment, and prognostic significance of psychiatric disorders in children in the United States, in *Mental Illness in the United States: Epidemiological Estimates of the Scope of the Problems*, ed. Dohrenwend, B. P., Dohrenwend, B. S., Gould, M., Link, B., Neugebauer, R., Wunsch-Hitzig, R., New York, pp. 9–44.

Gould, M., Wunsch-Hitzig, R., and Dohrenwend, B. (1981). Estimating the prevalence of childhood psychopathology: A critical review, *American Academy of Child Psychiatry*, *20*, 462–76.

Veroff, J., Kulka, R., and Douvan, E. (1981). *Mental Health in America: Patterns of Help Seeking From 1957–1976*, New York.

Robins, L., Helzer, J., Weissman, M., Orvaschel, H., Gruenberg, E., Burke, J., and Regier, D. (1984). Lifetime prevalence of specific psychiatric disorders in three sites, *Arch. Gen. Psychiatry.*, *41*, 949–58.

71. Mussen, P., Cogner, J., and Kagan, J. (1979). *Child Development and Personality*, 5th Edition, New York.

72. Chamove, A., Harlow, H., and Mitchell, G. (1967). Sex differences in the infant-directed behavior of preadolescent Rhesus monkeys, *Child Develop.*, *38*, 329–35.

73. Sapir, E. (1921). *Language: An Introduction to the Study of Speech*, New York.
Whorf, B. L. (1956). *Language, Thought and Reality*, Cambridge, Mass.

74. Hudson, R. A. (1980). *Sociolinguistics*, Cambridge.

75. Blount, B. (1975). Studies in child language: An anthropological view, *Amer. Anthropol.*, *77*, 580–600.

76. Luria, A. R., and Yudovich, F. J. A. (1959). *Speech and the Development of Mental Processes in the Child*, trans., Simon, J., London.

77. Lenneberg, E. (1967). *Biological Foundations of Language*, New York.
McNeill, D (1970). *The Acquisition of Language: The Study of Developmental Linguistics*, New York.
Slobin, D. I. (1971). Developmental psycholinguistics, in *A Survey of Linguistic Science*, ed, Dingwall, W. O., College Park Md.
Brown, R. (1973). *A First Language: The Early Stages*, Cambridge, Mass.
Vetter, D. K. (1980). Speech and language disorders, in *Child Development and Developmental Disabilities*, Gabel, S., and Erickson, M., Boston, pp. 303–20.

78. Roeper, T., and McNeill, D. (1973). Review of child language, *Annual Review of Anthropology*, *2*, pp. 127–37.

79. Miller, F. J. W., Court, S. D., Walton, W. S., and Knox, E. G. (1960). *Growing Up in Newcastle upon Tyne*, London.

80. Dennis, W., and Najarian, P. (1957). Infant development under environmental handicap, *Psychological Monographs*, *71*, 1–13.
Hess, R. (1970). Social class and ethnic influences on socialization, in *Carmichael's Manual of Child Psychology*, Vol. 2, ed. Mussen, P., 3rd ed., New York, pp. 457–558.

81. Bernstein, B. (1974). *Class, Codes and Control: Theoretical Studies toward the Sociology of Language*, New York.

82. Bernstein, B. (1960). Language and social class, *Brit. J. Sociol.*, *11*, 271–76.

83. Zigler, E., and Valentine, J., ed. (1979). *Project Head Start: A Legacy of the War on Poverty*, New York.

84. Labov, W. (1972). *Language in the Inner City: Studies in the Black English Vernacular*, Philadelphia.

85. Hess, R. D., and Torney, J. (1967). *Development of Political Attitudes in Children*, Chicago, Ill.

86. Coleman, J. S., Campbell, E. Q., Hobson, C. J., McPortland, J., Mood, A. M., Weinfeld, F. D., and York, R. L. (1966). *Equality of Educational Opportunity*, U.S. Department of Health, Education and Welfare, Office of Education, Washington, D.C.
Coleman, J., Heffer, T., and Kilgore, S. (1982). *High School Achievement: Public, Catholic, and Other Private Schools Compared*, New York.

87. Dennis, N., Henriques, F., and Slaughter, C. (1960). *Coal Is Our Life*, London.

88. **Jolly, H.** (1968). Play and the sick child, *Lancet*, 2, 1286–7.
89. **Lowenfeld, M.** (1935). *Play in Childhood*, London.
    Huizinga, J. (1949). *Homo Ludens: A Study of the Play-Element in Culture*, London.
90. **Freud, S.** (1924). *Beyond the Pleasure Principle*, London.
    Henrick, I. (1945). Work and the pleasure principle, in *The Yearbook of Psycho-Analysis*, New York.
91. **Watson, W.** (1950). *Children in Fife*, unpublished M. Sc. thesis, Cambridge University, Cambridge.
92. **Groos, K.** (1901). *The Play of Man*, trans, Baldwin, W. L., London.
93. **Klein, M.** (1932). *The Psycho-Analysis of Children*, London.
94. **Piaget, J.** (1932). *The Moral Judgement of the Child*, trans., Gabain, M., London.
95. **Bossard, J. H. S.** (1945). *The Sociology of Child Development*, New York.
96. **Gomme, A. B.** (1894). *Traditional Games of England, Scotland and Ireland*, London.
    Opie, I., and **Opie, P.** (1959). *The Lore and Language of School Children*, London.
97. **Tanner, J. M.** (1962). *Growth at Adolescence*, 2nd ed., Oxford.
98. **Acheson, R. M.**, and **Hewitt, D.** (1954). Oxford Child Health Survey: Stature and skeletal maturation in the pre-school child, *Brit. J. Prev. Soc. Med.*, 8, 59–65.
    Acheson, R. M., Kemp, F. H., and **Parfait, J.** (1955). Height, weight and skeletal maturity in the first five years of life, *Lancet*, 1, 691–2.
    McGregor, I. A., Billewicz, W. Z., and **Thomson, A. M.** (1961). Growth and mortality in children in an African village, *Brit. Med. J.*, 2, 1661–66.
99. **Pless, I.**, and **Roghmann, K.** (1971). Chronic illness and its consequences: Observations based on three epidemiologic surveys, *J. Pediatr.*, 79, 351–59.
    Pless, I. and **Pinkerton, P.** (1975) *Chronic Childhood Disorder: Promoting Patterns of Adjustment*, London.
    Stein, R., and **Jessop, D.** (1984). Relationship between health status and psychological adjustment among children with chronic conditions, *Pediatrics 73*, 169–74.
100. **Fagin, C. M.** (1969). Mothers and children in hospital, *Brit. Med. J.*, 2, 311–12.
101. **U.S. Dept. of Health and Human Services** (1982). *Health: United States*, Hyattsville, Md.
102. **Sabbeth, B.**, and **Leventhal, J.** (1984). Marital adjustment to chronic childhood illness: A critique of the literature, *Pediatrics*, 73, 762–68.
103. **Hamovitch, M. B.** (1964). *The Parent and the Fatally Ill Child*, Los Angeles, Calif.
104. **Davis, F.** (1963). *Passage Through Crisis: Polio Victims and Their Families*, New York.
105. **Leeson, J.** (1960). A study of six young mentally handicapped children and their families, *Med. Offr.*, 104, 311–14.
    Cartwright, A. (1964). *Human Relations and Hospital Care*, London.
106. **Glaser, B.**, and **Strauss, A.** (1965). *Awareness of Dying*, Chicago, Ill.
107. **Bowlby, J., Ainsworth, M., Boston, M.**, and **Rosenbluth, D.** (1956). The effects of mother-child separation: A follow-up study, *Brit. J. Med. Psychol.*, 29, 211–47.
    Saenger, G. (1961). *Follow-up Study of Former Blythedale Patients*, New York.
108. **Koos, E. L.** (1946). *Families in Trouble*, New York.
109. **Shere, M.** (1957). The socio-emotional development of the twin who has cerebral palsy, *Cerebr. Palsy Rev.*, 17, 16–18.
110. **Schaffer, H. R.** (1964). The too cohesive family: A form of group pathology, *Int. J. Soc. Psychiat.*, 10, 266–75.
111. **Cowen, E. L., Underberg, R. P.**, and **Verillo, T.** (1961). *Adjustment to Visual Disability in Adolescence*, New York.

Lorenz, G. (1968). Attitude Towards Racial Desegragation among the Blind and Patterns of Consensus between Blind and Sighted Relatives, unpublished Ph.D thesis, Columbia University, New York.

112. Sommers, V. (1944). *The Influence of Parental Attitudes and Social Environment on the Personality Development of the Adolescent Blind*, New York.

113. Richardson, S. A., Hastorf, A. H., Goodman, N., and Dornbusch, S. M. (1961). Cultural uniformity in reaction to physical disabilities, *Amer. Sociol. Rev.*, 26, 241–7.
    Goodman, N., Richardson, S. A., Dornbusch, S. M., and Hastorf, A. H. (1963). Variant reactions to physical disabilities, *Amer. Sociol. Rev.*, 28, 429–35.

114. Richardson, S. A., Hastorf, A. H., and Dornbusch, S. M. (1964). The effects of physical disability on a child's description of himself, *Child Develop.*, 35, 894–907.

115. Ladieu, G., Adler, D., and Dembo, T. (1948). Studies in adjustment to visible injuries: Social acceptance of the injured, *J. Soc. Issues*, 4, 55–61.
    Barker, R. G., Adler, D., and Dembo, T. (1948). Studies in adjustment to visible injuries: Social acceptance of the injured, *J. Soc. Issues*, 4, 28–34.
    Wright, B. A. (1960). *Physical Disability—A Psychological Approach*, New York.

116. Richardson, S. A. (1963). Some social psychological consequences of handicapping, *Pediatrics*, 132, 291–7.
    Richardson, S. A. (1963). Psychosocial and cultural deprivation in psychobiological development: Psychosocial aspects, in *Deprivation in Psychobiological Development*, Pan American Health Organization, *Science Publications*, No. 134.

117. Goffman, E. (1963). *Stigma*, Englewood Cliffs, N.J.

118. Korsch, B., and Barnett, H. L. (1961). The physician, the family and the child with nephrosis, *J. Pediat.*, 58, 707–15.

119. Hathaway, K. B. (1943). *The Little Locksmith*, New York.

120. Susser, M. W. (1968). *Community Psychiatry: Epidemiologic and Social Themes*, New York, pp. 299–321.

121. Palmer, W. T., and Pirie, D. (1958). Survey of pupils in schools for physically handicapped in London, *Brit. Med. J.*, 2, 1326–8.

122. Tizard, J. (1966). *Community Services for the Mentally Handicapped*, London.
    Hagberg. B. (1979). Epidemiological and preventative aspects of cerebral palsy and severe mental retardation in Sweden, *Eur. J. Pediatr.*, 130, 71–78.
    Kiely, J., Paneth, N., Stein, Z., and Susser, M. (1981). Cerebral palsy and newborn care. I. Secular trends in cerebral palsy, *Devel. Med. Child Neurol.*, 23, 533–38.
    Kiely, J., Paneth, N., Stein, Z., and Susser, M. (1981). Cerebral palsy and newborn care. II. Mortality and neurological impairment in low-birthweight infants, *Devel. Med. Child Neurol.*, 23, 650–59.
    Paneth, N. Kiely, J., Stein, Z., and Susser, M. (1981). Cerebral palsy and newborn care. III. Estimated prevalence rates of cerebral palsy under differing rates of mortality and impairment of low-birthweight infants, *Develop. Med. Child Neurol.*, 23, 801–17.

123. Narayanan, H. (1981). A study of the prevalence of mental retardation in Southern India, *Int. J. Mental Health*, 10, 28–36.
    Hasan, Z., and Hasan, A. (1981). Report on a population survey of mental retardation in Pakistan, *Int. J. Mental Health*, 10, 23–27.

124. Stein, Z., and Susser, M. (1980). The less developed world: Southeast Asia as a paradigm, in *Mental Retardation and Developmental Disabilities: An Annual Review*, ed. Wortis J., New York, pp. 220–40.

125. Lucas, W. P., and Pryor, H. B. (1935). Range and standard deviations of certain physical measurements in healthy children, *J. Pediat.*, 6, 533–45.

Marshall, W. (1978). Puberty, in *Human Growth, Volume 2: Postnatal Growth*, ed. Falkner, F., and Tanner, J., New York, pp. 141–82.

126. Hersov, L. A. (1960). Persistent non-attendance at school, *Child Psychol. Psychiat., 1*, 130–6.

Hersov, L. A. (1960). Refusal to go to school, *Child Psychol. Psychiat., 1*, 137–45.

Hersov, L. A. (1976). School refusal, in *Child Psychiatry-Modern Approaches*, ed. Rutter, M., and Hersov, L. A., London, pp. 455–86.

127. Bergner, L., and Susser, M. W. (1970). Low birthweight and prenatal nutrition: An interpretive review, *Pediatrics, 46*, 946–66.

Susser, M., Marolla, F., and Fleiss, J. (1972). Birthweight, fetal age and perinatal mortality, *Amer. J. Epi.* 96, 197–204.

128. Berry, W. T. C., and Cowin, P. J. (1954). Conditions associated with the growth of boys, 1954 *Brit. Med. J., 1*, 847–51.

Boyne, A. W. (1960). Secular changes in the stature of adults and the growth of children, with special reference to changes in intelligence of 11 years olds, in *Human Growth*, ed. Tanner, J. M., Oxford, pp. 97–120.

129. U.S. National Center for Health Statistics (1978). Skeletal maturity of youths 12–17 years: Racial, geographic area, and socioeconomic differentials, *Vital and Health Statistics*, Series 11, Number 167, Hyattsville, Maryland, pp. 38–40.

130. Scottish Council for Research in Education (1953). *Social Implications of the 1947 Scottish Mental Survey*, XXXV, London.

Stein, Z. A., and Susser, M. W. (1970). Mutability of intelligence and the epidemiology of mild mental retardation, *Rev. Educ. Res., 40*, 29–48.

131. Clarke, A. D. B., Clarke, A. M. and Reiman, S. (1958). Cognitive and social changes in the feebleminded: Three further studies, *Brit. J. Psychol.* 49, 144–57.

Stein, Z. A., and Susser, M. W. (1960). Families of dull children. Part IV. Increments in intelligence, *J. Ment. Sci., 106*, 1311–19.

132. Bullough, V. (1981). Age at menarche: A misunderstanding, *Science, 213*, 365–66.

Tanner, J. M. (1982). Menarcheal age, *Science, 214*, 604–6.

Wyshak, G., and Frisch, R. *(1982). Evidence for a secular trend in age of menarche, New Engl. J. Med., 306*, 1033–35.

133. Douglas, J. W. B. (1964). *The Home and the School*, London.

Douglas, J. W. B., Ross, J. M., and Simpson, H. R. (1965). The relation between height and measured educational ability in school children of the same social class, family size and stage of sexual development, *Hum. Biol., 37*, 178–86.

Tanner, J., and Eveleth, P. (1975). Variability between populations in growth and development at puberty, in *Puberty, Biologic and Psychological Components*, ed. Berenberg, S., Leiden, 256–323.

134. Khosla, T., and Lowe, C. R. (1968). Height and weight of British men, *Lancet, 1*, 742–5.

135. Kark, E. (1943). Menarche in South African Bantu girls, *S. Afr. J. Med. Sci., 8*, 35–40.

Burrell, R., Healy, M., and Tanner, J. (1961). Age at menarche in South African Bantu school girls living in the Transkei Reserve, *Human Biology, 33*, 250–61.

136. Douglas, J. W. B. (1966). The age of reaching puberty: Some associated factors and some educational implications, *Sci. Basis Med.*, London, pp. 91–105.

137. Belmont, L., Stein, Z., and Susser, M. W. (1975). Comparison of associations of birth order with intelligence test score and height, *Nature, 255*, 54–56.

138. Lee, J. A. H. (1957). An association between social circumstances and appendicitis in young people, *Brit. Med. J., 1*, 1217–19.

Registrar General (1960). *Statistical Review of England and Wales, 1958*, H.M.S.O., London.

139. Parlee, M. B. (1980). Changes in moods and activation levels during the menstrual cycle in experimentally naive subjects, *Psychology of Women Quarterly*, 7, 119–31.

140. Parlee, M. B. (1981). Gaps in behavioral research on the menstrual cycle, in *The Menstrual Cycle: Research and Implications for Women's Health, Vol. 2*, ed. Lomnenich, P., New York, pp. 45–53.

141. Kerr, M. (1958). *The People of Ship Street*, London.

142. Kinsey, A. C., Pomeroy, W. B., and Martin, C. E., (1948). *Sexual Behavior in the Human Male*, Philadelphia.

143. Kolodny, R., Masters, W. H., and Johnson, V.E., eds. (1979). *Textbook of Sexual Medicine*, Boston.

144. Kinsey, A. C., Pomeroy, W. B., Martin, C. E. and Gebhard, P. H. (1953). *Sexual Behavior in the Human Female*, Philadelphia.

145. Parsons, T. (1951). *The Social System*, Glencoe, Ill.

146. Himmelweit, H. T., Halsey, A. H., and Oppenheim, A. N. (1952). The views of adolescents on some aspects of the social class structure, *Brit. J. Sociol.*, 3, 148–72.

147. Morris, T. (1957). *The Criminal Area*, London.

148. Tizard, B., Hughs, M., Carmichael, H., and Pinkerton, G. (1983). Children's questions and adults' answers, *J. Child Psychol. Psychiat.*, 24, 269–81.

149. Tizard, B., Hughs, M., Pinkerton, G., and Carmichael, H. (1982). Adults' cognitive demands at home and at nursery school, *J. Child Psychol. Psychiat.*, 23, 105–16.

150. Kantor, M. B. (1965). Some consequences of residential and social mobility for the adjustment of children, in *Mobility and Mental Health*, ed. Kantor, M. B., Springfield, Ill, pp. 86–122.
Werkman, S., Fouley, G. K., Butler, C., and Quayhagen, M. (1981). The psychological effects of moving and living overseas, *J. Amer. Acad. Child Psychiat.*, 20, 645–57.

151. Schofield, M. (1965). *The Sexual Behaviour of Young People*, Boston.

152. Reiss, I. (1966). The sexual renaissance: A survey and analysis, *J. Soc. Issues*, 22, 123–37.

153. Kohn, M. (1969). *Class and Conformity: A Study of Values*, Homewood, Ill.

154. Merton, R. K. (1949). Social structure and anomie, in *Social Theory and Social Structure*, Glencoe, Ill.

155. Floud, J. (1954). The educational experience of the adult populations of England and Wales as at July 1949, in *Social Mobility in Britain*, ed. Glass, D. V., London.

156. Zussman, J. V. (1978). Relationship of demographic factors to parental discipline techniques, *Dev. Psych.*, 14, 685–86.

157. Myers, J. K., and Roberts, B. H. (1959). *Family and Class Dynamics in Mental Illness*, New York.

158. Ministry of Labour (1957). *Enquiry into Household Expenditure 1953-54*, H.M.S.O., London.
Citizens Boards of Enquiry into Hunger and Malnutrition in the United States (1968). *Hunger U.S.A.*, Washington, D.C.

159. Douglas, J. W. B., and Blomfield, J. M. (1958). *Children Under Five*, London.

160. Scottish Council for Research in Education (1953). *Social Implications of the 1947 Scottish Mental Survey*, XXXV, London.

161. Arnold, F., Bulatao, R., Buripakdi, C., Chung, B. Fawcett, J., Iritani, T., Lee, S., and Wu, T. (1975). *The Value of Children: A Cross-National Study*, Vol. 1, Honolulu.

162. Greenwood, M., and Yule, G. U. (1914). On the determination of size of family, and of the distribution of characters in order of birth, J. Roy. Statist. Soc., 77, 179–99.
    Haldane, J. B. S., and Smith, C. A. (1948). A simple exact test for birth-order effect, Ann. Eugen., 14, 117–24.
    Slater, E. (1962). Birth order and maternal age of homosexuals, Lancet, 1, 69–71.
163. MacMahon, B., and Pugh, T. F. (1970). Epidemiology: Principles and Methods, Boston.
164. Barker, D. J. P., and Record, R. G. (1966). The presence of disease and birth order: A comment on the Greenwood-Yule method, J. Roy. Statist. Soc., 16, 13–16.
    Barker, D. J. P., and Record, R. G. (1967). The relationship of the presence of disease to birth order and maternal age, Amer. J. Hum. Genet., 19, 433–49.
165. Hare, E. H., and Price, J. S. (1969). Birth order and family size: Bias caused by changes in birth rate, Brit. J. Psychiat., 115, 647–57.
166. Erlenmeyer-Kimling, L. (1969). The problem of birth order and schizophrenia: A negative conclusion, Brit. J. Psychiat., 115, 659–78.
167. MacMahon, B., Record, R. G., and McKeown, T. (1951). Congenital pyloric stenosis: An investigation of 578 cases, Brit. J. Soc. Med., 5, 185–92.
168. Schachter, S. (1963). Birth order, eminence and higher education, Amer. Sociol. Rev., 28, 757–68.
169. Altus, W. D. (1966). Birth order and its sequelae, Science, 151, 44–49.
    Warren, J. R. (1966). Birth order and social behaviour, Psychol. Bull., 65, 38–49.
    Belmont, L. (1977). Birth order, intellectual competence, and psychiatric status, J. Indiv. Psychol., 33, 97–104.
170. Belmont, L., and Marolla, F. A. (1973). Birth order, family size, and intelligence, Science, 182, 1096–1101.
    Breland, H. M. (1974). Birth order, family configuration, and verbal achievement, Child Development, 45, 1011–19.
171. Schooler, C. (1972). Birth order effects: Not here, not now!, Psychol. Bull., 78, 161–75.
    Belmont, L., Wittes, J., and Stein, Z. (1980). The only child syndrome: Myth or reality, in Human Functioning in Longitudinal Perspective, ed. Sells, S., Crandall, R., Roff, M., Strauss, J., and Pollin, W., 251–59.
172. Gerard, H. B., and Rabbie, J. M. (1961). Fear and social comparison, J. Abnorm. Soc. Psychol., 62, 586–92.
    Sampson, E. E., and Hancock, F. T. (1967). An examination of the relationship between ordinal position, personality, and conformity: An extension, replication, and partial verification, J. Pers. Soc. Psychol., 5, 398–407.
173. Fortes, M. (1938). Social and psychological aspects of education in Taleland, Memorandum XVII, London.
174. Freud, S. (1919). Totem and Taboo, trans. Brill., A., London.
175. Fortes, M. (1949). The Web of Kinship among the Tallensi, London.
176. Raum, O. F. (1940). Chaga Childhood, London.
    Wilson, M. (1951). Good Company: A Study of Nyasukusa Aga Village, London.
    Gluckman, M. (1954). Rituals of Rebellion in South East Africa, Manchester.
    Eisenstadt, S. N. (1956). From Generation to Generation: Age Groups and Social Structure, London.
177. Erikson, E. H. (1963). Childhood and Society, New York.
178. Allcorn, D. H. (1955). The Social Development of Young Men in an English Industrial Suburb, unpublished Ph.D. thesis, Manchester University, Manchester.

179. **Krohn, M., Massey, J., Skinner, W., and Lauer, R.** (1983). Social bonding theory and adolescent cigarette smoking: a longitudinal analysis, *J. Hlth. Soc. Behav., 24,* 337–49.
180. **Thrasher, F. M.** (1927). *The Gang,* Chicago.
    Whyte, W. F. (1943). *Street Corner Society,* Chicago.
    Hollingshead, A. (1949). *Elmstown's Youth,* New York.
    Reiss, A. J., Jr. (1951). Unravelling juvenile delinquency. II. An appraisal of the research methods, *Amer. J. Sociol., 62,* 115–20.
    Turner, M. L., and Spencer, J. C. (1955). Spontaneous youth groups and gangs, in *Culture and Mental Health,* ed. Opler, M. K., New York.
181. **Langner, T., McCarthy, E., Gersten, J., Simcha-Fagan, O., and Eisenberg, J.** (1979). The family research project, in *Research in Community and Mental Health, Volume 1,* ed. Simmons, R. Greenwich, Connecticut, pp. 143–81.
    Glueck, S., and Glueck, E. T. (1950). *Unravelling Juvenile Delinquency,* Cambridge, Mass.
182. **Rutter, M.** (1979). *Changing Youth in a Changing Society: Patterns of Adolescent Development and Disorder,* London.
183. **Burt, Sir Cyril** (1952). *The Young Delinquent,* 4th ed., London.
    Ferguson, T. (1952). *The Young Delinquent in his Social Setting,* London.
    Mays, J. B. (1954). *Growing Up in a City,* Liverpool.
    Mannheim, H., and Wilkins, L. T. (1955). *Prediction Methods in Relation to Borstal Training,* H.M.S.O., London.
184. **Eisner, V., and Tzuyemura, H.** (1965). Interactions of juveniles with the law, *Publ. Hlth. Rep., 80,* 681–91.
    Power, M. (1965). An attempt to identify at first court appearance those at risk of becoming persistent juvenile offenders, *Proc. Roy. Soc. Med., 58,* 704–5.
    Power, M. (1966). Families before the courts, *Ann. Rev. Res. Child Care Ass.,* pp. 1–12.
185. **United Nations** (1955). *Report of the First United Nations Congress on Prevention of Crime and Treatment of Offenders,* London, H.M.S.O.
186. **Hopper, K., and Guttmacher, S.** (1979). Rethinking suicide: Notes toward a critical epidemiology, *Intl. J. Hlth. Serv., 9,* 417–38.
187. **National Center for Health Statistics** (1983). *Monthly Vital Statistics Report, 32,* 4.
188. **Mandell, W., and Ginzburg, H. M.** (1976). Youthful alcohol use, abuse, and alcoholism, in *Social Aspects of Alcoholism,* ed. Kissim, B., and Begleiter, H., New York, pp. 167–204.
    Kandel, D., Single, E., and Kessler, R. (1976). The epidemiology of drug use among New York State high school students: Distribution, trends, and change in rates of use, *Amer. J. Publ. Hlth., 66,* 43–53.
    Kandel, D. (1982). Epidemiological and psychosocial perspectives on adolescent drug use, *J. Am. Acad. Child. Psychiat., 21,* 328–47.
189. **Ford, C. S., and Beach, F. A.** (1951). *Patterns of Sexual Behaviour,* New York.
190. **Marshall, D. S., and Suggs, R.** eds. (1971). *Human Sexual Behavior: Variations in the Ethnographic Spectrum,* New York.
    Ortner, S., and Whitehead, H. eds. (1981). *Sexual Meanings,* Cambridge.
    Herdt, G. (1981). *Guardians of the Flutes: Idioms of Masculinity,* New York.
191. **Gagnon, J., and Simon, W.** (1973). *Sexual Conduct: The Sources of Human Sexuality,* Chicago.
192. **Faderman, L.** (1981). *Surpassing the Love of Men,* New York.

193. **Weeks, J.** (1981). *Sex, Politics and Society: The Regulation of Sexuality Since 1800*, London and New York.
194. **Chilman, C.** (1980). *Adolescent Sexuality in a Changing American Society: Social Psychological Perspectives*, Bethesda, Md.
195. **Laws, J. L.,** and **Schwartz, P.** (1977). *Sexual Scripts: The Social Construction of Female Sexuality*, Chicago, Ill.
196. **Kagan, J.,** and **Moss, H.** (1962). *Birth to Maturity, A Study in Psychological Development*, New York.
197. **Simon, W.,** and **Gagnon, J.** (1969). Psychosexual development, *Transaction, 6,* 9–17.
198. **Rainwater, L.** (1966). Some aspects of lower class sexual behavior, *J. Soc. Issues, 22,* 96–108.
199. **Rubin, L.** (1976). *Worlds of Pain*, New York.
200. **Udry, J. R.** (1966). *The Social Context of Marriage*, Philadelphia.
201. **Reiss, I. L.** (1965). Social class and premarital sexual permissiveness: A re-examination, *Amer. Sociol. Rev., 30,* 747–56.
202. **Reiss, I. L.** (1960). *Premarital Sexual Standards in America*, New York.
203. **Zelnik, M.,** and **Kantner, J.** (1980). Sexual activity: Contraceptive use and pregnancy among metropolitian area teenagers 1971–1979, *Family Planning Population, 12,* 5.
    Zelnik, M., Kantner, J., and **Ford, K.** (1981). *Sex and Pregnancy in Adolescence*, Beverly Hills, Calif.
204. **National Center for Health Statistics** (1983). Advance report of final natality statistics. 1981, *Monthly Vital Statistics Report, 32,* 9, Supplement, Hyattsville, Maryland.
    National Center for Health Statistics (1984). Trends in teenage childbearing, *Vital and Health Statistics*, Series 21, No. 41, Hyattsville, Md.
205. **Nag, M.** (1962). *Factors Affecting Human Fertility in Nonindustrial Societies: A Cross-Cultural Study*, New Haven.
206. **Westoff, C. F.,** and **Ryder, N. B.** (1969). Recent trends in attitudes towards fertility control and in the practice of contraception in the United States, in *Fertility and Family Planning, A World View*, ed. Behram, S. J., Corsa, L., and Freedman, R., Ann Arbor, Mich, pp. 388–412.
207. **Jones, W. C., Meyer, H. J.,** and **Borgatta, E. F.** (1962). Social and psychological factors in status decisions of unmarried mothers, *Marr. Fam. Liv., 24,* 224–30.
    Illsley, R., and **Gill, D.** (1968). Changing trends in illegitimacy, *Soc. Sci. Med., 2,* 415–33.
208. **National Center for Health Statistics** (1978). Characteristics of births, *Vital and Health Statistics*, Series 21, No. 30, Hyattsville, Md.
209. **Anderson, E. W., Kenna, J. C.,** and **Hamilton, M. W.** (1960). A study of extra-marital conception in adolescence, *Psychiat. et Neurol. (Basel), 139,* 313–62.
210. **Belmont, L., Cohen, P., Dryfoos, J., Stein, Z.,** and **Zayac, S.** (1980). Maternal age and children's intelligence, in *Teenaged Parents and Their Offspring*, eds., Scott, K., Field, T., and Robertson, E., New York, pp. 177–94.

12

Old age:
the phase of replacement

The chances of longevity determine the scale and nature of the health and social problems that attend old age in each society. In turn, the longevity of populations is closely related to their mode of economic and social life. Social organization has led to longer life in humans, through collective action in producing and distributing food, and through the protection conferred on individuals by bonds of kinship and community. In Chapter 3 we noted that in a primitive environment the risk of death at each age after the first years remains more or less constant, and the special vulnerability of old people in the population emerges only with the elimination of causes of death in childhood and early life. A modal age at death appears, and aging in populations then shows itself as a sharp decline in survival beyond the modal age of death. In recent times the change in this direction has been rapid, as can be seen in the population of any industrialized country (see Figure 3.8). Table 12.1 shows the mortality rates in Britain and the United States at ages over 65 years, the substantial mortality sex ratio in favor of women, and the rate of the annual change; an accelerated decline appeared in the more recent years. Increasingly, the male disadvantage in mortality has produced a deficit of men in the older age-groups (see Table 12.2).

The number of the young in any population is an outcome of the birthrate (1), but the number of the old is an outcome of the survival of those who are born. Thus in the United States the population has been relatively young and in Britain relatively old because of high and low birthrates respectively, but in both there are large numbers of old people. In Britain the proportion of persons over the age of 65 has risen over the last 100 years from less than 5 per cent to more than 10 per cent, and may yet rise to 15 or 20 per cent. In the United States between 1850 and 1980 the proportion of total population over the age of 65 rose from 3 per cent to 11 per cent (2).

The mean age reached in particular conditions is thus an ecological phenomenon. Populations begin to show a modal or most common age at death only under favorable conditions, although the Biblical allocation of three score years and ten is evi-

515

Table 12.1a Age-specific death rates per 1000 at ages 65 years and over: England and Wales, and the United States, 1977

	65–	70–	75–	80–	85+	All 65+ age adjusted
England & Wales						
Male	38.9	62.3	96.5	142.4	232.2	72.1
Female	19.2	32.1	54.9	97.1	188.6	42.5
United States						
Male	34.7	53.2	81.5	113.6	173.0	60.3
Female	16.9	27.7	47.4	73.9	135.4	34.9

Table 12.1b Age-specific mortality sex ratios at ages 65 years and over: England and Wales, and the United States, 1977

	65–	70–	75–	80–	85+	All 65+
England & Wales	2.03	1.94	1.76	1.47	1.23	1.70
United States	2.05	1.92	1.72	1.54	1.28	1.73

Table 12.1c Average annual change in death rates at ages 65 years and over, England and Wales, and the United States

	1950–1977 (%)	1968–1977 (%)
England & Wales		
Male	−0.3	−1.0
Female	−1.0	−1.0
United States		
Male	−0.3	−1.5
Female	−1.3	−2.3

Source: Adapted from various tables, National Center for Health Statistics (1982). Changes in mortality among the elderly, United States, 1940–78, *Vital and Health Statistics*, Series 3, No. 22, Hyattsville, Maryland.

Table 12.2 Percentage of total population in older age groups, by sex: United States 1950 and 1976

	1950		1976	
Age-group	Men	Women	Men	Women
60 —	11.8	12.5	13.1	16.8
65 —	7.7	8.6	9.0	12.3
70 —	4.5	5.2	5.5	8.1
75 —	2.3	2.8	3.1	5.0
80 +	0.3	0.5	0.6	1.2

Source: U.S. Bureau of the Census. *Current Population Reports,* Series P-25, Nos. 311, 519, 614, 643, and 704. Taken from reference (5).

dence that man has long recognized *specific* age, meaning an age at death character-istic of a species. In an optimum environment specific age may be presumed to approach a "physiological" limit. This "physiological" specific age is approached by individuals in numbers that vary with environment. Even in relatively harsh environ-ments some individuals attain extreme ages, but in more favorable environments the number who do so is much increased. The modal age around which their deaths occur might be thought of as the "ecological" specific age. In contemporary industrial soci-eties, the modal age of death (ignoring newborn infants) is in the neighborhood of 75 to 80 years (3).

The maximum specific age for individuals probably falls between 105 and 110 years. The greatest authenticated life-span is said to be 120 years, and 109 in Britain. Old Parr was credited with 152 years, a record matched in the traditions of many societies. Many traditional claims do not meet rigorous criteria, such as documentary proof of birth and death and of individual identity. Identity is important, because the life-spans of individuals of the same name are often compounded. In contemporary societies noted for supposed longevity, as in the Caucasus and the Andes, age is accorded high prestige. In such circumstances, as in Ecuador, exaggeration of age has been demonstrated (4).

Extension of average life expectancy, in the light of the probable specific age limit, is a reasonable possibility. During the past century however, older age-groups have had the minor share in the considerable increase in survival in industrial societies (see Figure 12.1). This appears in the relative terms of the proportion of increased life expectancy at younger and older ages, and more sharply, in the absolute terms of years of life gained. Thus in the U. S. from 1900 to 1976, life expectancy *at birth* increased from 49.2 to 72.8 years (48 per cent) and at age 65, from 11.9 to 16 years (34 per cent) (5). While the general increase in longevity at older ages over the past half century is not to be ignored, direct evidence that describes in terms of health the quality of the years that have been added is scarce. We cannot be sure that there has been much improvement in the health of the greater number of survivors into old age in recent times as compared with the health of the fewer survivors of the past; opinions go in both directions (6).

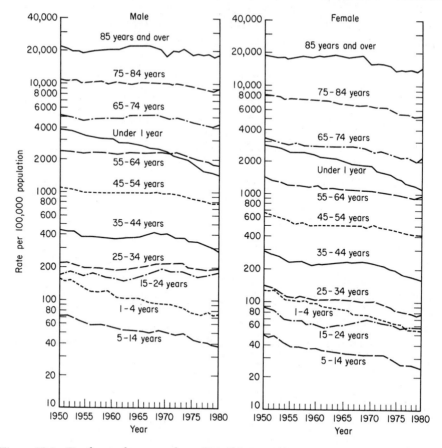

Figure 12.1 Death rates by age and sex: United States, 1950–1980. *Source:* National Center for Health Statistics (1983). *Monthly Vital Statistics Report,* vol. 32, No. 4, Supplement, p. 2.

In assessing this situation, a great deal depends on the type of measure and the type of analysis used. Much disease in old persons is inapparent, and denial of illness or disability, sickness and handicap among them is common. Different measures of outcome and of frequency must be expected to yield different results. In the United States, the recent decline in general mortality and in specific causes of death such as coronary heart disease and stroke is shared by the aged, and the decline may indicate a decline in incidence from these chronic and fatal diseases among them. On the other hand, the decline in mortality could indicate increased survival and lengthened duration of prevalent disease, since there is as yet no indication of a decline in the prevalence of disability. Because a decline in incidence could be balanced and masked by increasing survival, such countervailing changes can coexist with stable prevalence rates. Contrary trends may coexist also in the depiction of changes over time. We showed in Chapter 2 that cohort analysis can reveal the waning of mortality when period analysis exhibits an apparently rising trend.

Public attention has been drawn to the medicated survival of incapacitated and demented old people, but the overall level of disability at older ages might well be less than in the past. Despite uncertainties, there is reason to think that research and application in public health might extend the average length of life and improve the quality of health among the aged. However imperfectly, mortality reflects morbidity, and we know that in the United States mortality is greater than it need be. Death rates in the United States—after a long decline—still stand above the levels attained by the country with the lowest rate in each age-group, not excepting the oldest. Earlier projections of life expectancy, however, have had to be revised upward in the light of the unanticipated decline in deaths dating from the late 1960s. In the few years 1968 to 1975, age adjusted mortality rates declined by 15 per cent: diseases of the heart 20 per cent (Fig. 12.2); cerebrovascular disease or stroke 25 per cent (Fig. 12.3); accidents 19 per cent; and influenza and pneumonia 28 per cent. Death rates from malignancies continued to increase for males, although not for females (Figure 12.4), this being largely the residual effect of smoking on lung cancer (see Chapter 4). Overall, there was a resulting increase in life expectancy at age 65 years of 1.3 years or 9 per cent, of which one-half was owed to diseases of the heart and one-fifth to stroke (7). The hypothetical elimination of cardiovascular-renal diseases would, in 1976, have been expected to add 11.4 years to life expectancy at age 65 years (5).

Room for further improvement certainly exists, especially from the control of causal factors involved in multiple disorders. The elimination of adverse factors with multiple effects like smoking, alcohol, or poor nutrition is bound to produce a combined effect greater than the simple sum of the effects of each factor on each disorder, because the impact of each factor on the competing causes of death that remain when a single disorder has been prevented is simultaneously reduced. No specific cause of death, it is true, has been found in as many as one-third of a series of autopsies on persons aged 85 years and older (8). Furthermore, as we have been at pains to demonstrate, disease, disability, and death do not fall equally upon all the strata of any society, and their onset may be avoided, postponed, or advanced. The chances of an individual vary with socioeconomic status, marital status, and other aspects of social position. Death rates are higher, life expectancy is shorter, and the disabling chronic disease common among the aged is much more prevalent among lower income groups and the lower social classes than among the higher (see Figure 12.5 for disabilities). Likewise, the health disadvantage of older American nonwhites as compared with whites (see later discussion and Tables 12.7 and 12.14) is almost certainly attributable to their socioeconomic position.

In interpreting prevalence and mortality data, the possibility must be allowed that some of the difference between social classes may be the consequence rather than the cause of disability. For example, downward social mobility may follow chronic disability and inflate the rates for the poorer classes. In Britain, longitudinal mortality studies of representative national cohorts identified at the census have demonstrated that unrecognized effects of social selection and mobility contribute substantially to

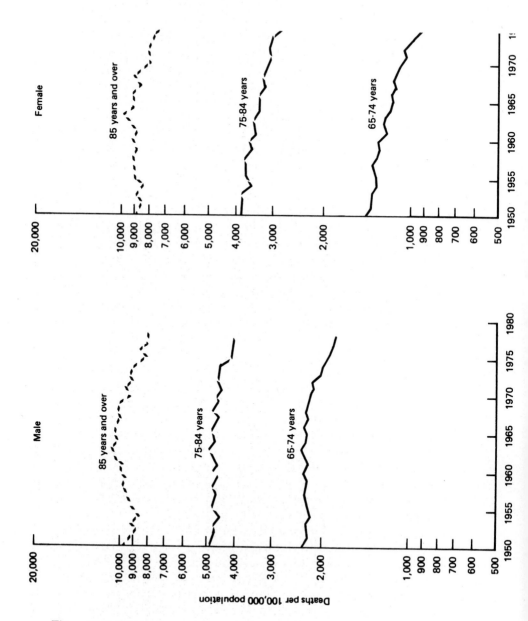

Figure 12.2 See caption at right

social variation in mortality (9). The advantage and disadvantage in health and disease that attach to social position appear at birth and are present at each stage of the life-cycle, however, and it seems unlikely that downward social mobility of disabled persons could alone produce the large difference between social classes.

When major killing and disabling diseases are considered, the known variations in incidence with environment are great enough to make the hope of prevention a reasonable one to entertain. Variations with environment in longevity, in health in old age, and in the specific causes of death argue that public health action could attain throughout society at least the rates that exist under optimum conditions at the present time. Some will argue that prevention of particular diseases may not add a great deal to the mean life expectancy of old people, because other pathologies may substitute for those that are avoided; above we have indicated the contrary arguments about the favorable potential that might reside in the elimination of adverse factors with multiple effects. At the least, prevention can surely add to the life expectancy and the quality of life for social groups now at a disadvantage. The way will thereby be cleared for research into deceleration of the aging process itself (10).

Age as a status

Seen as an attribute of individuals at a point in time, any particular age is like a measure of prevalence; it describes an existing condition. Age serves as an index at many levels at once. It is a physiological indicator with a set of functional accompaniments, and these can help to describe and predict the physical state of the organism.

The functional accompaniments of chronological age are closely tied to it, although not all are invariant. Those that manifestly affect appearance or performance, like grey hair or a shuffling gait or impaired mental state, also affect the individual's social status. Social status is bound up with physiological status. Since age, like sex, has social, psychological, and biological meaning, and no simple criteria exist that fully encompass these meanings, a public health task of epidemiology and social science is to disentagle these elements of the life stages, in order to reveal which can be modified and improved.

The various social and individual criteria by which old age, in particular, is defined well illustrate the complexity of the age variable. Old age, socially defined, can be taken as that portion of the life-span demarcated as old by the norms of a particular society. These norms are perceived differently across social groups, even within a single society. Among social groups, being "old" is a relative matter, a particular and not an absolute and universal state (11).

Kinship societies give regularity to life stages by *rites de passage*. Industrial societies have few *rites de passage*. For the old, however, fixed ages for retirement from

---

Figure 12.2 Death rates among persons 65 years of age and over for diseases of heart, by age and sex: United States, 1950–1978. *Source:* National Center for Health Statistics (1982) Changes in mortality among the elderly: United States, 1940–1978, *Vital and Health Statistics*, Series 3, Number 22, Hyattsville, Maryland, p. 7.

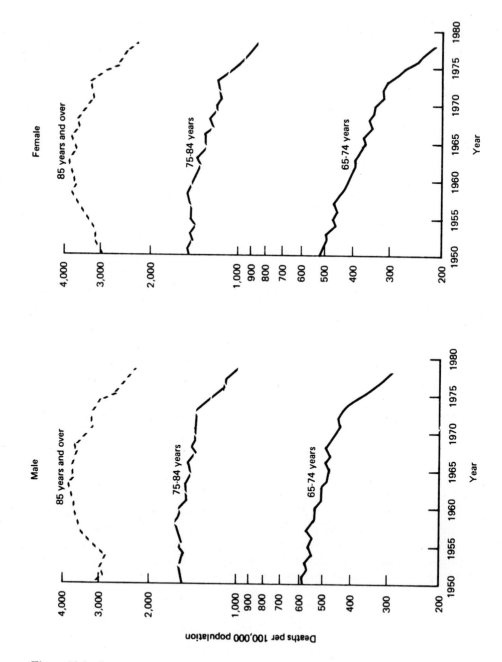

Figure 12.3 See caption at right.

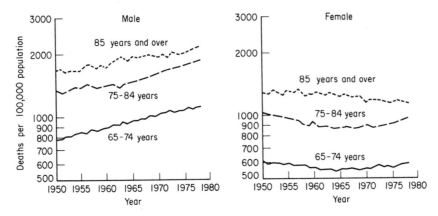

Figure 12.4 Death rates among persons 65 years of age and over for malignant neoplasms, by age and sex: United States, 1950–1978. *Source:* Changes in mortality among the elderly: United States 1940–1978, National Center for Health Statistics *Vital and Health Statistics,* Series 3, Number 22, Hyattsville, Maryland, p. 8.

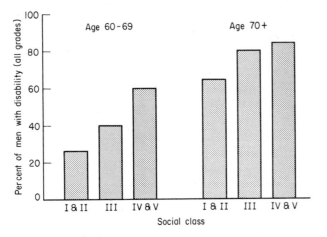

Figure 12.5 Prevalence of disability among older men, by social class. Percentage of men with disability (all grades). *Source:* Adapted from Edwards, F., McKeown, T., and Whitfield, A. G. W. (1959). Incidence of disease and disability in elderly men, *Brit. J. Prev. Soc. Med.,* *13,* 51–8; based on 641 men in Birmingham, England; as cited by Susser, M. W. (1969) Aging and the field of public health, in *Aging and Society,* Vol. II, eds. Riley, M. W., Riley, J. W., and Johnson, M. E., Russell Sage foundation, New York, p. 132.

Figure 12.3 Death rates among persons 65 years of age and over for cerebrovascular diseases, by age and sex: United States, 1950–1978. *Source:* National Center for Health Statistics (1982) Changes in mortality among the elderly: United States 1940–1978, *Vital and Health Statistics,* Series 3, Number 22, Hyattsville, Maryland, p. 11.

work and the drawing of pensions introduce regularities that mark the displacement of employees from their occupations, and their entry into a phase of social replacement. (The commonly used age of 65 years is owed to Otto von Bismarck in Germany. He chose this age for his Old Age, Sickness, and Pensions Law of 1889, the first "social security" system, in the belief that the number of survivors would not entail an undue burden for the state. In Britain Lloyd George adopted this age for men upon the introduction of old age pensions in 1911, but set the age for women at 60 years (12).) Within an industrial society, the manner of entry into this phase has depended on occupation; self-employed persons and professionals in practice may elect their time, while persons with skills in demand may continue in related work. Unskilled manual workers can expect retirement willy-nilly.

The social definition of old age thus rests on a more or less abrupt transition from one life stage to another, and the taking up of new sets of social roles as old ones are relinquished. In contemporary societies old age ordinarily involves a decrement in social status. The most productive and powerful social, occupational, and domestic roles are given up. However, as long as functional capacities persist, the final phase of life may yet become one of continuing development rather than one of abrogation.

The performance of social roles depends ultimately on the physical and mental integrity of the particular individual. In clinical terms, old age may be recognized by changes in skin, hair, physique, and physiological function (see Figure 12.6). Psychological changes in attitudes, memory, speed of comprehension and approaches to problem-solving appear to accompany the physical changes. Taken together, these changes are ultimately deteriorative in relation to the earlier years, and in the last phase of life, present knowledge offers only the prospect of organic decline.

On the other hand, although each complex of signs that underlies the social, psychological, or physical dimension of aging is interconnected with the others, the signs vary in time of onset and may be out of phase with one another, as in earlier stages of growth and development. In the matter of mental performance, on average, verbal abilities and so-called "crystallized intelligence" improve or remain stable unless undermined by physical or mental illness; abilities that depend on speed and so-called "fluid intelligence" tend to decline (13). Thus the rate of aging in these several dimensions is often asynchronous; since social roles and states of mind are not entirely limited by physical condition, each provides independent opportunities for environmental change or intervention to retard the process of deterioration (14).

The process of aging

On reaching the age of 80, E. M. Forster wrote that aging was an acute experience that he had got over at about the age of 35. Old age is a state or condition of a human being at a given time; aging is a process taking place through time. A person in the *state* of old age embodies the outcome of a *process* of interaction through the life course between the environment and the individual constitution.

Aging in individuals can be defined as a deteriorative process through which the resistance of the organism to the pressures of the environment progressively diminishes, until it can no longer withstand them and dies (3). Resistance against the forces of mortality is greatest in the hardy prepubescent phase, and it declines thereafter. A

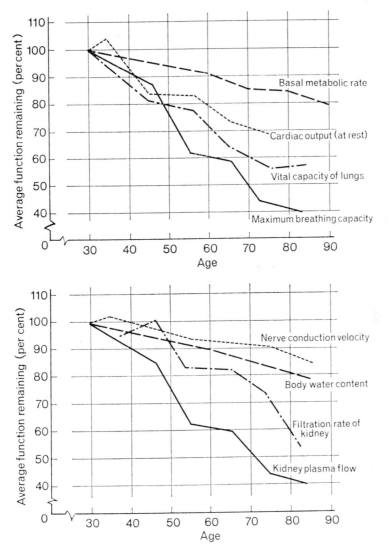

Figure 12.6 Estimates of the decline of physiological functioning after age 30. Percentage changes with age. The average value for each function at age 30 is taken as 100 per cent. *Source:* Adapted from Shock, N. W. (1962). The physiology of aging, *Scientif. Amer., 206,* 100–10; as cited in Riley, M. W., and Foner, A., eds. (1968). *Aging and Society,* Vol. I, Russell Sage Foundation, New York, p. 231.

combination of factors contributes to the senile change, and these may include the exhaustion of such irreplaceable structures as neurones, and the increasingly imperfect repair of accumulated injuries. However, senescence also reflects more fundamental "morphogenetic" processes that control the development of form in the organism through differentiation and growth of cells. Some biologists consider that the inevitable accompaniment of morphogenesis and development is a progressive loss of the capacity for growth and repair, and the eventual failure of the homeostatic mechanisms of the body. In other words, senescence is the corollary of growth and development. These developmental processes can be presumed to arise in the course of evolution.

The "fitness" of a species results from the evolutionary forces that act to determine survival of offspring in the reproductive phase of the life-cycle. The postreproductive phase that is becoming dominant in our society was not subject to these forces. Although this phase could have contributed indirectly to the survival of progeny and consequently to natural selection, such a phase hardly existed in the previous evolutionary history of primates and early humans (15). In one formulation, among many theories addressing different levels of organization, aging may be seen as the outcome of morphogenesis deferred to the backwater of the postreproductive phase, or as the outcome of an accumulation of injurious genetic effects deferred to this phase (3,10). Its social importance in contemporary society lies in the emergence of a phase of independence in the cycle of family development and in the extension of the phase of replacement.

A number of processes therefore interact to produce senescence, whether it is regarded as beginning in embryonic life with the differentiation of cells, or at puberty with the decline in resistance to the forces of mortality, or in the late twenties with the first detectable decline in specific physiological functions. No single intrinsic aging mechanism has yet been discovered, although many have been proposed. The culmination is death, but neither the state of old age nor the process of senescence has a single distinctive pathology, and most if not all individuals who die in extreme old age are found to harbor several potentially lethal disorders, commonly neoplastic and cardiovascular. Function declines throughout the body, usually more prominently in one or the other system, often the central nervous system or the cardiovascular system (see Figure 12.6). In this light it appears that, when every avenue for isolating and controlling environmental factors has been explored, a certain undetermined minimum of disorders will have to be ascribed to the biological aging process.

One cannot deny that in industrialized western societies, deterioration is the social as well as the psychological and biological connotation of aging. Once across the threshold of old age—ill-defined and changeable though that may be—the perception of the public is one of decrement in capabilities, roles, status, and prestige. The epidemiological data on disease and impairment in population groups reinforce this perception. Yet among individuals, and no less among groups, there are many departures from these perceived norms.

Social roles have most plasticity; thus several men in their eighties and others in their thirties have led contemporary societies. Generational effects have a powerful impact on the social history of the life course. The Great Depression of the early 1930s, for example, left its imprint on the subsequent careers of those exposed to it at a particular stage of adult life, as compared with cohorts born just before or just after (16). A demographic view of three birth cohorts (see Table 12.3), underlines the dramatic changes in the kind of environment and life-chances experienced by successive generations.

The psychological component displays plasticity too; artists and scientists have been

Table 12.3 A demographic perspective on the childhood, adulthood, and old age characteristics of three cohorts (United States)

Cohort Characteristics	Cohort of		
	1870	1900	1930
A. _Childhood_			
Size when aged 5–9 (in '000s)	6480	9761	10684
% rural when 5–9	78	59	51
% distribution by no. of siblings:			
0–1	6	14	29
2–3	14	25	34
4+	80	61	37
% with parent who died (before the child reached age 15)	27	22	11
% distribution by no. of school years completed:			
less than 8	44	28	8
8 to 11	42	45	25
12 and over	14	27	67
B. _Adulthood_			
Size when aged 25–29 (in '000s)	6529	9834	10804
% foreign-born when aged 25–29	17	11	3
% rural when aged 25–29	47	37	28
% distribution of males by occupation when aged 35–39			
White-collar	NA	31	44
Blue-collar (nonfarm)	NA	52	53
Farm	NA	17	3
Marital status of females:			
% never married by age 50	10	8	5
% divorced by age 40–44 (of those ever-married)	NA	11	21
% distribution of females by children ever born:			
0	23	28	13
1–3	36	51	52
4+	41	21	35
C. _Old Age_			
Size when aged 65–69 (in '000s)	3807	6992	9023
% of initial cohort surviving to age 65:			
Males	37	50	63
Females	42	62	77
% foreign-born when aged 65–69	21	13	7
Sex ratio when aged 65–69	99	81	80
Average no. of yrs. of life remaining at age 65:			
Males	11.7	13.7	?
Females	12.8	17.1	?
% of males in labor force when aged 65–69	69	42	25
Ratio of age-groups 70+/65–69, when cohort is aged 65–69	1.4	1.8	2.4

Source: Uhlenberg, P. (1979). Demographic change and problems of the aged, in _Aging from Birth to Death: Interdisciplinary Perspectives,_ ed. Riley, M. W., Boulder, Colorado, pp. 160–61. (Adult cohort inflated by migration.)

creative in their eighties as in their twenties. Among groups, appropriate analysis points to gain as well as to loss in different aspects of mental performance, as noted above. Verbal ability seems to be more strongly related, through most of life, to education and to intellectual enviroment than it is to age itself. Thus among those now living, birth cohort is a more powerful determinant of mental performance than age, and this relationship is best related to the education experiences of successive cohorts. The plasticity of mental performance is further demonstrated by the positive relationship of intellectual flexibility to the complexity of an individual's occupation, a factor that might explain some of the decided advantage long ago demonstrated in the performance of intellectual and academic over manual workers in old age (17).

From common observation, we can say that the physical component, while variable, has less plasticity in the developmental timetable. Yet with individuals as with groups, for each level of organization and each element within each level, the pace of change and the trajectory through the life-cycle may not be the same. For example, sexual activity tends to decline, especially among men, for social as well as physiological reasons, yet some evidently enjoy an increment with advancing age (18). Among successive cohorts, too, physique varies markedly at given ages. This is well documented in measures of height, of body weight, and of obesity. Morbidity and mortality, we emphasize once more, similarly vary greatly across cohorts.

Development and aging are indissolubly linked by the chronological idea at the core of the aging construct. Aside from chronology, no unique criterion marks the onset of the downward trajectory of the unidirectional aging process. For measures and indices we must either forge a compound of multiple criteria, or use singular criteria limited to some narrow dimension of change with aging.

Morbidity, mortality, and disability

The relations of mortality to age, together with the uses of period and generation or cohort analysis in establishing those relations, were outlined in an earlier chapter (see Chapter 2). Morbidity, as well as mortality, can be considered as a measure of senescence, and it rises steeply with age; this appears in prevalence surveys, and in the incidence of medical consultations, hospital admissions, absence from work through sickness, and unemployment. General practitioners devote proportionately more time to the care of old people than of the young (19). Morbidity and mortality for common diseases in the United States at ages over 65 years are shown in Tables 12.4 and 12.5.

Prevalence studies of men over 70, however, have not always shown a consistent rise in disease with increasing age. Thus, in a survey of old men on the lists of general practitioners in Birmingham, England, high rates of bronchitis, hypertension, coronary artery disease, arthritis, hernia, and peptic ulcer were found, but none of these increased regularly with age except for arthritis, which is not lethal. For lethal conditions, this irregularity is probably the result of the high rates of mortality and of admission to institutions amongst the sick at these ages, and the survival in the community of those who are relatively healthy. The cross-sectional survey that examines a residual population at one point in time cannot reveal these losses of less healthy persons, for they accumulate over a period of time.

Table 12.4   Primary diagnoses of noninstitutionalized persons age 65 and older, United States

Diagnosis	By discharge from short-stay hospitals (%)	By office-based physicians (%)
Diseases of the circulatory system	30.2	26.5
Hypertension	1.3	8.8
Acute myocardial infarction	2.7	—
Chronic ischemic heart disease	9.6	8.5
Cerebrovascular disease	6.2	—
Diseases of the nervous system & sense organs	5.5	10.4
Diseases of the central nervous system	0.8	—
Conditions of the eye	—	6.6
Cataract	3.0	—
Diseases of the musculoskeletal system	5.0	9.4
Arthritis	2.5	6.7
Diseases of the respiratory system	8.5	8.7
Acute upper respiratory infections (except influenza)	0.8	2.8
Pneumonia, all forms	2.9	—
Diseases of the digestive system	13.1	5.1
Ulcer	1.5	—
Inguinal hernia	1.4	—
Cholelithiasis	1.4	—
Endocrine, nutritional, and metabolic	3.5	4.9
Diabetes mellitus	2.4	3.9
Diseases of the genitourinary system	7.5	4.7
Hyperplasia of prostate	2.3	—
Accidents, poisoning, violence	8.7	4.5
Fractures, all sites	4.9	1.3
Neoplasms	10.5	4.0
Malignant	9.4	—
Benign or unspecified	1.2	—
Diseases of the skin	1.2	3.5
Mental Disorders	2.1	3.5
Infective and parasitic diseases	1.3	1.7
Diseases of the blood & blood-forming organs	1.2	—
Symptoms of ill-defined conditions	0.9	3.3
Special conditions & exams without illness	0.3	1.5
Other diagnoses	—	1.5

Source: Ouslander, J. G., and Beck, J. C. (1982). Defining the health problems of the elderly, *Ann. Rev. Publ. Hlth.*, 3, 55–83.

This problem is therefore a particular one of prevalence studies. It was shown in Chapter 3 that the sharp rise with age in prevalence of chronic disabling illness contrasts with the decline in acute disabling illness; from the age of 40, chronic illness has a greater prevalence than acute. Incidence rates, uninfluenced by the duration of illness, present a different picture; acute disabling illnesses exceed the chronic except in the age-groups over 75 (see Figures 3.5 and 3.6). Explanations other than the difference in measures must also be entertained. When the incidence of a disease

Table 12.5 Causes of death for United States population 65 years and older in 1974 (percentage of total deaths)

Specific cause	Women	Men	Both sexes
Diseases of the heart	45.1	44.3	44.7
Malignant Neoplasms	15.1	18.6	16.8
Cerebrovascular diseases	16.5	11.7	14.1
Influenza and pneumonia	3.2	3.4	3.3
Arteriosclerosis	3.0	1.9	2.5
Diabetes mellitus	2.7	1.6	2.2
Injuries	1.9	2.1	2.0
Motor vehicle injuries	0.3	0.6	0.5
All other injuries	1.6	1.5	1.5
Bronchitis, emphysema, asthma	0.7	2.4	1.5
Cirrhosis of the liver	0.5	0.9	0.7
Suicide	—	0.5	—
All other	11.3	12.7	12.3

Source: Ouslander, J. G., and Beck, J. C. (1982). Defining the health problems of the elderly, *Ann. Rev. Publ. Hlth.*, 3, 55–83.

changes through time, the changing distribution between cohorts appears in a cross-sectional analysis as a changing distribution with age.

The lack of precision in the use of terms relating to disease and its consequences adds to difficulties of interpretation. Questions about operational definitions must constantly be asked in assessing the literature. The disablement of sickness, which implies an incapacity for carrying out social roles, is a more general and inclusive measure of

Table 12.6 Percent of persons in age groups 65 and over unable to perform personal tasks on their own: England, 1976

	Age-groups				
	65–69	70–74	75–79	80–84	85 and over
Bath oneself	4	12	20	33	51
Wash oneself	1	1	2	5	7
Get to lavatory	°	1	3	5	6
Get in and out of bed	1	1	3	4	5
Feed oneself	°	°	1	2	2
Shave (men); do hair (women)	1	1	3	4	4
Cut own toenails	13	21	35	42	57
Get up and down stairs	2	4	10	13	19
Get around house or flat	°	1	2	5	6
Go out of doors on own	4	10	17	24	49
Use public transport	5	9	15	24	38

° Less than 0.5 per cent.

Source: Adapted from Hunt, A. (1978). The elderly: Age differences in the quality of life, *Population Trends, 11,* 14.

Table 12.7 Percent of persons in age-groups 65 and over reporting difficulty with common personal tasks, by age and race: United States, 1975[a]

Personal tasks	Whites				Blacks			
	65—	70—	75—	80+	65—	70—	75—	80+
Walking stairs	15	19	25	39	37	42	50	58
Getting about the house	4	4	6	13	9	10	19	19
Washing and bathing	5	5	8	14	10	8	19	26
Dressing, putting on shoes	5	5	8	16	15	8	17	23
Cutting toenails	10	19	24	37	30	28	41	54

[a] Excludes bedfast persons.

Source: Adapted from Shanas, E. (1980). Self-assessment of physical function: White and black elderly in the United States, in *The Epidemiology of Aging: Second Conference*, ed. Haynes, S. G., and Feinleib, M., NIH Pub. No. 80-969, Washington, D.C., p. 278.

health than is a particular functional disability. A functional disability, in turn, may be a more inclusive measure of health than a structural and physiological impairment of a particular limb, organ, or tissue, or than a specific disease (diagnosis) that causes impairments. On the other hand, one specific disease may give rise to several particular impairments and functional disabilities.

Tables 12.6 and 12.7 show the universal rapid decline with age in the proportion who remain able to perform personal tasks. A scale of "activities of daily living" (ADL) has been devised and widely used to measure functional disabilities. This scale, taken as an endpoint instead of death, has been applied in life table analysis to estimate the expectancy for continued independent daily living, rather than the usual expectancy for years of life remaining. Unsurprisingly, this expectancy for independent living is less the greater the age. The poor too, on this index as on all others, are at a distinct disadvantage in all age groups under study. Men and women do equally well at 70 years and over, although women under 70 have an advantage (Table 12.8).

Table 12.8 Active life expectancy (remaining years of independent ADL) among noninstitutionalized elderly people in Massachusetts, 1974

Age-group (yrs)	Average remaining active life (years)			
	Men	Women	Poor	Nonpoor
65–	9.3	10.6	8.1	10.5
70–	8.2	8.0	6.8	8.3
75–	6.5	7.1	6.1	6.9
80–	4.8	4.8	4.4	4.8
≥85	3.3	2.8	2.5	3.1

Source: Adapted from Katz, S., Branch, L. G., Branson, M. H., Papsidero, J. A., Beck, J. C., and Greer, D. S. (1983). Active life expectancy, *New Eng. J. Med., 309,* 1220.

Table 12.9   Percentage of total remaining years of life that are independent among noninstitutionalized elderly men and women in Massachusetts, 1974

	Independent years remaining (%)[a]	
Age-group (yrs)	Men	Women
65–69	71	54
70–74	69	50
75–79	68	54
80–81	65	49
≥85	51	36

[a]Percentage of independent years remaining equals "active life expectancy" divided by life expectancy.

Source: Katz, S., Branch, L. G., Branson, M. H., Papsidero, J. A., Beck, J. C., and Greer, D. S. (1983). Active life expectancy, *New Eng. J. Med.*, *309*, 1221.

But the proportion of the total remaining years of life that can be expected to be active and independent is much greater for men than for women; women can expect as many active years as men, but those years are more likely to end in death for men and survival with disability for women (Table 12.9). The loss of independent activity is not always permanent; until 85 years of age, about a quarter of all those not active at one point in time had recovered 15 months later (Table 12.10).

Thus the prevalence of a variety of measures of function and disability indicates that underlying medical problems are steadily accentuated with increasing age, and especially beyond the mid-seventies. Like the poor, blacks are markedly worse off and here, as in many other instances, race is a surrogate for poverty and the insults of a life course of accumulated disadvantage (Table 12.7; Figure 12.5). Beyond the mid-70s mental disorders as well as physical disorders begin to create severe problems. They limit the capacity for self-care as well as that for seeking care. Community surveys indicate that all forms of psychosis together affect almost 10 per cent of persons aged 65 years and older. Some of these are reversible depressions, not infrequently misdiagnosed as neurological or organic brain syndromes or senile dementia. Senile dementia and presenile dementia (Alzheimer's disease)—depending on the

Table 12.10   Return of function at 15 months follow-up among dependent noninstitutionalized elderly people in Massachusetts, 1974

Age-group (yrs)	Initially dependent (no. of persons)	Proportion with return of independence at 15 months
65–74	52	.31
75–84	42	.26
≥85	23	.04

Source: Katz, S., Branch, L. G., Branson, M. H., Papsidero, J. A., Beck, J. C., and Greer, D. S. (1983). Active life expectancy, *New Eng. J. Med.*, *309*, 1222.

Table 12.11 Physical mobility of elderly people in England, 1976
(per cent age-groups 65 and over)

Physical mobility	Men			Women		
	65	75	85 and over	65	75	85 and over
Bedfast permanently	—	—	2	—	1	2
Housebound permanently	2	7	15	2	7	20
Usually goes out with assistance	2	4	16	7	14	31
Usually goes out unaided	96	89	67	91	78	47

Source: Adapted from Hunt, A. (1978) The elderly: Age differences in the quality of life, *Population Trends, 11,* 13.

inclusiveness of the definition—may affect more than 5 per cent of persons over 65, and as many as 25 per cent of persons in their eighties, with an estimated incidence in the ninth decade of perhaps 5 per cent per year (20).

In old age, the capacity for movement becomes a yardstick of general health and disability. After the age of 75 an increasing proportion of old persons suffer restricted physical mobility, and after 80 many are confined to their homes and have difficulty even in getting about the house (Tables 12.6, 12.7 and 12.11). This decline in physical mobility arises from a number of causes that are all common to old age, including potentially lethal failures of the heart, lungs, and brain. Nonlethal causes assume importance in the seventies, such as diminution in the sensorium, in muscle power, and in joint movement, and the mundane disorders of urinary incontinence and of painful and poorly tended feet. All of these restrictions on mobility are mediated by situation, including cultural expectations and physical facilities to meet special needs. The fear of negotiating traffic often restricts the aged to their homes, and there they may be further restricted by steep stairs.

In survivors over 80, mental disturbance, incontinence of bladder and bowel, and blindness and deafness all show a sharp rise. Persons of that age run a particular risk from falls, for these readily cause injuries and fractures, especially in the frail osteoporotic bones of elderly women. In turn such fractures accelerate the advent of death. Old people suffer from "drop attacks," sudden disturbances of the mechanisms that maintain upright posture, and from poor vision and hearing, vertigo, and postural hypertension, as well as muscular weakness; together these cause many falls (21).

In old age the individual often perceives the burden of illness as more of a threat than death. Sickness is consistently more frequent in women than in men; in contrast, the death rates of old men are much higher than those of old women (see Table 12.1). In the United States among people 65 years and over, for every two men approximately three women survive; at 85 years and over, for every man more than two women survive (see Table 12.12). In Britain, for each man who has currently survived into the eighties there are approximately two women, and for each man who has survived into the nineties, three. In the United States the result of women's superior survival, combined with their lower age at marriage, is an average of eleven years of widowhood (22).

Hypotheses to explain the greater morbidity and lesser mortality of women include

Table 12.12   Sex ratios (males per 100
females) in the United States at ages 65
years and over: 1950, 1970, and projected to
1980

Age-group (yrs)	1950	1970	1980
65–	89.5	72.0	68.2
75–	82.6	63.3	56.2
85–	70.0	53.2	44.7

Source: Adapted from United States Bureau of the Census, *Current Population Reports*, Series P-25, Numbers 311, 519, 614, 643, and 704. Taken from reference (5).

biological sex differences and a greater propensity for women—because of socialization, values about work and family, or the demands of child care—to adopt the sick role. Among older women, their greater morbidity is possibly a consequence of selective mortality, in that the fewer men who survive to old age are healthy and constitutionally tough. This explanation accords reasonably well with the congruence in independent life expectancy between men and women and the incongruence in total life expectancy between them (see Tables 12.8, 12.9). In Salford, England, among old people who entered any form of psychiatric care for the first time, a similar pattern was found. More women than men became chronically disabled, but the difference was almost exactly made up by the greater number of men who died (23). Such selection probably accounts for the divergence between the sexes in social and geographic mortality patterns. After the age of 65 years in Britain, marked differences in the mortality of different social groups persist among men but not among women.

Thus, women survive into old age in greater numbers than men and are more often sick; women present the greater problem for health care, and men the greater problem for prevention. These disparities in morbidity and mortality between men and women in old age reflect both the constitutional and the role differences between men and women. Environmental hazards expose the sexes unequally by virtue of their different occupations and recreations. In addition, the differing demands of the social roles ascribed to men and women, and even to boys and girls, set different thresholds for complaints, and also for the exemptions accorded to each sex with the sick role. In the working phase, men carry a heavier load of severe and fatal illness than women. In contrast, women in paid work have been found to make more complaints of minor illnesses, to be more often absent from work, and to receive more medical care than men (24).

Vitality in old age of individuals of both sexes is an outcome of acquisitions in earlier life. Vitality flows not only from genetic and sexual constitution, but also from culture and education, all of which influence physique and personality and life experience. Family endowment helps to determine the possible life-span of individuals, and also some of the illnesses of old age, probably including, for instance, senile dementia (25). Culture and education contribute notably to social circumstances, health, and the distribution of intellectual capacities in old age. The relationship to education of problems of health and poverty is illustrated by responses in a representative sample survey in the United States in the 1970s (see Table 12.13). Education confers a lifelong and cumulative intellectual advantage. We noted above that individuals in intellectual and academic occupations retain their intellectual capacities into old age to a much greater extent than do individuals in manual occupations that make fewer intellectual demands, and that the steady increase in the exposure to schooling of successive cohorts (see Table 12.3) can explain the apparent decline in IQ scores with age seen in cross-sectional studies of old people.

The balance between these constitutional and environmental influences may be expected to change as people grow old. For extrinsic factors become more important in some instances, less in others. Widowhood seems to have sharper effects among the young than the old (26), and cigarette smoking and blood cholesterol too are more clearly related to coronary heart disease in the young than in the old (see Chapter 4). Organic brain disorders are much more prominent as causes of mental disorder among the old than the young. At the greatest ages, as among octogenarians, the relationship of social background factors to mortality diminishes. Insofar as such factors could be tested across the social spectrum found at these advanced ages among veterans of the Spanish-American War and among retired members of the United Automobile Workers, they were not predictive of survival (27).

Social dependence

Where primary prevention aimed at avoiding the onset of disorder altogether is not possible, we look to the methods of secondary prevention. These methods aim at the early detection of a disorder, with the object of intervening to stem its progress soon enough to abort or alleviate its effects. In terms of disease, incipient social dependence arising out of deteriorating health presents a suitable target for secondary prevention. In terms of disability and the roles of handicap and sickness, however, to avoid or defer the onset of dependence is primary prevention.

The state of social dependence or its imminence is a central problem in preventive medicine, for dependence is a source of economic, social, and mental strain for the affected person and for all on whom the person depends. No one at any age can ever

Table 12.13   The prevalence in the United States in 1975 of "very serious" problems of health and poverty by education (percentages)

Problem	College 4+ years	High school/some college	Less than high school
Health	9	14	26
Poverty	3	8	20

Source: Harris, L. and Associates, Inc. (1975). *The Myth and Reality of Aging in America*, Washington, D.C.

be independent of society, but the social dependence of old age has distinguishing features that are akin to those of the role of chronically sick or handicapped persons at any age. Thus, dependence in the elderly is likely to progress unless death supervenes; dependent old persons are often permanently exempt from normal social responsibilities, and it is recognized that they need continuing help and must be cared for. Society accepts a legal obligation to provide for them and many children feel a moral obligation to do so (28). Old people are in the phase of replacement; their children are dispersed and have founded new elementary families of their own. As parents, they have discharged their formal and many informal responsibilities. When parents become socially dependent, responsibilities are reversed, and in some societies are enforced by legal and customary sanctions.

Social dependence is a condition in which the individual is in varying degree unable to perform social roles and individual functions that will ensure a means of subsistence. The incidence and the effects of social dependence vary with the type of dependence as well as with the social setting. Inability to continue as a wage-earner may cause financial dependence. In the home, bodily incapacity may cause domestic dependence and call for assistance from others for such basic activities as dressing, bathing, feeding and evacuation. In the extreme, the individual may sink into dependence on mechanical medical devices for the continued physiological function of cardiovascular, respiratory, or renal systems. Information about the distribution of these various forms of dependence is scarce. Not surprisingly, disability (inability to work, restricted mobility) and impairment (memory loss for recent events, electrocardiographic signs of coronary heart disease, diastolic hypertension, hypercholesterolemia, obesity) as well as the perception of illness are sensitive and specific predictors of subsequent mortality (29).

Soon or late, dependency inevitably ends with death. The person who does not die suddenly makes a last transition from the state of sickness to the state of dying. Physicians and nurses face many uncertainties in dealing with the dying. Physicians may be called on to predict the timing of an unpredictable event for relatives who expect precise information. When death is probable or certain, physicians must judge how to tell a patient of his or her imminent demise. Often these tasks are evaded by physicians, and nurses may be left to deal with them alone (30).

To prevent dependence in the face of the large and growing numbers of old people at risk, health services must seek an economy of means. They must search out disabilities, or incipient disabilities, to stem the progress of disorders. They must command effective treatment and know when and in what circumstances it may be useful to intervene. For these purposes services must identify the groups that are at highest risk, discover the events and time periods that commonly precede the decline into dependence, and recognize those circumstances that are dangerous to independence and those that favor it. Not only sickness and disability but also retirement, bereavement, social isolation, and the absence of social support are circumstances in old age that can be potentially critical for continued function. These circumstances might serve to mark out persons who require help in retaining independence and avoiding the further crisis of admission to institutional care. We shall examine each of these social circumstances in turn.

Sickness and dependence

Physical and mental incapacity due to disease are the overriding causes of social dependence. Disabilities we have noted rise sharply in the late seventies, and so too do the failures in social function that follow. Some measure of the prevalence of social dependence arising from organic causes is given, for example, by the survey of men over 70 in Birmingham, England, referred to above (31). In the clinical judgments of the general practitioners who assessed them, for men aged 70 to 74 years domestic help was necessary for 25 per cent, nursing that called on technical skills for 5 per cent, and nursing that involved care for the person for about 2 per cent. For men aged 80 to 84 years, the need for each service was at least twice as great.

Sickness in old age, because it is so disabling, poses a constant threat of dependence (see Table 12.14). Failures of physiological function, diminished resistance to disease, and pathological changes tend to be cumulative and enduring, so that a large part of sickness at this time is either fatal, or chronic and recurring. For instance, the excess of deaths during spells of cold or heat or during persistent fogs is concentrated among the old, like deaths from influenza epidemics; these types of epidemic fatality are uncommon among the young and healthy. In Britain, hypothermia (a reduction in core body temperature) was found in 10 per cent of a national random sample of old people, with an excess among the poorest who received supplementary pensions; many houses were poorly heated because of fuel costs. In the United States, by far the highest risk of death from accidental hypothermia occurs among black males over 75 years of age; the homeless on the streets of American cities are especially vulnerable (32).

Illness and disability in old people readily initiate a cycle of decline into chronicity. They may be obliged to take to bed, and in so doing promote decalcification of bone that results in accelerated osteoporosis and fragility with increased risk of fractures, and also in the formation of kidney stones because of altered mineral metabolism.

Table 12.14   Illness and use of doctors in persons aged 65 and over, by age and sex, United States, 1975[a]

	Men (%)	Women (%)
Ill in bed in past year		
Whites	21	27
Blacks	33	44
Saw doctor within past month		
Whites	30	33
Blacks	35	48

[a]Excludes bedfast persons.

Source: Adapted from Shanas, E. (1980). Self-assessment of physical function: White and black elderly in the United States, in *The Epidemiology of Aging: Second Conference*, ed. Haynes, S., and Feinleib, M., NIH Pub. No. 80-969, Washington, D.C., p. 280.

Osteoporosis is increasingly prevalent in postmenopausal women. The wasting of skeletal muscle among the old who are confined to bed adds to their difficulties in maintaining an upright posture when they get up, and impairs the stability of their osteoar-
thritic joints and their strength for everyday living. The blood circulates sluggishly in
their legs because of muscular inactivity, so that there is a high risk of venous thrombosis, and of fatal pulmonary embolism to the lung arising from these thrombi. The
raised fatality rate following hip fractures in old people is to be expected where repercussions are so many. The consequences are measured in the occupation of hospital
beds. In Britain, people over 65 years of age occupy one-half of all hospital beds, those
over 75 years, one-third (33).

The well-being of aged patients is therefore tenuous, and subject to attack by a
combination of adverse factors that accelerate deterioration and dependence. Anxiety
and ensuing depression must be expected in old sick people who go in fear of these
formidable effects, which they observe in their peers. The tenacity with which old
people try to fulfill their accustomed roles in the face of disability can be seen as a
response to a conscious or unconscious recognition of the threat to their independence.

Although older people have been reported to be more likely than younger to see
advantages in being sick, the old are especially unlikely to adopt the sick role even
when it is fitting. Herein lies a cause for medical concern. In the United States, for
example, studies of Spanish-American War veterans in their eighties found a much
larger proportion reported symptoms than had made use of the free facilities for medical care available to them. In the United States generally, more than 6 out of 10
persons whose health was rated poor by physicians gave themselves a favorable health
rating, and similar results were found in a British survey (34,35). The maintenance
of normal social roles in the face of disease can be regarded as socially and psychologically to the good. Self-ratings of health among the elderly have been shown to
predict subsequent morbidity, over and above what is to be expected from the objective ratings of health made by others (29). On the other hand, the failure of old people
to seek care is in conflict with their objective medical needs, and can well frustrate
efforts to arrest the progress of incipient disorders or to cure established ones.

Since chronic disorders occur frequently among old people, early detection of those
conditions amenable to treatment could be an important preventive technique. The
risks of deterioration emphasize the need for intervention whenever it can be effective. Relief of the organic basis for perceived ill-health can be expected to improve
both health and morale, because there is an interplay between morale and disease;
self-awareness of ill-health in old people is associated with low morale and feeling old.
Many of the physical and mental disorders that underlie the disabilities of old people
are amenable to treatment, and some are reversible. For instance, vision can be corrected and false teeth fitted; prostates that cause problems of urinary continence can
be removed, feet can be cared for, depressive psychosis relieved, and the outcome of
stroke ameliorated (36).

To rely only on the demand for services will be unhelpful in the early detection of
disorders and will underrepresent need, since many old persons do not seek care for
illness or impairment. Poverty, limited education, and social isolation occur together
with old age to exacerbate this discrepancy between demand and need. The deter-

minants of low demand are to be found in the perceptions and beliefs among old people that lead to fatalism, negative views of health and medical services, and pride in independence; in the social causes of these modes of perception and belief; and in the unsubtle treatment (if not outright rejection) that old people meet from relevant agencies.

In the United States Title XVIII of the Social Security Amendments Act of 1965 (Medicare) was a belated recognition of the need for health services to cope with the burden of disease and the slender resources of the rising number of old people. The Medicare Act provides financial support for all old people; it does so in the manner of health insurance schemes but is paid for out of Social Security funds. The Act is not sufficient in itself to promote case-finding and the early detection of disease. Indeed, services more comprehensive and far-reaching than those available through Medicare, as British experience with the National Health Service shows, often fail to bring poor and isolated old people into medical care. To obtain participation, special efforts in communication and education in health matters must be made, for old people tend to be less oriented towards prevention than the young (37). At the same time, the service agencies themselves need to recognize the barriers to participation created by their own administrative organization, social structure, and organizational culture.

Retirement

Retirement is a landmark in progress through life, an overt sign that an individual has entered the phase of social replacement. For many individuals in our society, retirement is also a first step towards social dependence. Full social responsibility is no longer demanded when the obligation to work ceases. The imminence of dependence is recognized by the community, and the governments of industrial societies provide pensions to alleviate the financial side of dependence among the old.

More even than most aspects of old age, retirement is a product of society. Detailed examination of retirement legislation indicates a variety of motives among legislators. In part these have been humanitarian. In part, some American writers argue, motives have been overwhelmingly determined by requirements for sustaining the efficiency of workers and relieving unemployment (38). Qualifying ages for pensions are set by government, while other large-scale organizations typically impose retirement at a defined age, which has the effect of keeping open the channels of promotion for the young. During the twentieth century, these circumstances have much reduced the proportion of old men able voluntarily to continue in employment. Those older men who have been able to continue in their usual occupations have tended to be self-employed, or to work in smaller and more flexible organizaitons, and to belong to higher occupational classes (39).

In the United States by 1978, fewer than 30 per cent of men aged 65 to 69 were in the labor force, compared with about 46 per cent in 1960. Of the remaining 70 per cent, a majority reported that retirement was voluntary. A proportion were voluntarily working part-time. Nonetheless, mandatory retirement applies to somewhat more than half of all retiring males. Attitudes towards retirement are heavily influenced by the social context in which retirement occurs. In a 1968 national survey in the United States, for instance, among an estimated 54 per cent whose retirement was mandatory, 30 per cent retired early, and the remaining 24 per cent at the mandatory age. It was inferred that only 2.8 per cent of the total were both capable of continuing and did not wish to retire when obliged to do so (40). Since that time, the law has changed. Retirement cannot be mandated before 70 years of age, and in the future mandatory retirement may be abolished altogether. From the 1968 data, one would not expect these changes to produce marked effects. Subsequent national sample surveys contradict that impression. About one-third of retired older Americans claimed they would return to work if they could, and not much fewer than half (45 per cent) said they had not wished to retire (41).

Political and economic factors, such as the rising concern with the budgetary demands of social security, play a large part in the form national policy takes. Aside from personal desire, therefore, continued employment in old age depends on an array of economic, social, and individual physical factors—on the state of the labor market and on the financial needs of the family, as well as on physical capacity for manual work and mental capacity for nonmanual work. A proportion of men over the age of 65—perhaps more than a third—take up new work, frequently in occupations of lower status. The lesser importance that society still attaches to the work of women outside the home appears in the lesser proportion of women over the age of 65 who are in employment. In Britain only one in ten were working. In the United States a similar but lesser disparity exists (42,43).

Apart from the qualifying age for pensions and mandatory retirement, detailed evidence about other causes of retirement is sparse. Whether old people continue at work is strongly related to their physical fitness. The Birmingham survey—admittedly in the 1950s—considered that 67 per cent of the men over 70 in Social Class I were fit to work, but only 20 per cent of the men of this age in Social Class V (31). Data cited earlier in this chapter indicate that nothing has changed in this regard. Among those who do retire—with remarkable consistency in studies spanning three decades—failing health is the chief reason given for not continuing in work (44).

Thus the causes of retirement are a legitimate health question. It is not a simple question, and the nature of appropriate action requires discriminating study. Although men most often say they would continue to work for financial reasons, working into old age is commonest in occupations with high earnings where financial deprivation can only be relative and not absolute. Men in these occupations not only enjoy far better health than the poorly paid, but the satisfactions they gain from work and their commitment to it are likely to be greater.

There is, then, no single cause of retirement but a configuration of factors. One analyst sums up the causes as health, regulations, and money; that is, people retire because they have to (for health or mandated reasons) or because they can afford to. Even this simplification admits of several variables (45). Failing health is certainly an important cause, even among those who give other reasons. Year by year disease takes an increasing toll among the workforce, as we have seen it does for the population at large (46). The culling of less healthy workers leaves a healthier residue. This process produces the so-called "healthy worker" effect so apt to confound studies by unwary researchers who discover no ill-effects of occupational exposures among workers but have not included those who have already dropped out. The culling is not an entirely even process; eligibility for pensions and benefits are set in terms of duration of employment and age, and in turn eligibilities become turning points for decisions about retirement.

By no means all old men who are fit to work are in fact at work. This underemployment is not necessarily desired. Economic need, social support, social values, and psychic resources can all be expected to influence the mindset. In general, retired working-class men who follow some occupation have described themselves as happier and more content than men who do not (47). On the other hand, they are also healthier, and across two millennia Galen's aphorism reminds us that the health of body and mind go together. Ill-health is probably the most important factor in depressed mental performance among old people, and it is the likely common factor underlying the associations of work and satisfaction among the elderly.

General attitudes towards retirement fluctuate, often in tune with the effects of the economy on income. While for a period attitudes were becoming more favorable and accepting, attitudes later turned unfavorable with an increased concern over the effects of inflation. Of men who retire, at least two out of every three wage and salary workers say they retire by their own decision. A rising minority say that they prefer leisure to work, and most who continue in work give the chief reason as financial.

The effect of retirement conceived as a psychosocial stressor is, like the causes of retirement, a significant health question. Because ill-health can cause retirement, the effects of retirement on health can best be tested by longitudinal studies that control for the state of health before retirement (48). Most competent studies show, on the average, little effect of retirement on death or mobidity rates (49). Yet in apparent contradiction, case studies report that the sudden discontinuity in a major role brought about by retirement can accompany social maladjustment and acute emotional disturbance (50). This may be because averages may not reveal effects that exist only at the outer limits of a distribution, or only in special groups and special situations, or it may be an artifact because "cases" are by virtue of that status selected for being disturbed.

Throughout his adult life a man's occupational status tends to dominate his activities and aspirations. Occupation determines his social standing, wealth, and place of residence, as well as his productive contribution to society. For some men the sudden and irretrievable loss of this role is a kind of social death; not only has his work ended but so also has a major interest in life. Retirement is an unfolding process, which begins with anticipation of the event. A number of studies describe characteristic patterns of psychological response that follow the event. Retired old persons are said at first to enjoy a "honeymoon" phase, during which they tend to seek relaxation, and to exercise that free choice of activities that constitute the myth of retirement. Some men find psychological means to deny, at least temporarily, the reality of the fact that they are now deprived of a productive function. Later there follows for some a phase of "disenchantment": a period of turmoil, marked by anxiety and depression, an increase in somatic symptoms and preoccupation with the self, and feelings of inadequacy and irritability. The duration of this period varies between individuals, but often persists for many months, when it either subsides as the old person adjusts to his dependent role, or develops into a chronic failure of adjustment. With the development of a structured routine, phases of "reorientation" and stability can succeed disenchantment. In a phase of "termination"—marked by a return to work or more often by illness and disability—the retirement state becomes irrelevant (51).

As noted, large-scale surveys offer few findings to confirm such dramatic effects of the transition into retirement. Retired men do seem less adjusted to life than those at work. At the same time, since the retired are comparatively less healthy, worse off, and of lower social status, this social selection alone may account for their poorer adjustment. The most dissatisfied among the retired are those who are poor and in bad health. Longitudinal study, however, supports the notion of a phase of "disenchantment" after retirement. A shift in affect does tend to occur among retired people, though the shift is towards a state of mild dissatisfaction rather than dejection or despair. Feelings of deprivation are most common when there is reluctance to retire, and when retirement has serious financial consequences. Three years and more after retirement among blue-collar workers in the United States, both a decline in satisfaction and an increase in illness were observed; in Norway a raised mortality rate was observed (52).

The importance of occupational roles to individuals varies from one social class to another and consequently the effects of retirement can be expected to differ. Thus, the theory that there is a progressive disengagement from active social roles among old people, accompanied by a relatively painless reorientation to the roles appropriate to the phase of replacement, may have more validity in some classes than in others (53,54). The Kansas study on which the theory was based used a sample limited to middle-class, independent old people (53). By contrast, manual workers who rely solely on state pensions to sustain them in retirement may be thrust into near poverty; often their incomes are cut by more than half. In a national survey in the United States, although the proportion who said they had not wished to retire was 45 per cent overall, it was 61 per cent among those with incomes below $3000 (41).

The loss of earning power alters status, roles, and relations within the family, and more particularly in those families with segregated conjugal roles. The adjustment of conjugal and other familial relations when a husband is confined to the home is often a painful process in these families. The husband impinges on the domestic sphere of the wife, in which she is dominant; he may come to feel himself "in the way" or "not wanted" at home, at the same time as he has lost his friends and associates at work. His dependent role may be underlined by the presence of sons whose earnings now become the main prop of the family. The transition may be easier when men are able to take on domestic chores, for instance, when the wife is infirm and unable to perform them.

Joint-role families may find adjustment easier, but some reordering of relations is inevitable, except perhaps in those few extreme cases where both husband and wife are financially independent. This easier adjustment may help to mitigate disenchantment, although it cannot wholly substitute for an active productive role. Voluntary retirement from work at an early age as a matter of choice by men who are wealthy enough to do so is another matter, for they are free to follow some other occupation, and to use their leisure in the pursuit of new experience.

The anomalous position of old men in an industrial society, it has been thought, is reflected in rates of suicide (55). In England and Wales in the age groups from adolescence to the mid-thirties, for example, there is an approximately twofold suicide rate among men compared with women (a ratio that increased somewhat in the mid-1970s). After a convergence in middle life (with rates for women only a third higher than for males in the mid-1970s), the rates for the sexes diverge again in the seventh decade; the rates for men continue to rise, while at 75 years of age and over, those for women begin to decline. Again, suicide rates (and psychiatric hospital admissions) have declined during times of war, and likewise seem to serve as an indication of morale and the dissipation of anomie (56, 57).

Other factors in the environment may override or obscure such effects; the frequency of suicide, like disease, is volatile. In England and Wales in the period 1961–1974, a steady decline in suicides after the mid-thirties was closely related to the agents available: after 1963, the carbon monoxide content of town gas was reduced to nonlethal levels. This decline in suicide rates was most marked in men over 65 years of age, so that the male excess in that age-group also declined, from 110 per cent in the years around 1960 to only 65 per cent in the years around 1970 (57).

Retirement impinges on women as a group less than men, for paid work outside the home is still a supplement to the domestic life of many married women. When a woman has a number of married children, and a close-knit social network, she continues to function as the focal point of the network, and in giving help and advice with the rearing of her grandchildren. Even if her social network is dispersed, she retains her customary domestic duties. In either case, the continuity of her accustomed roles into old age provides her with social stability and probably with psychological security, and tends to strengthen her position relative to her husband.

By contrast, those women who have followed an occupation throughout their lives on retirement can be expected to experience the same social effects as men. In earlier generations, such women often achieved higher education and a professional career, but did not marry (58). The main factor in determining the effect of retirement on the individual, one may conclude, is the type of occupation followed and its economic and social significance.

Industrial society has not yet found how best to use the services of old people retired from their regular occupations. Cross-national studies show that the value placed on the status of the aged varies with the degree to which societies are modernized, as measured by the proportion of the labor force in agriculture, literacy, and education. A sharp devaluation of aging is found in societies in a stage of early modernization compared with traditional societies. The notably low status of the aged with early modernization may be transitional because they fare somewhat better in highly modernized societies (59).

In many tribal societies the services of the relatively few old people are used effectively, and many remain productive and socially important; they are the main source of knowledge and tradition in the absence of permanent records; they act as intermediaries between their fellows and the supernatural; and they often serve as counselors from the wisdom of experience (60). In changing societies, the prestige of the aged role evidently declines as accumulated knowledge preserved in an oral tradition loses relevance for the social situation in which younger generations find themselves. In a Mexican village observed over some 35 years, the elders were appreciated so long as they continued to function in their accustomed social and occupational roles, but their counsel was not sought out and their status was accepted rather than prized. Younger persons held most of the municipal offices (61). In highly differentiated industrial society the problem of old people is difficult because their number is greater, and has grown rapidly as large-scale industrial organization has developed. No suitable system has yet been devised to accommodate aged workers to the new forms of economic and productive organization, or to make these flexible enough both to retain the services and to meet the special needs of older workers.

In brief, retirement comes as a blow to some, as a release to others. Responses are affected by anticipatory attitudes, and by material and social consequences, and thus depend upon the individual's position in society and the life history that was the precursor. While retirement does not of itself seem to reduce the level of participation in available social roles, with the loss of occupation it reduces by at least one the number of roles available. The men most likely to continue in work are those who can exercise the choice to do so, are healthy, and gain satisfaction from work. For those who do retire, the transition marks their entry into a social category for which the risks of sickness and death are higher than for others, whether or not the transition itself heightens such risks. By retirement, men declare themselves as appropriate targets for some form of health screening procedure.

Bereavement

At any age bereavement is likely to be a major crisis in the life of the individual. In old age the crisis foreshadows the death of the survivor, and the loss may add to other disincentives to active readjustment. Partners who have survived together into old age have achieved an habitual distribution of roles and duties in domestic relations and in social relations outside the home, and their personal relations move in deep and customary grooves. The continuity of these relations provides each partner with emotional and personal security. Bereavement results in a drastic change, even if the dead partner was languishing, and the surviving spouse is faced with the necessity of readjusting to new situations at an age when transitions are not easily made.

The psychological response to the transition is likely to be one of grief. Acute grief, studied in the special circumstances of a disaster, has produced a characteristic reaction (62). Distressing sensations of the body such as tightness of the throat, choking and shortness of breath, sighing, empty feelings in the stomach, weakness, and "mental pain" occur in waves lasting 20 minutes to an hour. There may also be a sense of unreality and emotional distance from others, and a preoccupation with the image of the dead person, both in thought and dream. Eventually restless, unorganized activity is accompanied by loss of the habits of social intercourse, such as conversing and sharing enterprises with others. A sense of resentment and hostility may enter all personal relations, or be directed against a specific person, not uncommonly the physician who cared for the patient before death. However, bereavement may not be so openly complained of, nor grief expressed (63).

The psychological effects of grief and the social problems of bereavement are often resolved through the rituals of mourning, which provide a social mechanism for adjustment to the new situation (64). This resolution does not follow invariably, and some reactions may persist or lead to morbid states (65). Bereavement is sometimes followed by depression, apathy, and retardation, or by hostility and withdrawal and progressive social isolation. As with the social aspects of any disorder, however, the attributes found in hospital patients may be related to selection for hospital admission as much as to the disorder itself. Bereavement is such a factor in selection, for it may throw a surviving but already dependent person on the charge of state agencies, while other equally ill persons are maintained by their spouses in their own homes.

In a previous chapter we discussed the association of widowhood with high death rates, with suicide, and with entry into psychiatric care. Although these results and others support those case studies that have described emotional reactions of bereavement (26,66), they have not established a clear risk for old age; indeed, it seems probable that the most severe consequences may occur among younger persons. Whatever the psychological effects of bereavement on the aged may be, the social effects mark a step towards displacement from previous roles and towards the eventual possibility of social dependence and institutional care. As is self-evident from the distribution of the sexes at older ages (see Table 12.12), these are predominantly problems of women.

Widowhood, like retirement, can serve as a marker for routine health screening. A simple procedure to identify vulnerable persons makes use of the official certificates attesting the death of a spouse. Among bereaved women with deficient social support, randomized intervention with a psychiatrist providing support over a three-month period produced a significant improvement, a year after the bereavement, over those left to their own devices. The effect was especially notable in that subgroup lacking social support. (No data are given that distinguish age-groups or, indeed, that indicate tests for confounding by age (67).) Critical facets of the bereavement experience, one may reasonably infer, are the consequences for the social as well as the psychological state of the persons affected, and the availability of the social support that may alleviate them.

Social support

Isolation. Social networks serve their several functions—to provide a resource, in emergency or need, for material as well as for affective support; to test and mould perceptions of reality through mutual interaction; to affirm a scheme of values, statuses, and roles—in the phase of replacement as they do in earlier phases of the family cycle discussed in previous chapters. Isolation can be defined in terms of the absence of these functions. Social isolation has been under indictment as an adverse factor in psychosocial adjustment since ecological studies discovered associations with schizophrenia, with certain mental disorders of the aged, with suicide and attempted suicide (55,68). The condition of isolation is well suited to test the stability of an individual's values and norms of behavior, since these are no longer sustained by interaction and the continued reinforcement of what others expect.

Isolation has three distinct aspects: physical isolation in separate households; social isolation through separation from social contacts and social services; and emotional isolation arising from subjective feelings of loneliness and desolation (69). These three elements do not necessarily coincide, although they often do. Physical isolation does not always imply social isolation, particularly when old people have close-knit social networks. Many such have relatives living nearby. Psychological isolation also, although it occurs more frequently with physical and social isolation, does not always coincide with them. Some people prefer a withdrawn or house-centered life. Conversely, old people may live in a household with others and yet complain of loneliness; a bereavement is the most common antecedent of such feelings.

In medical care the two significant elements of isolation are the social and the emotional or subjective. The social isolation of people who cannot care for themselves may lead to rapid deterioration in their living conditions, in diet and nutrition, and consequently in their physical and emotional state. The extremes of social distress in industrial societies are found in old people who are socially isolated and have reached this deteriorated state, which frequently precipitates admission to an institution. Involuntary social isolation comes about through the coincidence of a number of conditions. The chief of these are first, advanced age, which is associated with restricted physical mobility and the loss through death of spouse and peers; second, the single state and thereby the absence of children who could provide support; and third, the withdrawal from previous social relations that follows retirement.

In certain instances, social isolation can be a voluntary withdrawal from interaction and participation in reciprocal roles; this may be the characteristic life-style of a minority. Because so many women now reach an advanced age, the main problem of social isolation arises with them, particularly when they are single or widows. In the late 1950s in Stockport, Lancashire, twice as many widows as widowers over the age of 80 lived alone, mainly because of the higher death rate among men: only 10 per cent of old women lived with their husbands, against 40 per cent of old men who lived with their wives. Old persons who were socially isolated were in the main in better health than those who lived with others, as might be expected, for their isolation indicated that they had not fallen into the dependence that often follows ill-health. On the other hand, they had fewer resources to command, and their living conditions were generally worse than those who could draw on social support (70).

The facts of demography and longevity have exaggerated these circumstances of the 1950s. Isolation in old age is an outcome of the demographic life history of an individual, which in turn is an expression of the cycles of both the family of origin and the family of procreation. Figure 12.7a illustrates the situation in Britain in 1980 for the average man and wife who married in 1920. Figure 12.8b projects the same analysis to 2005 for a couple who married in 1950 (71). Isolation is the obverse of social interaction and social support, and the attenuation of support available to the couple of the 1950 marriage on entering their 80s is plainly evident. The projections take into account the effects of the employment of men and women on the availability of support.

To turn to the psychological aspects of isolation among the aged, the function of social networks in mediating the stress of experience and its effects on well-being,

(a)

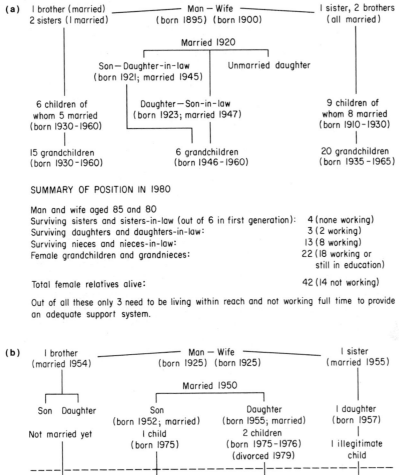

SUMMARY OF POSITION IN 1980

Man and wife aged 85 and 80
Surviving sisters and sisters-in-law (out of 6 in first generation):   4 (none working)
Surviving daughters and daughters-in-law: 3 (2 working)
Surviving nieces and nieces-in-law: 13 (8 working)
Female grandchildren and grandnieces: 22 (18 working or still in education)

Total female relatives alive: 42 (14 not working)

Out of all these only 3 need to be living within reach and not working full time to provide an adequate support system.

(b)

```
    I brother ───────── Man ─ Wife ───────── I sister
    (married 1954)    (born 1925) (born 1925)   (married 1955)

                       Married 1950

  Son   Daughter        Son             Daughter        I daughter
                   (born 1952; married)  (born 1955; married)  (born 1957)
  Not married yet       I child          2 children           I illegitimate
                     (born 1975)      (born 1975-1976)          child
                                       (divorced 1979)

─────────────────────── Projected to the year 2000 ───────────────────────

  3 grandchildren    No further         I child           Lost contact
                     children        (married 1995)
                                      I unmarried child
```

SUMMARY OF POSITION IN 2005

Man and wife aged 80
Surviving sisters and sisters-in-law: 2 (both retired)
Surviving daughters and daughters-in-law: 2 (I working)
Surviving nieces and nieces-in-law: 3 (all working)
Female grandchildren and grandnieces: 4 (in education)

Total female relatives alive: 11 (3 not working)

Therefore, all surviving nonworkers would have to live within reach to provide support system.

Figure 12.7 Cohort family structure in Britian: *a.* averaged up to 1980; *b.* averaged up to 2005. *Source:* Eversley, D. (1982). Some new aspects of aging in Britain, in *Aging and Life Course Transitions: An Interdisciplinary Perspective,* ed. Hareven, T. K., and Adams, K. I., New York, p. 257.

suggested by numerous studies, has proved difficult to establish securely. It may be that networks act as a buffer against adversity under some conditions and not others, and that these conditions are still to be defined. As we noted for widowhood, certain stressors seem less productive of effects on mental health and mortality among older than among younger people. Whether the absence of detectable effects of stressors among the elderly should be ascribed to anticipatory preparation for the inevitable, to successful denial and adaptation, to disengagement and detachment, or to other factors is a matter for speculation (45,53,72). In those instances in which networks have affective consequences for the aged, the elements of network function that contribute most are still to be discovered.

For example, in 400 elderly poor residents of three Connecticut cities, psychosocial variables measured at entry to a longitudinal study were associated with subsequent mortality (73). Two variables reflected states of mind: "religiousness" and "happiness" predicted reduced risk, mainly among persons in poor health at the outset. A third variable reflected social networks: presence of living offspring predicted reduced risk independent of other factors. What elements of networks—material, psychological or social—this finding portends one cannot say. A sense of psychological isolation, in the form of intense feelings of loneliness, was elicited in 5 per cent of all old people of pensionable age in a study of Bethnal Green in the East End of London. These feelings were common in socially isolated persons, and the factors associated with loneliness and with social isolation were similar. More generally, the number of significant others available to old persons has been found to correlate with measures of psychological well-being (74). Many socially isolated persons do not complain of loneliness, however, and pursue with equanimity the limited social intercourse to which they are accustomed.

The association of physical and social isolation with feelings of loneliness, low levels of activity, inadequate nutrition, and poor living conditions brings a vulnerable group into focus for public health attention. At the same time the very isolation of these people makes them relatively inaccessible to services. They are infrequent users of health and caretaking agencies (33), except at that late stage when admission to an institution is the only recourse. Effective health care for this social category of isolated people requires a special effort of caretakers, not only to mobilize resources but to reach them.

The place of institutions. The state of health and the risk of death vary markedly according to residential location and household arrangements. Much of the variation can be explained by movement from one setting to another because of failing health and needs for social support. This "health-related mobility" largely accounts for the fact that within institutions the single have the lowest mortality, the widowed intermediate levels, and the married the highest levels. This pattern contrasts with its mirror image found in the community at large (9).

A frequent end-point of the process leading to dependence is admission to an institution. This point is reached when the burden of caring for an old person outweighs available domestic support. Physical criteria alone are not sufficient to assess the health and supportive needs of old people in a community. The social circumstances in which the enfeeblement of age overtakes individuals, and the support available to them from kin and others, determines not only their need for social services but also, in part, their need for medical care. Their circumstances affect their reactions to the advent of sickness, retirement, isolation, and bereavement; and these events in turn affect the capacity of old people for social independence and survival, and the social support available to them.

The marital status of an adult helps to indicate the kind of household he or she lives in and therefore the extent of family support that might be available in a crisis. Table 12.15 shows the marital state and living arrangements for older persons in the United States in 1979, and Table 12.16 shows living arrangements in England in 1976. The inference we can draw from studies of the marital state of old people in institutions is, as we might expect, that persons admitted are likely to have only a minimum of family support available. In geriatric and mental hospitals, and in welfare homes, there is an excess of single men, single women, and widowers in that order of magnitude, which becomes more marked in older age-groups. In Britain about 3 per cent of all persons of pensionable age are in institutions, and in the United States about 7 per cent (75,76). The domestic and social relations of the remainder are clearly of importance in understanding their need for care.

The preference that people in our society show for an independent household does not decrease with age (47,76). Old people continue to live in their own households, even when widowed. The capacity to maintain themselves independently again varies with physical and mental state, and with the kind of support spouses, relatives, or

Table 12.15 Marital status and living arrangements of the elderly, by age and sex, United States, 1979 (percent distribution within age-groups)

Marital status and living arrangements	Males (age in yrs)			Females (age in yrs)		
	65 and over	65–74	75 and over	65 and over	65–74	75 and over
A. Marital status						
Single	5.4	5.6	4.9	6.1	6.0	6.2
Married, spouse present	74.6	78.4	66.9	36.9	46.9	20.9
Married, spouse absent	2.6	2.9	2.0	1.6	1.9	1.0
Widowed	14.1	9.3	24.0	52.2	41.2	69.7
Divorced	3.3	3.9	2.2	3.3	4.0	2.2
B. Living arrangements						
Head of a household	92.6	93.4	90.8	51.1	45.2	60.5
Head of a primary family	76.6	80.2	69.3	8.8	8.5	9.2
Primary individual	16.0	13.2	21.5	42.3	36.7	51.3
Living alone	15.4	12.7	20.8	41.0	35.4	50.1
Other	0.6	0.5	0.7	1.2	1.3	1.2
Not head of a household	7.4	6.6	9.2	48.9	54.8	39.5
In families	5.7	4.7	7.7	47.8	53.6	38.5
Secondary individual	1.8	1.9	1.6	1.1	1.2	1.0

Source: Adapted from United States Bureau of the Census (1980). Marital status and living arrangements: March 1979, *Current Population Reports*, Series P-20, No. 349, Tables 1 and 6.

Table 12.16 Type of household in which elderly people live: England, 1976 (percent distribution in age-groups)

	Males			Females		
Type of household	65–	75–	85 and over	65–	75–	85 and over
One elderly person alone	14	20	27	34	47	50
Elderly married couple only	64	60	31	41	21	5
Elderly siblings only	1	1	6	3	6	2
Others, one elderly person only	12	11	18	13	21	27
Others, more than one elderly person	10	8	18	10	6	16

Source: Adapted from A. Hunt (1978). The elderly: Age differences in the quality of life, *Population Trends, 11,* 11.

others can provide. Although many old unmarried people live alone, a large proportion form couples with siblings or other relatives, or with friends. The ranks of those living alone are constantly recruited from the widowed, if they do not have the support of an unmarried child. The widowed without available children to support them sometimes renew contact with siblings, and thus find a substitute for a spouse. Old people combine with others in a number of types of household; an old married couple may live alone, or with unmarried children, or with married children if there is a housing shortage or sufficient space.

The continuing independence of these households is related to the economic resources as well as the physical capacity of their members. The poorest areas, and those with the greatest proportion of people living in one-person households, give rise to the highest rates of suicide, and of admissions to mental hospitals among the aged as well as among younger persons (68,77). Old couples, whether they are spouses or a pair of siblings or friends, sometimes continue to care for each other well into the eighties. Their independence may be preserved by the efforts of only one of the couple, in which case a temporary failure of function in that one may lead to the collapse of the pair and a simultaneous need to support both. The same results can follow the temporary disablement of a young person sharing a household with an old person, for instance, an unmarried child whose strength and earnings support both himself or herself and an indigent parent.

Social networks in old age. The economic resources of a household are fundamental to its survival. Some old people can afford to pay for services that preserve their independence, whether or not there is a supportive social network available to them. For the majority of old people in poorer circumstances, the external relationships of members of the household take on large significance, for the present system of state agencies does not nearly meet the needs of old people whose powers are declining but who continue to live in independent households. In Britain, where local authorities provide daily help, probably none provide for all those known to need it, and the known form but a part of the population in need. In the face of inflation old-age pensions barely provide subsistence. Nutrition suffers, and social relationships are damaged or lost through the lack of money needed to maintain reciprocity in relations—that is, for bus and train fares, friendly gatherings, teas and entertainments, and gifts for grand-children. In these circumstances kinship relations become a major factor in helping old people to maintain their independent households (47,78). Several studies demonstrate the role of relatives in providing care for old people who are in fact socially dependent and thereby prevented from falling a charge upon the community.

The functioning of a social network as a means of material and social support for old people is influenced by economic and social factors inherent in the structure of industrial society. During the phase of dispersal, the occupational status gained by children, and the kind of marriages they make, will influence the content of social relations between themselves and their parents. The extent to which they will be able to assist their parents when they become dependent will also be influenced by the particular phase of their own family's developmental cycle in which the parental need arises. Hence, the social networks of old people will be largely determined by the extent to which their own children and siblings have become socially and residentially mobile, and will tend to differ according to their own occupations and social class.

Old people with close-knit contained networks built round a core of relatives are most likely to have immediate attention and support both materially and socially. In contained networks a continuous and localized series of relationships has been built up between successive generations, with reciprocity of domestic and personal services. In these close-knit networks, the illness or death of one member can be compensated by the services of another; hence a daughter-in-law can offer the services usually provided by a daughter, or an unmarried child can take on the domestic role of a spouse. When old people can no longer reciprocate services, however, this sometimes makes them less willing to accept help and their relatives less willing to offer it. The loss of ability to reciprocate is a sign of the onset of dependence, a reversal of roles that members of proximate generations may find difficulty in accepting for various reasons—economic, social, and moral. Nevertheless, in many working-class areas the services provided by relatives enable old people to continue living independently, even at advanced ages.

Early British studies described patterns of relationships that are seemingly widespread and persisting where material resources are lacking. Similar patterns of domestic reciprocity exist among urban people living in poverty in the United States (79). In the nature of things, however, small modern families cope better with dependence when the need for support is acute and short lived than when it is chronic and sustained. The newly widowed can expect help from kin during the initial crisis—in arranging funerals, cooking, cleaning, and other tasks—but less thereafter. In a Chicago study, fresh engagement of the widowed in family affairs was not much evident; on the contrary, relations with in-laws tended to fall away (80).

Some aspects of the supportive functions of dispersed social networks appeared in a study of a well-to-do suburb of Greater London (81). In this suburb almost as many old people lived with or near their children as in working-class Bethnal Green. However, an age difference appeared. In the suburb, there was a marked increase in the number of old people who lived with their children after the age of 70; this appeared to follow those events associated with the onset of dependence, mainly bereavements and physical and mental illness. The difficulties of adjusting to the reversal in lifelong roles sometimes led to dispute and conflict between the persons involved, between mothers and daughters for instance, whose responsibilities in the household were uneasily divided. They then tended to interpret each other's behavior in psychological terms. The nocturnal habits and the paranoid trend of ideas of some old people on the verge of dementia were neither understood nor readily tolerated, and were ascribed to quirks of personality.

A number of old people have no effective social networks, and as a result are socially isolated; more than 25 per cent of all persons of pensionable age live alone and, in various studies, at least, 10 per cent have had very infrequent social contact. In a San Francisco study, isolated old people were considered in two classes, lifelong isolates and recent isolates, and the majority of extreme isolates proved to have been solitary through most of their lives (82). The trends of demography, employment, and social mobility ineluctably increase social isolation, and diminish the social support available to the elderly (see Figures 12.7 and 12.8). The unmarried elder daughter of earlier times has disappeared as a member of the household of elderly parents; most members of households of both sexes work when they can; as a result of geographic dispersion, the direct contact achievable by a walk has been largely replaced, for those who can afford them, by contacts achieved by motor vehicles and telephones; households are smaller; and the increase in divorce and serial monogamy disperses the obligations of the couples involved and strains their financial resources (71).

The support rendered by old people's social networks is nonetheless still a resource that health agencies do well to recognize. In most industrial societies, and in most parts of the United States at the present time, there is little reason to think that the health and welfare services that support the poorer classes—often limited in scope—are adequate to the task. Independent old people do not favor institutional life, although once they are inmates they may become more accepting or resigned. If one judges by many accounts of institutions, such negative attitudes are well founded (83). For although they vary a great deal in the kind of care and facilities they provide, institutions have in common a comprehensiveness that often envelops all the activities of the individual. The impact of their social structure and culture on the social behavior of residents is inevitably powerful and potentially damaging (84). Indeed, the type of care provided may be sufficient to influence survival. One British study found that the survival of old people in residental homes was related to the ratio of staff to residents on an index of the quality of care. A study of elderly people within and outside institutions, however, does not support the hypothesis that institutional living induces inmates to take up the sick role. Sickness, measured from self-assessments, correlated with reports of objective indicators no more strongly in the the community than in institutions. Possibly the results were confounded by variations in self-assessments of sickness; relative to the severe levels of sickness of their reference groups within the institutions, residents may not have judged themselves very ill (85).

Endpoint

Sickness, retirement, bereavement, and social isolation are critical facts of old age. Each may mark a step towards displacement from social roles and toward eventual social dependence and death. This last phase of life, so beset with difficulties, has always presented a special challenge to human beings who, uniquely among animals, are aware of their own mortality. Each society treats in its own way the social and psychological problems of the phase preliminary to death.

The evolution of contemporary industrial societies has been too rapid for the solutions of even a century ago to remain effective. The number of people now reaching old age is so much greater than before that in a population sense old age represents virtually a new phase of life. Contemporary society has recognized this evolution, but social institutions have not coped with its problems. Even an innovation so radical for the United States as the Medicare legislation—which gives persons over 65 years of age access to medical care for acute needs irrespective of means—is but a partial solution to the overall problem of health care for the aged. Some 25 million people were enrolled in 1979. But payment for most long-term or custodial care is prohibited under Medicare, and for the long-term care provided by the Medicaid program only the very poor qualify. Public provision for the critical requirements of prevention and rehabilitation is minimal (86).

Old age poses dilemmas for social policy. Some of these are typical of any group defined by handicap, dependence, or deprivation. Particularist solutions, applied to the ascribed status defined by chronological age and directed to specific needs, only reinforce the adverse sentiments and stereotypes attached to old age in Western industrial societies. Notably in the United States, independence and self-reliance are valued, dependence stigmatized as undignified and shameful. Yet aged persons need help especially when they sink into dependence.

Universalist solutions that do not discriminate by age or other personal attributes are a means of avoiding such problems (87). Universalistic policies make health care available to everyone regardless of age, provide social support at home to avoid institutionalization according to need and regardless of age, maintain income above a threshold level instead of giving social security pensions for the aged and disabled, and confer the right to continue in employment given the capability and will to do so. Such policies are not without cost. For example, if retirement does not apply to all who reach an ascribed threshold age, then other criteria may be needed to end the achieved status of employment. Criteria that identify incompetence resulting from deteriorating powers or outmoded skills may well be less objective, more easily manipulated, and more readily taken as a mark of failure.

Large-scale organization of economic and productive resources in industrial societies has brought the amenities of life within the reach of millions, and the specialization of roles that has accompanied large-scale organization has expanded the possibilities of personal development for all. Industrial societies have moved towards Herbert Spencer's ideal of individuation (88). These possibilities have not been fully realized, and many people cannot avail themselves of the opportunities for individuation because of economic deprivation and educational blocks inherent in the economic and social system. Individuation, too, exacts its own price; insecurity is generated by increased personal responsibility shouldered in isolation from others and in competition with them, by the rapid change in social norms, and by the maintenance of social relations with different persons in many fields of activity (89). Industrial societies need to invent new roles to adapt to their changing demographic forms, and to satisfy the needs of all their members. They must also invent new forms of service and care, for nowhere are these sufficient.

References

1. **Coale, A. J.** (1965). Birth rates, death rates and rate of growth in human populations, in *Public Health and Population Change*, ed. Sheps, M. C., and Ridley, J. C., Pittsburgh. **Keyfitz, N.** and **Flieger, W.** (1968). *The Analysis of Vital Data*, Chicago.
2. **U.S. Bureau of the Census** (1976). *Historical Statistics of the United States, Colonial Times to the Present*, Washington, D.C.
    U.S. Bureau of the Census (1983). America in transition: An aging society, *Current Population Reports*, Series P-123, No. 128, Washington, D.C.
3. **Comfort, A.** (1979). *The Biology of Senescence*, 3rd ed., London.
4. **Mazess, R. B.,** and **Forman, S. J.** (1979). Longevity and age exaggeration in Vilcamba, Ecuador, *J. Gerontology, 34*, 94–98.
5. **Siegel, J. S.** (1980). Recent and prospective demographic trends for the elderly population and some implications for health care, in *Epidemiology of Aging: Proceedings of the Second Conference*, ed., Haynes, S. G., and Feinleib, M., U.S. Dept. of Health and Human Services, NIH Pub. No. 801–967, pp. 289–316.
6. **Susser, M.** (1975). Demography of aging—Discussant's perspective, in *Epidemiology of Aging, Summary Report and Selected Papers from a Research Conference*, ed., Ostfeld, A. M. and Gibson, D. C., Dept. of Health, Education and Welfare, DHEW Pub. No. (NIH) 75-711, p. 83–96.
    Gruenberg, E. M. (1977). The failure of success. *Milbank Mem. Fund Qtly. 55*, 3–24.
    Schatzkin, A. (1980). How long can we live? A more optimistic view of potential gains in life expectancy, *Amer. J. Pub. Hlth., 70*, 1199–1200.
    Fries, J. F. (1980). Aging, natural death, and the compression of morbidity, *New Eng. J. Med., 303*, 130–35.
    Schneider, E. L., and **Brody, J. A.** (1983). Aging, natural death, and the compression of morbidity: Another view, *New Eng. J. Med., 114*, 854–55.
    Fries, J. F., Nesse, R. M., Schneider, E. L., and **Brody, J. A.** (1984). [Letters on aging, natural death and the compression of morbidity], *New Eng. J. Med., 310*, 659–60.
7. **Tsai, S. P., Lee, E. S.,** and **Kautz, S. A.** (1982). Changes in life expectancy in the United States due to declines in mortality, 1968–75. *Amer. J. Epid. 116*, 376–84.
8. **Kohn, R. R.** (1982). Cause of death in very old people, *J. Amer. Med. Assoc., 247*, 1792–97.
9. **Fox, A. J.,** and **Goldblatt, P. O.** (1982). *Longitudinal Study: Sociodemographic Mortality Differentials*, Office of Population Censuses and Surveys, H.M.S.O., London.
10. **Medawar P. B.** (1952). *An Unsolved Problem in Biology*, London.
    Hayflick, L. (1975). Current theories of biological aging, *Federation Proceedings 34*, 9–13.
    Sacher, G. A. (1977). Life table modification and life prolongation, in ed. Birren, J. E., Hayflick, L., and Finch, C. W., *Handbook of the Biology of Aging*, New York.
    Cutler, R. G. (1981). Life-span expansion, in *Aging: Biology and Behavior*, ed. McGaugh, J. L., and Kiesler, S. B., New York, pp. 31–76.
11. **Susser, M.** (1968). Aging and the field of public health, in ed., Riley, J. W., and Johnson, M. E., *Aging and the Practicing Professions*, New York, pp. 114–60.

12. **Bunbury, H.** ed. (1957). *Lloyd George's Ambulance Wagon, Being the Memoirs of William J. Braithewaite 1911-1912*, London.
13. **Vernon, P. E.** (1955). The psychology of intelligence and G, *Bull. Brit. Psychol. Soc.*, 26, 1-14.
    Jarvik, L. F., Eisdorfer, C., and **Blum, J. E.** (1973). *Intellectual Functioning in Adults.* New York.
14. **Susser, M.** (1981). Environment and biology in aging: Some epidemiological notions in *Aging: Biology and Behavior*, ed. McGough, J. L., and Kiesler, S. B., New York, pp. 77-96.
15. **Washburn, S. L.** (1981). Longevity in primates, in *Aging: Biology and Behavior* ed. McGaugh, J. L., and Kiesler, S. B., New York, pp. 11-29.
16. **Uhlenberg, P.** (1978). Changing configurations of the life course, in *Transitions: The Family and the Life Course in Historical Perspective*, ed., Hareven, T. L., New York
    Guillemard, A-M., (1982). Old age, retirement and the social class structure: Toward an analysis of the structural dynamics of the latter stage of life, in *Aging and Life Course Transitions: An Interdisciplinary Perspective*, ed. Hareven, T. K., and Adams, K. J., New York, pp. 221-44.
17. **Welford, A. T.** (1957). Methodological problems in the study of changes in human performance with age, in *Methodology of the Study of Aging*, Vol. 3, ed. Wolstenholme, G. E. W., and O'Connor, C. M., London.
    Schaie, K. W., and **Parham, I. A.** (1977). Cohort-sequential analyses of adult intellectual development, *Developmental Psychology*, 13, 649-53.
    Botwinick, J. (1978), *Aging and Behavior*, 2nd ed., New York.
    Kohn, M. L., and **Schooler, C.** (1979). The reciprocal effects of the substantive complexity of work and intellectual flexibility: A longitudinal assessment, in *Aging From Birth to Death: Interdisciplinary Perspectives*, ed. Riley, M. W., Boulder, Colorado, pp, 47-76.
    Baltes, P. B., and **Willis, S. L.** (1979). Life-span developmental psychology, cognitive functioning and social policy, in *Aging From Birth to Death: Interdisciplinary Perspectives*, ed. Riley, M. W., Boulder, Colorado, pp. 15-45
18. **Christianson, M. A.,** and **Gagnon, J. H.** (1965). Sexual behavior in a group of older women, *J. Gerontol.*, 20, 351-56.
    Pfeiffer, E., Verwoerdt, A., and **Wang, H.** (1968). Sexual behavior in aged men and women, *Arch. Gen. Psychiat.*, 19, 753-58.
19. **Office of Population Censuses and Surveys** (1977). *The General Household Survey*, H.M.S.O., London.
    Office of Population Censuses and Surveys (1978). Morbidity Statistics from General Practice 1971-1972, Second National Study, *Studies on Medical and Subject Population*, No. 36, H.M.S.O., London.
    Cartwright, A. (1981). *General Practice Revisited: A Second Study of Patients and their Doctors*, London.
    [See also data from; National Center for Health Statistics, *Data from the Health Interview Survey*, Series 10; and Office of Population Censuses and Surveys, *Hospital Inpatient Enquiry*, Morbidity Series MB4, H.M.S.O., London.]
20. **Katzman, R.** (1976). The prevalence and malignancy of Alzheimer's disease, *Arch. Neurol.*, 33, 217-18.
    Gruenberg, E. M. (1980). Epidemiology of senile dementia, in *Epidemiology of Aging; Proceedings of the Second Conference*, ed. Haynes S. G., and Feinleib, M., U.S. Dept. of Health and Human Services, NIH No. 80-969, pp. 91-104.

Mortimer, J. and Schuman, L. M. (1981). *The Epidemiology of Dementia*, New York and Oxford.

21. Sheldon, J. H. (1960). On the natural history of falls in old age, *Brit. Med. J.*, 2, 1685–90.

    Hogue, C. (1980). Epidemiology of injury in older age, in *Epidemiology of Aging*, eds. Haynes, S. G., and Feinleib, M., U.S. Dept. of Health and Human Services, Proceedings of the Second Conference, NIH Pub. No. 80-967, pp. 127–38.

22. **National Center for Health Statistics** (1982). Changes in mortality among the elderly: United States, 1940–78, *Vital and Health Statistics*, Series 3, Number 22, Hyattsville, Maryland.

23. Susser, M., Stein, Z. A., Mountney, G., and Freeman, H. L. (1970). Chronic disability following mental illness in an English city: Part I. Prevalence, *Soc. Psychiat.*, 5, 69–76.

24. Logan, W. P. D, and Brooke, E. M. (1957). The survey of sickness, 1943–52, *Studies on Medical and Population Subjects*, No. 12, H.M.S.O., London.

    Cartwright, A., and Jeffreys, M. (1958). Married women who work: Their own and their children's health, *Brit. J. Prev. Soc. Med.*, 12, 159–71.

    Hinkle, L. E., Redmont, R., Plummer, N., and Wolff H. G. (1960). An examination of the relation between symptoms, disability and serious illness, in two homogenous groups of men and women, *Amer. J. Publ. Hlth*, 50, 1327–36.

25. Kallman, F. J., and Sander, G. (1949). Twin studies in senescence, *Amer. J. Psychiat.* 106, 29.

    Dubin, L. I., Lotka, A. J., and Spiegelman, M. (1949). *Length of Life: A Study of the Life Table*, New York.

    Sjogren, T., Sjogren, H., and Lindgren, A. G. H. (1952). Morbus Alzheimer and Morbus Pick: A genetic and patho-anatomical study, *Acta Psychiat. Scand. Suppl*, 22.

26. Jacobs, S., and Ostfeld, A. (1977). An epidemiological review of the mortality of bereavement, *Psychosomatic Medicine*, 39, 344–57.

    Susser, M. (1981) Widowhood: A situational life stress or a stresssful life event, *Amer. J. Pub. Hlth.*, 71, 793–95.

27. Richardson, A. H. (1973). Social and medical consequences of survival among octogenarians: United automobile worker retirees and Spanish-American war veterans, *J. Gerontol.*, 28, 207–15.

28. Riley, M. W., and Foner, A. (1968). *Aging and Society: An Inventory of Research Findings*, Vol. I, New York, pp. 550–54.

29. Maddox, G. L., and Douglass, E. B. (1968). Self-assessment of health: A longitudinal study of elderly subjects, *J. Hlth. Soc. Behav.*, 14, 87–93.

    Palmore, E. P. (1969). Physical, mental and social factors in predicting longevity, *Gerontologist*, 9a, 103–8.

    Palmore, E. P. (1969). Predicting longevity A follow-up controlling for age, *Gerontologist*, 9b, 247–50.

    Hodkinson, H. M., and Exton-Smith, A. N. (1976). Factors predicting mortality in the elderly in the community, *Age and Aging*, 5, 110–15.

    Botwinick, J., West, R., and Storandt, M. (1978). Predicting death from behavioral test performance, *J. Gerontol.*, 33, 755–62.

    Ouslander, J. G., and Beck, J. C. (1982). Defining the health problems of the elderly, *Ann. Rev. Pub. Hlth.*, 3, 55–83.

    Abramson, J. M., Gofin, R., and Peritz, E. (1982). Risk markers for mortality among elderly men in Jerusalem, *J. Chron. Dis.*, 35, 565–72.

Mossey, T. H., and Shapiro, E. (1982). Self-noted health: A predictor of mortality among the elderly, *Amer. J. Pub. Hlth.*, 72, 800–8.

30. Glazer, B., and Strauss, A. (1965). *Awareness of Dying*, Chicago.
    Bowling, A., and Cartwright, A. (1982). *Life After a Death: A Study of the Elderly Widowed*, London.

31. Edwards. F., McKeown, T., and Whitfield, A. G. W. (1959). Incidence of disease and disability in elderly men, *Brit. J. Prev. Soc. Med.*, 13, 51–58.
    Edwards, F., McKeown, T., and Whitfield, A. G. W. (1959). Contributions and demands of elderly men, *Brit. J. Prev Soc. Med*, 13, 59–66

32. Fox, R. H., Woodward, P. M., Exton-Smith, A. N., Green, M. F., Donnison, D. V., and Wicks, M. H. (1973). Body temperatures in the elderly: A national study of physiological, social, and environmental conditions. *Brit. Med. J.*, 1, 200–6.
    Rango, N. (1984). The social epidemiology of exposure-related hypothermia deaths in the United States: 1970–1979, *Am. J. Publ. Hlth.*, 74, 1159–60.

33. **Department of Health and Social Security** (1978). *A Happier Old Age*, H.M.S.O., London.

34. Suchman, E. A., Philips, B. S. and Streib, G. F. (1958). An analysis of the validity of health questionnaires, *Social Forces*, 36, 223–32.
    Freeman, H. E., Richardson, A. H., Cummins, S. F. and Schnaper, H. W. (1966). Use of medical resources by Spancos. I. Extent and sources of medical care in a very old population, *Amer. J. Publ. Hlth.*, 56, 1530–39.

35. Sheldon, J. H. (1948). *The Social Medicine of Old Age*, London.

36. Adams, G. F. (1965). Prospects for patients with strokes with special reference to the hypertensive hemiplegic, *Brit. Med. J.*, 2, 253–59.
    Exton-Smith, A. N. (1977). Rehabilitation of the elderly, in ed. Mattingly, S., *Rehabilitation Today*, London.

37. Kutner B., Fanshel, D., Togo, A. M., and Langner, T. S. (1956). *Five Hundred Over Sixty: A Community Survey on Aging*, New York.
    Freidson, E., and Feldman, J. J. (1958). The public looks at dental care, *J. Amer. Dent. Assn.*, 57, 325–35.
    Shanas, E. (1962) *The Health of Older People: A Social Survey*, Cambridge.
    Gergen, K. J., and Back, K. W. (1966). Aging and the paradox of somatic concern, in ed. Simpson H. I., and McKinley, J. C., *Social Aspects of Aging*, Durham, N.C., pp. 322–34.
    Riley, M. W., and Foner, A. (1968). *Aging and Society*, Vol. I, *An Inventory of Research Findings*, New York, pp. 317–23.
    Shanas, E. G. (1980). Self-assessment of physical function: White and black elderly of the United States, in ed. Haynes, S. G., and Feinleib, M. *Epidemiology of Aging: Proceedings of the Second Conference*, U.S. Dept. of Health and Human Services, NIH Pub. No. 80-969, pp. 269–86.

38. Graebner, W. (1980). *A History of Retirement: The Meaning and Function of an American Institution, 1885–1978*, New Haven.

39. Riley, M. W. and Foner, A. (1968). *Aging and Society*, Vol. I, *An Inventory of Research Findings*, New York, pp. 40–63.
    Clark, R. L., and Spengler, J. J. (1980). *The Economics of Individual and Population Aging*, New York.

40. Reno, V., and Zuckert, C. (1971). Benefit levels of newly retired workers: Findings from the survey of new beneficiaries, *Soc. Sec. Bull.*, 34, 3–31.

Schulz, J. H. (1979). The economics of mandatory retirement. *Intl. Gerontol.*, Winter, 1–10.

41. **Harris, L., and Associates** (1976). *The Myth and Reality of Aging in America*, Washington, D.C.

42. **Central Statistical Office** (1982). *Social Trends, 13*, H.M.S.O., London.

43. **U.S. Department of Commerce and Bureau of the Census** (1980). *Social Indicators, III*, Washington, D.C.

44. **Ministry of Pensions and National Insurance** (1954). *Reason Given for Retiring or Continuing at Work,,* H.M.S.O., London.
    Palmore E. (1964). Retirement patterns among aged men: Findings of the 1963 survey of the aged, *Soc. Sec. Bull.*, 27, 3–10.

45. **Barfield, R. E., and Morgan, J. N.** (1978). Trends in satisfaction with retirement, *Gerontologist*, 18, 19–23.

46. **Richardson, I. M.** (1956). Retirement: A socio-medical study of 244 men, *Scot. Med. J.*, 1, 381–91.
    Carp, F. M. (1977) Retirement and physical health, in ed. Kasl, S. V., and Reichsman, F., *Advances in Psychosomatic Medicine: Vol. 1. Epidemiological Studies in Psychosomatic Medicine*, Basel and New York.

47. **Townsend, P.** (1957). *The Family Life of Old People*, London.

48. **Myers, R. J.** (1954). Factors in interpreting mortality after retirement, *J. Amer. Statist. Assn.* 49, 499–509.
    Thompson, W. E., Streib, G. F., and Kosa, J. (1960) The effect of retirement on personal adjustments: A panel analysis, *J. Gerontol.*, 15, 165–69.

49. **Streib, G. F.** (1965) *Longitudinal Study of Retirement, Final Report to the Social Security Administration*, Washington, D.C.
    Thompson, W. E. and Streib, G. F. (1958) Situational determinants: Health and economic deprivation in retirement. *J. Soc. Issues*, 14, 18–34.
    Streib, G. F., and Scheider, C. J. (1971). *Retirement in American Society: Impact and Process*, Ithaca, N.Y.
    Friedmann, E. A., and Orbach, H. L. (1974). Adjustment to retirement, in *American Handbook of Psychiatry*, vol. 1, ed. Arieti, S., New York, pp. 609–45.
    MacBride, A. (1976). Retirement as a life crisis: Myth or reality? A review, *Can. Psychiat. Assoc. J.*, 21, 547–56.
    Rowland, K. F. (1977). Environmental events predicting death for the elderly, *Psycholog. Bull.*, 84, 349–72.
    Ekerdt, D. J., Baden, L., Bossé, R., and Dibbs, E. (1983). The effect of retirement on physical health, *Amer. J. Pub. Hlth.*, 73, 779–83.
    Ekerdt, D. J., Bossé, R., and Goldie, C. (1983). The effect of retirement on somatic complaints, *J. Psychosomat. Res.* 27, 61–7.

50. **Tyhurst, J. S.** (1957). The role of transition states, including disasters, in mental illness, in *Symposium on Preventive and Social Psychiatry*, Washington, D.C.
    Margolis, B. L., and Kroes, W. H. (1974). Work and the health of man, in *Work and the Quality of Life: Resource Papers for Work in America*, ed. S. O'Toole, Cambridge, Mass.

51. **Atchley, R. C.** (1976). *The Sociology of Retirement*, New York.

52. **Martin, J. and Doran, A.** (1966). Evidence concerning the relationship between health and retirement, *Sociol. Rev.*, 14, 329–43.
    Stokes, R. G., and Maddox, G. L. (1967). Some social factors on retirement adaptation, *J. Gerontol.*, 22, 329–33.

Riley, M. W. and Foner, A. (1968). *Aging and Society*, Vol. I, *An Inventory of Research Findings*, New York, pp. 453–58.

53. Cumming, E. and Henry, W. E. (1961) *Growing Old: The Process of Disengagement*, New York.

54. Havighurst, R. J. (1957). The social competence of middle-aged people. *Genet. Psychol. Monog.*, 56, 297–375.

Havighurst, R. J., Neugarten, B. L. and Tobin, S. S. (1964) Disengagement, personality, and life satisfaction in the later years, in *Age With a Future*, ed. Hansen, P. F., Proceedings of the Sixth International Congress of Gerontology, Copenhagen and Philadelphia, pp. 419–24.

55. Sainsbury, P. (1955). *Suicide in London: An Ecological Study*, London.

56. Durkheim, E. (1951; orig. pub. 1897). *Suicide: A Study in Sociology*, trans., Spaulding, J. A., and Simpson, G., New York.

Murphy, H. B. M. (1961). Social change and mental health, in *Causes of Mental Disorders: A Review of Epidemiological Knowledge*, New York, pp. 280–329.

57. Adelstein, A., and Mardon, C. (1976). Suicides 1961–74, *Population Trends*, 2, 13–18.

Hopper, K., and Guttmacher, S. (1979) Rethinking suicide: Notes toward a critical epidemiology, *Inter. J. Hlth. Serv.*, 9, 417–38.

National Center for Health Statistics (1983). *Monthly Vital Statistics Report*, Vol. 31, No. 13.

World Health Organization (1983). *World Health Statistics Annual*, Geneva.

58. Young, K. (1947). *Personality and Problems of Adjustment*, London.

Glass, D. V., ed. (1954). *Social Mobility in Britain*, London.

59. Palmore, E. P., and Manton, K. (1974). Modernization and status of the aged: International correlations, *J. Gerontology*, 29, 205–210.

Bengtson, V. L., Downs, J. J., Smith, D. H., and Inkeles A. (1975). Modernization, modernity, and perceptions of aging: A cross-cultural study, *J. Gerontol.*, 30, 688–95.

60. Simmonds, L. W. (1945). *The Role of the Aged in Primitive Society*, New York.

Hammer, J. H. (1972). Aging in a gerontocratic society: The Sidamo of southwest Ethiopia, in *Aging and Modernization*, ed. Cowgill, D. O. and Holmes, L. D., New York, pp. 15–30.

Holmes, L. D. (1972). The role and status of the aged in a changing Samoa, in *Aging and Modernization*, ed. Cowgill, D. O., and Holmes, L. D., New York, pp. 73–87.

Shelton, A. J. (1972). The aged and eldership among the Ibo, in *Aging and Modernization*, ed. Cowgill, D. O. and Holmes, L. D., New York, pp. 31–49

61. Foster, G. M. (1981). Old Age in Tzintzuntzan, Mexico, in *Aging: Biology and Behavior*, ed. McGaugh, J. L., and Kiesler, S. B., New York, pp. 115–40.

62. Lindemann, E. (1944). Symptomatology and management of acute grief, *Amer. J. Psychiat.*, 101, 141–48.

63. Marris, P. (1958). *Widows and Their Families*, London.

64. Gennep, A. van (1960; first pub. 1909). *The Rites of Passage*, trans. Vizedom, B. B., and Caffee, G. L., London.

65. Freud, S. (1925). Mourning and melancholia, in *Collected Papers*, Vol. IV, London.

Klein, M. (1948). Mourning and its relation to manic depressive states, in *Contributions to Psycho-analysis*, 1921–1945, London.

66. Clayton, P. J. (1974). Mortality and morbidity in the first year of widowhood, *Arch. Gen. Psychiat.*, 30, 747–50.

Helsing, K. S., Szklo, M., and Comstock, G. W. (1981). Factors associated with mortality after widowhood, *Amer. J. Pub. Hlth.*, 71, 801–9.

67. **Raphael, B.** (1977). Preventive intervention with the recently bereaved, *Arch. Gen. Psychiat.*, *34*, 1450–54.
68. **Faris, R. E. L.,** and **Dunham, H. W.** (1939). *Mental Disorders in Urban Areas: An Ecological Study of Schizophrenia and Other Psychoses*, New York.
    Gruenberg, E. M. (1954). Community conditions and psychoses of the elderly, *Amer. J. Psychiat.*, *110*, 888–96.
69. **Firth, R.** (1956). *Two Studies of Kinship in London*, London.
70. **Brockington, C. F.,** and **Lempert, S. M.** (1965). *The Social Needs of the Over-80's*, Manchester.
71. **Eversley, D.** (1982) Some new aspects of aging in Britain, in *Aging and Life Course Transitions: An Interdisciplinary Perspective*, ed. Hareven, T. K., and Adams, K. J., New York, pp. 245–66.
72. **Lazarus, R. S.,** and **Golden, G. Y.** (1981). The function of denial in stress, coping, and aging, in *Aging: Biology and Behavior,* ed. McGaugh, J. L., and Kiesler, S. B., New York, 283–307
73. **Zuckerman, D. M., Kasl, S. V.,** and **Ostfeld, A. M.** (1984). Psychosocial predictors of mortality among the elderly poor: The role of religion, well-being and social contacts, *Amer. J. Epi.*, *119*, 410–23.
74. **Moriwaki, S. Y.** (1973). Self disclosure, significant others and psychological well-being in old age, *J. Hlth. Soc. Behav.*, *14*, 226–32.
75. **Department of Health and Social Security** (1977). *On the Side of the Public Health*, Report of the Chief Medical Officer of the Department of Health and Social Security, H.M.S.O., London.
76. **Ermisch, J.** (1982). Demographic changes and housing and infrastructure investment, in *Population Change and Social Planning*, ed. Eversley, D. and Köllman, W., London, pp. 270–324.
    U.S. Bureau of the Census and Dept. of Commerce (1982). *Statistical Abstract*, 1982–83, Washington, D.C.
77. **Parsons, T.** (1949). Age and sex in the social structure of the United States, in *Personality in Nature, Society and Culture*, ed. Kluckhohn C., and Murray, H. A., London.
    Hunt, A. (1978). The elderly: Age differences in the quality of life, *Population Trends*, *11*, 10–15.
    Townsend, P. (1979). *Poverty in the United Kingdom: A Survey of Household Resources and Standards of Living*, Berkeley.
78. **Hunt, A.** (1978). *The Elderly at Home*, H.M.S.O., London.
79. **Stack, C.** (1974) *All Our Kin*, New York.
    Cantor, M. H. (1979). The informal support system of New York's inner city elderly: Is ethnicity a factor? in *Ethnicity and Aging: Theory, Research, and Policy*, ed. Gelfand, D. E., and Kutzik, A. S. New York, pp. 153–74.
    Susser, I. (1982). *Norman Street: Poverty and Politics in an Urban Neighborhood*, New York and Oxford.
80. **Schenkman, W., Glick, I., Weiss, R.,** and **Powkes, C.** (1973). *The First Years of Bereavement in Widowhood in an American City*, Cambridge.
    Lopata, H. Z. (1978). Contributions of extended families to the support systems of metropolitan area widows: Limitations of the modified kin network, *J. Marr. Fam.*, *40*, 355–64.
81. **Willmott, P.,** and **Young M.** (1960). *Family and Class in a London Suburb*, London.
82. **Lowenthal, M. F.** (1964). Social isolation and mental illness in old age, *Amer. Sociol. Rev.*, *29*, 54–70.

83. **Townsend, P.** (1962). *The Last Refuge: A Survey of Residential Institutions and Homes for the Aged in England and Wales*, London.

Vladeck, B. C. (1980). *Unloving Care: The Nursing Home Tragedy*, New York.

84. **Goffman, E.** (1961). *Asylums*, New York.

Bennett, R., and **Nahemov, L.** (1965). Institutional totality and criteria of social adjustment in residence for the aged, *J. Soc. Issues, 21,* 44–78.

Bennett, R. (1980). *Aging, Isolation and Resocialization*, New York.

85. **Bennett, A. E., Deane, M., Elliott, A.,** and **Holland, W. W.** (1968). Care of old people in residential homes, *Brit. J. Prev. Soc. Med., 22,* 193–98.

86. **Kelman, H. R.** (1980). The underdevelopment of evaluative research on health services for the elderly in the U.S., *Int. J. Health Services 10,* 501–11.

Callahan, J. J., Diamond L. D., Jr., Giele J. Z., and **Morris, R.** (1980). Responsibility of families for their severely disabled elders, *Health Care Finance Review, 1,* 29–48.

Gibson, R. M., and **Waldo, D. R.** (1981). National health care expenditures, *Health Care Finance Review, 3,* 1–54.

Somers, A. R. (1982). Long-term care for the elderly and disabled: A new health priority, *New Engl. J. Med., 307,* 221–26.

87. **Etzioni, A.** (1976). Old people and public policy, *Social Policy, 7,* 21–29.

88. **Spenser, H.** (1899). *System of Synthetic Philosophy, Principles of Biology*, London, Vol.2, Part 6, Chapter 12.

89. **Fromm, E.** (1942). *The Fear of Freedom*, London.

Author and citation index

Subject index